# PHYSICIAN ASSISTANT BOARD REVIEW

## PANCE CERTIFICATION
## AND PANRE RECERTIFICATION

# PHYSICIAN ASSISTANT BOARD REVIEW

## PANCE CERTIFICATION AND PANRE RECERTIFICATION

### FOURTH EDITION

**JAMES VAN RHEE,** MS, PA-C, DFAAPA

Chair of Assessment and Remediation, Touro Physician Assistant Program
Associate Professor
New York, NY
United States

**JONATHAN KILSTROM,** MPAS, PA-C, NRP

Yale Physician Assistant Online Program
Assistant Professor Adjunct
New Haven, CT
United States

**STEPHANIE NEARY,** MPA, MMS, PA-C

Director of Didactic Education, Yale Physician Assistant Online Program
Assistant Professor Adjunct
New Haven, CT
United States

**MARY RUGGERI,** MEd, MMSc, PA-C

Alumna, Yale Physician Assistant Online Program
Austin, TX
United States

ELSEVIER

Elsevier
1600 John F. Kennedy Blvd.
Ste 1800
Philadelphia, PA 19103-2899

PHYSICIAN ASSISTANT BOARD REVIEW
PANCE CERTIFICATION AND PANRE RECERTIFICATION, FOURTH EDITION       ISBN: 978-0-323-93420-6

---

**Notice**

---

Previous editions copyrighted 2016, 2010, and 2006.

Senior Content Development Manager: Somodatta Roy Choudhury
Content Strategist: Lauren Willis/James T. Merritt
Senior Content Development Specialist: Priyadarshini Pandey
Publishing Services Manager: Shereen Jameel
Project Manager: Vishnu T. Jiji
Senior Designer: Renee Duenow

Printed in India

Last digit is the print number:   9   8   7   6   5   4   3   2   1

Working together
to grow libraries in
developing countries

www.elsevier.com • www.bookaid.org

*Thanks to all the physician assistant students and physician assistants who have attended my board review courses over the years; without all of you this book would not have been possible, and thank you for all the suggestions that helped make the book better.*

**James Van Rhee**


*Thank you to my mentors and all the students I have worked with over the years who have helped me become a better educator and clinician. You humble and inspire me, and I learn more from you all every day.*

**Jonathan Kilstrom**


*To the fellow educators who continue to make this work fun and the group of students who give us our purpose. To my husband and daughters, who continue to support and inspire me along the way.*

**Stephanie Neary**


*To my mentors, colleagues, and students, thank you for your support and dedication to this profession—you make work fun and inspire me daily. To my family, I love you to pieces.*

**Mary Ruggeri**

# PREFACE TO THE FOURTH EDITION

As stated in the preface of the previous editions, many physician assistants view the Physician Assistant National Certifying Exam (PANCE) and Physician Assistant National Recertifying Exam (PANRE) with fear and trepidation. I hope that the previous editions of this book have helped you in preparing for these exams.

As with the previous editions, there are sample questions at the end of each chapter. These questions are to assist you in your retention of the material. These questions, while not typical of those found on the examinations, are here to make sure you understand some of the major points and concepts. There are still several tables, charts, graphs, diagrams, and color plates in the book to enhance your learning.

There have been some additions to this edition:

- The online examination has been reviewed and updated. These questions will provide you with a "real-life" experience of taking the examination.

- There is one additional chapter in the book. The professional practice chapter covers topics such as medical ethics, informatics, communication, public health, and risk management to name a few.

I would like to thank all the people who have made comments related to previous editions of the book and made note of areas that needed corrections. Although every author hopes that their book is perfect from the start, the truth is improvements can be made only with the help of the reader. A special thanks to all my past students at Western Michigan University, Wake Forest University, Northwestern University, and Yale University, all who have been more than happy to make note of one of their instructor's errors.

I wish you the best in your studies as you prepare for these examinations.

**James Van Rhee, MS, PA-C, DFAAPA**

# CONTENTS

Color Plate Section follows the Front Matter

1 Cardiovascular System *1*

2 Pulmonary System *32*

3 Gastroenterology System *53*

4 Musculoskeletal System *85*

5 Endocrine System *112*

6 Eyes, Ears, Nose, and Throat System *129*

7 Neurologic System *154*

8 Reproductive System *175*

9 Infectious Disease *204*

10 Psychiatry/Behavioral Science *230*

11 Dermatologic System *254*

12 Hematologic System *282*

13 Genitourinary and Renal Systems *302*

14 Pediatrics *322*

15 Pharmacology *351*

16 Laboratory Medicine *380*

17 Professional Issues *394*

18 Test-Taking Strategies *397*

Appendices

1 Adult Preventive Health Guidelines *402*

2 U.S. Preventive Services Task Force Screening Guidelines for Common Diseases *403*

3 Cranial Nerves and Function *404*

4 Common Signs in Medicine *405*

5 Poisoning Antidotes *406*

6 Normal Laboratory Values *407*

Index *411*

# COLOR IMAGES

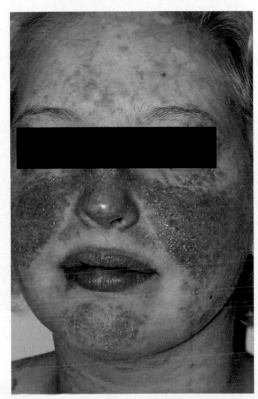

**Plate 1** Facial rash in systemic lupus erythematosus (SLE). *(With permission from Bolognia JL, Lorizzo JL, Rapini RP [2003]. Dermatology. Edinburgh: Mosby, pg. 603, Fig. 43.4.)*

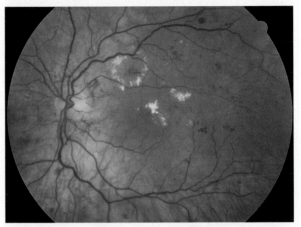

**Plate 2** Diabetic retinopathy. *(With permission from Goldman I [2008]. Cecil's Textbook of Medicine, 23rd ed. New York: Churchill Livingstone, pg. 2858, Fig. 449-15.)*

**Plate 3** Rubeola. *(With permission from Bolognia JL, Lorizzo JL, Rapini RP [2003]. Dermatology. Edinburgh: Mosby, pg. 1259, Fig. 81.6.)*

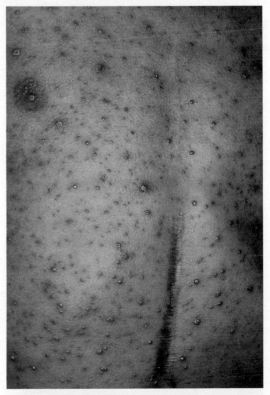

**Plate 4** Chickenpox. *(With permission from Bolognia JL, Lorizzo JL, Rapini RP [2003]. Dermatology. Edinburgh: Mosby, pg. 1242, Fig. 80.11A.)*

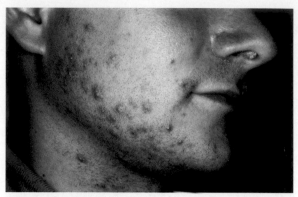

**Plate 5** Acne. *(With permission from Bolognia JL, Lorizzo JL, Rapini RP [2003]. Dermatology. Edinburgh: Mosby, pg. 533, Fig. 38.6.)*

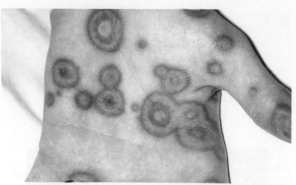

**Plate 6** Erythema multiforme. *(With permission from White GM, Cox NH [2002]. Diseases of the Skin: A Color Atlas and Text. Edinburgh: Mosby, pg. 116, Fig. 8.28.)*

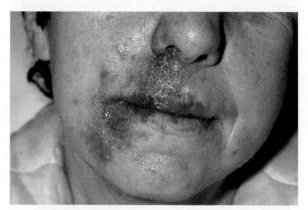

**Plate 7** Impetigo. *(With permission from White GM, Cox NH [2002]. Diseases of the Skin: A Color Atlas and Text. Edinburgh: Mosby, pg. 323, Fig. 20.2.)*

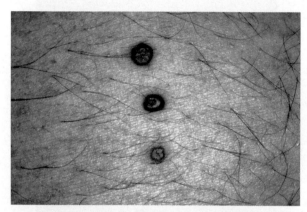

**Plate 8** Molluscum contagiosum. *(With permission from Bolognia JL, Lorizzo JL, Rapini, RP [2003]. Dermatology. Edinburgh: Mosby, pg. 1267, Fig. 81.12A.)*

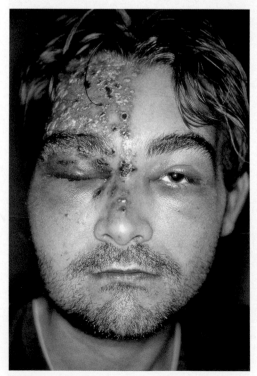

**Plate 9** Herpes zoster. *(With permission from Bolognia JL, Lorizzo JL, Rapini RP [2003]. Dermatology. Edinburgh: Mosby, pg. 1243, Fig. 80.12A.)*

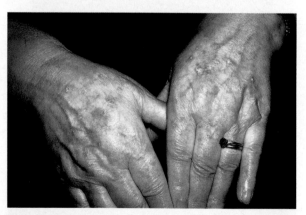

**Plate 10** Actinic keratosis. *(With permission from Bolognia JL, Lorizzo JL, Rapini RP [2003]. Dermatology. Edinburgh: Mosby, pg. 1681, Fig. 109.2.)*

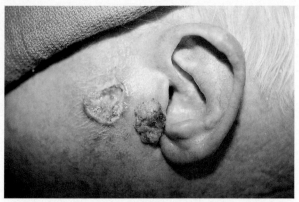

**Plate 11** Basal cell carcinoma. *(With permission from Miller RG, Ashar BH, Sisson SD [2008]. The Johns Hopkins Internal Medicine Board Review 2008–2009. Philadelphia: Mosby Elsevier, pg. 593, Fig. 66.20.)*

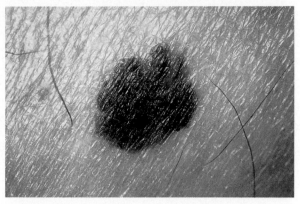

**Plate 12** Melanoma. *(With permission from Bolognia JL, Lorizzo JL, Rapini RP [2003]. Dermatology. Edinburgh: Mosby, pg. 1793, Fig. 114.6.)*

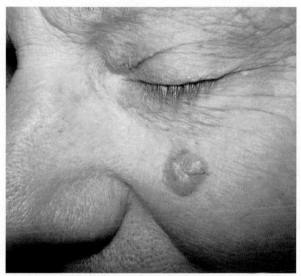

**Plate 13** Squamous cell carcinoma. *(With permission from White GM, Cox NH [2002]. Diseases of the Skin: A Color Atlas and Text. Edinburgh: Mosby, pg. 474, Fig. 29.55.)*

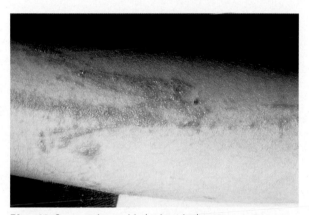

**Plate 14** Contact dermatitis (poison ivy). *(With permission from Bolognia JL, Lorizzo JL, Rapini RP [2003]. Dermatology. Edinburgh: Mosby, pg. 227, Fig. 15.1.)*

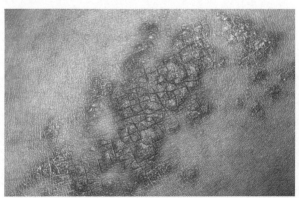

**Plate 15** Lichen planus. *(With permission from White GM, Cox NH [2002]. Diseases of the Skin: A Color Atlas and Text. Edinburgh: Mosby, pg. 68, Fig. 5.2c.)*

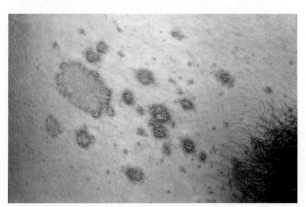

**Plate 16** Pityriasis rosea. *(With permission from White GM, Cox NH [2002]. Diseases of the Skin: A Color Atlas and Text. Edinburgh: Mosby, pg. 66, Fig. 4.44a.)*

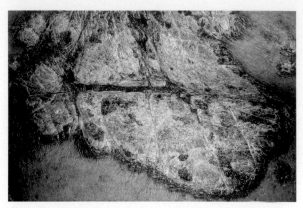

**Plate 17** Psoriasis. *(With permission from Bolognia JL, Lorizzo JL, Rapini RP [2003]. Dermatology. Edinburgh: Mosby, pg. 129, Fig. 9.1.)*

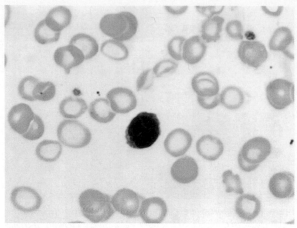

**Plate 18** Microcytic cells. *(With permission from Hoffman R, Benz EJ Jr, Shattil SJ, et al [2000]. Hematology: Principles and Practice, 3rd ed. New York: Churchill Livingstone, color plate 155.14.)*

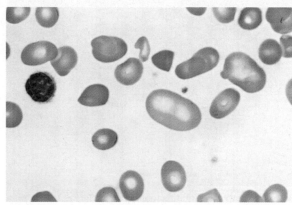

**Plate 19** Macrocytic cells. *(With permission from Hoffman R, Benz EJ Jr, Shattil SJ, et al [2000]. Hematology: Principles and Practice, 3rd ed. New York: Churchill Livingstone, color plate 155.15.)*

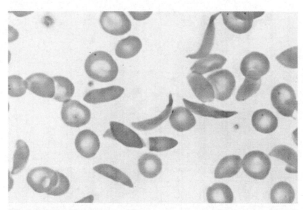

**Plate 20** Sickle cells. *(With permission from Hoffman R, Benz EJ Jr, Shattil SJ, et al [2000]. Hematology: Principles and Practice, 3rd ed. New York: Churchill Livingstone, color plate 155.23.)*

## EXAMINATION BLUEPRINT TOPICS

**CARDIOMYOPATHY**
Dilated
Hypertrophic
Restrictive

**CONDUCTION DISORDERS**
Atrial fibrillation/flutter
Atrioventricular block
Bundle branch block
Paroxysmal supraventricular tachycardia
Premature beats
Sick sinus syndrome
Ventricular Tachycardia
Ventricular fibrillation/flutter

**HEART FAILURE**
General
Clinical Manifestations
Diagnosis
Treatment

**HYPERTENSION**
Essential
Secondary
Hypertensive emergencies

**HYPOTENSION**
Cardiogenic shock
Orthostatic/postural

**LIPID DISORDERS**
Hypercholesterolemia
Hypertriglyceridemia

**ISCHEMIC HEART DISEASE**
Acute myocardial infarction
Angina pectoris

**VASCULAR DISEASE**
Acute rheumatic fever
Aortic aneurysm
Aortic dissection
Arterial embolism/thrombosis
Chronic/acute arterial occlusion

Giant cell arteritis
Phlebitis/thrombophlebitis
Venous thrombosis
Varicose veins

**VALVULAR DISEASE**
Aortic stenosis
Aortic regurgitation
Mitral stenosis
Mitral regurgitation
Mitral valve prolapse
Tricuspid stenosis
Tricuspid regurgitation
Pulmonary stenosis
Pulmonary regurgitation

**OTHER**
Acute/Subacute bacterial endocarditis
Acute pericarditis
Cardiac tamponade
Pericardial effusion

## CARDIOMYOPATHY

### I. DILATED
a. **General**
   i. Caused by malfunction of the myocardium.
   ii. Most common cause is idiopathic.
      1. Etiology may also be alcohol, myocarditis, ischemic heart disease, peripartum, or drugs (such as doxorubicin).
   iii. Cardiac dilation leads to right and left systolic dysfunction and then congestive heart failure.
b. **Clinical Manifestations**
   i. Most common first symptom is exertional intolerance.
   ii. Other signs and symptoms are same as congestive heart failure.
      1. Include dyspnea, orthopnea, and edema in the lower extremities.
      2. Atypical chest pain may also be noted.
   iii. Physical examination reveals an $S_3$ on cardiac auscultation, jugular venous distention (JVD) on neck inspection, and crackles noted on examination of the lungs.
      1. Mitral regurgitation may also be noted.
c. **Diagnosis**
   i. On electrocardiogram (EKG), nonspecific ST and T wave changes may be noted along with left bundle branch block (LBBB).
   ii. Chest x-ray film reveals cardiomegaly and pulmonary vascular congestion.
   iii. Echocardiogram reveals dilated chambers, thin left ventricular wall, and poor wall movement.
      1. Ejection fraction is decreased.
d. **Treatment**
   i. Withdraw offending agents, such as alcohol or drugs.

ii. Treatment of the congestive heart failure includes diuretics, sodium restriction, and digoxin to reduce symptoms.
  1. Angiotensin-converting enzyme (ACE) inhibitors are helpful unless contraindicated.
  2. Beta-blockers are indicated in patients with stable heart failure.
  3. Aldosterone antagonists should be added if still symptomatic after initiating ACE inhibitor and beta-blocker and an angiotensin receptor neprilysin inhibitor (ARNI) should be used in place of an ACE inhibitor or ARB.
iii. Implanted cardiac defibrillator and/or cardiac transplantation may be needed.

## II. HYPERTROPHIC
  a. **General**
    i. Most common cause of sudden death in young athletes.
      1. Due to ventricular tachyarrhythmias.
    ii. An autosomal dominant genetic cause seen in about 60% of cases. Abnormality has been noted on chromosome 14.
    iii. Pathogenesis.
      1. Hypertrophy of cardiac septum leads to left ventricular outflow obstruction and impaired diastolic filling.
      2. Impaired diastolic filling leads to pulmonary congestion.
  b. **Clinical Manifestations**
    i. Most patients are asymptomatic.
    ii. Most common presenting symptom is dyspnea on exertion (DOE).
      1. May also note angina and syncope.
    iii. Physical examination reveals mitral regurgitation, $S_4$, bifid carotid pulse, and prominent left ventricular impulse.
      1. Murmur of mitral regurgitation increases with Valsalva maneuver and decreases with handgrip and leg elevation.
  c. **Diagnosis**
    i. Echocardiogram makes diagnosis.
      1. Note septal wall thickness and ejection fraction are typically greater than 70%.
    ii. EKG reveals left ventricular hypertrophy (LVH).
  d. **Treatment**
    i. With presence of symptoms, treatment includes beta-blockers (propranolol) and calcium channel blockers (verapamil).
      1. Beta-blockers slow the heart rate and allow increased diastolic filling time.
      2. Calcium channel blockers improve ventricular compliance.
    ii. Implantable defibrillator if there is documented cardiac arrest, sustained ventricular tachycardia,

history of sudden death in one or more first-degree or close relatives 50 years of age or younger, LV wall greater than or equal to 30 mm, any recent syncope likely to have been caused by arrhythmia, LV apical aneurysm, or LV systolic dysfunction (EF less than 50%).
iii. Diuretics are used for fluid overload.

## III. RESTRICTIVE
  a. **General**
    i. Often caused by an infiltrative process.
      1. Such as amyloidosis, sarcoidosis, and hemochromatosis.
      2. May also be noted post radiation therapy and post open-heart surgery.
    ii. Pathogenesis.
      1. Myocardium changes lead to diastolic noncompliance with elevated filling pressures.
      2. Elevated filling pressures lead to pulmonary congestion.
  b. **Clinical Manifestations**
    i. Most common first symptoms are exertion intolerance and fluid retention.
      1. Signs of right-sided heart failure.
        (a) Elevated JVD.
    ii. On physical examination, a pronounced $S_4$ is noted along with mitral and tricuspid regurgitation.
  c. **Diagnosis**
    i. Echocardiogram reveals an ejection fraction between 25% and 50%, normal left ventricular wall thickness, and increased atrial size.
    ii. EKG reveals low-voltage QRS complexes and nonspecific ST-T wave changes.
    iii. Specific diagnosis made by tissue biopsy.
  d. **Treatment**
    i. Treat the underlying cause if possible. Heart transplant may be needed.
    ii. Diuretics are used to treat congestive heart failure.

# CONDUCTION DISORDERS

## I. ATRIAL FIBRILLATION/FLUTTER
  a. **Atrial Fibrillation**
    i. General
      1. Most common sustained arrhythmia in adults.
      2. Increased risk with increasing age.
      3. Increased risk of intraatrial clot formation.
      4. Etiologies include hypertension, coronary heart disease, myopathy, and hyperthyroidism.
    ii. EKG findings (Fig. 1.1)
      1. Rapid, irregular atrial rate of more than 400 beats/minute.
      2. Ventricular rate varies from 100 to 200 beats/minute.

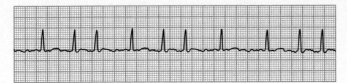

**Fig. 1.1** Atrial fibrillation.

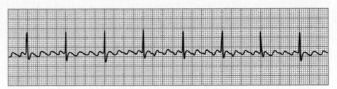

**Fig. 1.2** Atrial flutter.

3. RR interval is irregular.
4. Ventricular response is irregularly irregular.
5. Atrial fibrillation waves may be coarse, fine, and difficult to discern.

  iii. Treatment
1. Rate control is very important.
  (a) Rate control with beta-blockers (esmolol, metoprolol), calcium channel blockers (verapamil, diltiazem), or digoxin.
2. Anticoagulation is vital.
  (a) Long-term anticoagulation or antiplatelet therapy is needed.
  (b) Heparin is used acutely, and warfarin sodium (Coumadin) or direct-acting oral anticoagulant long-term.
  (c) Anticoagulant choice depends on $CHA_2DS_2$-VASc (**C**HF, **H**ypertension, **A**ge over 75 years [2 points], **D**iabetes, prior **S**troke or TIA [2 points], **V**ascular disease, **A**ge 65–74 years, **S**ex **c**ategory female) score.
    (i) One point for each condition, except age over 75 years and stroke, which get two points.
    (ii) Score of zero: treat with oral antiplatelet (aspirin) only.
    (iii) Score of 1: treat with oral anticoagulation or antiplatelet therapy, but preferably oral anticoagulation.
    (iv) Score greater than or equal to 2: treat with oral anticoagulation
3. Rhythm control.
  (a) Amiodarone is most effective, but side effects are common.
  (b) Cardioversion can be attempted if no sign of atrial clots.
  (c) Ablation therapy may be indicated in symptomatic paroxysmal disease.

**b. Atrial Flutter**
  i. General
1. Causes regular atrial rates from 250 to 400 beats/minute.
2. Symptoms include dizziness, palpitations, chest pain, and dyspnea.
3. Associated with chronic obstructive pulmonary disease (COPD), pulmonary embolism, thyrotoxicosis, and alcohol.

  ii. EKG findings (Fig. 1.2)
1. Present with a regular rhythm with sawtooth pattern of P waves in leads II, III, and aVF.
2. Ventricular response is 2:1 to 4:1.
  (a) Ventricular rates are then 100 to 150 beats/minute.

  iii. Treatment
1. Cardioversion should be attempted if no contraindications.
2. Acute treatment with beta-blockers (esmolol, metoprolol) and calcium channel blockers (verapamil, diltiazem) or ibutilide to control rate.
  (a) Long-term treatment with amiodarone, sotalol, quinidine, or procainamide.
3. If site of reentrant is known, catheter ablation can be attempted.

**c. Multifocal Atrial Tachycardia**
  i. General
1. Noted in patients with COPD or severe systemic illness.
  ii. EKG findings
1. Presence of multiple shaped (at least three different) P waves.
2. Differing PR intervals.
  iii. Treatment
1. Treat underlying cause.
2. Calcium channel blockers are agents of choice.
3. Avoid beta-blockers if lung disease present.

## II. ATRIOVENTRICULAR (AV) BLOCK
**a. General**
  i. AV block is defined as when some impulses are delayed or do not reach the ventricle.
  ii. Syncope may be noted.
**b. EKG Findings**
  i. First-degree block (Fig. 1.3).
1. Prolonged PR interval.
  (a) Greater than 0.2 second.

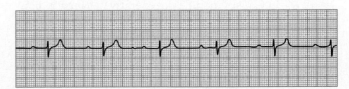

**Fig. 1.3** First-degree AV block.

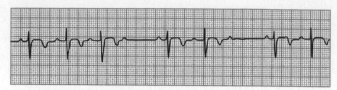

Fig. 1.4 Second-degree AV block: Wenckebach type.

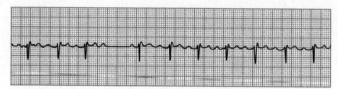

Fig. 1.5 Second-degree AV block: Mobitz type II.

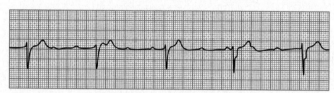

Fig. 1.6 Third-degree AV block.

   ii. Second-degree block.
     1. General.
       (a) Some P waves fail to produce a QRS complex.
     2. Mobitz type I (Wenckebach) block (Fig. 1.4).
       (a) Have a progressive increase in PR interval, until a P wave is blocked, and the cycle is repeated.
       (b) QRS duration is normal.
       (c) Causes include acute inferior wall myocardial infarction (MI), digitalis toxicity, and myocarditis.
     3. Mobitz type II block (Fig. 1.5).
       (a) Have a sudden block of a P wave with no change in PR interval.
       (b) QRS duration may be wide or narrow.
       (c) Causes include acute anterior wall myocardial infarct and calcification of aortic or mitral valve.
   iii. Third-degree block (Fig. 1.6).
     1. Occurs when atria and ventricles are controlled by different pacemakers.
     2. The atrial and ventricular rhythms are independent of each other.
     3. Causes include degenerative change in conduction system noted with aging, inferior or posterior infarcts, digitalis, and ankylosing spondylitis.
   iv. Table 1.1 summarizes EKG findings in arrhythmias and AV blocks.

**c. Treatment**
   i. Asymptomatic patients with first- or second-degree Mobitz type I AV block do not require treatment.
   ii. Correct any reversible causes.
   iii. Symptomatic patients may need to be treated with atropine or temporary pacing.
   iv. Permanent pacing may be needed.

## III. BUNDLE BRANCH BLOCK (BBB)
  **a. General**
   i. May develop after acute MI, cardiomyopathy, massive pulmonary embolism, or aortic stenosis; or may be normal.
   ii. Due to conduction delay in the right or left bundles.
     1. Represented by changes in the QRS complex.
   iii. Conduction across an accessory pathway can occur and leads to Wolff-Parkinson-White (WPW) syndrome.
     1. Patients with WPW are at greater risk for developing other cardiac arrhythmias.
  **b. EKG Findings**
   i. Right bundle branch block (RBBB) (Fig. 1.7A).
     1. QRS complex is wide.
       (a) QRS complex at least 0.12 second.
     2. An rSR in lead $V_1$.
     3. Wide terminal S wave in leads I and $V_6$.
     4. May note ST-T wave changes.
       (a) ST depression in $V_1$ and elevation in leads I and $V_6$.
   ii. LBBB (Fig. 1.7B).
     1. QRS complex is wide.
       (a) QRS complex at least 0.12 second.
     2. Upright and notched QRS complex in leads I and $V_6$.
     3. Mostly negative QRS in lead $V_1$.
     4. May note ST-T wave changes.
       (a) ST elevation in $V_1$ and depression in leads I and $V_6$.
   iii. Intraventricular conduction delay.
     1. QRS complex is wide.
     2. Lacks full criteria for either RBBB or LBBB signs on EKG.
   iv. WPW (Fig. 1.8).
     1. Preexcitation syndrome due to AV bypass tract through the bundle of Kent.
     2. QRS is wide.
     3. A delta wave is present at the start of the QRS complex.
     4. PR interval is short.
  **c. Treatment**
   i. Treat underlying cause.
   ii. In WPW, rate can be controlled with vagal maneuvers, adenosine, or verapamil. Medications

**TABLE 1.1**

**Rhythm Identification Flow Chart**

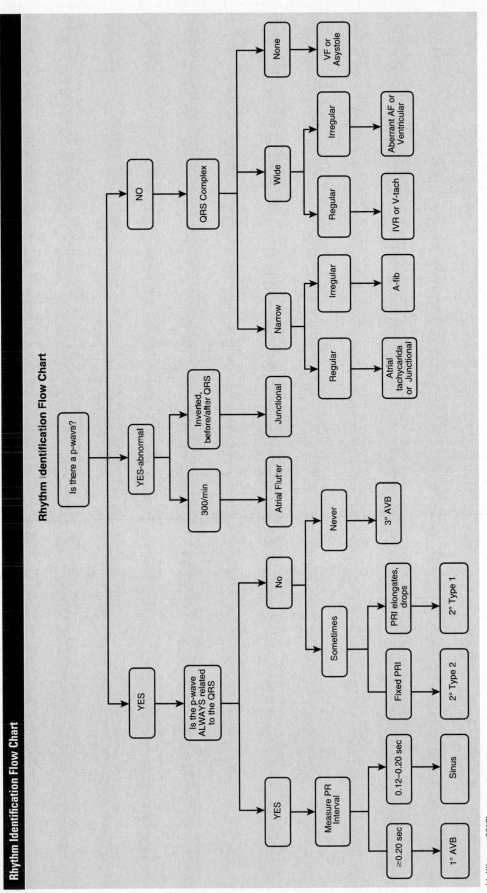

Rhythm Identification Flow Chart

*(J. Kilstrom, 2017)*

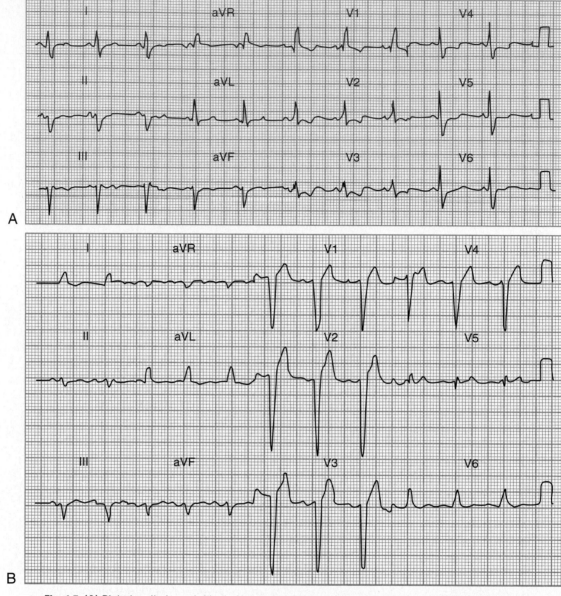

**Fig. 1.7 (A)** Right bundle branch block. Note wide QRS complex and rSR in lead $V_1$. **(B)** Left bundle branch block (LBBB). Note wide QRS complex and upright notched QRS complex in leads I and $V_6$.
*(From Goldman L, Ausiello D [eds]: Cecil Textbook of Medicine, 22nd ed. Philadelphia: WB Saunders, 2004:272, Fig. 50–54B.)*

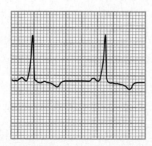

**Fig. 1.8** Wolff-Parkinson-White syndrome. Note delta wave, short PR interval, and wide QRS.

such as digoxin, beta-blockers or calcium channel blockers, which slow the heart rate, are contraindicated.

## IV. PAROXYSMAL SUPRAVENTRICULAR TACHYCARDIA
### a. General
   i. A reentry tachycardia.
   ii. Also called AV nodal reentry tachycardia (AVNRT).
   iii. Commonly noted in elderly patients with underlying heart disease.

iv. Patients may present with palpitations or anxiety.

**b. EKG Findings**

i. Ventricular rate is between 150 and 250 beats/minute, and rhythm is regular.

ii. Atrial activity is typically not seen.

**c. Treatment**

i. A vagal maneuver or antianxiety medication may be helpful.

ii. Drug of choice is adenosine.

1. Other rate-slowing medications (e.g., calcium channel blockers, beta-blockers, or digoxin) may be helpful.

## V. PREMATURE BEATS

**a. Premature Atrial Contractions**

i. General

1. Underlying rhythm interrupted by an early beat originating from the atria other than the sinoatrial node.

ii. EKG findings

1. Impulse is conducted with a narrow QRS complex, similar in appearance to normal sinus conducted beat, however p-wave morphology will appear different.

iii. Treatment

1. Treat underlying cause.

2. Antiarrhythmic drugs may be needed.

**b. Premature Ventricular Contractions (PVCs) (Fig. 1.9)**

i. General

1. Underlying rhythm interrupted by an early beat originating from the ventricles.

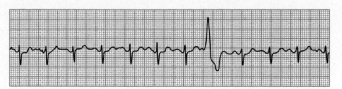

**Fig. 1.9** Premature ventricular contractions.

ii. EKG findings

1. Impulse conducted with a wide QRS complex, different from normal sinus conducted beat.

iii. Treatment

1. Treat underlying cause.

2. If noted in presence of acute ischemic heart disease, PVCs may lead to life-threatening ventricular arrhythmia.

3. Antiarrhythmic drugs may be needed. See Table 1.2 for list of antiarrhythmic drugs.

(a) Use of beta-blockers is common.

(b) Side effects are common.

## VI. SICK SINUS SYNDROME

**a. General**

i. Also called sinus node dysfunction.

ii. Abnormal cardiac impulse formation and propagation from the SA node prevent its pacemaker function.

iii. An uncommon syndrome that can lead to sinus arrest, sinus bradycardia, paroxysmal supraventricular tachycardia, and atrial fibrillation.

**TABLE 1.2**

| **Antiarrhythmic Drugs** | | | |
|---|---|---|---|
| **Class** | **Mechanism of Action** | **Drugs** | **Side Effects** |
| Ia | Sodium channel blocker | Quinidine Procainamide Disopyramide | Nausea, vomiting Quinidine: hemolytic anemia, thrombocytopenia, tinnitus Procainamide: drug-induced lupus |
| Ib | Sodium channel blocker | Lidocaine Mexiletine | Lidocaine: dizziness, confusion, seizures, coma Mexiletine: tremor, ataxia, rash |
| Ic | Sodium channel blocker | Flecainide Propafenone | Flecainide: nausea, dizziness |
| II | Beta-blocker | Propranolol Metoprolol | CHF, bronchospasm, bradycardia, hypotension |
| III | Prolonged action potential duration | Amiodarone Sotalol | Amiodarone: hepatitis, pulmonary toxicity, thyroid disease, peripheral neuropathy Sotalol: bronchospasm |
| IV | Calcium channel blocker | Verapamil Diltiazem | AV block, hypotension, bradycardia, constipation |

*AV*, Atrioventricular; *CHF*, congestive heart failure.

**b. Etiologies**

i. Often caused or worsened by medications, such as digitalis, calcium channel blockers, beta-blockers, and antiarrhythmics.

ii. Other etiologies include sarcoidosis, amyloidosis, and Chagas disease.

**c. Symptoms**

i. Stokes-Adams attacks (abrupt, transient loss of consciousness), dizziness, palpitations, chest pain, and shortness of breath may be noted.

**d. Diagnosis**

i. EKG results vary with bradyarrhythmias and tachybradyarrhythmias.

ii. EKG findings should be noted with symptoms.

**e. Treatment**

i. Pacemaker or medications for rate control.

## VII. VENTRICULAR TACHYCARDIA (VT) (FIG. 1.10)

**a. General**

i. Originates from below the bundle of His at a rate greater than 100 beats/minute.

ii. Precipitating causes include electrolyte imbalance, acid-base abnormalities, hypoxemia, MI, or drugs.

iii. Patients typically remain alert and stable with short runs of VT.

   1. If prolonged, patient may become hypotensive and develop myocardial ischemia.

iv. VT patients may become unstable.

   1. Syncope, palpitations, chest pain, dyspnea, and pulseless VT may be noted.

   2. Can cause sudden cardiac death.

v. Torsades de pointes.

   1. Polymorphic VT in which the QRS complexes change amplitude around an isoelectric axis (twisting of points).

   2. Drugs associated with torsades de pointes include the following:

     (a) Tricyclic antidepressants.

     (b) Erythromycin.

     (c) Clarithromycin.

     (d) Levofloxacin.

     (e) Ciprofloxacin.

     (f) Ondansetron.

     (g) Ketoconazole.

     (h) Haloperidol.

     (i) Disopyramide.

     (j) Sotalol.

     (k) Class I antiarrhythmics.

   3. May be caused by electrolyte abnormalities

     (a) Severe hypokalemia.

     (b) Hypomagnesemia.

   4. Long QT interval noted on EKG.

   5. Treatment includes removing any offending agents and use of antiarrhythmics.

**b. EKG Findings**

i. Rate greater than 100 beats/minute.

ii. QRS complex is wide.

**c. Treatment**

i. If VT lasts longer than 30 seconds, treatment is needed.

ii. Antiarrhythmic drugs, such as amiodarone or lidocaine should be used in stable patients.

iii. If patient becomes unstable, cardioversion is required.

iv. Empiric magnesium replacement should be considered if VT fails to terminate or worsens, especially in polymorphic VT.

## VIII. VENTRICULAR FIBRILLATION/FLUTTER

**a. Ventricular Fibrillation (Fig. 1.11)**

i. General

   1. Malignant arrhythmia with disorganized electrical activity leading to failure of cardiac contraction and failure to maintain cardiac output.

   2. Typically occurs in patients with ischemic heart disease and left ventricular dysfunction.

ii. EKG findings

   1. Irregular rhythm with an undulating low-amplitude baseline with no organized QRS complexes or T waves.

iii. Treatment

   1. Electrical defibrillation is required.

   2. Antiarrhythmics may also be beneficial.

**b. Ventricular Flutter**

i. General

   1. Very rapid, unstable form of VT.

   2. Typically progresses to ventricular fibrillation.

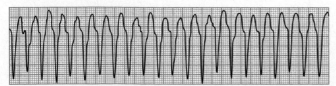

**Fig. 1.10** Ventricular tachycardia.

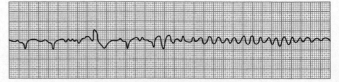

**Fig. 1.11** Ventricular fibrillation.

ii. EKG findings
   1. Sinus QRS complexes without distinct ST segment or T wave.
   2. Rate is from 240 to 280 beats/minute.
iii. Treatment
   1. Treat underlying cause.
   2. Electrical defibrillation is required.

# HEART FAILURE

## I. GENERAL

a. **Abnormal cardiac function leads to a decreased cardiac output that is not able to meet metabolic demands of the body.**
b. **Valvular heart disease, coronary artery disease, arrhythmias, hypothyroidism, high–cardiac output syndromes, and hypertension can lead to heart failure.**
   i. May be precipitated by reduction or discontinuing medications, increased sodium intake, anemia, infection, or pulmonary embolism.
c. **Systolic heart failure due to loss of contractile strength accompanied by ventricular dilation.**
   i. Will have a low ejection fraction.
d. **Diastolic heart failure due to impaired filling of ventricles with normal emptying capacity.**
   i. Will have a normal ejection fraction.

## II. CLINICAL MANIFESTATIONS

a. **Presenting symptoms include dyspnea, orthopnea, paroxysmal nocturnal dyspnea, fatigue, exercise intolerance, and edema.**
b. **Physical examination reveals a restless, dyspneic patient.**
   i. Neck examination reveals JVD.
   ii. Pulmonary examination reveals rales (crackles).
   iii. Cardiac examination reveals tachycardia, a displaced point of maximal impulse (PMI), and presence of an $S_3$ and $S_4$.
   iv. Abdominal and extremity examination reveals right upper quadrant tenderness, ascites, and peripheral edema.
   v. Laboratory tests show prerenal azotemia, elevated liver function tests, and elevated pro-B-natriuretic peptide.
      1. Complete blood count (CBC) and thyroid-stimulating hormone should be checked to rule out anemia and thyroid disease as potential causes of failure.
   vi. Chest x-ray film may reveal cardiomegaly and an increase in pulmonary vasculature (Fig. 1.12A and B).
      1. Pleural effusions may also be present.

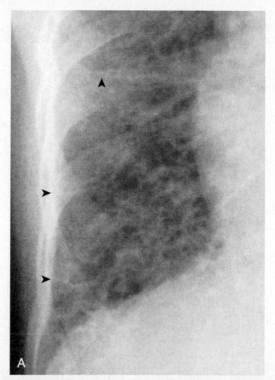

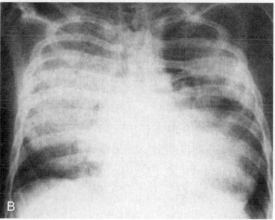

**Fig. 1.12** Chest x-ray in severe congestive heart failure. **(A)** Note Kerley B lines *(arrowheads)*. **(B)** Note cardiomegaly and increased pulmonary vascularity. *(From Grainger RG, Allison D, Adam A, Dixon AK [eds]: Diagnostic Radiology: A Textbook of Medical Imaging, 4th ed. London: Harcourt, 2001:874, Fig. 39.3A, B.)*

      2. Kerley B lines may be noted.
         (a) Due to fluid accumulation in the subpleural interlobular septa.
   vii. EKG may reveal LVH. Acute MI may also be noted.
   viii. Table 1.3 summarizes functional classification of heart failure.

## III. DIAGNOSIS

a. **Echocardiogram will reveal signs of systolic or diastolic dysfunction and decreased ejection fraction.**

**TABLE 1.3**

| Class | Definition |
|---|---|
| **Functional Classification of Heart Failure** | |
| I | No cardiac symptoms with ordinary activity |
| II | Cardiac symptoms with marked activity but asymptomatic at rest |
| III | Cardiac symptoms with mild activity but asymptomatic at rest |
| IV | Cardiac symptoms at rest |

## IV. TREATMENT

a. **Must treat the underlying cause, discontinue smoking, and control diet**
   i. Diet is low sodium, 1 g to 2 g daily.
b. **Pharmacologic Therapy**
   i. Goals are to control fluid retention, to control neurohormonal activation, and to control symptoms.
   ii. Diuretics are used to control fluid retention.
      1. Loop diuretics are drugs of choice in acute heart failure.
      2. Thiazide diuretics are used only in mild heart failure.
   iii. ACE inhibitors, which interfere with the renin-angiotensin system, are required of all patients with cardiac failure, unless contraindicated.
   iv. Vasodilators, including hydralazine and nitrates, are used when use of ACE inhibitors is not possible.
   v. Angiotensin receptor-neprilysin inhibitor (ARNI) should be used as a replacement for ACE-inhibitors in patients with heart failure and reduced EF who remain symptomatic on an ACE-inhibitor, beta-blocker, and mineralocorticoid inhibitor.
   vi. Beta-blockers (carvedilol, metoprolol) should be used in stable patients with left ventricular dysfunction, unless contraindicated.
   vii. Digitalis can improve symptoms and exercise tolerance by increasing cardiac contractility, in left-sided heart failure.
   viii. Other medications include oxygen and morphine.
   ix. Aspirin, nonsteroidal antiinflammatory drugs (NSAIDs), and calcium channel blockers should be avoided.

# HYPERTENSION

## I. ESSENTIAL

a. **General**
   i. Definition based in The Eighth Report of the Joint National Commission on Prevention, Detection,

**TABLE 1.4**

| Classification | Blood Pressure Levels |
|---|---|
| **Classification of Hypertension** | |
| Normal | <120 mm Hg systolic and <80 mm Hg diastolic |
| >60 years old | Systolic ≥150 mm Hg or diastolic >90 mm Hg |
| <60 years old | Systolic ≥140 mm Hg or diastolic >90 mm Hg |
| >18 years old with CKD or diabetes | Systolic ≥140 mm Hg or diastolic ≥90 mm Hg |

*CKD*, Chronic kidney disease.

**BOX 1.1**

**End-Organ Damage**

Left ventricular hypertrophy
Angina
Heart failure
Stroke
Chronic kidney disease
Peripheral artery disease
Retinopathy

Evaluation, and Treatment of High Blood Pressure (JNC VIII) guidelines (Table 1.4).
   ii. Incidence in the adult population is about 30%.
   iii. End-organ damage may occur to the brain, kidney, and heart (Box 1.1).
b. **Clinical Manifestations**
   i. Physical examination may be completely normal, except for elevated blood pressure.
      1. Physical examination should include evaluation of possible end-organ damage secondary to hypertension.
c. **Diagnosis**
   i. Based on two or more elevated blood pressure readings.
   ii. EKG may show LVH.
d. **Treatment**
   i. Lifestyle modifications.
      1. Weight loss.
      2. Limit alcohol intake.
      3. Regular aerobic exercise.
      4. Discontinue smoking.
      5. Reduce sodium intake.
      6. Reduce saturated fat and cholesterol intake.
   ii. Pharmacologic therapy.
      1. Initial therapy.
         (a) Non-Black patients over or under 60 years of age with or without diabetes are treated with a thiazide diuretic, ACE inhibitor, angiotensin II receptor blockers (ARB), or calcium channel blocker.

**TABLE 1.5**

| Treatment of Hypertension in Patients with Concomitant Disease | | | |
|---|---|---|---|
| **Concomitant Disease** | **Primary Choice** | **Secondary Choice** | **Avoid** |
| Angina | Beta-blockers<br>Calcium channel blockers | Diuretics<br>ACE inhibitors | |
| Diabetes | ACE inhibitors<br>$CA^{++}$ channel blockers | | Diuretics |
| Hyperlipidemia | ACE inhibitors<br>$CA^{++}$ channel blockers | | Diuretics<br>Beta-blockers |
| Congestive heart failure | Diuretics<br>ACE inhibitors<br>ARNI | | Beta-blockers<br>$CA^{++}$ channel blockers (verapamil) |
| Previous MI | Beta-blockers<br>ACE inhibitors | Diuretics<br>$CA^{++}$ channel blockers | |
| Chronic renal failure | Diuretics<br>$CA^{++}$ channel blockers | Beta-blockers<br>ACE inhibitors | |
| Asthma, chronic obstructive pulmonary disease | Diuretics<br>$CA^{++}$ channel blockers | ACE inhibitors | Beta-blockers |

*ACE*, Angiotensin-converting enzyme; *ARNI*, Angiotensin receptor-neprilysin inhibitors

(b) Black patients over or under 60 years of age with or without diabetes are treated with a thiazide diuretic or calcium channel blocker.

(c) Patients of any age with chronic kidney disease with or without diabetes are treated with ACE inhibitor or ARB.

(d) Other.

   i. Maximize first medication before adding a second, or

   ii. Add second medication before reaching maximum dose of first medication, or

   iii. Start with two medication classes separately or as a fixed-dose combination.

   iv. If patient is still not at blood pressure goal, consider added beta-blocker or aldosterone antagonist.

   v. Avoid the combined use of an ACE inhibitor and ARB.

2. Therapy options may vary with presence of comorbid conditions (Table 1.5).

## II. SECONDARY

a. **General**

  i. Defined as hypertension due to an identifiable cause.

  ii. Major etiologies include the following:

    1. Renovascular disease.

    2. Coarctation of the aorta.

    3. Primary aldosteronism.

    4. Cushing's syndrome.

    5. Pheochromocytoma.

    6. Obstructive sleep apnea.

    7. Renal parenchymal hypertension.

b. **Clinical Manifestations**

  i. Symptoms and laboratory results vary with etiology.

  ii. Table 1.6 shows clinical signs and symptoms.

**TABLE 1.6**

| Symptoms and Laboratory Findings in Secondary Hypertension | | |
|---|---|---|
| **Etiology** | **Clinical Signs and Symptoms** | **Evaluation** |
| Renovascular disease | Elevated serum creatinine | Captopril renogram<br>Magnetic resonance angiography of renal arteries |
| Coarctation of the aorta | Unequal pulses<br>Rib notching<br>Claudication | Magnetic resonance imaging |
| Primary aldosteronism | Hypokalemia<br>Metabolic alkalosis | Plasma renin and aldosterone |
| Cushing's syndrome | Truncal obesity | Plasma cortisol<br>Dexamethasone suppression test |
| Pheochromocytoma | Tachycardia<br>Polyuria<br>Headache<br>Diaphoresis | Plasma metanephrine and normetanephrine |
| Obstructive sleep apnea | Snoring<br>Obesity | Sleep study |
| Renal parenchymal | Elevated serum creatinine<br>Abnormal urinalysis | 24-hour urine for creatinine and protein<br>Renal ultrasound |

**c. Diagnosis**

    i. Based on finding of hypertension.

    ii. See Table 1.6 for evaluation testing.

**d. Treatment**

    i. Treat underlying cause.

    ii. Renovascular cause.

      1. Beta-blockers are used in patients with elevated renin.

      2. ACE inhibitors should be avoided in patients with bilateral renal artery stenosis.

      3. Diuretics used in combination with ACE inhibitors.

      4. Surgical revascularization.

## III. HYPERTENSIVE EMERGENCIES

**a. General**

    i. Potentially life-threatening situation.

    ii. Hypertension and symptoms of end-organ damage, such as retinopathy, cardiovascular or renal compromise, or encephalopathy.

    iii. Etiologies.

      1. Acute aortic dissection.

      2. Post coronary artery bypass graft.

      3. Acute MI.

      4. Unstable angina.

      5. Eclampsia.

      6. Head trauma.

      7. Severe burns.

    iv. Hypertension emergencies occur in 1% of hypertensive patients.

**b. Clinical Manifestations**

    i. Hypertension with end-organ disease.

**c. Diagnosis**

    i. Based on severely elevated blood pressure, greater than 220/140 mm Hg, and presence of headache, confusion, blurred vision, nausea and vomiting, seizures, grade II or IV hypertensive retinopathy, heart failure, and oliguria.

**d. Treatment**

    i. Requires immediate blood pressure reduction.

      1. Gradual decrease in blood pressure by no more than 25% in the first 1 to 2 hours of treatment and then 15% over the next 3 to 12 hours, to a target blood pressure of 170/100 mm Hg.

      2. Further decrease to a normal value over the next 48 hours.

    ii. Choice of agent varies with the cause.

      1. Nicardipine plus esmolol for patients with myocardial ischemia and infarction.

      2. Nicardipine for patients was ischemic stroke or intracerebral hemorrhage.

      3. Esmolol plus nicardipine for patients was aortic dissection.

      4. Oral clonidine can also be used for hypertensive urgency.

        (a) Sedation is common.

      5. Other options include captopril and nifedipine.

# HYPOTENSION

## I. CARDIOGENIC SHOCK

**a. General (Table 1.7 Shows Categories of Shock)**

    i. Tissue hypoperfusion due to decreased cardiac output (acute MI or end-stage heart failure).

    ii. Overall prognosis in cardiogenic shock is poor.

      1. Accounts for most deaths after acute MI.

    iii. Etiologies.

      1. Acute MI.

        (a) Pump failure.

        (b) Ventricular septal defect.

        (c) Ventricular rupture.

      2. Tachyarrhythmia.

      3. Valvular heart disease.

        (a) Acute mitral regurgitation.

        (b) Acute aortic regurgitation.

        (c) Aortic or mitral stenosis.

      4. Traumatic cardiac injury.

      5. Myocarditis.

**b. Clinical Manifestations**

    i. Hypotension.

      1. Defined as a systolic blood pressure less than 90 mm Hg or a decrease from baseline by more than 30 mm Hg.

    ii. Symptoms include altered mental status; cyanosis; oliguria; and cool, clammy extremities.

    iii. Physical examination reveals signs of hypoperfusion and hypovolemia.

    iv. Acute MI may be noted on EKG.

**c. Diagnosis**

    i. Echocardiogram is extremely helpful in diagnosing cardiogenic shock.

      1. May note left ventricular wall motion abnormalities and decreased left ventricular function.

**TABLE 1.7**

| Categories of Shock | | | |
| --- | --- | --- | --- |
| **Hypovolemic** | **Cardiogenic** | **Obstructive Noncardiogenic** | **Distributive** |
| Hemorrhage | Myocardial | Pericardial | Septic shock |
| Volume depletion |   dysfunction |   tamponade | Neurogenic |
| Extravascular | Valvular heart | Tension | Anaphylactic |
|   spacing |   defects |   pneumothorax | Drug induced |
| | | Severe pulmonary | |
| | |   embolism | |
| | | Left ventricular | |
| | |   outflow | |
| | |   obstruction | |

d. **Treatment**
  i. Adequate oxygenation and treatment of arrhythmias are especially important.
  ii. Improving blood pressure is critical.
    1. Intravenous (IV) fluids.
      (a) Trial of volume expansion is warranted.
    2. Vasopressor agents.
      (a) Norepinephrine is considered the most appropriate inotrope/vasopressor based on limited randomized clinical trials when compared to dopamine.
        i. Dopamine is still an acceptable option.
        ii. Increases systemic pressure and cardiac output.
      (b) Dobutamine can increase cardiac output but does not increase systemic blood pressure.
      (c) Risks of vasopressor drugs include aggravation of arrhythmias and increase in myocardial oxygen demand.
    3. Intra-aortic balloon pump.
      (a) Will increase diastolic coronary artery perfusion, decrease left ventricular afterload, improve cardiac output, and decrease myocardial oxygen demand.

## II. ORTHOSTATIC/POSTURAL

a. **General**
  i. May result in syncope that could be recurrent.
  ii. Defined as a fall in systolic blood pressure of 30 mm Hg or more or a fall in diastolic blood pressure of 10 mm Hg or more between recumbent and upright postures.
  iii. Etiologies include the following:
    1. Drugs.
      (a) Antipsychotic agents.
      (b) Diuretics.
      (c) Alpha-adrenergic blockers.
      (d) ACE inhibitors.
      (e) Alcohol.
      (f) Tranquilizers.
      (g) Vasodilators.
      (h) Methyldopa.
    2. Polyneuropathies.
    3. Parkinson's disease.
b. **Clinical Manifestations**
  i. Symptoms include change in mental status/confusion (secondary to cerebral hypoperfusion), weak pulse, cool extremities, tachypnea, and reduced urine output.
  ii. Physical examination reveals hypotension, tachycardia, and tachypnea.
c. **Diagnosis**
  i. Based on clinical findings.
d. **Treatment**
  i. Treat underlying cause; remove offending medications, if possible; and support blood pressure.

## LIPID DISORDERS

### I. HYPERCHOLESTEROLEMIA
a. **General**
  i. Linked to the development of atherosclerosis.
  ii. Due to elevations in low-density lipoprotein (LDL).
    1. Elevations of LDL are associated with increased risk of atherosclerotic heart disease.
    2. Elevations of high-density lipoproteins (HDL) are associated with a decreased risk of atherosclerotic heart disease.
  iii. Normal range for fasting lipids (Table 1.8).
  iv. Etiology.
    1. Familial hypercholesterolemia.
      a. Autosomal dominant disorder due to defective or absence of LDL receptors.
      b. See Table 1.9 for the Fredrickson phenotypes for hyperlipidemia.
    2. Nephrotic syndrome.
    3. Hypothyroidism.
    4. Obstructive liver disease.

**TABLE 1.8**

| Normal Range for Fasting Lipids | | | |
| --- | --- | --- | --- |
| Lipid | Acceptable (mg/dL) | Borderline (mg/dL) | Unacceptable (mg/dL) |
| Cholesterol | <200 | 200–239 | >240 |
| LDL | <130 (primary) <100 (secondary) | 130–159 130–159 | >160 >100 |
| HDL | ≥60 | 35–45 | <35 |
| Triglyceride | <150 | 150–500 | >500 |

*HDL*, High-density lipoprotein; *LDL*, low-density lipoprotein.

**TABLE 1.9**

| Fredrickson Phenotypes for Hyperlipidemia | | | |
| --- | --- | --- | --- |
| Type | Lipids Elevated | Subtype Elevated | Coronary Artery Disease Risk |
| I | Triglycerides | Chylomicrons | Normal |
| IIA | Cholesterol | LDL | Very high |
| IIB | Cholesterol and triglycerides | VLDL and LDL | Very high |
| III | Cholesterol and triglycerides | Beta-VLDL and LDL | Very high |
| IV | Triglycerides | VLDL | Varies |
| V | Triglycerides | VLDL and chylomicrons | Moderate |

*LDL*, Low-density lipoprotein; *VLDL*, very-low-density lipoprotein.

b. **Clinical Manifestations**
   i. Xanthomas noted on Achilles tendon, patellar tendon, and extensor tendons of the hand, as well as around the eyes.
c. **Diagnosis**
   i. Laboratory tests reveal elevated cholesterol (>200 mg/dL)
      1. Plasma cholesterol levels are typically greater than 300 mg/dL.
d. **Treatment**
   i. Dietary.
      1. Limit cholesterol intake to less than 300 mg/day.
      2. Limit total dietary fats to 30% and saturated fats to less than 10% of total calories.
   ii. Medications.
      1. Bile acid–binding agents.
         a. Bind bile acids/cholesterol and promote loss in the stool.
         b. Also increase LDL receptor expression, and directly remove LDL particles.
         c. Side effects include constipation and bloating.
         d. Agents can interfere with absorption of numerous medications, including glycosides, thiazides, warfarin, tetracycline, T₄, and iron salts.
      2. HMG-CoA reductase inhibitors (statins).
         a. Directly inhibits cholesterol biosynthesis.
         b. Side effects include myositis.
      3. Nicotinic acid (niacin).
         a. Inhibits release of lipoproteins from the liver.
         b. Side effects include flushing.

## II. HYPERTRIGLYCERIDEMIA

a. **General**
   i. Linked to the development of pancreatitis.
   ii. Due to elevations in very-low-density lipoprotein (VLDL) and chylomicrons.
   iii. Etiology.
      1. Familial hypertriglyceridemia
         a. Autosomal dominant disorder.
      2. Diabetes mellitus.
      3. Uremia.
      4. Sepsis.
      5. Obesity.
      6. SLE.
      7. Alcohol.
b. **Clinical Manifestations**
   i. Are typically asymptomatic and without signs of xanthomas.
   ii. May have signs and symptoms of pancreatitis.
   iii. Diagnosed with routine blood screening.

c. **Diagnosis**
   i. Marked elevations in triglycerides, normal or low LDL levels, and decreased levels of HDL cholesterol.
d. **Treatment**
   i. Treatment plan should begin with weight loss, increased physical activity, low-fat diet, andrestriction of alcohol.
   ii. Medications.
      1. Fibric-acid derivations.
         a. Reduce hepatic triglyceride production and increased HDL synthesis.
         b. Side effects include cholelithiasis and drug-induced hepatitis.
      2. Nicotinic acid.
      3. Fish oil.

# ISCHEMIC HEART DISEASE

## I. ACUTE MYOCARDIAL INFARCTION

a. **General**
   i. Myocardial necrosis brought on by ischemia.
   ii. Most deaths occur within 1 hour of onset of symptoms.
      1. Most deaths are caused by ventricular fibrillation.
      2. Rapid defibrillation can reverse ventricular fibrillation.
   iii. Box 1.2 lists risk factors for coronary atherosclerosis.
b. **Clinical Manifestations**
   i. Pain is retrosternal and is described as heavy, pressure-like, squeezing, or bandlike.
      1. Pain may radiate to the neck, jaw, or left arm.
      2. Pain typically lasts longer (20 minutes to several hours) than angina.
      3. Elderly patients or patients with diabetes may have acute MI that is painless.
      4. Watch for atypical presentation of pain.

**BOX 1.2**

| **Risk Factors for Coronary Atherosclerosis** |
|---|
| Hyperlipidemia |
| Hypertension |
| Increasing age |
| Obesity |
| Positive family history |
| Stress |
| Diabetes |
| Male gender |
| Sedentary lifestyle |
| Smoking |

ii. Associated signs and symptoms include nausea, vomiting, diaphoresis, dyspnea, and weakness.

iii. Physical examination reveals no specific findings that are diagnostic for acute MI.

1. Blood pressure may be elevated, an $S_4$ may be noted (due to a stiffened ventricle), and signs of heart failure may be evident.

2. Bradycardia may be noted in inferior wall infarcts, and tachycardia may be noted in large infarcts.

iv. Laboratory studies.

1. Myoglobin.
   (a) Detectable within 1 to 2 hours after acute MI.
   (b) Found in skeletal and cardiac muscle.
2. Creatine phosphokinase (CPK).
   (a) Total CPK correlates with infarct size.
   (b) CPK-MB is specific for cardiac muscle.
3. Troponin.
   (a) Not normally present in blood.
   (b) More sensitive and specific than CPK-MB
   (c) Elevated in acute MI.
   (d) Highly sensitive or fourth generation troponin assays (hs-cTnT) allow for detection of MI earlier, using the change in value over 3 hours.
4. Table 1.10 compares cardiac enzyme markers.
5. Other tests.
   (a) Leukocytosis may be noted on CBC.
   (b) A lipid profile should be obtained to determine if lipid-lowering therapy is indicated.
   (c) C-reactive protein is elevated.

v. EKG reveals ST elevation.

1. Table 1.11 summarizes acute MI damage patterns.

**c. Diagnosis**

i. Based on clinical and laboratory findings.

ii. Echocardiogram is obtained to evaluate global and regional cardiac function.

iii. Chest radiography may demonstrate signs of heart failure.

**TABLE 1.10**

| Cardiac Enzyme Markers in Acute Myocardial Infarction | | | |
| --- | --- | --- | --- |
| **Marker** | **Time to Appearance** | **Duration of Elevation** | **Note** |
| hs-cTnT | 1 hour | 7–14 days | Test of choice |
| Troponin I | 2–6 hours | 5–10 days | |
| Creatine kinase MB | 3–6 hours | 2–4 days | |
| Myoglobin | 1–2 hours | <1 day | Low specificity |

**TABLE 1.11**

| Locating Myocardial Damage | | | |
| --- | --- | --- | --- |
| **Affected Wall** | **EKG Leads** | **Artery Involved** | **EKG Leads Reciprocal Changes** |
| Inferior | II, III, aVF | RCA | I, aVL |
| Lateral | I, aVL, $V_5$, $V_6$ | Circumflex | $V_1$, $V_2$ |
| Anterior | $V_2$–$V_4$ | LAD | II, III, aVF |
| Posterior | $V_1$, $V_2$ | Posterior descending | |
| Apical | $V_3$–$V_6$ | LAD, RCA | None |
| Anterolateral | I, aVL, $V_4$–$V_6$ | LAD circumflex | II, III, aVF |
| Anteroseptal | $V_1$–$V_3$ | LAD | None |

*LAD,* Left anterior descending; *LCA,* left coronary artery; *RCA,* right coronary artery.

iv. Coronary angiography confirms location of injury and coronary vessel involved.

**d. Treatment**

i. Aspirin and $P2Y_{12}$ inhibitors should be given to all patients, unless contraindicated.

ii. Initial therapy.

1. Oxygen.
   (a) Only given if oxygen saturation is reduced.
2. Beta-blockers.
   (a) Control blood pressure and decrease probability of sudden cardiac death.
2. Nitroglycerin.
   (a) Used for coronary artery dilation.
3. Morphine.
   (a) Pain and blood pressure control.
4. Continuous EKG monitoring.

iii. Specific therapy.

1. Recanalization therapy.
   (a) Thrombolytic therapy.
      (i) Includes streptokinase and tissue plasminogen activator.
         (1) Major risk factors are bleeding and intracerebral hemorrhage.
         (2) Candidates for therapy include patients with ST elevation or new LBBB presenting within 12 hours of onset of symptoms and without contraindications.
         (3) Table 1.12 lists contraindications to thrombolytic therapy.
   (b) Primary percutaneous coronary intervention.
      (i) Mechanical recanalization by inflation of catheter-based balloon.
2. Antiplatelet therapy.
   (a) Aspirin.
      (i) Inhibits platelet aggregation and development of coronary thrombi.

**TABLE 1.12**

| Contraindications to Thrombolytic Therapy | |
|---|---|
| **Absolute** | **Relative** |
| Active bleeding/Bleeding disorders | Severe or uncontrolled hypertension |
| Prior hemorrhagic stroke/Other stroke within 3 months | Anticoagulation: therapeutic or elevated INR |
| Intracranial or spinal cord cancer | Old ischemic stroke |
| Suspected or known aortic dissection | Recent major surgery or trauma |
| | Recent internal bleeding |
| Significant head trauma within 3 months | Active peptic ulcer |
| | Pregnancy |

(b) Clopidogrel, prasugrel, or ticagrelor.
  (i) Has antiplatelet effects and is used in aspirin-allergic patients.
  (ii) Consider use for 9 to 12 months post-acute MI, particularly after stent placement.
(c) Glycoprotein IIb/IIIa receptor inhibitor (abciximab or eptifibatide).
  (i) Inhibits fibrinogen receptor and benefits high-risk patients by improving coronary artery patency.
3. Antithrombin therapy.
  (a) Heparin inactivates thrombin and factor X.
  (b) Used in combination with thrombolytic therapy.
4. Other.
  (a) Nitrates.
    (i) Induce vascular smooth muscle relaxation and reduce cardiac preload and afterload.
  (b) Beta-blockers.
    (i) Reduce heart rate, blood pressure, and myocardial contractility; stabilize the heart electrically.
      (1) Limit myocardial oxygen consumption.
      (2) Use metoprolol and carvedilol in patients with acute coronary syndrome and heart failure.

(c) ACE inhibitors.
  (i) Improve remodeling after acute MI.
  (ii) Avoid in presence of hypotension.
(d) Statins.
  (i) Start in hospital in all patients with acute coronary syndrome.
iv. Complications.
  1. Arrhythmias.
    (a) Ventricular.
    (b) Atrial fibrillation.
  2. Heart failure.
    (a) Left ventricular dysfunction.
    (b) Cardiogenic shock.
  3. Mechanical.
    (a) Papillary muscle rupture.
    (b) Left ventricular wall rupture.
    (c) Left ventricular aneurysm.
  4. Thromboembolic.
  5. Pericarditis: Dressler syndrome.

## II. ANGINA PECTORIS
### a. Stable
  i. General
    1. A symptom, pain that builds up rapidly in 30 seconds and disappears within 5 to 15 minutes.
      (a) Disappears more promptly if nitroglycerin is used.
    2. Is precipitated by activity and relieved by rest.
    3. Related to a fixed stenosis of one or more coronary arteries.
    4. See Table 1.13 for other etiologies of chest pain.
  ii. Clinical manifestations
    1. Pain presents as tightness and squeezing and is described as aching or dull discomfort.
      (a) Pain is midsternal with radiation to the neck, left shoulder, or left arm.
    2. Risk factors should be sought.
    3. Physical examination may be normal.
      (a) A transient $S_4$ or $S_3$ gallop may be noted.
    4. When the patient is pain-free, the EKG may reveal arrhythmia, prior MI, or LVH.
      (a) EKG obtained during or shortly after an episode of pain may reveal ST segment depression and T wave inversion.

**TABLE 1.13**

| Etiologies of Chest Pain | | | |
|---|---|---|---|
| **Cardiac** | | **Noncardiac** | |
| **Ischemic** | **Nonischemic** | **Cardiac** | **Noncardiac** |
| Coronary atherosclerosis | Anemia | Pericarditis | Gastrointestinal, esophagitis, gastroesophageal reflux disease, cholecystitis, peptic ulcer disease, pancreatitis |
| Coronary spasm | Sickle cell disease | Aortic dissection | Psychogenic, anxiety, panic, somatization |
| Cocaine induced | Hyperviscosity | | Pulmonary, pulmonary embolism, pneumothorax, pneumonia |
| Aortic stenosis | Hyperthyroidism | | Neuromuscular, costochondritis, herpes zoster |
| Hypertrophic cardiomyopathy | Adrenergic stimulation, hypoxia | | |

iii. Diagnosis
1. Exercise testing is used to detect myocardial ischemia.
   (a) Ischemia is indicated when ST segment depression of greater than 2 mm, during early stages of exercise, or during hypotension.
2. Perfusion scintigraphy testing.
   (a) Performed with exercise, adenosine, or dipyridamole injection.
   (b) Can localize sites of active ischemia.
   (c) Used in patients with baseline EKG changes.
3. Coronary angiography.
   (a) Required to exclude coronary artery disease with certainty.
iv. Treatment
1. General.
   (a) Smoking cessation.
   (b) Control hypertension.
   (c) Control diabetes.
   (d) Implement an exercise plan.
2. Reduce progression.
   (a) Manage lipids.
   (b) Antiplatelet medications.
      (i) Includes aspirin, clopidogrel, or warfarin.
   (c) Beta-blockers.
   (d) ACE inhibitors.
3. Control symptoms.
   (a) Beta-blockers.
   (b) Nitrates.
      (i) Excellent response to nitrates.
   (c) Calcium channel blockers.
4. Revascularization.
   (a) Includes percutaneous coronary interventions or coronary artery bypass graft.

**b. Unstable**
i. General
1. Diagnosed clinically when:
   (a) Patient has new-onset angina.
   (b) Patient has increasing angina.
   (c) Patient has angina occurring at rest.
2. An acute, nonocclusive thrombus is found in most cases.
   (a) Plaque rupture or erosion with overlying thrombus is the initiating mechanism.
ii. Clinical manifestations
1. Patient presents with dyspnea, palpitations, and fatigue.
2. Pain is located retrosternal or epigastric.
   (a) Described as pressure, burning, or squeezing pain.
   (b) May have associated nausea, shortness of breath, and diaphoresis.
      (i) These may be the only symptoms in elderly or diabetic patients.

3. Physical examination may be normal or may reveal an $S_4$ gallop, a mitral regurgitation murmur, and rales on lung examination.
4. EKG may be normal.
   (a) Nonspecific signs, such as transient ST changes and inverted T waves, may be noted.
5. Laboratory testing reveals normal cardiac enzymes.
iii. Diagnosis
1. Based on clinical findings.
2. Must rule out acute MI.
iv. Treatment
1. Reduce progression to or size of MI.
   (a) Antiplatelet medications.
      (i) Includes aspirin, $P2Y_{12}$ inhibitors, platelet glycoprotein IIb/IIIa receptor inhibitors, or heparin.
   (b) Beta-blockers.
   (c) ACE inhibitors.
2. Treatment of ischemic signs and symptoms.
   (a) Beta-blockers.
   (b) Nitrates.
      (i) Responds poorly to nitrates.
   (c) Calcium channel blockers.
3. Revascularization.
   (a) Includes coronary angioplasty or coronary artery bypass graft.

**c. Prinzmetal's Variant**
i. General
1. Pain occurs mainly at rest but may occur during exercise.
2. Pain may awaken patient in the morning.
   (a) Due to increased sympathetic activity.
3. Caused by occlusive spasm superimposed on a non-severe coronary artery stenosis.
4. Cardiac syndrome X is myocardial ischemia that occurs in patients with normal coronary arteries.
   (a) Due to disease of coronary microcirculation.
ii. Clinical manifestations
1. Pain is noted as above.
   (a) May be associated with Raynaud's phenomenon and migraine headache.
iii. Diagnosis
1. Diagnosed when transient ST segment elevation is documented during an episode of chest pain.
2. Coronary angiography, with injection of ergonovine or acetylcholine, can cause focal vasospasm.
iv. Treatment
1. Episodes respond well to nitrates and calcium channel blockers.

# VASCULAR DISEASE

## I. ACUTE RHEUMATIC FEVER

### a. General

i. Inflammatory disease that occurs as a response to an infection due to group A streptococci.
   1. Have exudative and proliferative inflammatory lesions on connective tissue, of the heart, joints, and subcutaneous tissue.

ii. Range of time from infection to onset of symptoms is 1 to 5 weeks.

iii. Mechanism is unknown.

iv. Peak incidence is in the 5- to 15-year age group.
   1. Rare in children younger than 4 years.

### b. Clinical Manifestations

i. Major manifestations (Jones criteria).
   1. Carditis.
      (a) Can involve the endocardium, myocardium, or pericardium.
      (b) Present with cardiac murmur, cardiomegaly, pericarditis, and congestive heart failure.
      (c) Cardiac murmur is an apical systolic murmur that is blowing and high pitched in nature.
   2. Polyarthritis.
      (a) Migratory arthritis that typically involves larger joints, knees, and ankles.
      (b) Synovial fluid reveals an increase in neutrophils, but no bacteria.
   3. Chorea.
      (a) Rapid, purposeless, involuntary movements, involving the face and extremities.
      (b) Speech is slurred; and the tongue, when protruded, retracts involuntarily.
   4. Erythema marginatum.
      (a) Erythematosus macule or papule that extends over the skin with central clearing.
   5. Subcutaneous nodules.
      (a) Firm, painless subcutaneous nodules that vary in size from a few millimeters to 2 cm.
      (b) Occur over bony surfaces and tendons of the elbows, knees, and wrists.

ii. Earliest manifestations include fever and joint involvement.
   1. Table 1.14 lists Jones criteria.

### c. Diagnosis

i. No laboratory tests are diagnostic for rheumatic fever.
   1. CBC reveals leukocytosis and an anemia of chronic disease.
   2. Sedimentation rate and C-reactive protein are elevated.

**TABLE 1.14**

| Jones Criteria for Diagnosis of Acute Rheumatic Fever | | |
| --- | --- | --- |
| **Major** | **Minor** | **Supporting** |
| Carditis | Arthralgia | Positive strep screen or throat culture |
| Polyarthritis | Fever | |
| Chorea | Prolonged PR interval | |
| Erythema marginatum | Laboratory findings: Increased erythrocyte sedimentation rate | Elevated or increasing ASO titer |
| Subcutaneous nodules | Increased C-reactive protein | |
| | Increased acute-phase reactants | |

*ASO,* Antistreptolysin-O.

ii. Documentation of a recent streptococcal infection is noted.
   1. Includes positive antistreptolysin-O (ASO), anti-DNase, or antihyaluronidase titers.

iii. Diagnosis is based on the Jones criteria.
   1. Two major or one major and two minor manifestations indicate a high probability of acute rheumatic fever.

### d. Treatment

i. Bed rest.

ii. Antibiotics do not modify the course of the disease but should be used to eradicate streptococcal infection if present.

iii. Antiinflammatory drugs suppress the signs and symptoms but are not curative.
   1. Major drugs include aspirin; corticosteroids if no response to aspirin.

iv. Decrease risk for disease by prevention with appropriate and timely treatment of streptococcal throat infections.

v. Secondary prevention of rheumatic fever, prevention of recurrent attacks; includes penicillin G or V or sulfadiazine.
   1. Erythromycin is used in the penicillin-allergic person.

## II. AORTIC ANEURYSM

### a. General

i. Pathologic dilation of the aorta.

ii. May involve any portion of the aorta, but abdominal aorta is the most common location.
   1. Abdominal aorta aneurysms are more common in men.

iii. Atherosclerosis is the major underlying cause.

iv. 90% of aortic aneurysms occur below the renal arteries.

### b. Clinical Manifestations

i. Most are asymptomatic.

ii. When symptoms are noted, they include a steady, gnawing hypogastric or low back pain.

iii. With rupture, the pain worsens; and blood pressure drops.

iv. On physical examination, a pulsatile abdominal mass may be noted.

c. **Diagnosis**

i. Ultrasound or computed tomography (CT) scan makes diagnosis.

1. Ultrasound is an excellent screening test.

(a) Screening recommended for males aged 65 to 75 years who have ever smoked.

2. Monitor change in aneurysm by CT scan.

d. **Treatment**

i. Goal is to reduce the risk for expansion and rupture.

ii. Serial imaging should be obtained to monitor size, and beta-blockers should be used to reduce aortic pressure.

1. Imaging should be done every 6 months for abdominal aortic aneurysm greater than 4 cm in size.

iii. Abdominal aortic aneurysm that is greater than 5.5 cm in size or that has undergone rapid expansion (>5 mm in 6 months) should be surgically repaired.

## III. AORTIC DISSECTION

a. **General**

i. Begins with a tear in the aorta intima; blood enters the media, dividing it into two layers.

ii. Increased risk in patients with Marfan syndrome.

iii. Peak incidence in patients without Marfan syndrome is age 60 to 80 years.

iv. Typically, patients have a history of hypertension.

b. **Clinical Manifestations**

i. Present with sudden, severe retrosternal pain, described as a tearing or sharp pain.

ii. Elevated blood pressure is common.

iii. Pulse deficits are common.

iv. Chest x-ray film may reveal an enlarged mediastinum.

c. **Diagnosis**

i. Magnetic resonance imaging (MRI) is the gold standard for diagnosis.

ii. Diagnosis also can be made via CT scan, aortograph, or transesophageal echocardiogram.

d. **Treatment**

i. Primary goal is to halt further progression of the dissection and to reduce the chance of rupture.

ii. Blood pressure control with a beta-blocker plus a vasodilator (esmolol plus nicardipine).

iii. Surgical repair is the definitive treatment.

## IV. ARTERIAL EMBOLISM/THROMBOSIS

a. **General**

i. Cause of acute arterial insufficiency.

ii. Arterial embolism secondary to atrial fibrillation/flutter, mitral stenosis, transmural infarct, trauma, hypercoagulable states, and post arterial procedures.

b. **Clinical Manifestations**

i. Patients present with acute onset of severe pain, diminished pulses, cold limbs, and cyanosis.

ii. Typically presents unilaterally.

iii. Physical examination reveals the 5 Ps as follows:

1. Pain.

(a) Constant and worse with any movement.

2. Pallor.

(a) Occurs first, followed by cyanosis.

3. Pulselessness.

(a) Associated with a cold limb.

4. Paresthesias.

(a) Caused by damage to peripheral nerves.

5. Paralysis.

(a) Due to damage to muscle and motor nerves.

c. **Diagnosis**

i. Echocardiogram obtained to evaluate for source of thrombus.

ii. Arteriogram to identify location.

d. **Treatment**

i. Heparin should be started immediately.

ii. Emergent embolectomy-thrombectomy is needed to restore blood flow.

iii. Complications include limb loss and compartment syndrome.

## V. CHRONIC/ACUTE ARTERIAL OCCLUSION

a. **General**

i. Decrease in 50% of arterial lumen will produce clinical symptoms, ischemia, and necrosis.

ii. Risk factors include smoking, hypercholesterolemia, diabetes, and hypertension.

iii. Most common cause is atherosclerosis.

iv. Lower extremities are the most common locations.

b. **Clinical Manifestations**

i. Patients may be asymptomatic due to collateral circulation.

ii. Major symptom is pain, followed by claudication.

1. The primary area involved is the calf.

2. Area of occlusion is distal to the site of claudication.

iii. Occlusion of certain vessels brings about certain conditions.

1. Carotid artery: transient ischemic attack.

2. Ophthalmic artery: amaurosis fugax.

**TABLE 1.15**

| Interpretation of Ankle/Brachial Index | |
| --- | --- |
| **Ankle/Brachial Index Result** | **Interpretation** |
| >1.0 | Normal |
| 0.5–0.9 | Arterial claudication |
| <0.4 | Severe arterial stenosis |

    iv. Physical examination reveals decreased peripheral pulses, bruits, ischemic skin changes, and painful ischemic ulcers.

  **c. Diagnosis**

    i. Ankle/brachial index can provide information regarding severity of disease.

      1. Table 1.15 summarizes interpretation of ankle/brachial index.

    ii. Doppler with ultrasound can be used to evaluate blood flow.

    iii. Arteriography is used to determine the location of occlusion.

  **d. Treatment**

    i. Pharmacologic therapies include the following:

      1. Cilostazol.

        (a) Phosphodiesterase inhibitor that suppresses platelet aggregation and is a direct arterial vasodilator.

      2. Antiplatelet agents.

        (a) Current data indicate antiplatelets result in only a modest or negligible improvement in claudication symptoms

      3. Heparin and warfarin have no therapeutic use.

    ii. Thromboendarterectomy can be used to repair diseased arteries.

    iii. Patient should be educated to stop smoking.

**VI. GIANT CELL ARTERITIS**

  **a. General**

    i. A granulomatous vasculitis that affects the temporal artery.

    ii. Typically affects patients older than 50 years.

    iii. Etiology is unknown.

    iv. May coexist with polymyalgia rheumatica.

  **b. Clinical Manifestations**

    i. Most common symptom is new onset of headache, located in the temporal region.

    ii. Jaw claudication, scalp tenderness, and visual disturbances are also noted.

      1. Transient vision loss or complete blindness may be noted.

    iii. On physical examination, enlargement, tenderness, and erythema of the artery may be noted.

      1. Bruit also may be present.

    iv. Laboratory testing reveals an elevated erythrocyte sedimentation rate (ESR), anemia, and leukocytosis.

  **c. Diagnosis**

    i. Diagnosis is made by biopsy of the artery.

  **d. Treatment**

    i. Corticosteroids should be started as soon as possible.

**VII. PHLEBITIS/THROMBOPHLEBITIS**

  **a. General**

    i. Inflammatory thrombosis involving the superficial veins of the lower extremity.

    ii. Associated with varicose veins, pregnancy, and catheter placement.

    iii. Septic thrombophlebitis is more common in patients who misuse intravenous drugs.

  **b. Clinical Manifestations**

    i. Vein is palpable and tender.

    ii. Induration, redness, and tenderness are localized along the course of the vein.

      1. A palpable cord is present.

    iii. There is no swelling of the extremity.

  **c. Diagnosis**

    i. Must rule out deep venous thrombosis (DVT).

    ii. Diagnosis based on clinical findings.

  **d. Treatment**

    i. Warm, moist compresses to the area.

      1. No restriction of activity is needed.

    ii. NSAIDs to relieve pain.

    iii. If septic thrombophlebitis, antibiotics are needed.

      1. Antibiotics should cover staphylococci.

**VIII. VENOUS THROMBOSIS**

  **a. General**

    i. DVT is the development of a clot in the deep veins of the extremities or pelvis.

    ii. Predisposing factors include venous stasis, activation of coagulation system, and vascular damage (Virchow's triad).

    iii. Risk factors for DVT are as follows:

      1. Prolonged immobilization.

      2. Postoperative, typically orthopedic procedures.

      3. Pelvic or extremity trauma.

      4. Oral contraceptives.

      5. Cancer.

      6. Hypercoagulable state.

      7. Pregnancy.

      8. Obesity.

      9. Smoking.

      10. Family history.

**b. Clinical Manifestations**
  i. Present with pain and swelling at the site and distal from the clot.
  ii. Physical examination may be normal.
     1. Homans sign—pain with dorsiflexion of the foot—may be positive but has low sensitivity and specificity for DVT.
**c. Diagnosis**
  i. Compression ultrasound, MRI, and venogram (rarely used) are diagnostic.
     1. Serial ultrasounds may be needed to confirm diagnosis.
  ii. D-dimer may be useful in ruling out thrombosis in patients with low probability for DVT.
**d. Treatment**
  i. Complications include pulmonary embolism.
  ii. Prophylaxis is required for all high-risk patients and includes the following:
     1. Low-molecular-weight heparin.
     2. Elastic stockings.
     3. Intermittent pneumatic leg compression.
  iii. Anticoagulation therapy is required.
     1. Direct-acting oral anticoagulants (DOACs).
     2. Warfarin.
        a. Intravenous unfractionated heparin or low-molecular-weight heparin is required acutely until warfarin levels are therapeutic.
           (a) Heparin is continued for at least 5 days and until warfarin levels are therapeutic.
              (i) Heparin-associated thrombocytopenia may occur within 5 to 10 days of starting heparin.
                 (1) Platelet count should be monitored.
           (b) With warfarin therapy, the international normalized ratio (INR) should be between 2 and 3 to be therapeutic.
           (c) DOAC and warfarin therapy is typically continued for 3 to 6 months in patients with reversible risk factors.
              (i) Indefinite therapy may be needed in high-risk patients.
     3. An inferior vena cava filter may be needed to prevent pulmonary embolism in patients with contraindications to anticoagulation.

## IX. VARICOSE VEINS
**a. General**
  i. Caused by incompetence of the saphenous vein.
     1. Due to increased intravascular pressure or defective valves.

  ii. Occur primarily in the superficial veins of the medial and anterior thigh, calf, and ankle.
  iii. Contributing factors include prolonged standing, pregnancy, and obesity.
     1. More common in females.
**b. Clinical Manifestations**
  i. Typically asymptomatic but may have local aching and fatigue.
  ii. Physical examination will reveal tortuous veins that are easily compressed.
**c. Diagnosis**
  i. Based on clinical findings.
**d. Treatment**
  i. Conservative management with elastic support stockings.
  ii. Surgical therapy consists of vein stripping or vein ligation.
  iii. Small varicose veins can be treated with a sclerosing agent.

# VALVULAR DISEASE

## I. AORTIC STENOSIS
**a. General**
  i. Symptoms due to left ventricular outflow obstruction leading to increased left ventricular pressure, muscle hypertrophy, and decreased ejection fraction.
  ii. More common in men than in women.
  iii. Etiology.
     1. Rheumatic inflammation.
     2. Congenital.
     3. Calcification/degeneration of valve.
**b. Clinical Manifestations**
  i. Symptoms include angina, syncope, dyspnea, and congestive heart failure.
  ii. Physical examination.
     1. Delayed carotid upstroke.
     2. Strong apical impulse.
     3. Narrowing pulse pressure.
     4. Loud, rough, systolic, diamond-shaped murmur.
        (a) Heard best at the base of the heart with radiation to the neck.
        (b) Associated with an ejection click.
**c. Diagnosis**
  i. Chest x-ray film reveals dilation of the ascending aorta and pulmonary congestion.
     1. Heart is boot shaped.
  ii. EKG reveals LVH and ST-T wave changes.
  iii. Doppler echocardiogram shows thickening of the left ventricular wall and valvular calcifications.
  iv. Diagnosis confirmed by cardiac catheterization.

### d. Treatment
    i. Strenuous activity should be avoided.
    ii. Treatment of congestive heart failure, if present, with diuretics and sodium restriction.
        1. ACE inhibitors are contraindicated.
    iii. Valve replacement is the treatment of choice in symptomatic patients.

## II. AORTIC REGURGITATION
### a. General
    i. Aortic insufficiency results in increased end-diastolic volume, ventricular dilation, leading to regurgitation.
    ii. Etiology.
        1. Hypertension.
        2. Ischemic heart disease.
        3. Infectious endocarditis.
        4. Syphilis.
        5. Collagen vascular disease.
        6. Marfan syndrome.
### b. Clinical Manifestations
    i. Symptoms include dyspnea on exertion, syncope, chest pain, and congestive heart failure.
    ii. Physical examination reveals the following:
        1. Wide pulse pressure.
        2. Bounding "water-hammer" pulses.
        3. Presence of an $S_3$.
        4. Displaced apical impulse, downward and to the left.
        5. Decrescendo, blowing diastolic murmur heard along left sternal border.
            (a) Low-pitched, apical diastolic murmur (Austin-Flint murmur).
### c. Diagnosis
    i. Chest x-ray film reveals LVH with or without signs of congestive heart failure.
    ii. Echocardiogram reveals left ventricular enlargement.
    iii. Cardiac catheterization confirms wide pulse pressure and evaluates left ventricular dysfunction.
### d. Treatment
    i. Congestive heart failure is treated with digoxin, diuretics, ACE inhibitors, and salt restriction.
        1. Long-term treatment with nifedipine and/or ACE inhibitors delays need for valve replacement.
    ii. Surgical valve replacement is required when signs of decompensation occur.
        1. Surgery should be performed when ejection fraction is less than 55%.

## III. MITRAL STENOSIS
### a. General
    i. Stenosis leads to increased atrial pressure and atrial enlargement, pulmonary congestion, pulmonary hypertension, and right-sided heart failure.
    ii. More common in women, between ages 25 and 45 years.
    iii. Etiology.
        1. Rheumatic fever.
        2. Congenital defect.
### b. Clinical Manifestations
    i. Symptoms include exertional dyspnea, orthopnea, and paroxysmal nocturnal dyspnea.
        1. Hemoptysis may occur secondary to pulmonary vessel rupture.
    ii. Physical examination.
        1. Prominent jugular A wave.
        2. Opening snap in early diastole.
        3. Soft, low-pitched, diastolic rumble heard best at the apex in the left decubitus position.
        4. A palpable right ventricular heave may be noted at the left sternal border.
### c. Diagnosis
    i. Echocardiogram and cardiac catheterization are diagnostic.
    ii. Chest x-ray film reveals left atrial enlargement and prominent pulmonary arteries.
    iii. EKG reveals left atrial enlargement or atrial fibrillation.
### d. Treatment
    i. Control atrial fibrillation and congestive heart failure.
    ii. Valve replacement or percutaneous transvenous mitral valvotomy is required in patients who respond poorly to medical treatment.

## IV. MITRAL REGURGITATION
### a. General
    i. Increased volume in left atrium from left ventricle leads to ineffective cardiac output.
    ii. Etiology.
        1. Ischemic heart disease.
        2. Rheumatic fever.
        3. Papillary muscle rupture.
        4. Chordae tendineae rupture.
        5. Calcification.
        6. Mitral valve prolapse.
        7. Systemic lupus erythematosus (SLE).
### b. Clinical Manifestations
    i. Symptoms include fatigue, dyspnea, orthopnea, and congestive heart failure.
    ii. Physical examination.
        1. Left ventricular lift or apical thrill.
        2. Holosystolic murmur at apex with radiation to the base or left axilla.
        3. $S_3$ may be present.
        4. Laterally displaced apical impulse.

c. **Diagnosis**
  i. Echocardiogram and cardiac catheterization.
  ii. EKG reveals LVH.
d. **Treatment**
  i. Treat congestive heart failure with digoxin, diuretics, ACE inhibitors, and salt restriction.
  ii. Valve replacement must be performed early and is the only definite treatment.

## V. MITRAL VALVE PROLAPSE
a. **General**
  i. More common in young females.
    1. Typically have a narrow anteroposterior chest diameter, low body weight, and hypotension.
b. **Clinical Manifestations**
  i. Symptoms include chest pain and palpitations.
  ii. Physical examination findings include mid to late click, which is heard best at the apex, and a crescendo, mid to late systolic murmur.
    1. Murmur worsens with Valsalva or standing.
c. **Diagnosis**
  i. Echocardiogram is diagnostic and reveals valve leaflets bulging posteriorly in systole.
d. **Treatment**
  i. Avoid stimulants.
  ii. Beta-blockers may be tried in symptomatic patients.

## VI. TRICUSPID STENOSIS
a. **General**
  i. Due to rheumatic heart disease or tricuspid valve replacement.
b. **Clinical Manifestations**
  i. Signs of right-sided heart failure.
  ii. Physical examination.
    1. Note a diastolic rumble along the left sternal border that increases with inspiration.
c. **Diagnosis**
  i. EKG reveals possible right atrial enlargement.
  ii. Echocardiogram is diagnostic and reveals an increased mean diastolic pressure gradient.
d. **Treatment**
  i. Treat heart failure as needed.
  ii. Valve replacement surgery.

## VII. TRICUSPID REGURGITATION
a. **General**
  i. Typically due to hemodynamic load in the right ventricle and not structural.
    1. Increases right atrial pressure, which leads to venous hypertension.
  ii. Etiology.
    1. Pulmonary hypertension.

2. Endocarditis.
  (a) Suspect in IV drug abusers.
3. Thyrotoxicosis.
b. **Clinical Manifestations**
  i. Symptoms are those of right-sided heart failure.
    1. Includes ascites, edema, and right upper quadrant pain.
  ii. Physical examination reveals hepatic enlargement, JVD, and a parasternal lift.
    1. Holosystolic murmur noted along left sternal border.
c. **Diagnosis**
  i. Diagnosis made by echocardiogram.
d. **Treatment**
  i. Treat underlying cause.
  ii. Surgery is rarely needed.

## VIII. PULMONARY STENOSIS
a. **General**
  i. A congenital disease due to fusion of the valve cusps.
  ii. Typically noted in childhood.
b. **Clinical Manifestations**
  i. Symptoms include angina and syncope.
  ii. Physical examination reveals an early systolic opening ejection click followed by a systolic ejection murmur, which radiates to the base.
c. **Diagnosis**
  i. Diagnosis made by echocardiogram.
d. **Treatment**
  i. If asymptomatic, no treatment is needed.
  ii. If symptoms are present, commissurotomy is needed.

## IX. PULMONARY REGURGITATION
a. **General**
b. **Clinical Manifestations**
  i. Signs and symptoms due to the underlying etiology.
  ii. Physical examination reveals a right ventricular lift, a second heart sound is widely split, and a systolic click may be noted.
    1. A murmur may or may not be noted.
c. **Diagnosis**
  i. RBBB is common on EKG.
  ii. Echocardiogram shows signs of pulmonary hypertension.
d. **Treatment**
  i. Treat the primary cause.

## X. TABLE 1.16 SUMMARIZES THE MAJOR VALVULAR DISEASES
## XI. TABLE 1.17 SUMMARIZES MANEUVERS ON VALVULAR MURMURS

**TABLE 1.16**

| Summary of Major Valvular Diseases | | | | |
|---|---|---|---|---|
| | **Aortic Stenosis** | **Mitral Stenosis** | **Aortic Regurgitation** | **Mitral Regurgitation** |
| Etiology | Rheumatic | Rheumatic | Endocarditis, Marfan syndrome | Mitral prolapse, endocarditis, papillary muscle dysfunction |
| Symptoms | Angina, syncope | Dyspnea, orthopnea, PND | Dyspnea, orthopnea, angina | Dyspnea, orthopnea, PND |
| Cardiac signs | Systolic ejection murmur, delayed carotid upstroke | Diastolic rumble, opening snap | Diastolic blowing murmur | Holosystolic apical murmur |
| EKG | LVH | RVH | LVH | LVH |
| Chest x-ray | Boot-shaped heart | Straight left heart border | Cardiac enlargement | Cardiac enlargement |

*EKG*, Electrocardiogram; *LVH*, left ventricular hypertrophy; *PND*, paroxysmal nocturnal dyspnea; *RVH*, right ventricular hypertrophy.

**TABLE 1.17**

| Maneuver Effects on Valvular Murmurs | | | | |
|---|---|---|---|---|
| | **Valsalva** | **Standing** | **Handgrip** | **Squatting** |
| Aortic stenosis | ↓ | ↓ | ↓ | ↑/↓ |
| Hypertrophic cardiomyopathy | ↑ | ↑ | ↓ | ↓ |
| Chronic aortic regurgitation | ↓ | ↓ | ↑ | ↑ |
| Chronic mitral regurgitation | ↓ | ↓ | ↑ | ↑ |
| Mitral valve prolapse | Move click and murmur closer to $S_1$ | Increase, lengthen duration | Move click and murmur closer to $S_2$ | Move click and murmur closer to $S_2$ |
| Mitral stenosis | ↓ | ↓ | ↑ | ↑ |

# OTHER

## I. ACUTE/SUBACUTE BACTERIAL ENDOCARDITIS
   a. **General**
      i. Infection of the endothelial surface of the heart and valves.
      ii. More common in elderly people and males.
      iii. Predisposing conditions that increase risk for endocarditis.
         1. Mitral valve prolapse.
         2. Degenerative valvular disease.
         3. IV drug abuse.
         4. Prosthetic valve.
         5. Congenital abnormalities.
      iv. Microorganisms that cause endocarditis vary with setting.
         1. Community acquired.
            (a) *Staphylococcus aureus.*
            (b) Viridans streptococci.
            (c) Enterococci.
         2. Nosocomial.
            (a) *S. aureus.*
            (b) *Staphylococcus epidermidis.*
            (c) Enterococci.
            (d) Fungal.
         3. Prosthetic valve.
            (a) *S. epidermidis.*
            (b) *S. aureus.*
            (c) Enterococci.
   b. **Clinical Manifestations**
      i. Symptoms include fever, chills, sweats, weakness, dyspnea, and weight loss.
      ii. Physical examination reveals the following:
         1. Petechiae.
         2. Osler's nodes.
            (a) Small, painful nodules on the palmar surface of the fingers and toes.
         3. Janeway lesions.
            (a) Hemorrhagic, nonpainful macules on the palms and soles.
         4. Splinter hemorrhages.
            (a) Non-blanching, linear brownish-red lesions in the nail beds, perpendicular to the growth of the nails.
         5. Roth's spots on funduscopic examination.
            (a) Retinal hemorrhages with pale centers.
         6. Cardiac murmur.
            (a) May be diastolic or systolic depending on valve involved.
         7. Splenomegaly.

iii. Laboratory tests reveal leukocytosis, elevated ESR, and hematuria.

c. **Diagnosis**
   i. Based on Modified Duke criteria.
      1. Major.
         (a) Two positive blood cultures for a microorganism that typically causes infective endocarditis.
         (b) Single positive blood culture for *Coxiella burnetti* or anti-phase IgG antibody titer greater than or equal to 1:800.
         (c) Endocardial involvement on echocardiogram or new regurgitation murmur.
      2. Minor.
         (a) Predisposing condition: cardiac or IV drug abuse.
         (b) Fever.
         (c) Vascular phenomena, including Janeway lesions and arterial emboli.
         (d) Immunologic phenomena, including Osler's nodes, Roth's spots, and a positive rheumatoid factor.
         (e) Positive blood culture not meeting the major criteria or serologic evidence of an active infection.
   ii. Definitive diagnosis with two major criteria or one major and three minor criteria.

d. **Treatment**
   i. Antibiotics are selected based on culture results but may need empirical treatment.
      1. Empirical treatment.
         (a) Native valve, community acquired, methicillin-resistant *S. aureus* (MRSA) unlikely.
            (i) Nafcillin plus penicillin plus gentamicin.
         (b) Hospital acquired, hemodialysis, suspected MRSA, or penicillin allergy.
            (i) Vancomycin plus gentamicin.
         (c) Prosthetic valve.
            (i) Vancomycin plus gentamicin plus rifampin.
            (ii) Valve may need to be replaced.
   ii. Antibiotics should be bactericidal; and therapy is prolonged, lasting 4 to 6 weeks.
   iii. Table 1.18 shows treatment options for infectious endocarditis.
   iv. Prevention.
      1. Required for select patients and for certain invasive procedures.
         (a) Antibiotics are typically given before the procedure so that peak level is at the time of the procedure.
      2. Needed for high-risk patients.
         (a) High-risk groups.
            (i) History of prosthetic valves.

**TABLE 1.18**

| Treatment Options for Infectious Endocarditis | |
|---|---|
| **Organism** | **Treatment** |
| Viridans streptococci | Penicillin G or ampicillin plus gentamicin, ceftriaxone plus gentamicin, or vancomycin |
| Enterococci | Ampicillin or penicillin G plus gentamicin or ampicillin plus ceftriaxone |
| *Staphylococcus aureus* | Nafcillin, oxacillin, or cefazolin |
| Methicillin-resistant *S. aureus* | Vancomycin or daptomycin |
| *Staphylococcus epidermidis* | Vancomycin plus gentamicin plus rifampin |

            (ii) Past history of endocarditis.
            (iii) Unrepaired congenital heart disease.
            (iv) Repaired congenital heart defect and prosthetic material or device, but only during the first 6 months after procedure.
            (v) Repaired congenital heart disease with residual defects.
            (vi) Cardiac transplantation recipients who develop cardiac valvulopathy.
      3. Invasive procedures include the following:
         (a) Dental procedures that involve manipulation of gingival tissue or the periapical region of the teeth or perforation of the oral mucosa, including routine cleaning.
         (b) Surgery involving respiratory mucosa (tonsillectomy, adenoidectomy, or bronchoscopy with biopsy).
         (c) Surgery on infected soft tissue or musculoskeletal tissue.
         (d) Surgery to place prosthetic heart valves or prosthetic intravascular or intracardiac materials.
      2. Antibiotic selection.
         (a) Oral therapy.
            (i) Amoxicillin.
            (ii) If penicillin allergy, can use cephalexin, azithromycin, clarithromycin, or doxycycline.
         (b) IV or IM therapy.
            (i) Ampicillin, ceftriaxone, or cefazolin.
            (ii) Penicillin allergy.
               i. Cefazolin or ceftriaxone.
            (iii) Surgery on infected tissue.
               i. Cefazolin or vancomycin.

## II. ACUTE PERICARDITIS
a. **General**
   i. Inflammation or infection of the pericardium.

    ii. Etiologies include the following:
      1. Viral: Coxsackie virus, echovirus, hepatitis B, and cytomegalovirus.
      2. Bacterial: *Staphylococcus*, *Streptococcus*, and tuberculosis.
      3. Post MI.
      4. Uremia.
      5. Malignancy: lung or breast metastases.
      6. Collagen vascular disease: SLE or rheumatoid arthritis (RA).
    iii. Constrictive pericarditis is thickening and fibrosis of the pericardium after an episode of acute pericarditis.

**b. Clinical Manifestations**
    i. Patients present with sharp, pleuritic chest pain that worsens with deep breathing, cough, or lying down.
      1. Pain improved with sitting and leaning forward.
    ii. Physical examination reveals a pericardial friction rub.
      1. Friction rub is diagnostic for pericarditis.

**c. Diagnosis**
    i. EKG reveals ST elevation in all precordial leads, except aVR, without reciprocal ST depression.
    ii. Cardiac enzymes are normal.
    iii. Echocardiogram reveals a pericardial effusion.

**d. Treatment**
    i. Treat underlying cause.
    ii. NSAIDs are used to treat pain and inflammation.
    iii. Steroids may be needed.
    iv. Constrictive pericarditis is treated with pericardiectomy.

## III. CARDIAC TAMPONADE

**a. General**
    i. Accumulation of fluid that results in an increase in pericardial pressure and impairs ventricular filling.
    ii. Typically a complication of pericardial effusion.

**b. Clinical Manifestations**
    i. Symptoms include hypotension, tachycardia, and dyspnea on exertion.
    ii. Physical examination reveals distended neck veins, indistinct heart sounds, narrow pulse pressure, and pulsus paradoxus.
      1. Pulsus paradoxus is present if a 10 mm Hg or more drop in blood pressure is noted with inspiration.

**c. Diagnosis**
    i. Echocardiogram is diagnostic for tamponade.

**d. Treatment**
    i. Pericardiocentesis by echocardiogram guidance.
    ii. Treat underlying cause.

## IV. PERICARDIAL EFFUSION

**a. General**
    i. Prolonged and severe inflammation leads to fluid accumulation around the heart.

**b. Clinical Manifestations**
    i. Small effusion causes no symptoms, whereas large effusions lead to cardiac tamponade.
    ii. Physical examination reveals diminished heart sounds.
      1. Friction rub may be noted if effusion is secondary to pericarditis.
    iii. Table 1.19 compares cardiac tamponade, pericarditis, and restrictive cardiomyopathy.

**c. Diagnosis**
    i. EKG reveals low-voltage QRS complexes and ST changes due to pericarditis.
    ii. Chest x-ray reveals an enlarged water-bottle–shaped heart.
    iii. Echocardiogram shows fluid between the layers of the pericardium.
      1. This is diagnostic for pericardial effusion.
    iv. Pericardiocentesis confirms the diagnosis.

**d. Treatment**
    i. If symptoms are severe, pericardiocentesis is required to remove the fluid.

**TABLE 1.19**

**Comparison of Tamponade and Pericarditis**

|  | Cardiac Tamponade | Constrictive Pericarditis | Restrictive Cardiomyopathy |
|---|---|---|---|
| Pulsus paradoxus | Positive | Negative | Negative |
| $S_3$ | Negative | Positive | Positive |
| $S_4$ | Negative | Negative | Positive |
| Cardiomegaly | Positive | Negative | Negative |
| Pericardial effusion | Positive | Negative | Negative |

## Cardiology Drugs

| Name | Mechanism | Therapeutic Use | Side Effects | Notes |
|------|-----------|-----------------|--------------|-------|
| Adenosine | Decreases conduction velocity | Antiarrhythmic (SVT) | Flushing<br>Chest pain<br>Hypotension | Very short duration of action |
| Amiodarone | Potassium channel blocker | Antiarrhythmic (atrial fibrillation, SVT, or VF) | Pulmonary fibrosis<br>Hyperthyroidism or hypothyroidism<br>Toxic liver<br>Photosensitivity<br>Blue skin discoloration | Full effects may take 6 weeks |
| Amrinone | Phosphodiesterase | CHF | | |
| Atenolol | Beta-blocker | Hypertension | Fatigue<br>Lethargy<br>Insomnia<br>Impotence<br>Hypotension | Rebound hypotension |
| Bretylium | Potassium channel blocker | Antiarrhythmic (VF or VT) | Postural hypotension | |
| Bumetanide | Inhibit Na/K/Cl transport in the ascending loop of Henle | CHF<br>Hypertension | Ototoxicity<br>Hyperuricemia<br>Hypovolemia<br>Hypokalemia | Rapid onset of action |
| Captopril | ACE inhibitor | CHF<br>Hypertension | Postural hypotension<br>Cough<br>Hyperkalemia<br>Altered taste | Should not be used in pregnancy |
| Clonidine | Alpha-2 agonist | Hypertension | Sedation<br>Dry nose | Does not worsen renal function |
| Digoxin | Enhances cardiac muscle contractility | CHF<br>Antiarrhythmic (atrial flutter, SVT) | Dysrhythmia<br>Nausea and vomiting<br>Headache<br>Confusion<br>Altered color perception | Not indicated in right-sided heart failure |
| Diltiazem | Calcium channel blocker | Antiarrhythmic<br>Angina<br>Hypertension | Hypotension<br>Constipation | Avoid in patients with depressed cardiac function |
| Disopyramide | Sodium channel blocker | Antiarrhythmic | Dry mouth<br>Urinary retention<br>Blurry vision<br>Constipation | |
| Dobutamine | Direct-acting catecholamine that is a beta-receptor agonist | CHF | Anxiety<br>Headache<br>Pulmonary edema | Use with caution in patients with atrial fibrillation |
| Enalapril | ACE inhibitor | CHF<br>Hypertension | Postural hypotension<br>Cough<br>Hyperkalemia<br>Altered taste | Should not be used in pregnancy |
| Esmolol | Beta-blocker | Antiarrhythmic | Fatigue<br>Lethargy<br>Insomnia<br>Impotence<br>Hypotension | Rebound hypotension |
| Flecainide | Sodium channel blocker | Antiarrhythmic | Dizziness<br>Blurred vision<br>Headache<br>Nausea | |
| Furosemide | Inhibits Na/K/Cl transport in the ascending loop of Henle | CHF<br>Hypertension | Ototoxicity<br>Hyperuricemia<br>Hypovolemia<br>Hypokalemia | Rapid onset of action |

*Continued*

## Cardiology Drugs—cont'd

| Name | Mechanism | Therapeutic Use | Side Effects | Notes |
|------|-----------|-----------------|--------------|-------|
| Hydralazine | Direct smooth muscle re-laxant | CHF<br>Hypertension | Headache<br>Nausea<br>Sweating<br>Lupus-like syndrome | |
| Hydrochlorothiazide | Increase sodium and water excretion | CHF<br>Hypertension | Hypokalemia<br>Hyperglycemia | |
| Isosorbide | Direct smooth muscle re-laxant | CHF<br>Angina | Headache | |
| Labetalol | Beta-blocker | Hypertension | Fatigue<br>Lethargy<br>Insomnia<br>Impotence<br>Hypotension | Rebound hypotension |
| Lidocaine | Sodium channel blocker | Antiarrhythmic (VT or VF) | Drowsiness<br>Slurred speech<br>Paresthesia<br>Confusion<br>Convulsions | |
| Lisinopril | ACE inhibitor | CHF<br>Hypertension | Postural hypotension<br>Cough<br>Hyperkalemia<br>Altered taste | Should not be used in pregnancy |
| Losartan | Angiotensin II Antagonist | Hypertension | Hypotension<br>Hyperkalemia | Fetotoxic |
| Metoprolol | Beta-blocker | Antiarrhythmic<br>Hypertension | Fatigue<br>Lethargy<br>Insomnia<br>Impotence<br>Hypotension | Rebound hypotension |
| Mexiletine | Sodium channel blocker | Antiarrhythmic | | |
| Minoxidil | Vasodilator (arterioles) | CHF<br>Hypertension | Reflex tachycardia<br>Edema<br>Hypertrichosis | |
| Nifedipine | Calcium channel blocker | Hypertension<br>Angina | Flushing<br>Headache<br>Hypotension<br>Edema<br>Constipation | |
| Nebivolol | Beta-blocker | Hypertension | Dizziness<br>Fatigue<br>Headache | Highly cardio selective |
| Nitroglycerin | Smooth muscle relaxant | Angina | Headache<br>Hypotension | |
| Prazosin | Alpha-blocker | Hypertension | First dose syncope<br>Reflex tachycardia | |
| Procainamide | Sodium channel blocker | Antiarrhythmic | SLE<br>Depression<br>Hallucination<br>Psychosis | |
| Propranolol | Beta-blocker | Antiarrhythmic (atrial flutter or fibrillation, SVT)<br>Angina<br>Hypertension | Fatigue<br>Lethargy<br>Insomnia<br>Impotence<br>Hypotension | Rebound hypotension |
| Quinidine | Sodium channel blocker | Antiarrhythmic (atrial flutter or fibrillation) | SA/AV blocks<br>Asystole<br>Nausea/Vomiting<br>Diarrhea | |

## Cardiology Drugs—cont'd

| Name | Mechanism | Therapeutic Use | Side Effects | Notes |
|------|-----------|-----------------|--------------|-------|
| Ramipril | ACE inhibitor | Hypertension | Postural hypotension<br>Cough<br>Hyperkalemia<br>Altered taste | |
| Sodium nitroprusside | Vasodilation | CHF<br>Hypertension emergency | Hypotension | Given IV only |
| Sotalol | Potassium channel blocker | Antiarrhythmic (VT) | Torsades de pointes | |
| Spironolactone | Inhibit sodium reabsorption and potassium secretion | Hypertension | Gynecomastia<br>Hyperkalemia<br>Nausea | |
| Timolol | Beta-blocker | Hypertension | Fatigue<br>Lethargy<br>Insomnia<br>Impotence<br>Hypotension | Rebound hypotension |
| Triamterene | Block Na-K exchange | Hypertension | Leg cramps<br>Increased BUN and uric acid | |
| Verapamil | Calcium channel blocker | Antiarrhythmic (atrial flutter, SVT)<br>Angina<br>Hypertension<br>Migraine headache | Hypotension<br>Constipation | Avoid in patients with depressed cardiac function |

*ACE,* Angiotensin-converting enzyme; *AV,* atrioventricular; *BUN,* blood urea nitrogen; *CHF,* congestive heart failure; *IV,* intravenous; *SA,* sinoatrial; *SLE,* systemic lupus erythematosus; *SVT,* supraventricular tachycardia; *VF,* ventricular fibrillation; *VT,* ventricular tachycardia.

# QUESTIONS

## QUESTION 1
Which of the following is a common physical examination finding in endocarditis?

A Displaced PMI
B Hepatomegaly
C Pericardial friction rub
D Splinter hemorrhages
E Pulsus paradoxus

## QUESTION 2
A 55-year-old patient presents with orthopnea and paroxysmal nocturnal dyspnea. On physical examination, jugular venous distention and pulmonary rales are noted. Which of the following laboratory tests would most likely be elevated in this patient?

A Thyroid stimulating hormone
B Brain natriuretic peptide
C Myoglobin
D D-dimer
E Renin

## QUESTION 3
A 35-year-old patient presents with chest pain that worsens with lying down. EKG reveals diffuse ST elevation in all the precordial leads. Which of the following is the most likely diagnosis?

A Dilated cardiomyopathy
B Subacute bacterial endocarditis
C Acute inferior wall infarct
D Acute pericarditis
E Aortic dissection

## QUESTION 4
Given the rhythm strip below, which of the following is the most likely diagnosis?

A Torsades de pointes
B Premature ventricular contraction
C Wolff-Parkinson-White syndrome
D Ventricular tachycardia
E Ventricular fibrillation

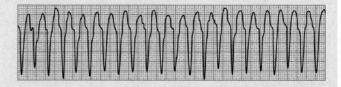

## QUESTION 5
A 65-year-old male with a history of benign prostatic hypertrophy develops hypertension. Which of the following would be the best treatment option for this patient's hypertension?

A Calcium channel blocker
B Alpha-blocker
C Beta-blocker
D ACE inhibitor
E Diuretic

*Continued*

## QUESTIONS—cont'd

### QUESTION 6

Which of the following conduction disorders increases the risk of intraatrial clot formation?

**A** Atrial fibrillation
**B** Ventricular tachycardia
**C** Ventricular fibrillation
**D** Premature atrial contractions
**E** Wolff-Parkinson-White syndrome

### QUESTION 7

Which of the following coronary arteries is typically involved in a lateral wall MI?

**A** Right coronary artery
**B** Circumflex artery
**C** Left anterior descending artery
**D** Left coronary artery
**E** Posterior descending

### QUESTION 8

A 72-year-old hypertensive male presents with chest pain. He describes the pain as a tearing pain. Which of the following would be the next best diagnostic test to further evaluate this patient?

**A** Ventilation perfusion scan
**B** Posteroanterior (PA) and lateral chest x-ray
**C** CT scan of the thorax
**D** Electrocardiogram
**E** Echocardiogram

### QUESTION 9

A patient presents with severe burning pain of the left lower extremity. On physical examination the extremity is cold and pale, and no pulses are noted. Which of the following would be most helpful in the further evaluation of this patient?

**A** D-dimer level
**B** Ankle/Brachial index
**C** Angiogram of the extremity
**D** Venous Doppler of the extremity
**E** Transesophageal echocardiogram

### QUESTION 10

A patient presents for a routine physical examination. On cardiac examination, a grade 2/6 holosystolic murmur is noted. It is heard best at the apex of the heart with radiation to the axilla. Which of the following is the most likely etiology of this murmur?

**A** Mitral stenosis
**B** Aortic stenosis
**C** Mitral insufficiency
**D** Aortic insufficiency
**E** Pulmonary stenosis

## ANSWERS

**1. D**
EXPLANATION: Physical examination findings in endocarditis include Osler nodes, Janeway lesions, splinter hemorrhages, Roth spots, and cardiac murmur. **Topic: Endocarditis**
☐ Correct ☐ Incorrect

**2. B**
EXPLANATION: The patient with congestive heart failure typically presents with dyspnea, orthopnea, paroxysmal nocturnal dyspnea, fatigue, and edema. On physical examination, jugular venous distention and pulmonary rales are noted. Laboratory evaluation will reveal prerenal azotemia, elevated liver function tests, and elevated brain natriuretic peptide. **Topic: Congestive heart failure**
☐ Correct ☐ Incorrect

**3. D**
EXPLANATION: In pericarditis, chest pain worsens with deep breathing, coughing, or lying down. EKG reveals ST elevation in all precordial leads without reciprocal ST depression. **Topic: Acute pericarditis**
☐ Correct ☐ Incorrect

**4. D**
EXPLANATION: Ventricular tachycardia presents with a rate greater than 100 beats/minute and a wide QRS complex.
**Topic: Conduction disorders**
☐ Correct ☐ Incorrect

**5. B**
EXPLANATION: The use of a single medication to treat two disorders is encouraged to decrease the risk of side effects. Alpha-blockers treat both hypertension and benign prostatic hypertrophy. **Topic: Hypertension**
☐ Correct ☐ Incorrect

**6. A**
EXPLANATION: Atrial fibrillation presents with an irregular rate with no visible P wave activity. Atrial fibrillation increases the risk of intraatrial clot formation and requires long-term anticoagulation. **Topic: Atrial fibrillation**
☐ Correct ☐ Incorrect

## ANSWERS—cont'd

**7.  B**

EXPLANATION: Lateral wall MI presents with EKG changes in leads I, aVL, $V_5$, and $V_6$. These changes correspond to occlusion of the circumflex artery.  ***Topic: Myocardial infarction***

☐ **Correct**   ☐ **Incorrect**

**8.  C**

EXPLANATION: Sudden searing or tearing chest pain in a hypertensive patient is most likely due to aortic dissection. CT scan of the chest is the immediate imaging study of choice; a transesophageal echocardiogram could also be used. ***Topic: Aortic dissection***

☐ **Correct**   ☐ **Incorrect**

**9.  C**

EXPLANATION: Arterial occlusion presents with pain, hyperesthesia, absence of pulses, and a pale, cool extremity. Angiography is the test of choice for making the diagnosis of arterial occlusion.  ***Topic: Chronic/Acute arterial occlusion***

☐ **Correct**   ☐ **Incorrect**

**10.  C**

EXPLANATION: People with mitral insufficiency present with a holosystolic murmur heard best at the apex of the heart. Patients with mitral stenosis and aortic insufficiency present with diastolic murmurs, those with aortic stenosis present with a systolic murmur heard best at the right sternal border, and those with pulmonary stenosis present with a systolic ejection murmur that radiates to the base of the heart.  ***Topic: Valvular disease***

☐ **Correct**   ☐ **Incorrect**

# CHAPTER 2
# PULMONARY SYSTEM

## EXAMINATION BLUEPRINT TOPICS

**INFECTIOUS DISORDERS**
Acute bronchitis
Influenza
Pneumonia
Tuberculosis

**NEOPLASTIC DISEASE**
Bronchogenic carcinoma
Carcinoid tumors
Metastatic tumors
Pulmonary nodules

**OBSTRUCTIVE PULMONARY DISEASE**
Asthma
Status asthmaticus
Bronchiectasis
Chronic bronchitis
Emphysema

**PLEURAL DISEASES**
Pleural effusion
Pneumothorax

**PULMONARY CIRCULATION**
Pulmonary embolism
Pulmonary hypertension
Cor pulmonale

**RESTRICTIVE PULMONARY DISEASE**
Idiopathic pulmonary fibrosis
Pneumoconiosis
Sarcoidosis

**OTHER**
Acute respiratory distress syndrome

## INFECTIOUS DISORDERS

### I. ACUTE BRONCHITIS
  a. **General**
    i. Inflammation of the large airways of the tracheobronchial tree.
    ii. Caused by infectious agents.
      1. Most frequently due to viruses.
        (a) Adenovirus.
        (b) Influenza A and B.
        (c) Coronavirus.
        (d) Rhinovirus.
        (e) Respiratory syncytial virus (RSV).
      2. Other causes include the following:
        (a) *Bordetella pertussis.*
        (b) *Mycoplasma pneumoniae.*
        (c) *Chlamydophila pneumoniae.*
    iii. Most prevalent during the winter and early spring.
    iv. Smoking is the most likely causative risk factor.
  b. **Clinical Manifestations**
    i. Major complaints are cough preceded by nasal congestion, sore throat, malaise, headache, and sneezing.
    ii. Cough often is productive and lasts greater than 5 days.
    iii. Fever is rare.
    iv. Physical examination reveals findings of upper respiratory tract infection.
      1. Lung examination may reveal rhonchi, crackles, or wheezing.
      2. No signs of lung consolidation.
    v. Chest x-ray film is normal.
  c. **Diagnosis**
    i. Based on clinical findings and negative chest x-ray.
  d. **Treatment**
    i. Supportive measures, including rest, antitussives, and oral hydration.
      1. Antitussives are not recommended in children.
    ii. Decongestants and inhaled bronchodilators may be helpful.
    iii. Macrolides are used in cases due to *Mycoplasma*, *Bordetella*, or *Chlamydophila.*

### II. INFLUENZA
  a. **General**
    i. Common respiratory infection caused by influenza A or B.
    ii. Spread by respiratory droplets.
    iii. Incubation period is from 1 to 4 days.
    iv. Outbreaks occur every fall and winter.
  b. **Clinical Manifestations**
    i. Present with abrupt onset of fever, chills, myalgias, headache, and a nonproductive cough.
      1. Coryza and sore throat are also common.
    ii. Physical examination often reveals tachycardia, fever, mild pharyngeal erythema, cervical adenopathy, and clear nasal drainage.

**c. Diagnosis**

i. Throat and nasal specimens for immunofluorescence or rapid antigen immunoassays can be used for rapid detection.

**d. Treatment**

i. Primarily supportive.

ii. Rimantadine and amantadine are not recommended for the treatment of influenzae owing to resistance development.

1. Both medications can lead to central nervous system side effects.

ii. Zanamivir, oseltamivir and peramivir are active against both influenza A and B.

1. Are neuraminidase inhibitors.

2. Side effects include bronchospasms with zanamivir and nausea and vomiting with oseltamivir.

iii. Baloxavir is Food and Drug Administration (FDA) approved for the treatment of uncomplicated influenza A and B infections.

1. Selective inhibitor of influenza cap-dependent endonuclease.

2. Side effects include diarrhea and bronchitis.

3. Mechanism of action is different than other so is useful as a part of a multidrug therapy for resistent disease.

iv. Prevention.

1. Mainstay of prevention is the inactivated influenza vaccine.

2. High-risk groups in need of vaccine include the following:

(a) Anyone over age 50.

(b) Nursing home/chronic care residents.

(c) History of chronic obstructive pulmonary disease (COPD) or cardiac disease.

(d) Chronic disease, such as diabetes, renal disease, or hemoglobinopathies.

(e) Pregnant women in their second or third trimester.

(f) Children, aged 6 months to 18 years.

(g) Groups in contact with high-risk patients.

3. Contraindications.

(a) Egg allergy.

i. History of egg allergy with hives only may receive any recommended influenza vaccine.

(b) Previous strong allergic reaction to influenza vaccine.

(c) Live, attenuated influenza vaccine (LAIV) should not be given to immunocompromised patients, pregnant patients, or those over 50 years of age.

(d) History of Guillain-Barré syndrome within 6 weeks of previous influenza immunizations.

v. Complications include bacterial pneumonia.

**TABLE 2.1**

| **Causes of Pneumonia** | | |
|---|---|---|
| **Bacterial** | **Viral** | **Fungal** |
| *Streptococcus pneumoniae* | Adenovirus | *Aspergillus* species |
| *Staphylococcus aureus* | Respiratory syncytial virus | *Candida albicans* |
| *Haemophilus influenzae* | Parainfluenza virus | *Cryptococcus neoformans* |
| **Anaerobes** | | *Histoplasma capsulatum* |
| *Bacteroides* species | Influenza A and B | *Coccidioides immitis* |
| *Peptostreptococcus* species | Rhinovirus | ***Rickettsia* species** |
| *Fusobacterium* species | Hantavirus | *Coxiella burnetii* |
| **Enterobacteriaceae** | Varicella-Zoster virus | *Rickettsia rickettsii* |
| *Escherichia coli* | Coronavirus | **Other** |
| *Klebsiella pneumoniae* | | *Mycoplasma pneumoniae* |
| *Enterobacter* species | | *Chlamydophila pneumoniae* |
| *Pseudomonas aeruginosa* | | *Chlamydia psittaci* |
| *Legionella pneumophila* | | *Mycobacterium tuberculosis* |
| *Actinomyces* species | | |
| *Nocardia* species | | |
| *Moraxella catarrhalis* | | |

**III. PNEUMONIA**

**a. Bacterial**

i. General

1. Due to microaspiration of oral contents, inhalation of small droplets, or hematogenous spread.

2. Etiologies: Table 2.1 shows common bacterial, viral, fungal, rickettsial, and other causes of pneumonia.

ii. Clinical manifestations

1. Symptoms include productive cough, dyspnea, pleuritic chest pain, and fever.

2. Rusty-colored sputum noted in infection due to *Streptococcus pneumoniae*.

3. Currant jellylike sputum noted in infection due to *Klebsiella pneumoniae*.

4. Nonspecific symptoms such as confusion, dehydration, loss of appetite, or failure to thrive may be noted.

5. Patients with aspiration pneumonia may present with foul-smelling sputum.

6. Physical examination.

(a) Tachypnea.

(b) Bronchial breath sounds, inspiratory crackles and egophony.

(c) Dullness to percussion.

(d) Decreased breath sounds.

7. Exposure history or underlying disease states may provide clues to etiology (Table 2.2).

iii. Diagnosis

1. Laboratory testing reveals leukocytosis and positive sputum Gram stain and culture.

**TABLE 2.2**

| Factors Related to Specific Etiologies | |
| --- | --- |
| **Factor** | **Etiology** |
| Alcohol Use Disorder | *Streptococcus pneumoniae* |
| | Gram-negative *bacilli*, such as |
| | *Klebsiella pneumoniae* |
| | Anaerobes |
| Aspiration | Anaerobes |
| | Gram-negative *bacilli* |
| Cystic fibrosis | *Pseudomonas aeruginosa* |
| | *Pseudomonas cepacia* |
| Exposure to bats | *Histoplasma capsulatum* |
| Exposure to birds | *Cryptococcus neoformans* |
| | *Chlamydia psittaci* |
| HIV/AIDS | *Pneumocystis jirovecii* |
| Intravenous drug use | *Staphylococcus aureus* |
| | Anaerobes |
| | Tuberculosis |
| Nursing home residence | *Streptococcus pneumoniae* |
| | Gram-negative bacilli |
| | *Haemophilus influenzae* |
| | Tuberculosis |
| Recent history of influenza | *Staphylococcus aureus* |
| | *Streptococcus pneumoniae* |
| | *Haemophilus influenzae* |
| Smoking, chronic obstructive pulmonary disease | *Streptococcus pneumoniae* |
| | *Haemophilus influenzae* |
| | *Moraxella catarrhalis* |

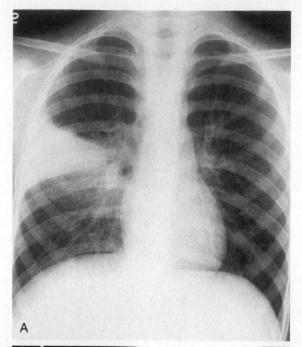

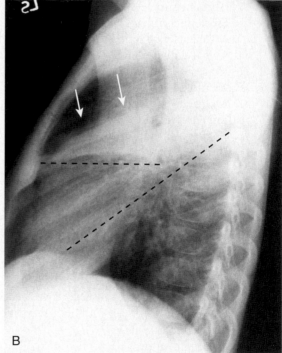

2. In patients with pneumonia, sputum Gram stain will contain fewer than 10 epithelial cells per low-power field and more than 25 white blood cells per low-power field.
3. Urine testing for legionella may be positive.
4. Chest x-ray film reveals five classic patterns.
   (a) Lobar pneumonia (Fig. 2.1).
      (i) Density that involves a distinct segment of the lung.
      (ii) Noted in infection due to *S. pneumoniae, Haemophilus influenzae*, and *Legionella* species.
   (b) Bronchopneumonia.
      (i) Patchy infiltrates involving multiple areas of the lung.
      (ii) Noted in infection due to *Staphylococcus aureus*, gram-negative bacilli, *Mycoplasma, Chlamydia*, and viruses.
   (c) Interstitial pneumonia.
      (i) Patients present with fine, diffuse, granular infiltrates.
      (ii) Noted in infection due to influenza, cytomegalovirus, and *Pneumocystis jirovecii*.

**Fig. 2.1** Chest x-ray pneumonia. **(A)** Right upper lobe pneumonia. **(B)** Infiltrate *(arrows)* above minor fissure *(horizontal dash line)* indicating right upper lobe pneumonia. The oblique line is the oblique fissure. Mettler FA Jr.: *Essentials of Radiology, 4th ed.* Philadelphia: Elsevier; 2019:65. Fig. 3.44. *(From Mettler FA: Essentials of Radiology, 2nd ed. Philadelphia: Elsevier Saunders, 2005:80, Fig. 3-44.)*

   (d) Lung abscess.
      (i) Present with loss of lung tissue and cavity formation.
      (ii) Noted in infection due to anaerobes.
   (e) Nodular lesions.
      (i) Multiple or single nodular lesions.

**TABLE 2.3**

| Empiric Treatment of Pneumonia | | | |
| --- | --- | --- | --- |
| **Community-Acquired Pneumonia, Inpatient** | **Community-Acquired Pneumonia, Outpatient** | **Aspiration (Community)** | **Aspiration (Hospital)** |
| Moxifloxacin | Amoxicillin | Ampicillin-sulbactam | Fluoroquinolone plus metronidazole |
| Levofloxacin | Amoxicillin/clavulanate | Ceftriaxone plus metronidazole | Ceftriaxone plus metronidazole |
| Ampicillin-sulbactam | Doxycycline | Cefotaxime plus metronidazole | Ticarcillin-clavulanate |
| Cefotaxime | Macrolide | | Piperacillin-tazobactam |
| Ceftriaxone | | | |
| Ceftaroline | | | |
| Doxycycline | | | |
| Macrolide | | | |

(ii) Noted in the infections due to histoplasmosis, coccidioidomycosis, and cryptococcosis.

iv. Treatment

1. Empiric therapy is based on most likely organism and clinical setting (Table 2.3).
2. See Fig. 2.2 for treatment protocol.

**b. Atypical**

i. General

1. Etiologies include the following:

(a) *M. pneumoniae.*

(i) Typically seen in patients younger than 40 years.

(ii) Higher incidence in fall and winter.

(b) *C. pneumoniae.*

(c) Viruses including adenovirus, parainfluenza, influenza A and B, and RSV.

ii. Clinical manifestations

1. Subacute disease with patients typically having symptoms for 7 to 10 days before seeking medical attention.
2. Symptoms are less severe than other forms of pneumonia.

(a) Cough is nonproductive.

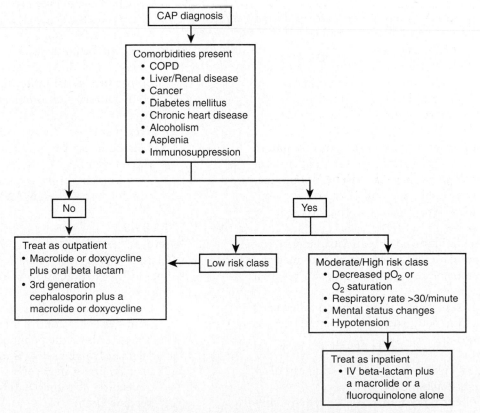

**Fig. 2.2** Community-acquired pneumonia (CAP) treatment.

(b) Patients also present with fever, malaise, and headache.

(i) Headache and sore throat are common in *Mycoplasma* and *Chlamydophila* infections.

iii. Diagnosis

1. Chest x-ray film in *Mycoplasma* and *Chlamydophila* infections reveals unilateral or bilateral patchy lower lobe infiltrates.
2. Rapid viral screens are available for detection of influenza.
3. Cold agglutinins test positive 1 to 2 weeks after infection with *Mycoplasma*.

iv. Treatment

1. Treat *Mycoplasma* and *Chlamydophila* with macrolides, tetracyclines, or fluoroquinolones.
2. Influenza treated with neuraminidase inhibitors.

(a) Prevention can be obtained with influenza vaccine.

c. **Fungal**

i. General

1. Includes *Histoplasma capsulatum* and *Coccidioides immitis*.
2. Histoplasmosis.

(a) More common in the midwestern (Ohio and Mississippi river valleys) and southeastern United States.

(b) A dimorphic fungus that is found in the soil.

(c) Infection is noted in cave explorers, from exposure to bat guano.

3. Coccidioidomycosis.

(a) More common in central California, Arizona, New Mexico, and Texas.

(b) A dimorphic fungus found in the soil and more common in the summer.

ii. Clinical manifestations

1. Histoplasmosis presents as a flu-like illness.

(a) Two weeks after exposure, patients develop high fever, headache, nonproductive cough, and dull chest pain.

(b) May disseminate to other parts of the body.

2. Coccidioidomycosis patients may be asymptomatic or present with fever, pleuritic chest pain, dry cough, and shortness of breath.

(a) Disease may disseminate to other parts of the body, such as the central nervous system.

iii. Diagnosis

1. Fungal culture or antigen testing can diagnose histoplasmosis.

(a) Chest x-ray film reveals a patchy infiltrate and mediastinal lymphadenopathy.

(b) Difficult to distinguish from sarcoidosis.

2. Coccidioidomycosis can be diagnosed by fungal culture.

(a) Eosinophilia may be noted.

(b) Sputum sample may reveal spherules.

(c) Multiple serologic tests are available.

3. Both organisms can be noted on silver stain.

iv. Treatment

1. Histoplasmosis.

(a) Itraconazole is the treatment of choice.

2. Coccidioidomycosis.

(a) Most cases resolve spontaneously.

(b) Disseminated or severe disease should be treated with itraconazole, fluconazole, or amphotericin B.

d. **Human Immunodeficiency Virus (HIV) Related**

i. General

1. Due to the fungus, *P. jirovecii*.
2. Patients typically have a CD4 count less than 200 cells/$\mu$L.

ii. Clinical manifestations

1. Patients present with gradual onset of fever, dry cough, dyspnea, weight loss, fatigue, and tachypnea.
2. Physical examination is typically normal for pulmonary complaints.

iii. Diagnosis

1. Lactate dehydrogenase (LDH) is elevated.
2. Gallium scan is positive, reveals increased uptake in the infected areas.
3. Gram stain is negative for bacteria. Gomori-Weigert silver stain on respiratory specimens will be positive.
4. Chest x-ray film may be normal or reveal diffuse interstitial infiltrates.

(a) A butterfly pattern may be noted.

iv. Treatment

1. Treatment of choice is trimethoprim-sulfamethoxazole or primaquine plus clindamycin.
2. Steroids can be given if severe respiratory compromise is present ($pO_2$ <70 mm Hg).

## IV. TUBERCULOSIS

a. **General**

i. Caused by *Mycobacterium tuberculosis*.

ii. Spread by aerosolization of contaminated respiratory secretions.

1. Organism reaches the alveolar surface, macrophages fail to control infection, and infection spreads via the pulmonary lymphatics to the hilar lymph nodes (Ghon complex).
2. From there, it may spread via the systemic circulation to other parts of the body or become latent.

(a) Reactivation occurs when macrophages can no longer contain the infection.

3. Only 10% of people infected will have clinical disease at some point in their lifetime.

   iii. HIV and acquired immune deficiency syndrome (AIDS) have contributed to the rise in tuberculosis infections.

b. **Clinical Manifestations**

   i. Pulmonary disease symptoms include cough, fever, and night sweats.

      1. Cough starts dry and becomes productive with hemoptysis.

      2. Weight loss is also noted.

   ii. Extrapulmonary disease symptoms depend on the site involved.

      1. Table 2.4 summarizes manifestations.

c. **Diagnosis**

   i. Chest x-ray is very important in making the diagnosis.

      1. Apices show fibronodular scarring that develops into fluffy and then cavitary lesions.

   ii. Sputum smears and culture are specific for making the diagnosis.

      1. Acid-fast smears identify mycobacteria, but are not species specific.

2. Cultures are the gold standard, but require 4 to 6 weeks to make the identification of the organism.

3. Nucleic acid amplification testing (NAAT-TB) can identify *M. tuberculosis* within hours of sputum processing.

   (a) The World Health Organization suggests NAAT-TB as the ideal initial test for diagnosis and resistance profiling in those whom pulmonary or extrapulmonary TB is suspected.

   iii. Tuberculin skin test or interferon gamma release assay (IGRA) used to identify latent disease.

      1. Intradermal tuberculin skin injection given and read 48 to 72 hours later.

         (a) Read induration only, not erythema.

         (b) Table 2.5 shows interpretation of tuberculin skin test.

      2. Becomes positive 4 to 5 weeks after infection.

      3. Use of bacille Calmette-Guérin (BCG) vaccine is not a contraindication to a tuberculin skin test.

         (a) In high-risk patients, the history of prior BCG vaccine should not alter the interpretation of the tuberculin skin test.

d. **Treatment**

   i. Treatment should be based on a patient-centered case management system with direct observation of therapy.

   ii. Multiple agents are needed to improve bacteria clearance and to decrease the development of drug resistance.

   iii. A four-drug regimen is recommended: isoniazid, rifampin, pyrazinamide, and ethambutol.

      1. Other drugs include rifapentine and streptomycin.

   iv. Preventive therapy for latent infection.

      1. Before treatment begins, active tuberculosis must be ruled out.

**TABLE 2.4**

| Clinical Manifestations of Extrapulmonary Tuberculosis | |
| --- | --- |
| **Organ System** | **Clinical Manifestations** |
| Bone | Lumbar spine pain in older patient with high dorsal pain in the young |
| Central nervous system | Fever, headache, vomiting, focal neurologic deficits |
| Disseminated | Fever, night sweats |
| Genitourinary | Hematuria, pyuria, routine culture negative |
| Lymphatic | Painless, unilateral cervical adenopathy |
| Pericardial | Substernal pain, signs of heart failure |

**TABLE 2.5**

| Interpretation of Tuberculin Skin Test | | |
| --- | --- | --- |
| **≥5 mm of Induration Is a Positive Test in the Following Groups** | **≥10 mm Is a Positive Test in the Following Groups** | **≥15 mm Induration Is a Positive Test in the Following Groups** |
| HIV positive<br>Contact with person with clinically active tuberculosis<br>Findings of old healed tuberculosis (fibrotic changes on chest x-ray film)<br>Organ transplant recipient<br>Other immunosuppressed patients | Recent arrivals from high prevalence countries<br>Intravenous drug abusers<br>Residents and employees in the following high-risk settings:<br>    Prisons and jails<br>    Nursing homes<br>    Hospitals<br>    Homeless shelters<br>Clinical condition that places patient at high risk<br>Children <4 years of age<br>Children exposed to adults in high-risk settings | No known risk factors for tuberculosis |

2. First-line drugs include isoniazid, rifampin, rifapentine, pyrazinamide, ethambutol, or streptomycin.
   (a) Drugs can be given daily, two times per week, or three times per week.
3. Patients should be monitored for signs of hepatitis.

# NEOPLASTIC DISEASE

## I. BRONCHOGENIC CARCINOMA

### a. General
   i. Lung cancer is the leading cause of cancer deaths in both men and women in the United States.
      1. Overall 5-year survival rate is 21%.
   ii. Arises from the respiratory epithelium cells.
   iii. Two subtypes.
      1. Non–small cell lung cancer (84%).
         (a) Adenocarcinoma (50%).
            (i) Noted in the periphery of the lung or central airway.
            (ii) Tumor cells contain mucins.
            (iii) Bronchoalveolar carcinoma is a subtype of adenocarcinoma.
               (1) Arises in the periphery of the lung.
         (b) Squamous cell carcinoma (13%).
            (i) Originates in the central airways.
         (c) Large cell carcinoma (1.3%).
      2. Small cell lung cancer (13%).
   iv. Risk factors.
      1. Smoking increases risk 10 times from baseline.
      2. Passive smoke exposure.
      3. Asbestos exposure increases risk 75 times from baseline.
         (a) Also linked to mesothelioma.
      4. Radiation therapy.
      5. Radon.
      6. Pulmonary fibrosis.

### b. Clinical Manifestations
   i. Clinically silent for most of the course of the disease, with symptoms appearing only late in the disease.
   ii. Symptoms include new cough, change in chronic cough, hemoptysis, chest pain, dyspnea, weight loss, and hoarseness.
   iii. Physical examination findings include wheezing due to airway obstruction, and findings due to various syndromes.
   iv. Other syndromes may present.
      1. Superior vena cava syndrome.
         (a) May be noted with local invasive disease.
         (b) Present with facial and neck swelling due to blockage of superior vena cava by local tumor.
      2. Horner's syndrome.
         (a) Due to disruption of cervical sympathetic nerves.
         (b) Present with unilateral facial anhidrosis, ptosis, and miosis.
      3. Pancoast's syndrome.
         (a) Due to tumor invading apex and superior sulcus and invasion of brachial plexus and cervical sympathetic nerves.
         (b) Patients present with arm and shoulder pain and signs of Horner's syndrome.

### c. Diagnosis
   i. Chest x-ray film may reveal pleural effusions and lung masses or nodules (Fig. 2.3).

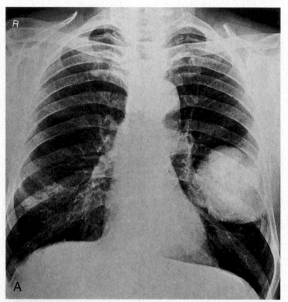

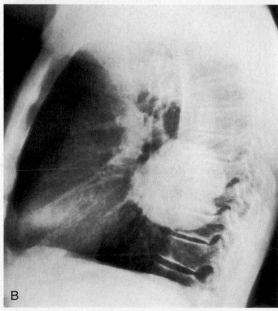

**Fig. 2.3 (A)** and **(B)** Bronchial carcinoma in left lower lobe. *(From Grainger RG, Allison D, Adam A, Dixon AK [eds]: Diagnostic Radiology: A Textbook of Medical Imaging, 4th ed. London: Harcourt, 2001:464, Fig. 22.1.)*

ii. Computed tomography (CT) scan is used to detect abnormalities in lymph nodes or metastases to surrounding structures.

iii. Sputum cytology, biopsy of lymph nodes, and tissue from bronchoscopy determine lung cancer cell type.

iv. Lung cancer tends to metastasize to lymph nodes, brain, bone, adrenal glands, and liver.

d. **Treatment**

i. Staging is required to predict prognosis and to determine appropriate therapy.

ii. Treatment varies with the subtype of lung cancer.

1. Non–small cell lung cancer is treated with surgery and offers the best chance for survival.

(a) Chemotherapy and radiation therapy are effective in combination with surgery.

(b) Targeted therapy using EGFR tyrosine kinase inhibitors for patients with *EGFR* mutation.

(c) Targeted therapy using ALK tyrosine kinase inhibitors in patients with *ALK-rearranged* lung cancers.

(d) Immune checkpoint inhibition using PD-1 or PD-L1 inhibitors.

2. Small cell lung cancer is treated with chemotherapy and radiation therapy.

iii. Prevention.

1. Smoking cessation is the most important strategy in the prevention of lung cancer.

2. Lung cancer screening using low-dose chest CT in adults 50 to 80 years who have a 20 pack-year smoking history and currently smoke or have quit within the past 15 years.

## II. CARCINOID TUMORS

a. **General**

i. Low-grade malignant neoplasms.

1. Slow growing and rarely metastasize.

2. Six times more common than bronchial gland carcinomas.

ii. Most cases are noted in patients younger than 60 years and equally common in males and females.

iii. Complications include bleeding and airway obstruction.

b. **Clinical Manifestations**

i. Symptoms include hemoptysis, cough, wheezing, and recurrent pneumonia.

ii. Carcinoid syndrome, with flushing, diarrhea, and hypotension, is rare.

c. **Diagnosis**

i. Chest x-ray film may show a solitary pulmonary nodule.

ii. CT scan is helpful in localizing the lesion and following its growth over time.

iii. Diagnosis is confirmed by biopsy.

iv. Octreotide scintigraphy is used to localize tumors.

d. **Treatment**

i. Surgical excision is treatment of choice; chemotherapy and radiation therapy are not helpful.

1. Prognosis is typically favorable.

## III. METASTATIC TUMORS

a. **General**

i. Due to spread of other malignant tumors to the lung, via vascular system or lymphatic system or via direct extension.

ii. Most any cancer can spread to the lung.

b. **Clinical Manifestations**

i. Symptoms are uncommon, but include cough, hemoptysis, and dyspnea.

ii. Most symptoms are related to the primary tumor.

c. **Diagnosis**

i. Chest x-ray and CT scan reveal multiple nodules.

ii. Diagnosis is confirmed by percutaneous needle biopsy or transbronchial biopsy.

iii. Positron emission tomography (PET) scans will show increased activity at the site of metastases.

d. **Treatment**

i. Management consists of treatment of primary tumor and pulmonary complications.

ii. Local resection of the tumors is available in selected cases.

## IV. PULMONARY NODULES

a. **General**

i. A nodule is a round or oval, sharply circumscribed lesion, up to 3 cm in diameter.

1. If larger than 3 cm, it is termed "a mass."

ii. A central cavity or calcification, with or without surrounding lesions, may be noted.

iii. One quarter of patients with bronchogenic carcinomas present with a solitary pulmonary nodule.

iv. Benign nature of the nodule is favored if the nodule is of small size (<2 cm in diameter), if it has smooth margins, if the patient is of a young age, and if there is an absence of symptoms.

b. **Clinical Manifestations**

i. Are asymptomatic or present with symptoms of the underlying malignancy.

c. **Diagnosis**

i. CT scan is obtained to determine location and effect on surrounding structures.

ii. Biopsy is used to determine whether a nodule is benign or malignant, or has an infectious etiology.

d. **Treatment**

i. All nodules must be monitored closely.

ii. All solitary nodules in patients older than 35 years should be considered potentially malignant.

iii. Resection is indicated in patients with a high probability of malignancy.

# OBSTRUCTIVE PULMONARY DISEASE

## I. ASTHMA

a. **General**

   i. Chronic respiratory disease with intermittent, reversible obstruction of the airways.

   ii. Three basic pathophysiologic changes are as follows:

      1. Airway inflammation.
      2. Airway obstruction.
      3. Airway hyperresponsiveness.

   iii. Disease classified based on frequency of symptoms.

b. **Clinical Manifestations**

   i. Most common symptoms include episodic wheezing, cough, chest tightness, and shortness of breath.

      1. Symptoms are typically more prevalent at night and most severe in the morning.

   ii. Physical examination reveals diffuse wheezing, tachypnea, tachycardia, and prolonged expiration.

      1. In severe cases, may note accessory muscle use, intercostal retractions, and distant breath sounds.

c. **Diagnosis**

   i. Laboratory testing may reveal elevated white blood cell count with eosinophilia.

   ii. Sputum examination reveals eosinophils, Curschmann's spirals (mucous casts of small airways) or Charcot-Leyden crystals.

   iii. Early in an asthmatic episode, the arterial blood gases may reveal respiratory alkalosis and hypoxia.

      1. A normalizing $Pco_2$ or development of respiratory acidosis indicates impending respiratory failure.

   iv. Pulmonary function testing shows an obstructive pattern.

      1. Improvement in pulmonary function tests noted after treatment with bronchodilators.
      2. Table 2.6 compares pulmonary function tests in obstructive and restrictive lung disease.

d. **Treatment**

   i. Based on classification of chronic asthma with addition of agents as severity increases (Table 2.7).

   ii. Acute exacerbations.

      1. Inhaled, short-acting beta-agonist is the first agent of choice.

**TABLE 2.6**

| Obstructive and Restrictive Patterns on Pulmonary Function Testing | | |
|---|---|---|
| **Measurement** | **Obstructive** | **Restrictive** |
| Vital capacity (VC) | Normal or decreased | Decreased |
| $FEV_1$ | Decreased | Normal or decreased |
| $FEV_{1\%}$ | <75% | Normal or increased |
| Residual volume (RV) | Normal or increased | Decreased |
| Total lung capacity (TLC) | Normal or increased | Decreased |
| RV/TLC | Increased | Normal or increased |

**TABLE 2.7**

| Classification of Chronic Asthma | | | |
|---|---|---|---|
| **Step** | **Classification** | **Frequency of Symptoms** | **Nocturnal Symptoms** |
| 1 | Mild intermittent | <2 times per week | <2 times per month |
| 2 | Mild persistent | >2 times per week | 3–4 times per month |
| 3 | Moderate persistent | Daily | >1 time per week, but not nightly |
| 4 | Severe persistent | Continuous | Often 7 times per week |

      2. This should be followed by oral or intravenous (IV) corticosteroids.
      3. Oxygen may also be required.

   iii. Exercise-induced asthma.

      1. A beta-agonist or cromolyn sodium is used 15 minutes before exercise.

   iv. Prevention.

      1. Decrease exposure to allergens.
      2. Avoid exposure to smoking.
      3. Annual influenza vaccine to reduce risk of influenza.

## II. STATUS ASTHMATICUS

a. **General**

   i. Unremitting asthma with rapidly increasing severity.

   ii. Respiratory failure develops due to two mechanisms.

      1. Diffuse bronchial obstruction leading to ventilation-perfusion mismatch and hypoxia.
      2. Respiratory muscle fatigue.

b. **Clinical Manifestations**

   i. Symptoms include acute onset of chest tightness, shortness of breath, and cough.

ii. Physical examination reveals tachycardia, tachypnea, cyanosis, use of accessory muscles, intercostal retractions, pulsus paradoxus, and absence of wheezing.

c. **Diagnosis**
   i. Laboratory findings include hypoxemia and hypercapnia.
   ii. Spirometry is very useful in assessment of status asthmaticus.
      1. Peak flow and forced expiratory volume in 1 second ($FEV_1$) will be decreased.
      2. Monitor peak flow or $FEV_1$ before and after treatment.
      3. Peak flow <200 L/minute or 50% decrease from baseline indicates severe obstruction.
   iii. Chest x-ray film reveals hyperinflation and increased anteroposterior diameter.

d. **Treatment**
   i. Treatment consists of the following:
      1. Oxygen.
         (a) Supplemental oxygen needed to raise oxygen saturation to greater than 90% (95% in pregnancy).
      2. Bronchodilators.
         (a) Aerosolized beta-adrenergic agonists to open airways.
            (i) Safe in pregnancy.
            (ii) Salmeterol, long-acting beta-adrenergic agonist. Not indicated in acute disease.

(b) Intramuscular epinephrine can be used, but side effects include tachycardia, increased myocardial oxygen requirement, and hypertension.
(c) Inhaled anticholinergics (ipratropium bromide) with a beta-agonist may enhance bronchodilation.
(d) Intravenous magnesium is also an effective bronchodilator.
      3. Corticosteroids.
         (a) IV or oral corticosteroids are recommended early in treatment.
         (b) Are safe in pregnancy and should not be withheld if needed.
         (c) Work by decreasing inflammation.
      4. Mechanical ventilation.
         (a) Indications include altered mental status, acute $CO_2$ retention, poor response to therapy, or impending respiratory muscle fatigue.
      5. Table 2.8 summarizes medication options in treatment of asthma.

III. **BRONCHIECTASIS**
   a. **General**
      i. Abnormal dilation of the large conducting airways.
      ii. Due to congenital structural abnormalities or acquired process.
         1. Congenital causes include cystic fibrosis and alpha-1-antitrypsin deficiency.

**TABLE 2.8**

| Asthma Medications | | | |
|---|---|---|---|
| **Drug** | **Classification** | **Side Effects** | **Notes** |
| Albuterol | Beta-adrenergic agonist | Tachycardia Hyperglycemia Hypokalemia | |
| Pirbuterol | Beta-adrenergic agonist | Tachycardia Hyperglycemia Hypokalemia | |
| Salmeterol | Beta-adrenergic agonist | Tachycardia Hyperglycemia Hypokalemia | Long-acting agent, not used for acute therapy |
| Terbutaline | Beta-adrenergic agonist | Tachycardia Hyperglycemia Hypokalemia | |
| Ipratropium bromide | Anticholinergics | No real side effects | Very useful in chronic obstructive pulmonary disease, helps dry secretions |
| Theophylline | Not established | Anorexia Nausea Abdominal pain Seizures Arrhythmias | Must monitor serum drug levels |

*Continued*

**TABLE 2.8**

| Asthma Medications—cont'd | | | |
|---|---|---|---|
| **Drug** | **Classification** | **Side Effects** | **Notes** |
| Aminophylline | Not established | Anorexia<br>Nausea<br>Abdominal pain<br>Arrhythmias | Must monitor serum drug levels |
| Beclomethasone dipropionate | Antiinflammatory agent | Osteoporosis<br>Edema<br>Increased appetite | Increased risk for oral candidiasis |
| Budesonide | Antiinflammatory agent | Osteoporosis<br>Edema<br>Increased appetite | Increased risk for oral candidiasis |
| Flunisolide | Antiinflammatory agent | Osteoporosis<br>Edema<br>Increased appetite | Increased risk for oral candidiasis |
| Fluticasone propionate | Antiinflammatory agent | Osteoporosis<br>Edema<br>Increased appetite | |
| Methylprednisolone | Antiinflammatory agent | Osteoporosis<br>Edema<br>Increased appetite | |
| Prednisone | Antiinflammatory agent | Osteoporosis<br>Edema<br>Increased appetite | |
| Triamcinolone | Antiinflammatory agent | Osteoporosis<br>Edema<br>Increased appetite | |
| Montelukast | Leukotriene inhibitor | Elevated liver function tests<br>Headache<br>Dyspepsia | |
| Zafirlukast | Leukotriene inhibitor | Elevated liver function tests<br>Headache<br>Dyspepsia | Will interfere with warfarin |
| Cromolyn sodium | Mast cell stabilizer | Sore throat<br>Cough<br>Mouth dryness | Has value only when used prophylactically |
| Nedocromil sodium | Mast cell stabilizer | Sore throat<br>Cough<br>Mouth dryness | Has value only when used prophylactically |
| Omalizumab | Monoclonal antibody | | Given as subcutaneous injection. Binds to IgE and prevents interaction with IgE receptor on mast cells and basophils |
| Mepolizumab | Monoclonal antibody | | Given as subcutaneous injection. Binds to IL-5 and prevents interaction with the receptor |
| Reslizumab | Monoclonal antibody | Black box warning for anaphylaxis | Given intravenously. Binds to IL-5 |

2. Acquired processes include viral and bacterial infections, foreign bodies, COPD, and tumors.

b. **Clinical Manifestations**
   i. Major symptom is cough, which is daily and productive with purulent sputum.
      1. Hemoptysis may accompany the cough.
   ii. As disease progresses, exercise intolerance, dyspnea, and weight loss may develop.
   iii. Physical examination reveals coarse crackles with wheezing.

c. **Diagnosis**
   i. Chest x-ray film reveals thickened bronchial walls.
      1. May be described as "tram tracks" or ring-like markings.
   ii. CT scan is the standard test for diagnosing disease.
      1. Shows failure of bronchi to taper and shows increased wall thickness.
      2. Also note signet-ring sign on airways projecting on end.

iii. Pulmonary function tests may be normal at first and may later develop an obstructive, restrictive, or combined pattern.

d. **Treatment**
   i. Treatment of the underlying cause is crucial.
   ii. Antibiotics for acute exacerbations.
   iii. Daily chest physiotherapy with postural drainage and chest percussion.
   ii. Inhaled bronchodilators.

## IV. CHRONIC BRONCHITIS

a. **General**
   i. A clinical diagnosis of excessive sputum production with chronic or recurring cough on most days for at least 3 months of the year for at least 2 consecutive years, in which other causes of chronic cough have been excluded.
   ii. Cigarette smoking is a major risk factor.
      1. Increases risk by 10 to 30 times over nonsmokers.

b. **Clinical Manifestations**
   i. Most common early symptom is exertional dyspnea. Three most common symptoms are dyspnea, chronic cough, and sputum production.
   ii. Physical examination reveals an overweight, cyanotic patient with pedal edema (blue bloater).
      1. Signs of right sided heart failure may be common.
      2. Becomes dyspneic almost immediately when lying flat.
      3. Digital clubbing is rare.
   iii. Table 2.9 shows a comparison of emphysema and chronic bronchitis.

c. **Diagnosis**
   i. Pulmonary function test reveals an obstructive pattern (see Table 2.7).
   ii. Arterial blood gases reveal mild to moderate hypoxemia with normal $Pco_2$.

**TABLE 2.9**

| Comparison of Emphysema and Chronic Bronchitis | | |
| --- | --- | --- |
| | **Emphysema** | **Chronic Bronchitis** |
| Description | "Pink puffer" | "Blue bloater" |
| Major complaint | Dyspnea | Chronic cough |
| Age at onset | After age 50 years | Late 30s and 40s |
| Body habitus | Thin | Overweight |
| Lung examination | No adventitious sounds | Rhonchi are present |
| Peripheral edema | Negative | Positive |
| Hemoglobin | Normal | Elevated |
| Blood gases | $Po_2$ normal or reduced $Pco_2$ elevated | $Po_2$ reduced $Pco_2$ normal or reduced |
| Chest x-ray film | Hyperinflated with flat diaphragms | Increased interstitial markings and normal diaphragms |

iii. Electrocardiogram (EKG) will be normal early in disease and later will develop right-axis deviation.
iv. Chest x-ray film may reveal cardiac enlargement, congestion, increased lung markings, and bronchial wall thickening.

d. **Treatment**
   i. Smoking cessation is the number one intervention.
   ii. First-line therapy is bronchodilators.
      1. Used to reverse bronchospasm.
      2. Improve symptoms, exercise tolerance, and $FEV_1$.
      3. Side effects include palpitations, tachycardia, nervousness, and hypertension.
   iii. Theophylline is a weak bronchodilator and is used as an adjunct with beta-agonists.
      1. Side effects include nausea, vomiting, tachycardia, hypertension, and tremor.
      2. Erythromycin, cimetidine, and ciprofloxacin may increase theophylline levels.
   iv. Corticosteroids can be helpful in reducing inflammation.
   v. Mucokinetics facilitate mucociliary clearance by decreasing viscosity of mucus.
   vi. Supplemental oxygen for patients with resting hypoxemia.
      1. Has been shown to improve survival and quality of life.
   vii. Vaccinations, including pneumococcal and influenza, are needed.

## V. EMPHYSEMA

a. **General**
   i. Defined as destructive changes to the alveoli walls and enlargement of air spaces.
      1. Affects lung parenchyma distal to terminal bronchioles.
   ii. Cigarette smoking is a major risk factor.
      1. Increases risk by 10 to 30 times over nonsmokers.
   iii. Alpha-1-antitrypsin should be suspected in patients who develop emphysema in their late 30s.
      1. Treatment consists of recombinant antiprotease replacement therapy.

b. **Clinical Manifestations**
   i. Three most common symptoms are dyspnea, chronic cough, and sputum production.
   ii. Physical examination reveals a thin patient with pursed-lip breathing and pink skin color (pink puffer).
      1. Table 2.9 shows a comparison of emphysema and chronic bronchitis.

c. **Diagnosis**
   i. Pulmonary function test reveals an obstructive pattern (see Table 2.7).
   ii. Arterial blood gases reveal severe hypoxemia and hypercapnia.

iii. Chest x-ray film may be normal or show over-inflation, flat diaphragm, and increased retrosternal space.

**d. Treatment**

i. Smoking cessation is the number one intervention.

ii. First-line medical therapy includes anticholinergic agents and short-acting beta-agonists.

1. Agents should be given on a regular basis.

2. Side effects for anticholinergic agents include dry mouth, skin flushing, blurry vision, tachycardia, and urinary retention.

3. Side effects for beta-agonists include nausea, vomiting, tachycardia, hypertension, and tremor.

iii. Theophylline is a weak bronchodilator and is used as an adjunct with anticholinergic agents.

1. Side effects include nausea, vomiting, tachycardia, hypertension, and tremor.

2. Erythromycin, cimetidine, and ciprofloxacin may increase theophylline levels.

iv. Corticosteroids can be helpful in reducing inflammation.

v. Supplemental oxygen for patients with resting hypoxemia.

1. Has been shown to improve survival and quality of life.

vi. Vaccinations, including pneumococcal and influenza, are needed.

# PLEURAL DISEASES

## I. PLEURAL EFFUSION

**a. General**

i. Pleural space lies between the lung and chest wall.

ii. Effusion is present when there is excess quantity of fluid in the pleural space.

iii. Mechanisms of pleural effusion development.

1. Increased hydrostatic pressure in microcirculation.
   (a) Seen in left-sided heart failure.
   (b) Most common cause of pleural effusions.

2. Decreased oncotic pressure in microcirculation.
   (a) Seen in hypoalbuminemia.

3. Decreased pressure in the pleural space.
   (a) Seen in collapsed lung.

4. Increased permeability in microcirculation.
   (a) Seen in pneumonia.

5. Impaired lymphatic drainage.
   (a) Seen in malignancy.
   (b) Most commonly noted in lung cancer, breast cancer, and lymphoma.

6. Movement of fluid from peritoneal space.
   (a) Seen in ascites.

iv. Must determine whether fluid is a transudate or exudate.

1. Transudates occur when systemic factors that control formation and absorption of pleural fluid are altered.
   (a) Causes include left-sided heart failure, nephrotic syndrome, and cirrhosis.

2. Exudates occur when local factors that control formation and absorption of pleural fluid are altered.
   (a) Causes include bacterial pneumonia, malignancy, viral infection, pancreatitis, and pulmonary embolism.

**b. Clinical Manifestations**

i. Symptoms include dyspnea, cough, and chest pain.

ii. Lung examination reveals decreased breath sounds, dullness to percussion, and absent tactile fremitus.

**c. Diagnosis**

i. Chest x-ray film reveals blunting of margins (Fig. 2.4).

1. Free pleural fluid can be demonstrated with a lateral decubitus film.

ii. Laboratory results.

1. Exudates meet at least one of the following criteria, while transudates meet none.
   (a) Pleural fluid protein-to-serum protein ratio greater than 0.5.
   (b) Pleural fluid LDH-to-serum LDH ratio greater than 0.6.
   (c) Pleural fluid LDH is more than two thirds the normal upper limit for serum.

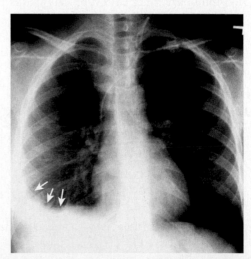

**Fig. 2.4** Moderate-sized, right-sided pleural effusion *(arrows)*. Note blunting of costophrenic angle. Mettler FA Jr. *Essentials of Radiology, 4th ed.* Philadelphia, Elsevier; 2019:86. Fig. 3.79A. *(From Mettler FA Jr. [ed]: Essentials of Radiology, 2nd ed. Philadelphia: Elsevier, 2004:107, Fig. 3-79A.)*

**d. Treatment**

    i. Thoracentesis can be diagnostic as well as therapeutic.

## II. PNEUMOTHORAX

**a. General**

    i. Due to the presence of air in the pleural space.

    ii. Clinical manifestations include sudden onset of dyspnea and pleuritic chest pain.

    iii. Physical examination reveals decreased or absent breath sounds, decreased tactile fremitus, and hyperresonant percussion.

    iv. Chest x-ray is essential to confirm the diagnosis and reveals a collapsed lung with loss of lung markings at the periphery.

**b. Types**

    i. Primary spontaneous.

        1. Occurs in the absence of underlying lung disease.

           (a) Seen most commonly in thin males aged 20 to 40 years.

        2. Typically due to rupture of pleural blebs and occurs almost exclusively in smokers.

        3. Recurrence is common.

        4. Treatment is simple aspiration or pleural abrasion to prevent recurrences.

    ii. Secondary spontaneous.

        1. Occurs in the presence of underlying lung disease, such as COPD, cystic fibrosis, lung malignancies, and necrotizing pneumonia.

        2. More life threatening.

        3. Treatment consists of a chest tube and use of a sclerosing agent.

    iii. Traumatic.

        1. Results from penetrating or nonpenetrating chest injuries.

        2. Treat with a chest tube unless the pneumothorax is very small.

    iv. Tension.

        1. Pneumothorax, in which the pressure in the pleural space is positive throughout the respiratory cycle.

           (a) Occurs most commonly during mechanical ventilation or pulmonary resuscitation.

        2. Life threatening due to positive pressure in thorax decreasing venous return and cardiac output.

        3. Physical examination reveals decreased or absent breath sounds on the affected side and shift of the mediastinum to the contralateral side.

        4. Chest x-ray film reveals collapsed lung with mediastinal and tracheal shift away from the pneumothorax (Fig. 2.5).

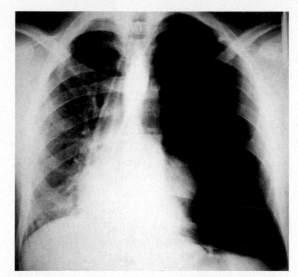

**Fig. 2.5** Tension pneumothorax on the left with mediastinal shift to the right. *(From Grainger RG, Allison D, Adam A, Dixon AK [eds]: Diagnostic Radiology: A Textbook of Medical Imaging, 4th ed. London: Harcourt, 2001:337, Fig. 16.44.)*

        5. Treatment consists of rapid placement of a large-bore needle into the pleural space through the second anterior intercostal space followed by chest tube placement.

## PULMONARY CIRCULATION

### I. PULMONARY EMBOLISM (PE)

**a. General**

    i. Most pulmonary emboli arise from venous thrombi in the deep veins of the lower extremities, followed by right-sided heart chamber, pelvic veins, and venous catheters.

        1. Emboli are usually multiple and bilateral and are typically found in the lower lobes.

    ii. Risk factors include the following:

        1. Hypercoagulable states.

        2. Pregnancy and oral contraceptives.

        3. Recent orthopedic, neurologic, or gynecologic surgery with general anesthesia.

        4. Recent major trauma.

        5. Atrial fibrillation.

        6. Right ventricular myocardial infarction.

        7. Immobilization.

        8. History of prior PE.

    iii. Pathophysiology.

        1. Total stoppage of blood flow to the distal lung leads to respiratory and hemodynamic changes.

           (a) Respiratory changes.

               (i) Development of an area of the lung that is ventilated but not perfused.

(ii) Pneumoconstriction leading to stoppage of pulmonary capillary flow.

(iii) Loss of surfactant, leading to alveolar collapse.

(b) Hemodynamic changes.

(i) Increased resistance to blood flow through the lung, which leads to acute right ventricular strain and decrease in cardiac output, as well as an increase in heart rate.

**b. Clinical Manifestations**

i. Clinicians must have a high index of suspicion.

ii. Symptoms include acute onset of dyspnea, pleuritic chest pain, cough, hemoptysis, syncope, calf/thigh swelling, and substernal chest pain.

iii. Physical examination reveals tachycardia and tachypnea.

1. In most patients, lung examination is normal.

2. In a massive PE, an $S_3$ may be noted.

**c. Diagnosis**

i. Laboratory results.

1. Arterial blood gases reveal an acute respiratory alkalosis, hypoxia, and hypocapnia.

2. EKG may show the classic $S_1Q_3T_3$ with or without a right bundle branch block (RBBB).

3. Chest x-ray film.

(a) Most abnormalities are nonspecific.

(b) May note Westermark's sign, an area of decreased pulmonary vascularity with a cutoff sign, or Hampton's hump, a shadow or density in contact with one or more pleural spaces corresponding to the lung segment involved.

4. Elevated D-dimer.

(a) Excellent test for ruling out pulmonary embolism in low-probability patients.

ii. Diagnosis is made with one of the following.

1. V/Q.

(a) Scoring system and percentage of patients with intermediate probability of pulmonary embolism.

(i) Normal: 6% PE rate.

(ii) Low probability: 16% PE rate.

(iii) Intermediate probability: 28% PE rate.

(iv) High probability: 88% PE rate.

(b) Limited use if other lung pathology is present.

2. Spiral CT scan.

(a) Increase use with 95% sensitivity for large PE and 75% sensitivity for subsegmental PE.

3. Pulmonary angiography.

(a) The gold standard for diagnosis.

(b) Very invasive with increased morbidity (5%) and mortality (<2%) rates.

**d. Treatment**

i. Prevention.

1. Includes early ambulation after surgery or delivery, heparin therapy for high-risk patients, or compression stockings.

ii. Anticoagulation.

1. Heparin is the gold standard for acute therapy.

(a) Low-molecular-weight heparin can be used.

(i) Less bleeding likely, and no laboratory monitoring is needed.

(b) Direct-acting oral anticoagulants (DOACs) can be used in hemodynamically stable patients.

2. Long-term therapy includes warfarin sodium (Coumadin) or DOACs.

3. Treat for at least 3 months.

4. Table 2.10 compares heparin and warfarin sodium.

iii. Pulmonary embolectomy.

1. Rarely needed except for large saddle emboli or patients with failed thrombolytic therapy.

iv. Thrombolytic therapy.

1. Should be used for high-risk or massive PEs with low risk of bleeding.

v. Vena cava filter.

1. Indications include absolute contraindication to anticoagulation, recurrence of PE or major bleeding while on anticoagulation, or septic emboli from a pelvic source.

**TABLE 2.10**

| Comparison of heparin and coumadin | | |
| --- | --- | --- |
| | **Heparin** | **Coumadin** |
| Mechanism of action | Catalyzes antithrombin III inactivation, allowing increased levels of activated coagulation factors in the blood | Inhibits vitamin K–dependent factors (II, VII, IX, X, and protein C and S) |
| Half life | 1–2 hours | 36 hours |
| Monitoring test | Partial thromboplastin time | Prothrombin time/INR |
| Side effects | Bleeding | Fetal toxic |
| | Overdose (treat with protamine sulfate) | Bleeding |
| | Heparin-associated thrombocytopenia | Overdose (treat with fresh frozen plasma or vitamin K) |
| Notes | Safe in pregnancy | Multiple drug interactions |
| | | Use contraindicated in pregnancy |

## II. PULMONARY HYPERTENSION

a. **General**
   i. Occurs when resistance to flow across the pulmonary vasculature increases.
   ii. Three groups based on pathophysiology.
      1. Precapillary.
         (a) Abnormality that leads to elevated pressures is located in the pulmonary arteries or arterioles.
         (b) Etiologies.
            (i) Pulmonary embolism.
            (ii) Congenital heart disease with pulmonary vascular disease.
               (1) Left-to-right shunts.
               (2) Ventricular septal defect.
               (3) Patent ductus arteriosus.
            (iii) Collagen vascular disease.
            (iv) Sickle cell anemia.
            (v) Portal hypertension.
            (vi) COPD.
            (vii) Diffuse interstitial lung disease.
            (viii) Cystic fibrosis.
      2. Passive.
         (a) Abnormality that leads to elevated pressure is due to diseases that increase pulmonary venous return.
         (b) Etiologies.
            (i) Left ventricular failure.
            (ii) Hypertension.
            (iii) Ischemic heart disease.
            (iv) Mitral stenosis.
            (v) Obstruction of major pulmonary veins.
      3. Reactive.
         (a) Patients have long-standing increased pulmonary venous pressure complicated by pulmonary arteriolar vasoconstriction.
         (b) Etiologies.
            (i) Mitral stenosis.
   iii. Primary pulmonary hypertension.
      1. Disease of unknown origin.
      2. Patients do not have pulmonary or cardiac disease.
      3. Patients present with exertional dyspnea without orthopnea, as well as syncope, chest pain, weakness, and palpitations.
      4. Physical examination.
         (a) Pulmonic ejection sound and flow murmur.
         (b) Hepatomegaly, peripheral edema, and ascites.
         (c) Right ventricular heave.
      5. Diagnosis confirmed by cardiac catheterization or pulmonary angiography.

b. **Clinical Manifestations**
   i. Patients with precapillary illness present with dyspnea, but no orthopnea, paroxysmal nocturnal dyspnea, or pulmonary edema.
      1. Physical examination reveals tachypnea with normal lung examination.
   ii. Patients with passive illness present with dyspnea, orthopnea, and paroxysmal nocturnal dyspnea.
      1. Physical examination reveals findings consistent with underlying etiology.
   iii. In reactive illness, patients present with severe dyspnea and markedly decreased exercise tolerance.

c. **Diagnosis**
   i. Chest x-ray film.
      1. Precapillary reveals right ventricular enlargement and prominent pulmonary arteries.
      2. Passive reveals prominent upper lobe pulmonary veins, increased density in the central lung fields, and Kerley B lines.
      3. Reactive reveals right ventricular enlargement and very prominent central pulmonary arteries.
   ii. EKG.
      1. Precapillary demonstrates right ventricular hypertrophy or right-axis deviation.
      2. Reactive demonstrates right ventricular hypertrophy.
   iii. Right heart catheterization or pulmonary angiography is needed to confirm diagnosis.
      1. Table 2.11 shows angiography results in pulmonary hypertension.

d. **Treatment**
   i. Treat the underlying cause.
   ii. Therapy based on the patient's functional status according to the NYHA/WHO classification.
      1. Nitric oxide pathway.
         a. Phosphodiesterase inhibitors.

**TABLE 2.11**

| Angiography Results in Pulmonary Hypertension | | | | |
| --- | --- | --- | --- | --- |
| Pressure Measurement | Normal | Precapillary | Passive | Reactive |
| Pulmonary artery pressure | 15 mm Hg | Increased | Increased | Increased |
| Left atrial pressure | 5 mm Hg | Normal | Increased | Increased |
| Pulmonary artery/left atrial pressure gradient | >12 mm Hg | <12 mm Hg | >12 mm Hg | |

b. Soluble guanylate cyclase stimulators.
2. Endothelin pathway.
   a. Endothelin receptor agonists.
3. Prostacyclin pathway.
   a. Prostacyclin analogs and prostacyclin receptor agonists.
ii. Acute pulmonary hypertension can be treated with prostaglandin (epoprostenol), nitrous oxide, or adenosine.
iii. Calcium channel blockers can be helpful in a select group of patients.
iv. Anticoagulation should be considered in all patients.
v. Reactive pulmonary hypertension is reversible with correction of underlying cause.
vi. Final treatment options include heart and heart-lung transplantation.

## III. COR PULMONALE

a. **General**
   i. Enlargement or dysfunction of the right ventricle due to pulmonary hypertension.
   ii. Most common cause is COPD.
      1. Other causes include the following:
         (a) Cystic fibrosis.
         (b) Diseases of pulmonary vasculature.
         (c) Primary pulmonary hypertension.
         (d) Acute massive PE.
         (e) Connective tissue disease.
         (f) Interstitial lung disease.
         (g) Malignant disease.
         (h) Sleep apnea syndromes.
b. **Clinical Manifestations**
   i. Patients present with symptoms of the underlying cause that leads to right ventricular hypertrophy and failure.
      1. Typically present with easy fatigability, increased dyspnea, exertional angina, and peripheral edema.
   ii. Physical examination reveals a dyspneic patient with central cyanosis, distended neck veins, parasternal lift, systolic murmur along left sternal border that changes with inspiration, and peripheral edema.
c. **Diagnosis**
   i. Arterial blood gases reveal hypoxia and hypercapnia.
   ii. EKG demonstrates right ventricular hypertrophy and prominent P waves in leads II, III, and aVF.
      1. Indicates right atrial enlargement.
   iii. Chest x-ray film reveals enlarged central pulmonary vessels and decrease in peripheral vessels.
      1. Described as pruning on chest x-ray film.

iv. Echocardiography, magnetic resonance imaging, or cardiac catheterization may be used to evaluate size and function of the right ventricle.
d. **Treatment**
   i. Treatment must focus on the underlying cause.
      1. In patients with COPD, this will include bronchodilators, beta-agonists, and antibiotics.
   ii. Oxygen may be needed but used with caution because many patients with cor pulmonale retain $CO_2$.
   iii. Vasodilators, such as hydralazine or calcium channel blockers, can be used to decrease pulmonary vascular resistance and to increase right ventricular stroke volume.
   iv. Diuretics may be needed for peripheral edema.

## RESTRICTIVE PULMONARY DISEASE

### I. IDIOPATHIC PULMONARY FIBROSIS

a. **General**
   i. A fibrosing interstitial pneumonia.
      1. Course is progressive with increasing fibrosis.
   ii. Patients typically present between ages 50 and 70 years.
      1. Very uncommon for patients to present symptoms before age 40.
   iii. Cigarette smoking is a strong link to this disease.
   iv. Etiology is unknown.
   v. Includes the following disorders:
      1. Acute interstitial pneumonia (AIP).
      2. Usual interstitial pneumonia (UIP).
      3. Nonspecific interstitial pneumonia (NSIP).
      4. Bronchiolitis obliterans with organizing pneumonia (BOOP).
      5. Table 2.12 compares various idiopathic interstitial pneumonias.
b. **Clinical Manifestations**
   i. Initial symptoms include exertional dyspnea (major symptom) and nonproductive cough.
   ii. Physical examination reveals tachypnea, clubbing, and fine bibasilar inspiratory crackles (Velcro rales).
c. **Diagnosis**
   i. Chest x-ray film reveals bilateral reticular opacities in the periphery and lower lobes.
   ii. Pulmonary function test reveals a restrictive pattern.
   iii. Lung biopsy is the gold standard for diagnosis.
d. **Treatment**
   i. There is no proven treatment.
      1. Mean survival after diagnosis is 3 years.

**TABLE 2.12**

### Comparison of Types of Idiopathic Interstitial Pneumonias

| Feature | AIP | UIP | NSIP | BOOP |
|---|---|---|---|---|
| Onset/age | Acute/50s | Insidious/60s | Subacute/50s | Acute or subacute/50s |
| Cigarette smoking | Unknown | Two thirds | Not known | One half |
| Mean survival | 1–2 months | 5–6 years | 18 months | Unknown |
| Steroid response | Poor | Poor | Good | Excellent |
| Complete recovery possible | Yes | No | Yes | Yes |

*AIP*, Acute interstitial pneumonia; *BOOP*, bronchiolitis obliterans with organizing pneumonia; *NSIP*, nonspecific interstitial pneumonia; *UIP*, usual interstitial pneumonia.

ii. Anti-inflammatory medications, mainly corticosteroids, are the mainstay of therapy.
   1. Corticosteroids are used to suppress chronic alveolitis.
   2. Therapy must be attempted for 3 months before effectiveness can be assessed.
   3. Corticosteroids can be combined with azathioprine or cyclophosphamide to improve response.
      (a) Table 2.13 lists common side effects of medications used in treatment of idiopathic pulmonary fibrosis.

**TABLE 2.13**

### Side Effects of Medications Used in Idiopathic Pulmonary Fibrosis

| Corticosteroids | Cyclophosphamide | Azathioprine |
|---|---|---|
| Water retention | Leukopenia | Leukopenia |
| Hyperglycemia | Thrombocytopenia | Anemia |
| Depression | Hemorrhagic cystitis | Thrombocytopenia |
| Osteoporosis | Nausea and vomiting | Nausea and vomiting |
| Peptic ulcer disease | | |

iii. Single lung transplantation should be considered in young patients.

## II. PNEUMOCONIOSIS
a. **General**
   i. Chronic lung disease caused by inhalation of dust particles through work exposure.
   ii. Smoking has an added detrimental effect.
   iii. Common disorders and features are described in Table 2.14.
b. **Clinical Manifestations**
   i. Obtaining occupational history is vital.
   ii. Most patients are asymptomatic.
   iii. As disease progresses, patients develop a mild productive cough and exertional dyspnea that may worsen to dyspnea at rest.
   iv. Physical examination is unremarkable early; patients later develop decreased breath sounds, rhonchi, wheezing, clubbing, cyanosis, and edema.
c. **Diagnosis**
   i. Chest x-ray film results vary with etiology.
      1. Later, these lesions become larger.

**TABLE 2.14**

### Comparison of Pneumoconioses

| Feature | Asbestosis | Coal Miner's Lung | Silicosis | Berylliosis |
|---|---|---|---|---|
| Material | Asbestos | Coal dust | Silica | Beryllium |
| Occupations | Asbestos millers<br>Brake lining workers<br>Insulators<br>Construction workers | Coal miners | Foundry workers<br>Glass makers<br>Pottery workers<br>Sandblasters | Aerospace<br>Electronics<br>Foundries<br>Nuclear reactors<br>Nuclear weapons<br>Telecommunications |
| Chest x-ray film | Pleural plaques | Small nodules in lower lung fields | Hilar node calcification (eggshell pattern) | Diffuse interstitial infiltrates and hilar adenopathy |
| Pulmonary function test pattern | Restrictive | Obstructive | Restrictive | Vary |
| Complications | Mesotheliomas | Caplan's syndrome | Lung cancer<br>Increased risk of tuberculosis | Unknown |
| Treatment | Supportive care plus steroids | Supportive care plus steroids | Supportive care plus steroids | Supportive care plus steroids, lifelong therapy needed |

ii. Pulmonary function tests reveal a mixed pattern depending on etiology.

**d. Treatment**

i. Further exposure to material should be avoided and smoking cessation is critical.

ii. Supportive therapy is the center of therapy; other options include pulmonary rehabilitation, inhaled beta-agonists, and oxygen.

## III. SARCOIDOSIS

**a. General**

i. Multisystem disorder characterized by alveolitis followed by epithelioid granulomas.

1. Associated with inclusion bodies such as Schaumann's bodies and asteroid bodies.

ii. Etiology is unknown.

iii. Disease is more common in young people (<40 years old), Black people, and females.

**b. Clinical Manifestations**

i. Symptoms include fatigue, weakness, weight loss, fever, and sweats.

ii. Most common organ system involved is the lungs.

1. Patients present with cough, wheezing, and dyspnea.

iii. Other systems involved include skin, gastrointestinal, cardiac, ocular, and nervous systems.

**c. Diagnosis**

i. Chest x-ray results are grouped by stages.

1. Stage I: Bilateral hilar adenopathy (Fig. 2.6).

2. Stage II: Bilateral hilar adenopathy with diffuse parenchymal infiltrates.

3. Stage III: Diffuse parenchymal infiltrates without bilateral hilar adenopathy.

4. Stage IV: Advanced fibrotic changes, primarily in the upper lobes.

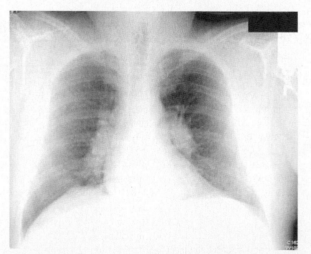

**Fig. 2.6** Sarcoidosis stage I. Note hilar adenopathy and normal lungs. *(From Mason RJ, Murray and Nadel's Textbook of Respiratory Medicine, 4th ed., London: Elsevier, 2005, Fig. 55-1.)*

ii. Angiotensin-converting enzyme (ACE) level is elevated in 40% to 80% of patients.

iii. Gallium scan is positive.

iv. Diagnosis based on history, chest x-ray findings, and biopsy results.

**d. Treatment**

i. Staging predicts the percentage of patients with resolution of disease.

1. Higher stage means lower percentage of resolution.

ii. The disease course is unpredictable.

iii. Antiinflammatory medications, including glucocorticoids, methotrexate, azathioprine, and infliximab.

# OTHER

## I. ACUTE RESPIRATORY DISTRESS SYNDROME

**a. General**

i. Form of noncardiac pulmonary edema as a result of acute damage to the alveoli.

ii. Definition involves three criteria.

1. Ratio of $Pao_2$ to $Fio_2$ less than or equal to 300 with PEEP greater than or equal to 5 cm $H_2O$.

2. Detection of bilateral pulmonary infiltrates on chest x-ray film.

3. Progressive dyspnea within 7 days of a known clinical insult.

iii. Etiologies.

1. Sepsis.

2. Aspiration.

3. Trauma.

4. Multiple blood transfusions.

5. Drugs.

6. Pneumonia.

7. Burns.

8. Pancreatitis.

9. Near-drowning.

**b. Clinical Manifestations**

i. Signs and symptoms include profound dyspnea, chest discomfort, and cough.

ii. Physical examination reveals tachypnea, intercostal retractions, tachycardia, elevated blood pressure, and crackles in both lungs.

**c. Diagnosis**

i. Arterial blood gases reveal hypoxia and respiratory alkalosis.

ii. Bronchoalveolar lavage shows an increased number of neutrophils and possibly eosinophils.

iii. Chest x-ray film may be normal initially, followed later by bilateral interstitial infiltrates within 24 hours.

1. White-out of lung fields can be seen in severe cases.

iv. Presence of pulmonary edema, high cardiac output, and a low pulmonary artery wedge pressure are characteristic.

**d. Treatment**

i. Ventilatory support, mechanical ventilation, is typically necessary.

1. Consider prone positioning.

ii. Treat the underlying cause.

iii. Fluid management is critical.

iv. Corticosteroids may be helpful in patients with increased eosinophils in bronchoalveolar lavage.

v. Patients must be treated with some form of deep venous thrombosis and stress ulcer prophylaxis.

vi. Overall mortality rate is approximately 30%.

# QUESTIONS

## QUESTION 1

Which of the following is the major symptom of idiopathic pulmonary fibrosis?

A Cervical adenopathy

B Pleuritic chest pain

C Exertional dyspnea

D Peripheral edema

E Hepatosplenomegaly

## QUESTION 2

Which of the following pulmonary function test results is typically noted in restrictive pulmonary disease?

A Decreased $FEV_1$

B Increased VC

C Increased RV

D Decreased TLC

E Increased forced vital capacity (FVC)

## QUESTION 3

A 60-year-old patient with a history of lung cancer presents with facial and neck swelling. Which of the following is the most likely diagnosis?

A Horner's syndrome

B Superior vena cava syndrome

C Pancoast's tumor

D Tumor lysis syndrome

E Sialadenitis

## QUESTION 4

A 25-year-old male presents with sudden onset of shortness of breath and chest pain. Physical examination reveals absent breath sounds on the entire right side. Which of the following is the treatment of choice?

A Heparin

B Chest tube

C Prostaglandin

D Corticosteroids

E Incentive spirometry

## QUESTION 5

An 18-year-old college student presents with a sudden onset of chills, myalgias, and a nonproductive cough. On physical examination, temperature is 102.3° F, pulse 114/minute, and respiratory rate 18/minute. Pharynx is erythematous without exudates. Lungs are clear. Which of the following is the treatment of choice?

A Albuterol

B Zanamivir

C Prednisone

D Amoxicillin

E Tetracycline

## QUESTION 6

High-risk groups, such as the elderly, patients with COPD, and children aged 6 to 24 months, should routinely receive which of the following yearly vaccines?

A Tuberculosis

B Tetanus

C Pertussis

D Influenzae

E Pneumococcal

## QUESTION 7

Which of the following is the most common cause of pneumonia in patients with a history of alcoholism?

A *Staphylococcus aureus*

B *Pneumocystis jirovecii*

C *Klebsiella pneumoniae*

D *Mycobacterium tuberculosis*

E *Pseudomonas aeruginosa*

## QUESTION 8

A 25-year-old patient presents with a nonproductive cough. The patient also notes headache and malaise, but denies shortness of breath, chest pain, or fever. Physical examination reveals a normal lung examination. Chest x-ray film reveals patchy infiltrates. Which of the following is the most likely diagnosis?

A Tuberculosis

B Sporotrichosis

C Blastomycosis

D Mycoplasmal pneumonia

E Pneumococcal pneumonia

*Continued*

## QUESTIONS—cont'd

### QUESTION 9
A 35-year-old Black female presents with complaints of a gradual worsening of exertional dyspnea associated with a mild dry cough. Physical examination is unremarkable. A chest x-ray reveals the presence of bilateral hilar adenopathy. Which of the following laboratory results is most likely in this patient?
A  Positive antinuclear antibody
B  Hypocalcemia
C  Elevated D-dimer
D  Decreased serum calcium
E  Elevated angiotensin-converting enzyme (ACE) level

### QUESTION 10
Which of the following is a major risk factor for the development of mesothelioma?
A  Smoking
B  Asbestos
C  Radon gas
D  Hantavirus
E  Epstein-Barr virus

## ANSWERS

**1.  C**
EXPLANATION: The major symptom of idiopathic pulmonary fibrosis is exertional dyspnea. *Topic: Restrictive pulmonary disease*
☐ Correct   ☐ Incorrect

**2.  D**
EXPLANATION: Restrictive pulmonary diseases typically present with decreased VC, RV, and TLC. FEV and FEV₁ may be normal. *Topic: Restrictive pulmonary disease*
☐ Correct   ☐ Incorrect

**3.  B**
EXPLANATION: Superior vena cava syndrome is commonly noted in patients with lung cancer and presents with facial and neck swelling. *Topic: Bronchogenic carcinoma*
☐ Correct   ☐ Incorrect

**4.  B**
EXPLANATION: Pneumothorax typically develops in thin males who present with decreased or absent breath sounds and sudden onset of dyspnea and pleuritic chest pain. Diagnosis is confirmed on chest x-ray film and is treated with chest tube placement to reexpand the involved lung. *Topic: Pneumothorax*
☐ Correct   ☐ Incorrect

**5.  B**
EXPLANATION: The patient presents with signs and symptoms consistent with influenza. Treatment of choice is zanamivir and oseltamivir. *Topic: Influenza*
☐ Correct   ☐ Incorrect

**6.  D**
EXPLANATION: Influenza vaccine should be given to high-risk groups. These groups include the elderly, nursing home residents, patients with a history of chronic diseases such as COPD or cardiac disease, patients who are pregnant, children aged 6 to 24 months, and persons in contact with high-risk patients. *Topic: Influenza*
☐ Correct   ☐ Incorrect

**7.  C**
EXPLANATION: In the alcoholic patient, the most common causes of pneumonia are *S. pneumoniae* and *K. pneumoniae*. *Topic: Pneumonia*
☐ Correct   ☐ Incorrect

**8.  D**
EXPLANATION: *Mycoplasma* pneumonia is seen most commonly in the young and patients who present with a nonproductive cough, malaise, myalgias, and headache. The pulmonary examination is typically normal, and the chest x-ray film reveals diffuse infiltrates. *Topic: Pneumonia*
☐ Correct   ☐ Incorrect

**9.  E**
EXPLANATION: Sarcoidosis is seen most commonly in Black females who present with dyspnea, malaise, and fever. Typical chest x-ray film findings include bilateral hilar and right paratracheal lymphadenopathy. ACE levels will be elevated. Hypercalcemia is noted in about 10% of cases. *Topic: Sarcoidosis*
☐ Correct   ☐ Incorrect

**10.  B**
EXPLANATION: Development of mesothelioma has been linked to asbestos exposure, radiation, and SV40 virus. Smoking and radon exposure have been linked to bronchogenic lung cancer, and Epstein-Barr virus has been linked to Burkitt's lymphoma. *Topic: Bronchogenic carcinoma*
☐ Correct   ☐ Incorrect

# CHAPTER 3

# GASTROENTEROLOGY SYSTEM

## EXAMINATION BLUEPRINT TOPICS

**ESOPHAGUS**
Esophagitis
Motility disorders
Mallory-Weiss tear
Neoplasms
Strictures
Varices

**STOMACH**
Gastroesophageal reflux disease
Gastritis
Neoplasms
Peptic ulcer disease

**GALLBLADDER**
Acute cholecystitis
Primary sclerosing cholangitis
Cholelithiasis

**LIVER**
Acute hepatitis
Chronic hepatitis
Neoplasms
Cirrhosis

Disorders of bilirubin metabolism

**PANCREAS**
Acute pancreatitis
Chronic pancreatitis
Neoplasms

**SMALL INTESTINE/COLON**
Appendicitis
Celiac disease
Constipation
Diverticular disease
Inflammatory bowel disease
Irritable bowel disease
Ischemic bowel disease
Malabsorption
Neoplasms
Obstruction
Polyps
Toxic megacolon

**RECTUM**
Anal fissure
Anorectal abscess/Fistula

Fecal impaction
Hemorrhoids
Neoplasms
Pilonidal disease
Polyps

**HERNIA**
Hiatal
Incisional (ventral)
Inguinal
Umbilical

**INFECTIOUS DIARRHEA**
Acute infectious diarrhea
Traveler's diarrhea
Nosocomial diarrhea

**NUTRITIONAL DEFICIENCIES**
Table 3.21 summarizes nutritional deficiencies

**FOOD ALLERGIES**

## ESOPHAGUS

**I. ESOPHAGITIS**
  **a. Infectious**
    i. General
      1. Occurs principally in immunocompromised patients.
      2. Most common agents include the following:
        (a) *Candida albicans*.
        (b) Herpes simplex.
        (c) Cytomegalovirus.
    ii. Clinical manifestations
      1. Odynophagia may be severe.
      2. Dysphagia, weight loss, and substernal chest pain are common.
      3. Esophageal candidiasis is associated with oral candidiasis.

      4. Herpes esophagitis is associated with oral herpetic lesions.
    iii. Diagnosis
      1. Barium swallow.
        (a) "Shaggy" mucosa suggests *Candida*.
        (b) Many small, volcanic-shaped ulcers suggest herpes.
        (c) Large, deep linear ulcers suggest cytomegalovirus.
      2. Endoscopy
        (a) A biopsy is required to make the definitive diagnosis.
        (b) *Candida* reveals many small, white-yellow plaques on the mucosa.
        (c) Herpes reveals many vesicles that ulcerate to form small, shallow, volcanic-shaped ulcers.

(d) Cytomegalovirus reveals multiple, large, shallow, often linear ulcers typically at lower esophagus.

iv. Treatment
1. *Candida* esophagitis.
   (a) Oral fluconazole or itraconazole.
   (b) If IV therapy is needed, use caspofungin, micafungin, or amphotericin B.
   (c) Amphotericin B is recommended in pregnancy.
2. Herpes esophagitis.
   (a) Oral or intravenous (IV) acyclovir.
   (b) Valacyclovir or famciclovir are also possible, or IV foscarnet for resistant disease.
3. Cytomegalovirus esophagitis.
   (a) First choice is IV ganciclovir or IV foscarnet.

**b. Medication-Induced**
i. General
1. Common in elderly patients or any patient not taking medication correctly.
2. Common drugs include the following:
   (a) Doxycycline/tetracycline.
   (b) Potassium chloride.
   (c) Vitamin C.
   (d) Nonsteroidal antiinflammatory drugs (NSAIDs)/aspirin.
   (e) Quinidine.
   (f) Alendronate.
   (g) Iron.
ii. Clinical manifestations
1. Characterized by sudden onset odynophagia accompanied by dysphagia.
2. Endoscopic appearance is of a discrete ulcer.
iii. Treatment
1. Stop the offending agent, switch to liquid form of the medication, and treat with sucralfate suspension.

**c. Radiation**
i. General
1. Occurs from radiation to the chest at levels exceeding 3000 cGy.
ii. Clinical manifestations
1. Can develop severe esophagitis and ulcerations.
2. Concomitant chemotherapy with cytotoxic agents can potentiate the injury.
3. Patients present with substernal chest pain, odynophagia, and dysphagia.
iii. Treatment
1. Nutritional supplement.
2. Delay radiation if possible.
3. Sucralfate suspension.
4. Topical anesthetics (lidocaine).
5. Antacid therapy.

**II. MOTILITY DISORDERS**
**a. General**
i. May present with chest pain, dysphagia, or both.
ii. Dysphagia is with solids and liquids.
iii. Types of dysphagia.
1. Oropharyngeal.
   (a) Due to neuromuscular disorders of the oropharynx or skeletal muscle of the esophagus.
   (b) Difficulty in bolus transfer to esophagus, nasal regurgitation, or coughing with swallowing.
   (c) Etiologies include stroke, Parkinson's disease, amyotrophic lateral sclerosis, multiple sclerosis, and myasthenia gravis.
   (d) Procedure of choice for diagnosis is the modified barium swallow with video fluoroscopy.
2. Esophageal.
   (a) Due to disease of the smooth muscle of the esophagus.
   (b) No difficulty with transfer of bolus, regurgitation, or coughing.
   (c) Characterized by difficulty swallowing several seconds after initiating a swallow. Sensation of food getting stuck in the esophagus.
   (d) Etiologies include stricture, cancer, and Schatzki's ring.
3. Dysphagia with only solids.
   (a) Consider achalasia, diffuse esophageal spasm, and scleroderma.
4. Dysphagia with solids and liquids.
   (a) Procedure of choice for diagnosis is manometry to evaluate peristaltic and sphincter function.

**b. Achalasia**
i. General
1. Most common esophageal motor disorder.
2. Etiology is unknown.
   (a) Degeneration of nerves in Auerbach's plexus, vagus nerve, and swallowing center.
   (b) Leads to increase in lower esophageal sphincter (LES) pressure, incomplete relaxation of the LES with swallowing, and aperistalsis in the esophagus.
ii. Clinical manifestations
1. Dysphagia of liquids and solids is the primary problem.
2. Regurgitation of retained material is common.
iii. Diagnosis

1. Barium swallow shows a dilated esophagus, air fluid level, delayed esophageal emptying, and a smooth, tapered "bird's-beak" deformity at the LES (Fig. 3.1).
2. Confirm by esophageal manometry showing elevated LES pressure.

iv. Treatment
1. Myotomy.
2. Endoscopic injection of botulinum toxin or pneumatic dilation.

c. **Diffuse Esophageal Spasm**

i. General
1. Uncommon disorder.
2. Signs and symptoms are intermittent.
3. Associated with degeneration of Auerbach's plexus.

ii. Clinical manifestations
1. Patients present with chest pain, dysphagia, or both.
2. Pain can be precipitated by drinking cold liquids.

iii. Diagnosis
1. Barium swallow shows prominent, spontaneous, non-propulsive, tertiary contractions.
2. Gives a "corkscrew" or "rosary-bead" esophagus appearance on barium swallow.

3. Manometry reveals excessive simultaneous contractions of the distal esophagus.

iv. Treatment
1. Supportive and empirical.
2. Smooth muscle relaxants: nifedipine, isosorbide.
3. Antidepressants: trazodone, imipramine.
4. Relaxation exercises, biofeedback, or counseling.

## III. MALLORY-WEISS TEAR

a. **General**

i. One of the major causes of upper gastrointestinal (GI) bleeding.
ii. Occurs in the distal esophagus at the gastroesophageal (GE) junction.
iii. Typically occurs after a bout of vomiting or retching.
iv. Bleeding occurs when tear involves the underlying venous or arterial plexus.
v. Increased risk in patients with portal hypertension.

b. **Clinical Manifestations**

i. Typically, middle-aged males who present with painless hematemesis.
1. Frequently follows episodes of vomiting after drinking alcohol.

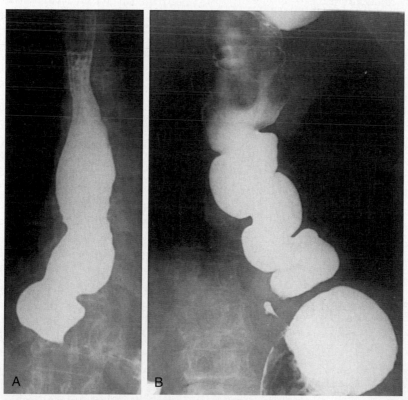

**Fig. 3.1** Achalasia. (A) Note the bird's-beak deformity. (B) Note marked distortion of the esophagus.
*(From Feldman M: Sleisenger and Fordtran's Gastrointestinal and Liver Disease, 7th ed. Philadelphia: WB Saunders, 2002: 578, Fig. 32.9.)*

### c. Diagnosis
   i. Endoscopy is the procedure of choice.
      1. Appears as an elongated or elliptical ulcer at the GE junction.

### d. Treatment
   i. Most tears stop bleeding spontaneously.
   ii. Endoscopic clipping, band ligation and thermal coagulation may be needed.
      1. Avoid thermal coagulation in patients with portal hypertension or esophageal varices, which may worsen bleeding.
   iii. Complications include rebleeding.

## IV. NEOPLASMS
### a. General
   i. Predominantly affects patients between 50 and 70 years of age.
   ii. Two types of cancer.
      1. Adenocarcinoma: typically involves the distal esophagus.
      2. Squamous cell: typically involves the middle or distal esophagus.
      3. Table 3.1 lists esophageal cancer risk factors.

### b. Clinical Manifestations
   i. Most common presenting symptom is progressive dysphagia.
      1. First solids, then liquids.
   ii. Also present with odynophagia, chest pain, weight loss, and anorexia.

### c. Diagnosis
   i. Initial workup includes barium esophagram, which shows narrowing of the lumen at the tumor site and dilation proximal to the tumor.
   ii. Confirm diagnosis with upper endoscopy with biopsy.

### d. Treatment
   i. Squamous cell treated with chemoradiation and surgery.
   ii. Adenocarcinoma is treated with surgery or chemotherapy because it is not sensitive to radiation.
   iii. Overall 5-year survival rate is less than 20%.

**TABLE 3.1**

| Esophageal Cancer Risk Factors | |
|---|---|
| **Adenocarcinoma** | **Squamous Cell Carcinoma** |
| Alcohol consumption | History of radiation therapy |
| Barrett's esophagus and gastro-esophageal reflux disease | Smoking |
| History of colon cancer | Achalasia |
| Obesity | Alcohol consumption |
| Smoking | |

## V. STRICTURES
### a. General
   i. Include esophageal webs and rings, as well as diverticula.
      1. Webs and rings are thin diaphragm-like structures that interrupt the esophageal lumen.

### b. Disorders
   i. Cervical esophageal webs.
      1. More commonly found in females and often associated with iron deficiency anemia (Plummer-Vinson syndrome).
      2. Major complaint is intermittent solid food dysphagia.
      3. Signs of iron deficiency may also be present.
      4. Cine-esophagography is the study of choice for diagnosis.
      5. Web is often ruptured during endoscopic examination; therefore the procedure may be curative.
   ii. Lower esophageal ring (Schatzki's ring).
      1. Common cause of intermittent solid food dysphagia.
      2. Tends to occur when patients are eating quickly.
      3. Barium esophagram is the diagnostic tool.
      4. Treatment includes dilation of the ring.
   iii. Zenker's diverticulum.
      1. Outpouching of the posterior pharyngeal constrictor muscle in the back of the pharynx.
      2. Pathogenesis is unknown.
      3. Many people are asymptomatic but may present with dysphagia and regurgitation.
      4. Spontaneous regurgitation of food ingested several hours previously is characteristic of a large Zenker's diverticulum.
      5. Barium esophagram is used to make the diagnosis.
      6. Endoscopic and nasogastric tube placement are contraindicated because of the risk of perforation.
      7. Treatment consists of surgery.

## VI. VARICES
### a. General
   i. Venous collaterals that develop as a result of portal hypertension.
      1. Causes include pre-hepatic thrombosis, hepatic disease, post sinusoidal disease, alcoholic liver disease, and viral hepatitis.
   ii. Typically have massive upper GI bleeding and history of chronic liver disease and cirrhosis.

### b. Clinical Manifestations
   i. Symptoms include hematemesis, melena, hematochezia, and dizziness.

ii. Manifestations of cirrhosis and portal hypertension may be noted.

iii. Elevation in liver enzymes and bilirubin with low albumin and cholesterol, and elevated prothrombin time (PT) are noted.

c. **Diagnosis**
   i. Endoscopy is the test of choice for diagnosis.

d. **Treatment**
   i. Medical therapy.
      1. IV vasopressin.
      2. IV nitroglycerin.
      3. IV octreotide.
      4. Balloon tamponade.
      5. Antibiotic prophylaxis.
      6. Vitamin K in cirrhotic patients with abnormal prothrombin time.
   ii. Endoscopic therapy.
      1. Endoscopic hemostasis is the treatment of choice and includes the following:
         (a) Variceal band ligation.
         (b) Endoscopic sclerotherapy is seldom used in clinical practice.
   iii. Complications.
      1. Bleeding stops spontaneously in more than 50% of patients.
      2. Increased mortality in patients with continued bleeding.
      3. Uncontrolled bleeding can lead to hemorrhage and death.

# STOMACH

## I. GASTROESOPHAGEAL REFLUX DISEASE (GERD)
a. **General**
   i. A process that refers to the effortless movement of gastric contents from the stomach to the esophagus.
   ii. Affects men more than women and is more common in White populations than Black.
   iii. Develops when acid content of the stomach refluxes into the esophagus and remains long enough to overcome the resistance of the esophageal epithelium.
      1. Due to increased frequency of transient LES relaxations.
      2. Etiologies include nicotine, alcohol, caffeine, peppermint, chocolate, and drugs (anticholinergics, calcium channel blockers, and nitrates).

b. **Clinical Manifestations**
   i. Recurrent heartburn is the hallmark symptom.
   ii. Alarm symptoms include dysphagia, GI bleeding, or weight loss.
      1. If present, consider stricture or adenocarcinoma.

iii. Extraesophageal symptoms.
      1. Include pharyngitis, ear pain, gingivitis, laryngitis, chronic cough, asthma, and aspiration pneumonia.

c. **Diagnosis**
   i. History of recurrent heartburn and a positive response to acid-suppression drugs.
   ii. Specific testing is reserved for patients with alarm symptoms.
      1. Upper GI endoscopy.
         (a) Detects grossly abnormal reflux.
      2. Esophageal pH monitoring.
         (a) The gold standard for identifying reflux.
      3. Bernstein's test.
         (a) Establishes GERD as a cause of symptoms.

d. **Treatment**
   i. Consists of lifestyle modifications and drug therapy.
   ii. Table 3.2 shows lifestyle modifications.
   iii. Table 3.3 lists drug therapy.

## II. GASTRITIS
a. **General**
   i. Inflammation of the gastric mucosa.
   ii. Etiologies.
      1. *Helicobacter pylori*.
      2. Autoimmune.
         (a) Pernicious anemia is a late complication of autoimmune gastritis.
      3. Environmental: alcohol, burns, or mechanical ventilation.
      4. Chemical: bile, NSAIDs.

b. **Clinical Manifestations**
   i. Epigastric pain with bleeding or asymptomatic bleeding.
   ii. Nausea and vomiting.

c. **Diagnosis**
   i. *H. pylori*.
      1. Detect by serology testing, urea breath test, or stool antigen testing.

**TABLE 3.2**

| Lifestyle Modifications for Gastroesophageal Reflux Disease |
| --- |
| Avoid bedtime snacks |
| Avoid chocolate, peppermint, coffee, tea, colas, and citrus fruit juices |
| Decrease dietary fat |
| Decrease meal size |
| Elevate head of bed 6 inches |
| Stop alcohol consumption |
| Stop smoking |

**TABLE 3.3**

| Drug Therapy in Gastroesophageal Reflux Disease | | |
| --- | --- | --- |
| **Drug Therapy** | **Mechanism** | **Example** |
| Antacids | Buffer HCl and increase lower esophageal sphincter pressure | Mylanta |
| Barriers | Viscous mechanical barrier and buffer HCl | Aluminum hydroxide |
| H$_2$ receptor antagonists | Decrease HCl secretion | Cimetidine Famotidine |
| Prokinetics | Increase lower esophageal sphincter pressure and increase gastric emptying | Bethanechol Metoclopramide |
| Proton pump inhibitors (PPIs) | Decrease HCl secretion and gastric volume | Omeprazole Lansoprazole Rabeprazole |

*HCl,* Hydrochloric acid.

    ii. Endoscopy.
       1. Note erosions and petechial hemorrhages.
  **d. Treatment**
    i. *H. pylori:* antibiotics and proton pump inhibitor (PPI).
    ii. Discontinue drugs (NSAIDs).
    iii. Medical therapy with PPI or H$_2$ antagonists.

**III. NEOPLASMS**
  **a. General**
    i. Predominantly malignant, with a majority of them being adenocarcinoma.
    ii. Occur typically in the 50- to 70-year-old age group and is rare before age 30 years.
    iii. Etiologic factors include the following:
       1. Environmental.
         (a) *H. pylori.*
         (b) Dietary: excess salt, nitrates/nitrites, and deficiency in fresh fruit and vegetables.
       2. Genetic.
         (a) Blood group A.
       3. Predisposing conditions.
         (a) Chronic gastritis.
         (b) Pernicious anemia.
         (c) Large gastric adenomatous polyps.
         (d) Chronic peptic ulcer.
  **b. Clinical Manifestations**
    i. Early in the disease, the patient is asymptomatic.
    ii. Later symptoms include bloating, dysphagia, epigastric pain, weight loss, or early satiety.
       1. Food or antacids do not relieve the epigastric pain.
    iii. Physical examination may be unremarkable.
       1. Later in the disease, the patient becomes cachectic, and an epigastric mass may be noted.
       2. Patients may show signs of metastatic disease.

         (a) Hepatomegaly and jaundice due to liver metastases.
         (b) Lymph node involvement in the left supraclavicular region (Virchow's node) or periumbilical nodes (Saint Mary Joseph's node).
  **c. Diagnosis**
    i. Upper endoscopy with biopsy.
  **d. Treatment**
    i. Survival rate varies greatly by stage, location and histologic features.
    ii. Surgical resection provides the highest chance for cure.
    iii. Somewhat responsive to chemotherapy.
    iv. Radiation therapy is ineffective alone, but combined with chemotherapy it has been shown to improve survival.

**IV. PEPTIC ULCER DISEASE**
  **a. General**
    i. Most common causes are *H. pylori* and NSAIDs.
    ii. Unusual cause is a gastrinoma (Zollinger-Ellison syndrome).
       1. Tumor that secretes excess amounts of gastrin, by the stomach G cells, and gastric acid hypersecretion.
       2. Leads to multiple ulcers.
       3. Diarrhea is common.
       4. Tumors located in the pancreas and duodenum.
       5. Laboratory studies reveal markedly elevated serum gastrin levels.
       6. Gastrin levels are increased in patients on H2 blockers and PPIs.
       7. Other causes of elevated gastrin levels include pernicious anemia, chronic gastritis, renal failure, and hyperthyroidism.

**TABLE 3.4**

| Symptoms in Gastric and Duodenal Ulcers | | |
| --- | --- | --- |
| **Symptom** | **Gastric Ulcer** | **Duodenal Ulcer** |
| Epigastric pain | +++ | +++ |
| Nocturnal pain | + | +++ |
| Pain relief with food | + | ++ |
| Episodic pain | + | ++ |
| Bloating/Belching | ++ | ++ |
| Anorexia/Weight loss | ++ | + |
| Nausea/Vomiting | +++ | ++ |

+, Rare; ++, common; +++, likely.

**TABLE 3.5**

| Treatment of *Helicobacter pylori* Infection |
| --- |
| **Triple Therapy** |
| A proton-pump inhibitor BID, plus |
| Amoxicillin 1 g BID, or metronidazole 500 mg BID, plus |
| Clarithromycin, 500 mg BID |
| **Three- and Four-Times-Daily Triple Therapies** |
| Bismuth subsalicylate 524 mg QID, plus |
| Tetracycline, 500 mg QID, plus |
| Metronidazole, 500 mg TID |
| **Quadruple Therapies** |
| Proton pump inhibitor BID, plus |
| Bismuth subsalicylate, 2 tablets QID, plus |
| Tetracycline, 500 mg QID, plus |
| Metronidazole, 250 mg QID |

*BID*, Twice a day; *QID*, four times a day; *TID*, three times a day.

8. Treatment is with maximum dose PPIs and surgery.

**b. Clinical Manifestations**
  i. Burning, epigastric pain worse on empty stomach or at night.
  ii. May also present with GI bleeding.
  iii. On examination, may note epigastric tenderness with deep palpation.
  iv. Symptoms vary with source—gastric versus duodenal.
    1. Table 3.4 compares gastric and duodenal ulcers.

**c. Diagnosis**
  i. Upper GI endoscopy.
    1. Important to biopsy gastric ulcers because of risk for cancer.
    2. Duodenal ulcers are almost never malignant, so biopsy is not needed.
  ii. Barium contrast studies.
  iii. Gastrin levels are indicated in intractable ulcer disease for possible Zollinger-Ellison. syndrome.
  iv. Tests for *H. pylori* include the following:
    1. Rapid urease test: requires endoscopy.
    2. Histology: requires endoscopy.
    3. Culture: requires endoscopy.
    4. Urea breath test: useful for initial diagnosis and follow-up.
    5. Stool antigen test: useful for initial diagnosis and follow-up.
    6. Serologic testing: unsuitable for follow-up.

**d. Treatment**
  i. Antisecretory drugs.
    1. $H_2$ receptor antagonists.
    2. PPIs.
    3. Synthetic prostaglandin.
  ii. Antimicrobial therapy.
    1. Treatment requires multiple drug therapy.
    2. Table 3.5 lists treatment options.
  iii. Stop NSAIDs, if possible.
  iv. Surgery.

    1. Usually seen in cases of intractable or persistent disease.
    2. Procedures include the following:
      (a) Truncal vagotomy and pyloroplasty.
      (b) Highly selective vagotomy without pyloroplasty.
  v. Complications.
    1. Hemorrhage.
      (a) Peptic ulcer disease is the most common cause of upper gastrointestinal bleeding.
    2. Perforation.
      (a) Patients typically present with abrupt onset of severe abdominal pain followed by signs of peritoneal inflammation.
    3. Gastric outlet obstruction.

# GALLBLADDER

**I. ACUTE CHOLECYSTITIS**
  **a. General**
    i. Due to sustained obstruction of the cystic duct.
  **b. Clinical Manifestations**
    i. Pain is severe, located in the right upper quadrant, and will last longer than 6 hours.
    ii. On examination, there is right upper quadrant tenderness with positive Murphy's sign.
    iii. Fever may be present.
    iv. Laboratory tests reveal a leukocytosis and mild elevation in liver function tests (LFTs).
  **c. Diagnosis**
    i. Ultrasonography.
      1. Detects stones, gallbladder wall thickening (>4–5 mm), edema (double-wall sign), or pericholecystic fluid.

(a) Pericholecystic fluid is highly specific for acute cholecystitis and not chronic disease.

2. Hepatobiliary scintigraphy.

(a) Uses a radioactive isotope to detect obstruction of cystic duct.

(b) Failure of the isotope to appear in the gallbladder in 4 hours is highly specific for acute cholecystitis.

### d. Treatment

i. Laparoscopic cholecystectomy.

ii. Open cholecystectomy.

iii. Broad-spectrum antibiotics: beta-lactam/beta-lactam inhibitor or third-generation cephalosporins plus metronidazole.

iv. Pain control: NSAIDs or opioids.

## II. PRIMARY SCLEROSING CHOLANGITIS

### a. General

i. Idiopathic disorder of the biliary system.

ii. Associated with ulcerative colitis.

iii. Cancer of the biliary system can develop.

### b. Clinical Presentation

i. Fatigue, anorexia, indigestion and pruritus.

ii. Elevated alkaline phosphatase.

### c. Diagnosis

i. Endoscopic retrograde cholangiopancreatography (ERCP) or transhepatic cholangiogram.

### d. Treatment

i. Ursodeoxycholic acid.

ii. Ciprofloxacin for acute bacterial cholangitis.

iii. Liver transplant.

## III. CHOLELITHIASIS

### a. General

i. Two types of stones.

1. Cholesterol.

2. Pigmented.

ii. Risk factors.

1. Increasing age.

2. Female sex.

3. Pregnancy.

4. Estrogens.

5. Obesity.

6. Indigenous Americans.

7. Cirrhosis.

8. Hemolytic anemia.

### b. Clinical Manifestations

i. Most are asymptomatic.

ii. In symptomatic patients, the clinical features can vary.

1. Episodic pain.

(a) Due to intermittent obstruction of the cystic duct.

(b) Pain is in the upper right quadrant with radiation to right side of back or right shoulder.

(i) Pain can be nocturnal.

(c) Pain is described as wavelike, cramping pain that develops between 15 minutes and 2 hours after eating a fatty meal.

(d) Pain may last up to 4 hours with concomitant nausea and vomiting.

(e) Physical examination is normal between episodes; and, during episode, right upper quadrant tenderness is noted.

2. Complications.

(a) Acute cholecystitis.

(b) Common bile duct stones.

(c) Pancreatitis.

(d) Cholangitis.

### c. Diagnosis

i. Ultrasonography.

1. Has more than 95% sensitivity in detecting gallstones.

ii. Oral cholecystography.

1. Useful in providing information on gallbladder function.

iii. Computed tomography (CT)/Magnetic resonance imaging (MRI).

iv. ERCP.

v. Hepatobiliary scintigraphy.

1. Not useful in detecting stones but useful in patients with acute cholecystitis.

### d. Treatment

i. If asymptomatic and patient is healthy, the gallstones should be left alone.

ii. Surgical therapy.

1. Laparoscopic cholecystectomy.

2. Open cholecystectomy.

iii. Nonsurgical therapy.

1. Ursodeoxycholic acid.

(a) Stones >1.5 cm or pigmented stones are not responsive to treatment via this method.

2. Extracorporeal shock wave lithotripsy.

# LIVER

## I. ACUTE HEPATITIS

### a. General

i. Caused by five different viruses.

ii. Routes of spread include fecal–oral, parenteral, and sexual.

iii. Table 3.6 summarizes viral hepatitis.

### b. Clinical Manifestations

i. Incubation period: virus can be detected, but laboratory tests are normal.

1. Patient is asymptomatic.

**TABLE 3.6**

| Comparison of Causes of Acute Viral Hepatitis | | | | | | |
|---|---|---|---|---|---|---|
| Hepatitis Virus | Genome | Spread | Incubation Period | Fatality Rate | Chronic Rate | Antibody |
| A | RNA | Fecal–Oral | 25 days | 1% | None | Anti-HAV |
| B | DNA | Parenteral–Sexual | 75 days | 1% | 5% | Anti-HBs<br>Anti-HBc<br>Anti-HBe |
| C | RNA | Parenteral | 50 days | <0.1% | 80% | Anti-HCV |
| D | RNA | Parenteral–Sexual | 30–150 days | 2%–10% | 5% | Anti-HDV |
| E | RNA | Fecal–Oral | 35 days | 1% | None | Anti-HEV |

*HAV*, Hepatitis A virus; *HBs*, hepatitis B surface; *HBc*, hepatitis B core; *HBe*, hepatitis B envelope; *HCV*, hepatitis C virus; *HDV*, hepatitis D virus; *HEV*, hepatitis E virus.

ii. Preicteric phase: symptoms include malaise, nausea, decreased appetite, and vague abdominal pain.
   1. Viral specific antibodies start to appear.
   2. Serum transaminases start to elevate.
iii. Icteric phase: symptoms worsen, and jaundice appears.
   1. Serum transaminases reach their peak.
      (a) Ten times the upper limit of normal.
   2. Urine darkens in color, and stool becomes lighter in color.
c. **Diagnosis**
   i. Serology results vary with each virus.
   ii. Table 3.7 summarizes serology testing in acute hepatitis.
d. **Treatment**
   i. Symptomatic treatment, with avoidance of alcohol and sexual contact.
   ii. Virus specific
      1. Hepatitis A.
         (a) Hepatitis A virus (HAV) vaccine.
         (b) Postexposure prophylaxis with immune globulin for household and intimate contacts.
         (c) HAV vaccine and immune globulin can be used concurrently.
      2. Hepatitis B.

(a) Hepatitis B virus (HBV) vaccine.
   (i) First dose recommended at birth.
(b) Postexposure prophylaxis with hepatitis B immune globulin (HBIG) and hepatitis B vaccine.
   (i) Recommended for newborns and patients with parenteral exposure.
3. Hepatitis C.
   (a) Direct-acting and host-targeting antiviral agents.
4. Hepatitis D.
   (a) No specific treatment, but hepatitis B vaccine can prevent infection with hepatitis D.
5. Hepatitis E.
   (a) No specific treatment.

## II. CHRONIC HEPATITIS
a. **General**
   i. All have chronic inflammatory injury of the liver that can lead to cirrhosis and end-stage liver disease.
   ii. There are multiple causes.
      1. Chronic hepatitis B, D, and C.
      2. Autoimmune hepatitis.
      3. Drug-induced chronic hepatitis.
      4. Wilson's disease.

**TABLE 3.7**

| Serology Testing for Acute Hepatitis | | | | |
|---|---|---|---|---|
| Diagnosis | Screening Assays | Duration | Antibodies | Note |
| Hepatitis A | Anti-HAV immunoglobulin M | 4 weeks to 10 months | Anti-HAV | HAV in stool before onset of symptoms |
| Hepatitis B | HBsAG<br>Anti-HBc immunoglobulin M | 5–25 weeks<br>6–52 weeks | HBeAG<br>Anti-HBe | |
| Hepatitis C | Anti-HCV | Onset 8 weeks | | |
| Hepatitis D | HBsAG | | Anti-HDV | Seen only in presence of hepatitis B |
| Hepatitis E | History | | Anti-HEV | |

*HAV*, Hepatitis A virus; *HBc*, hepatitis B core; *HBe*, hepatitis B envelope; *HBeAG*, hepatitis B envelope antigen; *HBsAG*, hepatitis B surface antigen; *HCV*, hepatitis C virus; *HDV*, hepatitis D virus; *HEV*, hepatitis E virus.

   iii. Chronic hepatitis B and C can cause cirrhosis and hepatocellular carcinoma.

**b. Clinical Manifestations**

   i. Clinical symptoms are typically nonspecific, intermittent, and mild.

   ii. The most common symptom is fatigue.

   iii. On physical examination, the most common finding is liver tenderness.

**c. Diagnosis**

   i. Laboratory results reveal elevated serum transaminases and little or no elevation in alkaline phosphatase.

      1. Serum transaminases are elevated one to five times normal.

   ii. Table 3.8 lists diagnostic testing for chronic hepatitis.

   iii. Diagnosis is based on histologic appearance of the liver.

**d. Treatment**

   i. Varies with specific cause.

      1. Chronic hepatitis B.

         (a) Pegylated interferon-alpha.

         (b) Oral nucleoside analogues such as lamivudine, adefovir, entecavir, tenofovir, and telbivudine.

         (c) Avoid all immunosuppressive drugs.

      2. Chronic hepatitis D.

         (a) Therapy is difficult, but prolonged treatment with peginterferon alfa-2b results in some improvement.

      3. Chronic hepatitis C.

         (a) Direct-acting and host-targeting antiviral agents.

         (b) Most common cause of liver transplant.

      4. Autoimmune.

         (a) Will have a rapid clinical response to corticosteroids.

            (i) Prednisone with azathioprine can be used.

      5. Drug induced.

         (a) Discontinue the involved drug.

      6. Wilson's disease.

         (a) Copper chelation improves survival but does not reverse cirrhosis.

**III. NEOPLASMS**

**a. General**

   i. Metastatic tumors are the most common malignant tumors of the liver.

      1. The most frequent primary tumors to spread to the liver include GI (colon, stomach, and pancreas), lung, and breast.

      2. Prognosis is poor, with mean survival only 6 months.

   ii. Most common primary malignancy of the liver is hepatocellular carcinoma.

      1. A complication of chronic liver disease and cirrhosis.

         (a) Causes include hepatitis C infection, alcohol usage, and hemochromatosis.

**b. Clinical Manifestations**

   i. Present with abdominal pain, palpable abdominal mass, and constitutional symptoms.

   ii. Can also have signs of obstructive jaundice.

   iii. Primary hepatocellular carcinoma can metastasize to the lymph nodes and lung.

**c. Diagnosis**

   i. Alpha-fetoprotein (AFP) is elevated in up to 70% of hepatocellular carcinoma cases.

      1. AFP plus ultrasound are excellent for screening.

   ii. CT/MRI scan will reveal the lesions of both primary and metastatic liver carcinoma.

   iii. Diagnosis is confirmed by biopsy.

**d. Treatment**

   i. Prevention is most important.

   ii. For primary disease, resection or transplantation may be indicated.

      1. Systemic chemotherapy and radiation therapy are of limited value.

**IV. CIRRHOSIS**

**a. General**

   i. Liver cirrhosis represents the end stage of chronic liver disease.

      1. Due to chronic wound healing in the liver after chronic damage.

   ii. Table 3.9 shows causes of cirrhosis.

   iii. Table 3.10 summarizes metabolic diseases of the liver.

**b. Clinical Manifestations**

   i. Symptom onset is often insidious and includes weakness, fatigue, weight loss, anorexia, and abdominal pain.

   ii. Physical examination reveals jaundice, ascites, edema, and dermatologic changes.

**TABLE 3.8**

| Diagnostic Tests for Chronic Hepatitis | |
| --- | --- |
| **Diagnosis** | **Screening Test** |
| Chronic hepatitis B | HbsAg (Hepatitis B surface antigen) |
| Chronic hepatitis C | Anti-HCV (Anti-hepatitis C virus) |
| Chronic hepatitis D | Anti-HDV (Anti-hepatitis D virus) |
| Autoimmune hepatitis | ANA (Antinuclear antibody) |
| Drug-induced disease | Medication history |
| Wilson's disease | Ceruloplasmin |

## TABLE 3.9

### Causes of Cirrhosis

**Alcohol Abuse**

**Viral Hepatitis**

Hepatitis B
Hepatitis D
Hepatitis C

**Metabolic Disorders**

Hemochromatosis
Wilson's disease
Alpha-1-antitrypsin deficiency
Cystic fibrosis

**Autoimmune Hepatitis**

Biliary disorders
Sclerosing cholangitis
Primary biliary cirrhosis

**Drugs and Toxins**

Carbon tetrachloride
Dimethylnitrosamine
Methotrexate
Amiodarone

     1. Dermatologic changes include spider angiomas, telangiectasias, palmar erythema, purpura, and signs of feminization.
   iii. Laboratory results vary depending on the cause.

1. Screening tests include LFTs, iron studies, renal function, ceruloplasmin, complete blood count (CBC), viral hepatitis serology markers, antinuclear antibodies, AFP, and ammonia level.
2. In cirrhosis low albumin, elevated LFTs, and prolonged PT are common.
3. Laboratory findings are often normal or minimally abnormal in early compensated cirrhosis.
4. Table 3.11 summarizes the uses of LFTs.

  **c. Diagnosis**
    i. Abdominal ultrasound to evaluate liver size, shape, and composition.
    ii. Liver biopsy.
  **d. Treatment**
    i. Treat the underlying cause and prevent and treat complications.
      1. Abstain from alcohol.
      2. Autoimmune hepatitis: treat with immunosuppressive therapy (corticosteroids and azathioprine).
      3. Hemochromatosis: frequent phlebotomies.
      4. Wilson's disease: a chelating agent (penicillamine).
      5. Primary biliary cirrhosis: a bile acid, ursodeoxycholic acid.
    ii. Liver transplantation is the treatment of choice for end-stage liver disease.

## TABLE 3.10

### Metabolic Diseases of the Liver

| Disease | Inheritance | Clinical | Laboratory | Treatment |
|---|---|---|---|---|
| Alpha-1-antitrypsin | Recessive | Chronic obstructive pulmonary disease<br>Cirrhosis | ↓Alpha-1-antitrypsin level<br>Phenotyping | Transplantation |
| Wilson's disease | Autosomal recessive | Kayser-Fleischer rings<br>Cirrhosis | ↑Copper level<br>↓ Ceruloplasmin | Copper chelation with penicillamine |
| Hemochromatosis | Autosomal recessive | Abdominal pain<br>Hepatomegaly<br>Cirrhosis | ↑Hepatic iron index<br>↑Ferritin | Phlebotomy<br>Iron chelation with deferoxamine |

## TABLE 3.11

### Liver Function Tests

| Name | Normal Range | Utilization |
|---|---|---|
| Aspartate aminotransferase (AST) | 0–40 IU/L | Hepatocellular damage |
| Alanine aminotransferase (ALT) | 0–40 IU/L | Hepatocellular damage |
| Alkaline phosphatase | 25–100 IU/L | Cholestatic hepatobiliary disease |
| γ-Glutamyltransferase | 5–30 U/L | Cholestatic hepatobiliary disease |
| Total bilirubin | 0.5–1.2 mg/dL | Metabolite clearance |
| Ammonia | 10–65 mmol/L | Metabolite clearance |
| Prothrombin time | 18–22 sec | Hepatic synthesis function |
| Albumin | 3.5–4.5 g/dL | Hepatic synthesis function |
| Alpha-fetoprotein | <20 ng/dL | Tumor marker for hepatocellular carcinoma |

iii. Complications include the following:
   1. Jaundice: due to failure to break down bilirubin.
   2. Variceal bleeding: due to portal hypertension.
   3. Ascites: due to portal hypertension and hypoproteinemia.
      (a) Treat with diuretics, sodium restriction, paracentesis.
   4. Spontaneous bacterial peritonitis.
      (a) Treat with third-generation cephalosporins.
   5. Encephalopathy.
      (a) Treat with lactulose and/or rifaximin to reduce ammonia-producing intestinal flora.
   6. Hypersplenism: leads mainly to thrombocytopenia, but also anemia and neutropenia.

## V. DISORDERS OF BILIRUBIN METABOLISM (TABLE 3.12)

# PANCREAS

## I. ACUTE PANCREATITIS
a. **General**
   i. Inflammatory disease of the pancreas.
   ii. Etiology.
      1. Gallstones (45% of cases).
      2. Alcohol (20% of cases).
      3. Metabolic: hyperlipidemias (chylomicronemia, hypertriglyceridemia, or both), hypercalcemia
      4. Drugs/Toxins.
         (a) Major drugs involve the immunosuppressants (azathioprine), didanosine (DDI), thiazide diuretics, angiotensin-converting enzyme (ACE) inhibitors, and estrogens.
      5. Infections: mumps, cytomegalovirus, SARS-CoV-2.
      6. ERCP.
   iii. Due to activation of digestive enzymes and autodigestion.
b. **Clinical Manifestations**
   i. Patients typically present with abdominal pain, nausea, and vomiting.
   ii. Pain is constant, located in the midepigastric region with radiation to the mid back.
   iii. Abdominal examination results vary from minimal tenderness to marked generalized rebound tenderness with guarding.
   iv. Bowel sounds may be diminished.
   v. In severe necrotizing pancreatitis, may note large ecchymoses on the flanks (Grey Turner's sign) or periumbilical (Cullen's sign).
c. **Diagnosis**
   i. Laboratory results.
      1. Elevated serum amylase and lipase.
         (a) Elevated serum amylase noted the first 6 to 12 hours with a decrease in levels over 3 to 5 days.
         (b) Elevated serum lipase noted first 8 hours, peak at 24 hours, with decreasing levels over 8 to 14 days.
         (c) Amylase and lipase are also elevated in intestinal injury/obstruction, biliary stone, and renal failure.
      2. Other laboratory test findings.
         (a) Leukocytosis.
         (b) Mild hyperglycemia.
         (c) Hypocalcemia.
         (d) Elevated serum bilirubin, alkaline phosphatase, and transaminases.
         (e) Elevated urinary assay of trypsinogen activation peptide (TAP).
   ii. Ultrasound/CT scan.

**TABLE 3.12**

### Disorders of Bilirubin Metabolism

| Feature | Crigler-Najjar Syndrome Type I | Crigler-Najjar Syndrome Type II | Gilbert's Syndrome | Dubin-Johnson Syndrome | Rotor's Syndrome |
|---|---|---|---|---|---|
| Incidence | Very rare | Uncommon | Up to 12% of population | Uncommon | Rare |
| Total bilirubin (mg/dL) | 15–45 | 5–25 | ≤4 | 2–5 | 3–7 |
| Liver function tests | Normal | Normal | Normal | Normal | Normal |
| Pharmacologic response | No response to phenobarbital | Phenobarbital reduces bilirubin by ≤75% | Phenobarbital reduces bilirubin to normal | Increased bilirubin with estrogens | |
| Clinical features | Kernicterus in infancy | Kernicterus with fasting | None | Occasional hepato-splenomegaly | None |
| Inheritance | Recessive | Recessive | Recessive | Recessive | Recessive |
| Treatment | Phototherapy | Phenobarbital | None | Avoid estrogens | None |

1. Ultrasound may note the presence of gall-stones and pancreatic edema.
2. CT scan is used to evaluate the extent and local complications.
    iii. ERCP.
       1. Not useful in diagnosing acute pancreatitis but useful for the diagnosis and treatment of persistent bile duct stones.
       2. ERCP may also increase the risk for developing pancreatitis.
  d. **Treatment**
    i. Must establish severity of pancreatitis to predict course and risk for complications.
    ii. Ranson's criteria are commonly used.
       1. Patients with fewer than two criteria have a 1% mortality rate.
       2. Presence of three or more criteria predicts a complicated clinical course.
       3. Table 3.13 summarizes Ranson's criteria.
    iii. Main goal is supportive care.
       (a) Maintain fluid balance.
       (b) No oral fluids or food until abdominal pain resolved.
          (i) Nutritional support (enteral or parenteral) needed if NPO (nothing by mouth) for more than 5 to 7 days.
       (c) Pain control with opioids.
       2. If gallstones are present, cholecystectomy is indicated.
       3. Abstain from alcohol.
    iv. Complications.
       1. Local.
          (a) Pancreatic necrosis.
             (i) Noted in patients who worsen after initial improvement.
             (ii) Will develop signs of sepsis: fever, marked leukocytosis, and positive blood cultures.
             (iii) Treatment includes CT-guided aspiration of fluid, as well as antibiotics.

(1) Prophylactic antibiotics are not recommended in the prevention of necrotizing pancreatitis.
(2) If necrotizing pancreatitis is confirmed, imipenem or meropenem should be used.
       (b) Pseudocysts.
          (i) Noted in patients who show evidence of persistent pancreatitis.
          (ii) Develop only 2 to 4 weeks after episode of pancreatitis.
          (iii) Diagnosis made with ultrasound or CT scan.
          (iv) Small cysts will resolve without treatment; larger cysts require surgical drainage.
       2. Systemic.
          (a) Renal failure.
             (i) As a result of hypovolemia and decreased renal perfusion.
          (b) Respiratory failure.
             (i) May develop acute respiratory distress syndrome.
          (c) Splenic vein thrombosis.

## II. CHRONIC PANCREATITIS
  a. **General**
    i. Permanent and progressive damage to the pancreas.
       1. Intermittent attacks of acute pancreatitis.
    ii. Major cause is alcohol consumption.
  b. **Clinical Manifestations**
    i. Abdominal pain is the major symptom.
       1. Pain may improve as severity of pancreatitis worsens.
    ii. Other symptoms include weight loss, diarrhea and steatorrhea (secondary to malabsorption), and diabetes mellitus.
  c. **Diagnosis**
    i. Suggested by history and confirmed by measurement of pancreatic function.
       1. Assessment of pancreatic exocrine function.
          (a) 72-hour fecal fat.
          (b) Serum amylase and lipase may elevate during acute attacks, but will likely be normal otherwise.
          (c) Secretin or cholecystokinin stimulation tests.
       2. Assessment of pancreatic structure.
          (a) CT or MRI is recommended as an initial test for diagnosis.
          (b) Plain abdominal x-ray can be used to evaluate for calcification of the pancreas (present in 30% of patients).

**TABLE 3.13**

| Ranson's Criteria | |
| --- | --- |
| **On Admission** | **48 hours after Admission** |
| Age >55 years | Hematocrit decreases by >10%. |
| White blood cell count >16,000/mL | Blood urea nitrogen increases by >5 mg/dL. |
| Aspartate aminotransferase >250 U/L | Calcium <8 mg/dL |
| Lactate dehydrogenase >350 U/L | Arterial PO$_2$<60 mm Hg |
| | Base deficit >4 mEq/L |
| Glucose >200 mg/dL | Fluid sequestration >6 L |

(c) Fig. 3.2 shows x-ray film and CT scan of chronic pancreatitis.

(d) ERCP is the most sensitive and specific test for the diagnosis of chronic pancreatitis.

(e) Histology is the gold standard for diagnosis when imaging studies are inconclusive yet a strong clinical suspicion exists.

**d. Treatment**

   i. Avoidance of alcohol.

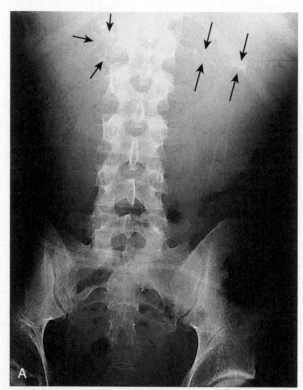

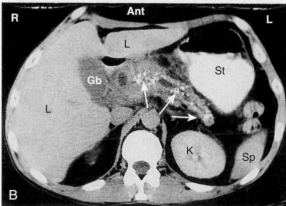

**Fig. 3.2** (A) Abdominal x-ray film of a patient with chronic pancreatitis. Note the calcifications *(arrows)*. (B) Abdominal CT scan of patient with chronic pancreatitis. Note calcifications in the pancreas *(arrows)*. *Ant,* anterior; *Gb,* gallbladder; *K,* kidney; *L,* left; *L,* liver; *R,* right; *Sp,* spleen; *St,* stomach. *(From Mettler FA: Essentials of Radiology, 2nd ed. Philadelphia: Elsevier Saunders, 2005: 171, Fig. 6-13.)*

   ii. Pain control.
     1. Opioids should be avoided if possible.
     2. Acetaminophen, NSAIDs, and multimodal pain management are preferred.

   iii. Management of pancreatic insufficiency.
     1. Pancreatic enzyme replacement used to control steatorrhea.
     2. $H_2$ blockers, PPIs, or sodium bicarbonate can be used to decrease the inactivation of lipase by acid and may decrease steatorrhea when used with enzyme replacement.
     3. Low-fat diet should be encouraged.

## III. NEOPLASMS

**a. General**

   i. Most common is ductal adenocarcinoma.
     a. Most common location is the head of the pancreas.
   ii. Fourth most common cause of cancer death.
   iii. Five-year survival rate is 2%–5%.
   iv. Risk factors include age, tobacco use, obesity, family history, chronic pancreatitis, diabetes mellitus, high intake of animal fat, and prolonged exposure to petroleum products.

**b. Clinical Manifestations**

   i. Early symptoms include nonspecific abdominal discomfort, nausea, vomiting, anorexia, and malaise.
   ii. Most common presenting symptoms are epigastric pain, obstructive jaundice, and weight loss.
     1. Typically found late in disease and associated with advanced disease.
   iii. On physical examination, a palpable and distended, nontender gallbladder may be noted (Courvoisier's sign).

**c. Diagnosis**

   i. CT scan of the abdomen is the test of choice for evaluation of possible pancreatic cancer.
   ii. Tumor marker CA-19-9 is elevated in pancreatic cancer.
     1. Not useful for early detection.

**d. Treatment**

   i. Surgical resection is the treatment of choice if no metastatic disease is present.
   ii. After resection, chemotherapy is indicated with 5-fluorouracil, gemcitabine, or gemcitabine with capecitabine and a modified FOLFIRINOX (5-fluorouracil, leucovorin, irinotecan, oxaliplatin) regimen with or without radiation therapy.
   iii. If not resectable, endoscopic stenting of the bile duct can relieve jaundice and biliary and gastric bypass may be considered.

# SMALL INTESTINE/COLON

## I. APPENDICITIS
  a. **General**
    i. Acute inflammation of the appendix, typically due to obstruction by a fecalith.
    ii. Most common in ages 10 to 30 years.
  b. **Clinical Manifestations**
    i. Patients first present with abdominal pain, colicky in nature, in the periumbilical or epigastric area.
    ii. Pain then becomes constant and more severe and localizes to the right lower quadrant.
    iii. Anorexia and nausea are common. Vomiting may be present.
    iv. Fever occurs late in the presentation or after perforation.
    v. On physical examination, tenderness is noted at McBurney's point, and rebound tenderness is present.
      1. Rovsing's, psoas, and obturator signs are positive.
  c. **Diagnosis**
    i. Laboratory tests reveal a leukocytosis with a left shift.
    ii. Urinalysis is typically normal; a few white and red blood cells may be noted.
    iii. Ultrasound or CT scan of the appendix will reveal a dilated appendix and thickened wall.
  d. **Treatment**
    i. Surgical removal of the appendix.
    ii. Conservative management with antibiotics for 7 days may be considered in patients with a non-perforated appendicitis.
    ii. Broad-spectrum antibiotics are needed if perforation is present.
  e. **See Tables 3.14 and 3.15 for other abdominal and non-abdominal causes of abdominal pain**

**TABLE 3.14**

### Abdominal Causes of Acute Abdomen Pain

| Disease | Location | Mode of Onset | Referred Pain | Nausea/Vomiting | Fever | Evaluation |
|---|---|---|---|---|---|---|
| Appendicitis | RLQ | Gradual | Yes | Yes | CT scan Ultrasound | |
| Diverticulitis | LLQ | Gradual | No | Yes | CT scan | |
| Ectopic pregnancy | RLQ LLQ | Sudden | No | No | Beta-HCG Ultrasound | |
| Endometriosis | RLQ LLQ | Intermittent | No | No | Laparoscopy | |
| Gallbladder | RUQ | Gradual | Right shoulder/ Scapula | Yes | No | Ultrasound |
| Biliary tract | | | Intermittent | Liver function tests | | |
| Gastritis | LUQ | Gradual | No | No | Clinical endoscopy | |
| Hepatic abscess | RUQ | Gradual | Right shoulder | No | Yes | Ultrasound CT scan |
| Hepatitis | RUQ | Gradual | No | No | Serology | |
| Intestinal obstruction | Diffuse RLQ | Sudden: high intestine Gradual: low intestine | Yes | No | Abdominal x-ray CT scan | |
| Mesenteric thrombus | Diffuse | Sudden | Yes | No | CT scan | |
| Pancreatitis | Epigastric RUQ | Gradual | Back-midline | No | Yes | Amylase Lipase Ultrasound CT scan |
| Peptic ulcer disease | RUQ | Intermittent, gradual | No | No | Endoscopy | |
| Peritonitis | Diffuse | Sudden | Yes | Yes | Clinical | |
| Renal stone | RLQ LLQ | Sudden | Groin Genitalia | Yes | No | Abdominal x-ray CT scan |
| Salpingitis (pelvic inflammatory disease) | RLQ LLQ | Intermittent, gradual | No | Yes | Ultrasound | |
| Splenic rupture | LUQ | Sudden | Left shoulder/ Scapula | No | No | CT scan |

*CT*, Computed tomography; *beta-HCG*, beta–human chorionic gonadotropin; *LLQ*, left lower quadrant; *LUQ*, left upper quadrant; *RLQ*, right lower quadrant; *RUQ*, right upper quadrant.

**TABLE 3.15**

### Nonabdominal Causes of Acute Abdominal Pain

Myocardial infarction
Pneumonia
Herpes zoster virus
Metabolic
    Diabetic ketoacidosis
    Uremia
    Addisonian crisis
Sickle cell crisis
Leukemia
Aortic aneurysm
Toxins
    Drugs
    Venoms
    Lead poisoning
Acute porphyria

## II. CELIAC DISEASE

**a. General**
i. Major cause of fat malabsorption.
ii. Malabsorption of fat-soluble vitamins (A, D, E, and K).
iii. Inability to digest gluten.

**b. Symptoms**
i. Greasy, oily, fatty diarrhea (steatorrhea).
ii. Restricted growth in infants.
iii. Weight loss.
iv. Abdominal distension.

**c. Physical Examination**
i. Dermatitis herpetiformis: vesicular skin rash on extensor surfaces of the body.
    1. Low sensitivity, occurring in less than 10% of patients with celiac disease, but is extremely specific.

**d. Diagnosis**
i. Positive IgA transglutaminase-2 (IgA TG2) antibody.
ii. Atrophy of duodenal folds and loss of intestinal villi on small bowel biopsy.
    1. Biopsy done to rule out small bowel lymphoma.

**e. Treatment**
i. Gluten-free diet: no wheat, rye, or barley.
    1. Oats are thought to be safe, but are often contaminated with other gluten-containing products in the manufacturing process.
ii. Dietary supplements as needed, especially early in the disease.

## III. CONSTIPATION

**a. General**
i. Perception of abnormal bowel movements.
    1. Two or fewer bowel movements per week are considered abnormal.
ii. Is more common in women and with advancing age.
iii. Table 3.16 shows causes of constipation.

**b. Clinical Manifestations**
i. Include bloating, abdominal pain or discomfort, stools difficult to pass, anal pain, and nausea.

**c. Diagnosis**
i. Screening for systemic disease with CBC, chemistry profile, and thyroid function.
ii. Further testing should be reserved for severe disease and for patients who have failed conservative treatment.
    1. Colonic transit study.
    2. Pelvic floor function.

**TABLE 3.16**

### Causes of Constipation

| Lifestyle | Medications | Structural | Systemic Disease |
|---|---|---|---|
| Low fiber | *Anticholinergics* | Perianal disease | *Metabolic/Endocrinologic* |
| Decreased fluid intake | Antidepressants | Obstruction lesions | Hypothyroidism |
| Poor toilet habits | Antihistamines | Colon strictures | Hypercalcemia |
| Inability to toilet | Antiparkinson drugs | | Renal failure (chronic) |
| Decreased exercise | *Antihypertensives* | | Diabetes |
| | Calcium channel blockers | | *Neurologic* |
| | Clonidine | | Spinal cord lesions |
| | *Cation-containing agents* | | Multiple sclerosis |
| | Iron | | Parkinson's disease |
| | Calcium | | Hirschsprung's disease |
| | Antacids | | Autonomic neuropathy |
| | Opiates | | *Other* |
| | Morphine | | Amyloidosis |
| | Codeine | | Depression |
| | | | Dementia |
| | | | Dermatomyositis |

### d. Treatment
i. Limit use of medications that cause constipation.
ii. Regular exercise and adequate hydration are also beneficial.
iii. Dietary modifications by increasing fiber intake.
iv. Drug therapy
1. Osmotic laxatives: magnesium hydroxide, polyethylene glycol.
   (a) Used to soften the stool by increasing secretion of water into the intestinal lumen.
   (b) Work within 24 hours of administration.
   (c) Non-absorbable sugars: lactulose or sorbitol.
      (i) May lead to cramping and bloating.
   (d) Saline laxatives: magnesium hydroxide.
      (i) Use caution in patients with renal failure owing to risk of hypermagnesemia.
2. Secreatgogues: lubiprostone, guanylcyclase C.
   (a.) Stimulate intestinal chloride secretion through activation of chloride channels.
   (b.) Tend to be cost prohibitive.
2. Emollient laxatives: mineral oil.
   (a) Work to promote stool softening.
   (b) Risk for aspiration pneumonitis.
3. Stimulant laxatives: senna or bisacodyl.
   (a) Useful in acute constipation.
   (b) Work within 6–12 hours with oral administration and 15–60 minutes with rectal administration.

## IV. DIVERTICULAR DISEASE
### a. Diverticulosis
i. General
1. Occurs when the vasa recta penetrates the circular muscle layers between the tenia coli.
2. Thought to be due to lack of fiber in the diet leading to increase in intraluminal pressure, but exact etiology is unclear.
ii. Clinical manifestations
1. Typically asymptomatic or may present with intermittent cramping abdominal pain in the left lower quadrant.
2. Physical examination may reveal mild left lower quadrant tenderness.
3. Laboratory studies are normal, and fecal occult blood is negative.
iii. Diagnosis
1. Often an incidental finding during screening colonoscopy.
2. Barium enema demonstrates multiple diverticula, typically involving the descending and sigmoid colon.
3. Avoid endoscopic examinations if diverticulitis is suspected.
iv. Treatment
1. Pain control and promoting regular bowel activity.
   (a) Increase in dietary fiber and decrease in dietary fat are recommended.
   (b) Avoidance of nuts and seeds is not indicated.
2. Surgery is not indicated in uncomplicated diverticulosis.

### b. Acute Diverticulitis
i. General
1. Perforation of a diverticulum causing acute infection.
2. Occurs in about 20% of patients with diverticulosis.
ii. Clinical manifestations
3. Present with gradual onset of left lower quadrant pain.
   (a) Pain persists and is accompanied by colonic spasms and loose bowel movements.
4. Anorexia, nausea, and vomiting may occur.
5. On physical examination, fever is noted with left lower quadrant tenderness.
iii. Diagnosis
1. Laboratory results reveal a leukocytosis, and urinalysis may show red and white blood cells.
2. Barium enema.
   (a) Note spasm and a sawtooth pattern of the involved segment.
   (b) Barium enema is a relative contraindication in acute diverticulitis.
3. CT scan.
   (a) Note inflammation of surrounding tissues, thickening of the bowel wall, abscess formation, and diverticula.
4. Endoscopic evaluation is contraindicated in acute diverticulitis.
iv. Treatment
1. Medical therapy.
   (a) Pain control.
   (b) Rehydration.
   (c) Clear liquid diet for 2–3 days.
   (d) Broad-spectrum antibiotics.
2. Surgical therapy.
   (a) Colectomy indicated in recurrent disease.
3. Complications.
   (a) Fistula formation.
   (b) Colonic obstruction.
   (c) Abscess formation.
   (d) Peritonitis.
   (e) Hemorrhage.

c. **Diverticular Hemorrhage**
  i. General
    1. About 10% of patients with diverticulosis will develop an acute hemorrhage.
    2. Diverticular hemorrhage accounts for 50% of the causes of lower GI bleeding.
  ii. Clinical manifestations
    1. Present with dark to bright red blood per rectum in moderate to large amounts.
    2. Typically, bleeding is painless.
    3. Hemoglobin and hematocrit may be normal at start.
  iii. Diagnosis
    1. Red blood cell scans.
    2. Endoscopic evaluation.
  iv. Treatment
    1. Most diverticular hemorrhages will stop spontaneously.
    2. Medical therapy.
      (a) Supportive with IV fluid administration.
      (b) Blood transfusions are typically needed.
    3. Surgical therapy.
      (a) Colectomy indicated after failed medical therapy.

## V. INFLAMMATORY BOWEL DISEASE

a. **Ulcerative Colitis**
  i. General
    1. Inflammation confined to the mucosa and submucosa.
    2. Confined to the colon.
    3. Equal distribution between males and females.
    4. Peak ages of onset are between 15 and 25 years and between 55 and 65 years.
    5. Cigarette smoking may reduce severity, but should not be encouraged.
  ii. Clinical manifestations
    1. Major symptom is bloody diarrhea.
    2. May have rectal or lower quadrant abdominal pain with fever.
    3. Urgency and fecal incontinence are also noted.
    4. Laboratory studies reveal leukocytosis, anemia, and an elevated erythrocyte sedimentation rate.
    5. Antineutrophil cytoplasmic antibody (ANCA) is positive.
    6. May have extraintestinal manifestations.
      (a) Arthritis.
      (b) Ankylosing spondylitis.
      (c) Hepatitis/Cirrhosis.
      (d) Sclerosing cholangitis.
      (e) Pyoderma gangrenosum.
      (f) Erythema nodosum.
      (g) Uveitis.

  iii. Diagnosis
    1. Pathology.
      (a) Inflammation begins in the rectum and extends proximally a certain distance and then stops.
      (b) A clear separation between inflamed and non-inflamed tissue is noted.
    2. Radiographic.
      (a) Barium enema reveals loss of haustra markings, narrowing of the lumen, and straightening of the colon.
    3. Endoscopy.
      (a) Note diffuse erythema with edema and loss of vascular pattern in the rectum.
      (b) Inflammation begins in the rectum and extends proximally.
  iv. Treatment
    1. General supportive care.
      (a) Antidiarrheal agents and nutritional support play a small role in ulcerative colitis.
    2. Aminosalicylates.
      (a) Not systemically absorbed but work in the lumen.
      (b) Can be given orally or via rectum.
    3. Corticosteroids.
    4. Immunomodulator.
      (a) Work by blocking lymphocyte proliferation and activation.
    5. Surgery.
      (a) Colectomy may be curative.
    6. Complications.
      (a) Toxic megacolon.
      (b) Increased risk for colon cancer.

b. **Crohn's Disease**
  i. General
    1. Inflammation extends through the intestinal wall from mucosa to serosa.
    2. Can appear in any part of the GI tract, but distal small bowel and colon are commonly affected.
    3. Equal distribution between males and females.
    4. Peak ages of onset are between 15 and 25 years and between 55 and 65 years.
    5. Cigarette smoking is strongly associated with the development of Crohn's disease.
  ii. Clinical manifestations
    1. The major presenting symptoms are abdominal pain, diarrhea, and weight loss.
    2. On physical examination, aphthous ulcer may be noted on the oral mucosa.
    3. Abdomen may be tender and perianal disease is common.

4. Laboratory studies reveal leukocytosis, anemia, vitamin $B_{12}$ deficiency, and an elevated erythrocyte sedimentation rate.
5. Anti-Saccharomyces cerevisiae antibody (ASCA) is positive.
6. May have extraintestinal manifestations.
   (a) Arthritis.
   (b) Ankylosing spondylitis.
   (c) Hepatitis/Cirrhosis.
   (d) Sclerosing cholangitis.
   (e) Pyoderma gangrenosum.
   (f) Erythema nodosum.
   (g) Uveitis.
7. Table 3.17 compares ulcerative colitis and Crohn's disease.

iii. Diagnosis
1. Pathology.
   (a) Inflammation leads to thickening of the bowel wall and cobblestone appearance on the mucosa.
   (b) Typically have rectal sparing from inflammation.
   (c) Typically, areas of inflammation are separated by normal tissue (skip lesions).
2. Radiographic.
   (a) Barium enema shows aphthous ulcers. When they deepen and enlarge, they give a cobblestone appearance.
   (b) Fistulas and strictures are common.

3. Endoscopy.
   (a) Aphthous ulcers are noted, giving the mucosa a cobblestone appearance.
   (b) Areas of normal mucosa are noted between areas of inflammation.

iv. Treatment
1. General supportive care.
   (a) Antidiarrheal agents and nutritional support play small roles in ulcerative colitis.
2. Aminosalicylates.
   (a) Are not systemically absorbed but work in the lumen.
   (b) Can be given orally or topically in the rectum.
3. Corticosteroids.
4. Immunomodulators.
   (a) Work by blocking lymphocyte proliferation and activation.
   (b) Azathioprine and 6-mercaptopurine are effective in treating Crohn's disease.
   (c) Drugs may cause leukopenia and increase risk for lymphoma.
5. Anti-TNF therapies.
   (a) Preferred first-line agents to induce remission.
   (b) Can be used with immunomodulators.
   (c) Infliximab or adalimumab are frequently used as first-line agents.
6. Antibiotics.
   (a) Used in the management of complications, such as abscess and perianal disease.
7. Surgery.
   (a) Used more conservatively because it is not curative; recurrence is common.
   (b) Segmental resection is most commonly performed.
8. Complications.
   (a) Abscesses and fistulas.
   (b) Intestinal obstruction.
   (c) Perianal disease.
   (d) Colon cancer.
      (i) Risk is less than that of ulcerative colitis, but greater than that of the general population.

## VI. IRRITABLE BOWEL DISEASE
a. General
   i. Greater incidence in females than males.
   ii. Typically present for care between ages 30 and 50 years.
   iii. Due to abnormality in motor function (smooth muscle) and disturbed sensation (visceral hypersensitivity).

**TABLE 3.17**

**Comparison of Ulcerative Colitis and Crohn's Disease**

| Feature | Ulcerative Colitis | Crohn's Disease |
|---|---|---|
| **Pathologic** | | |
| Rectal involvement | Always | Common |
| Fissures and fistulas | Never | Common |
| Skip lesions | Never | Always |
| Perianal disease | Never | Common |
| Granulomas | Occasional | Common |
| **Clinical** | | |
| Rectal bleeding | Always | Occasional |
| Malaise, fever | Occasional | Common |
| Abdominal pain | Occasional | Common |
| Abdominal mass | Never | Common |
| Fistulas | Never | Common |
| **Endoscopic** | | |
| Aphthous ulcers | Never | Common |
| Friable mucosa | Common | Occasional |
| Rectal involvement | Always | Common |
| Cobblestoning | Rare | Common |

**b. Clinical Manifestations**
  i. Chronic or recurrent abdominal pain is the major symptom.
    1. Described as postprandial cramps or discomfort.
    2. Pain is relieved by defecation.
  ii. Irregular defecation (diarrhea, constipation, or alternating between the two) is common.
  iii. Bloating, heartburn, and nausea without vomiting are also noted.
  iv. Physical examination may reveal abdominal tenderness.
  v. No alarm features such as weight loss, anemia, rectal bleeding, and nocturnal symptoms.

**c. Diagnosis**
  i. Based on history and after ruling out other causes of the symptoms. Rome criteria include 3 months of the following:
    1. Abdominal pain relieved by defecation or associated with a change in frequency and/or consistency of stool.
    2. And/or disturbed defecation.
      (a) Two or more of the following:
        (i) Altered stool frequency.
        (ii) Altered stool form.
        (iii) Altered stool passage.
        (iv) Passage of mucus.
    3. Bloating or abdominal distention.

**d. Treatment**
  i. Counseling and discussion of the disease with the patient are vital.
  ii. Avoid unnecessary medications that can cause constipation or diarrhea.
  iii. Dietary changes include increasing fiber intake and decreasing fat intake.
  iv. Antispasmodics may be helpful.
  v. Antidepressants are helpful in resistant cases.

**VII. ISCHEMIC BOWEL DISEASE**
  **a. General**
    i. Symptoms vary with location of the ischemia.
    ii. Blood flow to the GI tract.
      1. Celiac trunk supplies the liver, biliary tract, spleen, stomach, duodenum, and pancreas.
      2. Superior mesenteric artery supplies the duodenum, pancreas, small intestine, ascending colon, and part of the transverse colon.
      3. Inferior mesenteric artery supplies part of the transverse colon, descending colon, and rectum.
  **b. Acute Arterial Mesenteric Ischemia**
    i. General
      1. Patients typically have a history of heart disease and arrhythmias, congestive heart failure, recent myocardial infarction, or hypotension.
    ii. Clinical manifestations
      1. Sudden abdominal pain with abdominal tenderness on examination.
    iii. Diagnosis
      1. Laboratory results may reveal leukocytosis, metabolic acidosis, and elevated amylase.
      2. Abdominal x-ray film shows formless loops of small intestine, ileus, or "thumbprinting" of the small bowel or right colon secondary to submucosal edema/bleeding.
      3. CT with contrast is highly accurate at determining the presence of intestinal ischemia.
      4. Ultrasound or angiogram may be helpful.
    iv. Treatment
      1. Treat the underlying cause.
      2. Laparotomy is required to restore blood flow to the organ.
      3. Survival rate is low unless diagnosed early.
  **c. Ischemic Colitis**
    i. General
      1. The most common ischemic injury to the GI tract.
      2. Most patients are older than 60 years.
      3. Cause or trigger of most episodes is unknown.
    ii. Clinical manifestations
      1. Presents with sudden, mild, crampy, left lower abdominal pain; urge to defecate; and passage of bright red blood mixed with stool.
      2. Physical examination typically reveals only mild abdominal tenderness over the involved area of bowel.
    iii. Diagnosis
      1. If there are no signs of peritonitis, a colonoscopy should be performed.
      2. Barium studies reveal "thumbprinting."
      3. CT with contrast is highly accurate at determining the presence of intestinal ischemia.
    iv. Treatment
      1. Most symptoms resolve in 24 to 48 hours.
      2. Blood pressure maintenance is crucial.
      3. If no signs of peritonitis, then bowel rest, antibiotics, and supportive care.
      4. Resection of the colon is indicated if signs of peritonitis or gangrene are present.

**VIII. MALABSORPTION**
  **a. General**
    i. Refers to impaired transport across the mucosa.

ii. Pathophysiologically due to the following:
    1. Impaired luminal hydrolysis.
    2. Impaired mucosal function.
    3. Impaired removal of nutrients from the mucosa.

**b. Clinical Manifestations**
    i. Typically presents with steatorrhea.
      1. Stools are pale in color, bulky, and greasy.
      2. Diarrhea is watery and stools tend to float.
    ii. Abdominal distention and increased flatus.
    iii. Weight loss is common in severe malabsorption.
    iv. Other symptoms related to vitamin and mineral deficiency.

**c. Diagnosis**
    i. Tests for fat absorption.
      1. Qualitative or quantitative fecal fat.
        (a) Elevated in fat malabsorption disorders.
    ii. Tests for carbohydrate absorption.
      1. D-xylose test.
        (a) Low levels suggest mucosal dysfunction.
    iii. Tests for small bowel bacterial overgrowth.
      1. Glucose breath hydrogen test.
      2. Quantitative culture of jejunum aspirate.
    iv. Routine blood test.
      1. Includes CBC, chemistry profile, PT, vitamin $B_{12}$, folate, iron, and carotene.
    v. Radiology.
      1. Small bowel follow-through and CT scan are helpful in the evaluation, and results vary depending on the etiology.
    vi. Pathology.
      1. Biopsy of the small intestine is important in the evaluation process.

**d. Specific Disorders**
    i. Celiac sprue: see section on Celiac disease.
    ii. Small bowel bacterial overgrowth.
      1. Bacteria influence fat absorption by interfering with bile acids, and protein and carbohydrate absorption are affected secondary to mucosal damage.
      2. Diagnosis made by showing evidence of malabsorption and bacterial overgrowth.
      3. Treatment consists of antibiotics.
    iii. Disaccharidase deficiency.
      1. Classic disease is lactase deficiency.
      2. As patients age, there is loss of lactase activity.
      3. Diarrhea is profuse, and an osmotic gap may exist.
      4. Treatment is avoidance of the offending agent.

## IX. NEOPLASMS
**a. General**
    i. Adenocarcinoma makes up 98% of malignancies of the large intestine.

ii. Peak incidence is between ages 60 and 80 years.
iii. Risk factors include increasing age, first-degree relatives with colon cancer, inflammatory bowel disease, and diets high in fat and low in fiber.
iv. Screening.
    1. Fecal occult blood testing, flexible sigmoidoscopy, and colonoscopy are major approaches to cancer screening.
      (a) Starting at age 45 years, the average-risk patient should have occult blood testing done yearly, flexible sigmoidoscopy every 5 years, and colonoscopy every 10 years.
      (b) Patients with a single first-degree relative with colorectal cancer diagnosed at age 60 or older should begin screening at age 40.
      (c) Patients with two first-degree relatives with colorectal cancer or a single first-degree relative diagnosed with colorectal cancer before age 60 should begin screening at age 40 or 10 years younger than age at diagnosis of the youngest affected relative.
        i. Colonoscopy should be repeated every 5 years.

**b. Clinical Manifestations**
    i. May remain clinically silent for years.
    ii. Major symptoms suggestive of colon cancer are rectal bleeding, pain, and change in bowel habits.
    iii. Laboratory tests reveal occult blood positive stools and anemia.
    iv. Symptoms related to metastatic disease may also be present (hepatomegaly, bowel obstruction, and pulmonary complaints).

**c. Diagnosis**
    i. Colonoscopy with biopsy.

**d. Treatment**
    i. Surgical resection of tumor is the treatment of choice.
    ii. Radiation therapy and chemotherapy are also helpful in reducing local recurrence and distant metastasis.
    iii. Monitor response to treatment with carcinoembryonic antigen (CEA) levels.
      1. Normal is $<2.5$ $\mu$g/L.

## X. OBSTRUCTION
**a. Small Intestine**
    i. General
      1. Mechanical obstruction implies a physical barrier to the movement of intestinal contents.

(a) Paralytic ileus (adynamic ileus) refers to a disorder that has neurogenic disruption of peristalsis as the cause of failure to move intestinal contents forward. There is no mechanical obstruction.

2. Most common cause is adhesions, followed by neoplasms, hernias, intussusception, and volvulus.

(a) Volvulus is due to rotation of bowel loops around a fixed point.

(i) Typically, due to congenital abnormalities or adhesions.

(ii) Onset of obstruction is abrupt, and strangulation occurs rapidly.

ii. Clinical manifestations

1. Signs and symptoms vary with location of the obstruction.

(a) High: frequent vomiting, intermittent pain, and no distention.

(b) Middle: moderate vomiting, moderate distention, and intermittent crescendo, colicky abdominal pain.

(c) Low: feculent vomiting late in the course, marked distention, and variable pain.

2. If a patient has signs of shock, consider strangulation obstruction.

iii. Diagnosis

1. Abdominal x-ray films show a stepwise pattern of dilated small intestine with air-fluid levels.

(a) The colon typically shows lack of intestine gas.

(b) Fig. 3.3 shows abdominal x-ray findings in bowel obstruction.

iv. Treatment

1. Partial obstruction can be treated with decompression via a nasogastric tube.

2. Surgery should be considered with complete or strangulation obstructions.

**b. Large Intestine**

i. General

1. Most common location is the sigmoid colon.

2. Etiologies include carcinoma, diverticulitis, fecal impaction, and inflammatory disorders.

ii. Clinical manifestations

1. Deep, visceral, cramping pain that is referred to the hypogastrium is noted.

2. Constipation is common in complete obstruction.

3. Vomiting may occur late in the course.

4. Physical examination reveals abdominal distention and tympany.

(a) High-pitched tinkles with gurgles are noted on auscultation.

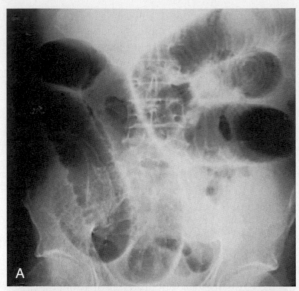

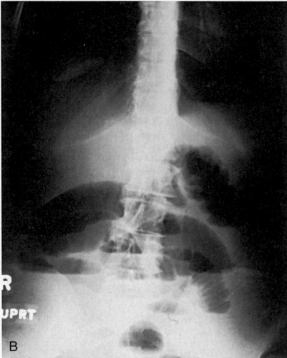

**Fig. 3.3** Small bowel obstruction. (A) Small bowel obstruction with dilated small bowel. (B) Note air-fluid levels in the bowels. *(From Feldman M: Sleisenger and Fordtran's Gastrointestinal and Liver Disease, 7th ed. Philadelphia: WB Saunders, 2002:2116, Fig. 109-2.)*

iii. Diagnosis

1. Abdominal x-ray film shows a dilated large intestine.

2. Barium enema will confirm diagnosis and identify the location.

iv. Treatment

1. First goal is decompression.

2. Surgery to remove the obstruction.

## XI. POLYPS

a. **Hereditary Nonpolyposis Syndrome (Lynch Syndrome)**

   i. Autosomal dominant inherited condition.

   ii. High incidence of colorectal, ovarian, and endometrial cancer.

   iii. Start screening at age 25 with colonoscopy every 1 to 2 years.

b. **Familial Adenomatous Polyps**

   i. Due to adenomatous polyposis coli (APC) gene.

   ii. Develop adenomas by age 35 and colon cancer by age 50.

   iii. Screening starts at age 12 with flexible sigmoidoscopy.

   iv. When polyps are found, perform colectomy.

c. **Gardner Syndrome**

   i. Colon cancer associated with multiple, soft-tissue tumors.

     1. Osteomas of the mandible are common.

   ii. Screening not recommended.

d. **Peutz-Jeghers Syndrome**

   i. Hamartomatous polyps in the large and small intestine with hyperpigmented spots.

     1. Melanotic spots on lips, buccal mucosa, and skin.

   ii. May present with abdominal pain.

   iii. Screening not recommended.

e. **See Table 3.18 for inherited colorectal cancer syndromes.**

## XII. TOXIC MEGACOLON

a. **General**

   i. A rare life-threatening complication of ulcerative colitis or infectious colitis.

b. **Clinical Manifestations**

   i. Signs of toxic colitis, including fever, tachycardia, abdominal distention, and signs of peritonitis.

c. **Diagnosis**

   i. Laboratory results may reveal leukocytosis.

   ii. Abdominal x-ray film shows a dilated colon, greater than 6 cm.

d. **Treatment**

   i. Aggressive fluid management.

   ii. IV steroids and broad-spectrum antibiotics.

   iii. If a patient fails to improve in 24 to 48 hours or there are signs of perforation, surgery is indicated.

# RECTUM

## I. ANAL FISSURE

a. **General**

   i. Due to a split in the anoderm distal to the dentate line.

     1. An ulcer is a chronic fissure.

     2. A skin tag (sentinel pile) is associated with a mature ulcer.

   ii. Fissures are most commonly caused during defecation of a large, firm stool.

b. **Clinical Manifestations**

   i. Present with severe anal pain and bleeding with defecation.

   ii. Blood is noted on the stool or toilet paper.

   iii. On physical examination, a linear tear with a white ulcerated base.

c. **Diagnosis**

   i. Diagnosis based on physical examination.

d. **Treatment**

   i. Stool softeners, bulking agents, and sitz baths are successful in healing fissures.

   ii. Internal anal sphincterotomy is required when conservative measures are not successful.

## II. ANORECTAL ABSCESS/FISTULA

a. **General**

   i. Abscess arises from infected anal crypt glands.

   ii. Fistula is a chronic manifestation of a rectal abscess.

b. **Clinical Manifestations**

   i. Causes severe continuous throbbing anal pain that is worse with ambulation and straining.

   ii. On rectal examination, the patient has a very tender mass palpable externally in the perianal area.

**TABLE 3.18**

| Inherited Colorectal Cancer Syndromes | | | | | |
| --- | --- | --- | --- | --- | --- |
| Syndrome | Histology | Distribution | Age Onset | Risk for Colon Cancer | Other |
| Familial polyposis | Adenoma | Large intestine | 8–30 years | 100% | Have 100s to 1000s of polyps in the large intestine |
| Gardner's syndrome | Adenoma | Large and small intestine | 8–30 years | 100% | Have extraintestinal manifestations |
| Peutz-Jeghers syndrome | Hamartoma | Large and small intestine | First decade | Slightly above average | Mucocutaneous pigmentation |

c. **Diagnosis**
  i. Diagnosis is made on physical examination.
d. **Treatment**
  i. Requires surgical drainage.
  ii. Complications.
    1. Infection may spread, resulting in tissue loss.
    2. May develop fistula-in-ano.

## III. FECAL IMPACTION
a. **General**
  i. May lead to obstruction of the large intestine.
  ii. Predisposing conditions include severe psychiatric disease, prolonged bed rest, neurogenic disease of the colon, spinal cord disease, and constipating medications.
b. **Clinical Manifestations**
  i. Patients may present with pelvic pain, diarrhea, nausea, vomiting, and abdominal distention.
  ii. On rectal examination, hard, dry stool is noted.
c. **Treatment**
  i. Enemas or digital disimpaction.
  ii. Long-term care includes maintaining soft stools.

## IV. HEMORRHOIDS
a. **General**
  i. Internal hemorrhoids arise above the dentate line.
  ii. External hemorrhoids arise below the dentate line.
  iii. Major risk factor is prolonged straining with defecation.
  iv. Internal hemorrhoids are classified based on the following:
    1. First degree: bleeding only.
    2. Second degree: bleeding and prolapse that reduce spontaneously.
    3. Third degree: bleeding and prolapse that require manual reduction.
    4. Fourth degree: bleeding with incarceration that cannot be reduced.
b. **Clinical Manifestations**
  i. Internal hemorrhoids do not cause pain, but cause bright red blood per rectum, mucus discharge, and rectal fullness.
  ii. External hemorrhoids cause sudden severe perianal pain and a perianal mass.
c. **Diagnosis**
  i. Diagnosed with anoscopy.
  ii. Rarely cause anemia; if anemia present, must rule out malignancy.
d. **Treatment**
  i. Medical management consists of dietary changes, stool softeners, bulking agents, and increased fluids.

  ii. Excisional hemorrhoidectomy may be needed for large hemorrhoids.

## V. NEOPLASMS
a. **General**
  i. Neoplasms of the anus are rare.
  ii. Located in anal canal or anal margin.
  iii. Risk factors include anogenital warts, history of pelvic cancer, and smoking.
  iv. Histologic types vary with location.
    1. Anal margin: squamous cell, basal cell, Bowen's disease, and Paget's disease.
    2. Anal canal: epidermoid carcinoma.
b. **Clinical Manifestations**
  i. May note rectal mass, bleeding, pain, discharge, itching, and tenesmus.
c. **Diagnosis**
  i. Diagnosis is made by biopsy.
d. **Treatment**
  i. Wide local excision of the mass.
  ii. Radiation and chemotherapy may be needed for large tumors or metastatic disease.

## VI. PILONIDAL DISEASE
a. **General**
  i. Increased disease in White males aged 15 to 40 years.
  ii. May be congenital or acquired.
    1. Increased risk in hirsute obese individuals.
b. **Clinical Manifestations**
  i. Present with small midline pits or abscesses near the midline of the coccyx or sacrum.
  ii. On examination, a suppurative or draining abscess is noted with hair protruding from the openings.
c. **Diagnosis**
  i. Based on physical examination.
d. **Treatment**
  i. Drainage and deroofing of the abscess.
  ii. Maintaining hygiene is important until the abscess heals.
  iii. Antibiotics are generally not indicated unless signs of cellulitis are present or the patient is immunocompromised or at high risk for endocarditis.

## VII. POLYPS
a. **General**
  i. Adenomatous polyps are common in the distal colon and rectum.
  ii. Neoplastic with malignant potential.
    1. Malignancy potential related to polyp size and level of dysplasia.
  iii. Common in elderly people.

b. **Clinical Manifestations**
   i. Patients are typically asymptomatic.
   ii. May have stool positive for occult blood or hematochezia.
c. **Diagnosis**
   i. Colonoscopy with biopsy is the gold standard.
   ii. Diagnosis made on endoscopic examination or barium studies.
d. **Treatment**
   i. Goal is removal or destruction of the polyp.
   ii. Follow-up colonoscopy timing depends on polyp histology and size.

# HERNIA

## I. HIATAL
a. **General**
   i. Two types: paraesophageal and sliding.
   ii. In paraesophageal hernias, all or part of the stomach herniates into the thorax.
      1. This occurs to the left of the nondisplaced GE junction.
   iii. Sliding hiatal hernias are due to decreased resting pressure in LES.
b. **Clinical Manifestations**
   i. Paraesophageal hernias are typically asymptomatic.
      1. If symptoms do occur, they are due to obstruction.
   ii. Sliding.
      1. Reflux is common and often worse when lying down.
      2. Nausea and vomiting are uncommon in adults but common in children.
      3. Dysphagia may also be noted.
c. **Diagnosis**
   i. Diagnosis made on upper GI series.
d. **Treatment**
   i. Surgical repair is indicated in paraesophageal hernias.
      1. In sliding hiatal hernias, surgery is indicated in persistent or recurrent symptoms.
         (a) Nissen fundoplication is the most effective surgery.
   ii. Medical treatment is indicated in sliding hiatal hernias.
      1. Prokinetic drugs, $H_2$ receptor blockers, or PPIs are indicated.

## II. INCISIONAL (VENTRAL)
a. **General**
   i. History of prior abdominal surgery.
   ii. Risk factors include poor surgical technique, wound infection, age, obesity, and placement of drains.
b. **Clinical Manifestations**
   i. Mass noted at site of prior surgery.
c. **Diagnosis**
   i. Diagnosis made on clinical findings.
d. **Treatment**
   i. Surgical repair to eliminate risk for obstruction.

## III. INGUINAL
a. **General**
   i. Indirect inguinal hernias are congenital hernias and typically present during the first year of life.
      1. May not appear until the patient is older, when the increased intraabdominal pressure and dilated internal inguinal ring allow abdominal contents to enter the cavity.
   ii. Direct inguinal hernias are acquired as a result of weakness of the transversalis fascia in Hesselbach's triangle.
b. **Clinical Manifestations**
   i. Most hernias produce no symptoms until a lump is noted in the groin.
   ii. With indirect hernias, some patients may note a dragging sensation or radiation of pain into the scrotum.
   iii. On physical examination, different results are noted.
      1. Direct.
         (a) When standing, the hernia appears as a symmetric, circular swelling at the external ring.
         (b) Disappears when the patient is supine.
      2. Indirect.
         (a) Descends into the scrotum.
         (b) Present as an elliptical swelling that does not reduce easily.
   iv. Tissue must be noted in the inguinal ring with coughing for the diagnosis of a hernia.
c. **Diagnosis**
   i. Based on clinical findings.
d. **Treatment**
   i. Indirect hernias are more likely to become incarcerated or strangulated.
   ii. Surgical repair is indicated.

## IV. UMBILICAL
a. **General**
   i. More common in adult females than males.
   ii. In adults, due to gradual loosening of the tissue around the umbilical ring.

1. In children, due to the umbilical ring not closing.
   iii. Predisposing factors include multiple pregnancies, ascites, obesity, and large intra-abdominal tumors.
   b. **Clinical Manifestations**
   i. Present as increasing mass at the umbilical ring.
   c. **Diagnosis**
   i. Based on clinical findings.
   d. **Treatment**
   i. In children, they will often obliterate spontaneously by 12 months of age.
   ii. Surgical repair indicated to avoid incarceration and strangulation.

# INFECTIOUS DIARRHEA

## I. ACUTE INFECTIOUS DIARRHEA
a. **General**
   i. Acute diarrhea is a sudden change in bowel habits, passage of increased number of stools, or decreased form for less than 2 weeks.
   ii. Table 3.19 compares inflammatory and noninflammatory infectious diarrhea.
   iii. Table 3.20 lists causes of infectious diarrhea.
b. **Clinical Manifestations**
   i. History very important and should include the following:
      1. Travel history.
      2. Foods eaten.
      3. Recent hospitalizations.
      4. Recent antibiotic usage.
      5. Exposure to others affected.
      6. Sexual history.
      7. Shellfish ingestion.
      8. Exposure to farm animals.
      9. Systemic disease.
      10. Immune status.
   ii. Physical examination to include vitals with orthostatics, skin turgor, and abdominal and rectal examinations.
c. **Diagnosis**
   i. Evaluation should include fecal white blood cell count, stool culture, stool for ova and parasites, *Clostridium difficile* toxin, and possible endoscopy.
d. **Treatment**
   i. Oral rehydration with World Health Organization Oral Rehydration Solution (WHO-ORS) or similar product.
   ii. Empirical antibiotic therapy.
      1. Most cases of infectious diarrhea resolve in 3 days without antibiotics.
      2. Antibiotics may prolong the duration of fecal excretion of the pathogen.
   iii. Symptomatic therapy.
      1. Antimotility agents such as diphenoxylate or loperamide.
      2. Avoid these agents if there is fever or bloody diarrhea.

## II. TRAVELER'S DIARRHEA
a. **General**
   i. Passage of three loose stools in a 24-hour period, with nausea and vomiting, tenesmus, or passage of blood or mucus in stool.
   ii. Transmitted by fecal–oral route.
   iii. Can occur up to 1 week after returning from travel.
   iv. Most cases are bacterial in etiology.
      1. Include enterotoxigenic *Escherichia coli* and *Shigella*, *Campylobacter*, *Aeromonas*, *Salmonella*, and *Vibrio* species.
b. **Clinical Manifestations**
   i. Symptoms vary with etiology.
   ii. May have high fever, bloody stools, nausea and vomiting, and leukocytosis.
c. **Diagnosis**
   i. Evaluation should be based on location of travel and possible etiologic agents.
      1. Could include fecal white blood cell count, stool culture, stool for ova and parasites, *C. difficile* toxin, and possible endoscopy.
   ii. Prevention.
      1. Instruct patients to refrain from drinking local water or eating fresh fruits and vegetables.
      2. Prophylactic measures include bismuth subsalicylate and the fluoroquinolones.

**TABLE 3.19**

| Inflammatory Versus Noninflammatory Infectious Diarrhea | | |
| --- | --- | --- |
| | **Inflammatory Diarrhea** | **Noninflammatory Diarrhea** |
| Clinical | Small-volume bloody diarrhea | Large-volume watery diarrhea |
| | Lower abdominal pain | Upper abdominal pain |
| | Fecal urgency | Nausea and vomiting |
| **Fecal leukocytes** | **Present** | **Absent** |
| Etiologies | *Shigella* species | *Vibrio* species |
| | *Campylobacter* species | *Giardia* species |
| | *Salmonella* species | Enterotoxigenic |
| | *Entamoeba histolytica* | *Escherichia coli* |
| | *Yersinia* species | Rotavirus |
| | *Clostridium difficile* | Norwalk agent |
| | Enteroinvasive *Escherichia coli* | *Staphylococcus aureus* |
| | | *Clostridium perfringens* |

**TABLE 3.20**

## Causes of Infectious Diarrhea

| Organism | Vehicle | Presentation | Treatment |
|---|---|---|---|
| **Viral** | | | |
| Rotavirus | Person to person | Vomiting followed by watery diarrhea Duration: 5–7 days | Volume replacement |
| Norwalk agent | Person to person | Duration: 1–2 days | Volume replacement |
| **Bacterial** | | | |
| Staphylococcus aureus | Mayonnaise-containing foods Cream-filled pies | Symptoms occur within 1–6 hours. Nausea, vomiting, abdominal pain, and then diarrhea Fever is rare | Supportive No role for antibiotics |
| Bacillus cereus | Fried rice Poorly refrigerated prepared foods | Symptoms occur within 1–6 hours for emetic form and within 8–16 hours for diarrheal form | Supportive |
| Clostridium perfringens | Canned foods | Onset within 24 hours Present with watery diarrhea and epigastric pain Resolves in 24 hours | Supportive |
| Vibrio cholerae | Water Seafood | Severe diarrhea and fluid loss Death can occur in 3–4 hours Stools are described as rice water | Fluid and electrolyte replacement Antibiotics, including tetracycline or doxycycline, are agents of choice |
| Vibrio parahaemolyticus | Shellfish | Diarrhea lasting 5 days | Supportive |
| Pathogenic Escherichia coli | Water (foreign travel) | Watery diarrhea, nausea, and abdominal cramping Diarrhea improves in 24 hours | Antibiotics, including trimethoprim-sulfamethoxazole or fluoroquinolones |
| Shigella species | Poultry Seafood Day care centers | Abdominal pain, fever, and multiple small-volume bloody diarrheas Length of disease: 7 days | Supportive Antibiotics, including trimethoprim-sulfamethoxazole or fluoroquinolones, will shorten duration of disease |
| Salmonella species | Poultry Eggs Reptiles | Bacteremia common High fever, headache, and abdominal pain | Antibiotics, including third-generation cephalosporins or fluoroquinolones |
| Campylobacter species | Poultry | Diarrhea and fever are common | Supportive Antibiotics (erythromycin) may be indicated in severe cases |
| Enterohemorrhagic Escherichia coli (O157:H7) | Undercooked beef | Can lead to development of hemolytic-uremic syndrome (HUS) in children Severe diarrhea, abdominal pain, nausea, and vomiting | Supportive Antibiotics may increase risk for HUS |
| Aeromonas species | Water | Watery diarrhea, vomiting, and mild fever | Trimethoprim-sulfamethoxazole is the drug of choice Protozoal |
| Entamoeba histolytica | Water | Tissue invasive and can infect other sites such as liver | Metronidazole |
| Giardia lamblia | Water with animal vector such as beaver | Diarrhea with mucus but no blood | Metronidazole |
| Cryptosporidium parvum | Water Day care | Associated with HIV Watery diarrhea, with nausea, abdominal cramps, and low-grade fever | Supportive Paromomycin may be considered |

d. **Treatment**
   i. Fluid replacement is vital. Monitor vital signs.
   ii. Antibiotics are used in moderate or severe disease.
      1. Antibiotics of choice are the fluoroquinolones.
   iii. Antidiarrheal agents can also be used to control symptoms.

## III. NOSOCOMIAL DIARRHEA

a. **General**
   i. Most common etiology is *C. difficile*.
      1. A gram-positive, toxin-producing, anaerobic organism.
   ii. Occurs most commonly after antibiotic or chemotherapy usage.
      1. Can appear up to 6 weeks after the antibiotic use.
   iii. A severe inflammatory response that can lead to pseudomembrane formation.

b. **Clinical Manifestations**
   i. Present with watery diarrhea and crampy abdominal pain.
   ii. On physical examination, a distended abdomen and diffuse tenderness may be present.

c. **Diagnosis**
   i. Positive for fecal leukocyte.
   ii. Positive for *C. difficile* toxin.
   iii. Endoscopic examination reveals colitis to pseudomembranes.

d. **Treatment**
   i. Discontinue the offending agent.
   ii. Avoid antimotility agents.
   iii. Antibiotics are typically required.
      1. Oral fidaxomicin or vancomycin is the drug of choice for non-severe disease.
      2. Oral vancomycin plus IV metronidazole is recommended for fulminant disease.

# NUTRITIONAL DEFICIENCIES

## I. TABLE 3.21 SUMMARIZES NUTRITIONAL DEFICIENCIES

# FOOD ALLERGIES

a. **General**
   i. Typically caused by proteins in milk, egg, wheat, soy, fish, shellfish, peanuts, and tree nuts.

**TABLE 3.21**

| Nutritional Deficiencies | | | | | | |
| --- | --- | --- | --- | --- | --- | --- |
| **Vitamin** | **Fat Soluble** | **Function** | **Deficiency** | **Toxicity** | **Source** | **Note** |
| Niacin (vitamin B$_3$) | No | NAD/NADP coenzyme | Pellagra | Flushing Hyperglycemia Liver damage | Fish, liver, meat, poultry, grains, eggs, milk | Lowers low-density and increases high-density lipoprotein cholesterol |
| Thiamine (vitamin B$_1$) | No | Neural conduction | Beriberi | Lethargy Ataxia | Pork, liver, organ meats, legumes, grains, wheat germ | |
| Vitamin A | Yes | Visual pigments, cell differentiation, gene regulation | Night blindness | Hepatocellular necrosis Intracranial hypertension | Liver, dairy, yellow and dark green leafy vegetables | Teratogenic early in pregnancy Toxic in large amounts |
| Riboflavin | No | Coenzyme | Cheilosis Glossitis Angular stomatitis | None | Milk and dairy, organ meats, green leafy vegetables | |
| Vitamin C | No | Antioxidant | Scurvy | Nausea Diarrhea | Citrus fruits Tomato | Decreased levels impair wound healing |
| Vitamin D | Yes | Calcium homeostasis, bone metabolism | Rickets Osteomalacia | Renal damage Hypercalcemia | Milk, liver, eggs, salmon, tuna | Toxic in large amounts |
| Vitamin K | Yes | Blood clotting | Hemorrhage | With IV administration, dyspnea and cardiovascular collapse can occur | Liver, oils, green leafy vegetable Synthesized by intestinal tract bacteria | Interferes with warfarin Toxic in large amounts |

*NAD*, Nicotinamide adenine dinucleotide; *NADP*, adenine dinucleotide phosphate.

ii. Shellfish, peanuts and tree nuts are the most common cause of food anaphylaxis in adults.

iii. Milk and egg allergies in atopic children often resolve by adulthood.

**b. Clinical Manifestations**

i. Signs and symptoms include urticaria, swelling of lips and tongue, dyspnea, dysphagia, and GI upset.

**c. Diagnosis**

i. Often a clinical diagnosis after the first episode of allergy.

ii. A combination of history, skin tests, and serum specific IgE tests can identify offending allergen.

**d. Treatment**

i. Avoidance of allergen.

ii. All patients should have access to self-administered epinephrine auto-injector for acute reactions.

## Drugs Used in Gastroenterology

| Drug Name | Mechanism of Action | Therapeutic Use | Side Effects |
|---|---|---|---|
| Cimetidine | $H_2$ receptor antagonist | PUD<br>GERD<br>Zollinger-Ellison syndrome | Headache<br>Dizziness<br>Diarrhea<br>Gynecomastia |
| Famotidine | $H_2$ receptor antagonist | PUD<br>GERD<br>Zollinger-Ellison syndrome | Headache<br>Dizziness<br>Diarrhea<br>Gynecomastia |
| Nizatidine | $H_2$ receptor antagonist | PUD<br>GERD<br>Zollinger-Ellison syndrome | Headache<br>Dizziness<br>Diarrhea<br>Gynecomastia |
| Ranitidine | $H_2$ receptor antagonist | PUD<br>GERD<br>Zollinger-Ellison syndrome | Headache<br>Dizziness<br>Diarrhea<br>Gynecomastia |
| Misoprostol | Analogue of prostaglandin E1 | NSAID-induced ulcers | Diarrhea<br>Nausea<br>Contraindicated in pregnancy |
| Lansoprazole | Binds to $H^+/K^+$-ATPase (proton pump) and suppresses $H^+$ secretion | Esophagitis<br>PUD<br>Zollinger-Ellison syndrome | Gastric carcinoid tumor<br>No drug interactions |
| Omeprazole | Binds to $H^+/K^+$-ATPase (proton pump) and suppresses $H^+$ secretion | EsophagitisPUD (Helicobacter pylori)<br>Zollinger-Ellison syndrome | Gastric carcinoid tumor<br>Multiple drug interactions: warfarin, phenytoin, and diazepam |
| Sucralfate | Binds with particles to form a barrier | Duodenal ulcers | Do not give with an $H_2$ antagonist. |
| Prochlorperazine | Phenothiazine—blocks dopamine receptors | Antiemetic | Hypotension<br>Restlessness<br>Extrapyramidal symptoms |
| Domperidone | Butyrophenone—blocks dopamine receptors | Chemotherapy-induced nausea and vomiting | Tardive dyskinesia<br>Extrapyramidal symptoms<br>Neuroleptic malignant syndrome |
| Droperidol | Butyrophenone—blocks dopamine receptors | Chemotherapy-induced nausea and vomiting | Tardive dyskinesia<br>Extrapyramidal symptoms<br>Neuroleptic malignant syndrome |
| Haloperidol | Butyrophenone—blocks dopamine receptors | Chemotherapy-induced nausea and vomiting | Tardive dyskinesia<br>Extrapyramidal symptoms<br>Neuroleptic malignant syndrome |
| Alprazolam | Enhances affinity for GABA receptors | Anticipatory vomiting | Drowsiness<br>Ataxia<br>Confusion |
| Lorazepam | Enhances affinity for GABA receptors | Anticipatory vomiting | Drowsiness<br>Ataxia<br>Confusion |
| Granisetron | Blocks 5-$HT_3$ receptors in periphery and brain | Chemotherapy and postoperative nausea and vomiting | Headache |

*Continued*

## Drugs Used in Gastroenterology—cont'd

| Drug Name | Mechanism of Action | Therapeutic Use | Side Effects |
|---|---|---|---|
| Ondansetron | Blocks 5-HT$_3$ receptors in periphery and brain | Chemotherapy and postoperative nausea and vomiting | Headache |
| Diphenoxylate | Opioid-like action on bowel and decreases peristalsis | Antidiarrheal | Drowsiness<br>Abdominal cramps<br>Dizziness<br>Toxic megacolon |
| Loperamide | Opioid-like action on bowel and decreases peristalsis | Antidiarrheal | Drowsiness<br>Abdominal cramps<br>Dizziness<br>Toxic megacolon |
| Bismuth subsalicylate | Decreases fluid secretion in bowel | Antidiarrheal | Salicylate toxicity<br>Black stools |
| Castor oil | Irritating to gut and promotes increased peristalsis; stimulates colon activity | Laxative | Atonic colon |
| Senna | Irritating to gut and promotes increased peristalsis; stimulates colon activity | Laxative | Atonic colon |
| Sodium phosphate | Saline cathartic | Laxative | Rare |
| Polyethylene glycol | Osmotic laxative | Colonic lavage | Nausea/Vomiting<br>Abdominal cramps |
| Lactulose | Osmotic laxative | Laxative | Nausea/Vomiting |
| Mineral oil | Stool softener, surface active agent | Laxative | Lipid pneumonitis<br>Decreased absorption of fat-soluble vitamins |
| Bethanechol | Cholinergic agonist, increased tone and motility of the bowel | Postoperative ileus | Cramping<br>Diarrhea<br>Salivation<br>Sweating<br>Urinary incontinence |
| Metoclopramide | Enhances motility and tone by stimulating acetylcholine releaseAntiemetic by blocking dopamine receptors | Antiemetic<br>Gastroparesis<br>Parkinsonism | GI cramping<br>Diarrhea |

*GABA*, γ-Aminobutyric acid; *GERD*, gastroesophageal reflux disease; *PUD*, peptic ulcer disease.

# QUESTIONS

## QUESTION 1
Which of the following is the most common presenting symptom of esophageal cancer?

A  Dysphagia
B  Regurgitation
C  Hoarseness
D  Lymphadenopathy
E  St. Mary nodule

## QUESTION 2
Which of the following is the most likely cause of a positive fecal leukocyte test?

A  External hemorrhoid
B  *Shigella* infection
C  *Giardia* infection
D  Viral infection
E  Rectal adenoma

## QUESTION 3
A 50-year-old male, with a long history of alcohol abuse, presents with epigastric pain. The pain radiates to the back. He also notes some nausea and vomiting. Laboratory testing reveals an elevated lipase level. Which of the following is the most likely diagnosis?

A  Pancreatitis
B  Cholecystitis
C  Hiatal hernia
D  Peptic ulcer disease
E  Hepatocellular carcinoma

## QUESTIONS—cont'd

### QUESTION 4

An 80-year-old patient presents with a 1-year history of constipation. The workup has been negative. What management option should be recommended to this patient?

A  Regular enemas and low-protein diet

B  Daily laxative and high-fat diet

C  Increased physical activity and daily multivitamin

D  Increased fluid intake and high-fiber diet

E  Daily glycerin suppository and high-carbohydrate diet

### QUESTION 5

What is the mechanism of action of omeprazole (Prilosec)?

A  Produces a viscous gel

B  Blocks $H_2$ histamine receptors

C  Blocks cholinergic receptors

D  Stimulates prostaglandin receptors

E  Inhibits $H^+/K^+$-ATPase proton pump

### QUESTION 6

Toxic megacolon is a common complication of which of the following disorders?

A  Ulcerative colitis

B  Cystic fibrosis

C  Diverticulosis

D  Crohn's disease

E  Colon cancer

### QUESTION 7

A 10-year-old boy develops fever, headache, and abdominal pain after playing with a pet snake. Later, he develops a bloody diarrhea. Which of the following is the most likely agent causing these symptoms?

A  *Campylobacter* species

B  *Shigella* species

C  *Salmonella* species

D  *Vibrio* species

E  *Aeromonas* species

### QUESTION 8

A 22-year-old patient presents with a 24-hour history of periumbilical pain. The pain has moved to the right lower quadrant, and he has developed nausea and anorexia. On examination, there is tenderness in the right lower quadrant. Which of the following is the most likely diagnosis?

A  Testicular torsion

B  Cholecystitis

C  Diverticulitis

D  Appendicitis

E  Pancreatitis

### QUESTION 9

Which of the following is indicated by the presence of antibody to hepatitis B surface antigen and antibody to hepatitis B core antigen?

A  Acute hepatitis B infection

B  Response to antiviral therapy

C  Previous hepatitis B infection

D  Chronic active hepatitis B infection

E  Previous hepatitis B vaccination

### QUESTION 10

Which of the following is the most appropriate treatment for stage I hemorrhoids?

A  Sclerotherapy

B  Hemorrhoidectomy

C  Increase dietary fiber

D  Rectal hydrocortisone

E  Rubber-band ligation

## ANSWERS

**1.  A**

EXPLANATION: The most common presenting symptom for esophageal cancer is dysphagia, first to solids and then liquids. Patients may also present with odynophagia, chest pain, weight loss, and anorexia. ***Topic: Esophagus: Neoplasms***

☐ Correct   ☐ Incorrect

**2.  B**

EXPLANATION: Presence of fecal leukocytes indicates the presence of inflammation in the colon. Causes of inflammatory diarrhea include *Shigella, Salmonella, Campylobacter, Entamoeba histolytica, Yersinia, C. difficile*, and enteroinvasive *E. coli*. ***Topic: Infectious diarrhea***

☐ Correct   ☐ Incorrect

*Continued*

## ANSWERS—cont'd

**3.  A**

EXPLANATION: Pancreatitis presents with epigastric pain that radiates through to the back. Nausea and vomiting are also common. Laboratory testing reveals an elevated amylase and lipase. *Topic: Acute pancreatitis*
☐ Correct  ☐ Incorrect

**4.  D**

EXPLANATION: Constipation, with no underlying cause, should be treated with conservative measures. These measures include regular exercise, adequate fluid intake, and increased dietary-fiber intake. *Topic: Constipation*
☐ Correct  ☐ Incorrect

**5.  E**

EXPLANATION: Omeprazole is a proton-pump inhibitor; it works by binding to $H^+/K^+$-ATPase and suppresses $H^+$ secretion. *Topic: Peptic ulcer disease*
☐ Correct  ☐ Incorrect

**6.  A**

EXPLANATION: Complications of ulcerative colitis include toxic megacolon. Fistulas and bowel obstructions are common complications of Crohn's disease. *Topic: Inflammatory bowel disease*
☐ Correct  ☐ Incorrect

**7.  C**

EXPLANATION: *Salmonella* infection presents with bloody diarrhea, high fever, headache, and abdominal pain. The vehicle of infection is poultry, eggs, and reptiles. *Topic: Infectious diarrhea*
☐ Correct  ☐ Incorrect

**8.  D**

EXPLANATION: Appendicitis begins as periumbilical pain that migrates to the right lower quadrant and is associated with nausea, vomiting, and anorexia. On physical examination, tenderness is noted in the right iliac region (McBurney's point). *Topic: Appendicitis*
☐ Correct  ☐ Incorrect

**9.  C**

EXPLANATION: The presence of antibodies to hepatitis B surface and hepatitis B core indicates previous hepatitis B infection. Antibodies to hepatitis B surface antigen (Anti-HBs) alone indicate previous hepatitis B vaccination. *Topic: Hepatitis*
☐ Correct  ☐ Incorrect

**10.  C**

EXPLANATION: Stage I hemorrhoids should be treated first with conservative methods, including increasing dietary-fiber and fluid intake. *Topic: Hemorrhoids*
☐ Correct  ☐ Incorrect

# CHAPTER 4
# MUSCULOSKELETAL SYSTEM

## EXAMINATION BLUEPRINT TOPICS

**DISORDERS OF THE SHOULDER**
Dislocations
Rotator cuff disorders
Separations

**DISORDERS OF THE FOREARM/WRIST/HAND**
Dislocations
Gamekeeper's thumb
Nursemaid's elbow (subluxation of the radial head)
Sprains (fingers)
Tenosynovitis

**DISORDERS OF THE BACK/SPINE**
Ankylosing spondylitis
Back strain/Sprain
Cauda equina syndrome
Herniated disk pulposus
Kyphosis/Scoliosis
Low back pain
Spinal stenosis
Thoracic outlet syndrome
Torticollis

**DISORDERS OF THE HIP**
Aseptic necrosis (osteonecrosis)
Dislocations

**DISORDERS OF THE KNEE**
Bursitis
Dislocations
Meniscal injuries
Sprains/Strains

**DISORDERS OF THE ANKLE/FOOT**
Dislocations
Sprains/Strains

**FRACTURES**
General
Types

**INFECTIOUS DISEASES**
Osteomyelitis
Septic arthritis

**NEOPLASTIC DISEASE**
Bone cysts
Bone tumors
Ganglion cysts
Osteosarcoma

**OSTEOARTHRITIS**
General
Clinical manifestations
Diagnosis
Treatment

**OSTEOPOROSIS**
General
Clinical manifestations
Diagnosis
Treatment
Screening

**COMPARTMENT SYNDROME**
General
Develops after the following
Clinical manifestations
Diagnosis
Treatment

**RHEUMATOLOGIC CONDITIONS**
Fibromyalgia
Gout/Pseudogout
Polyarteritis nodosa
Polymyositis/Dermatomyositis
Polymyalgia rheumatica
Reiter's syndrome
Rheumatoid arthritis
Systemic lupus erythematosus
Systemic sclerosis
Sjögren's syndrome

## DISORDERS OF THE SHOULDER

### I. DISLOCATIONS
  a. **General**
  i. Dislocation can be anterior or posterior.
    1. Anterior dislocation is most common.
  ii. Mechanism of action.
    1. Anterior: due to blow to an abducted, externally rotated, extended arm.
    2. Posterior: due to axial loading of an arm that is adducted and internally rotated or due to violent muscle contractions (seizures or electrocution).
  b. **Clinical Manifestations**
  i. Sensation of shoulder slipping out of joint when arm is abducted and externally rotated.

  1. Note severe pain with any movement of the shoulder.
  ii. With anterior dislocation, patient supports the arm in a neutral position.
    1. Apprehension test positive in anterior dislocation.
  iii. With posterior dislocation, patient holds the arm in adduction and internal rotation.
    1. Jerk test positive in posterior dislocation.
  iv. Evaluate for possible axillary nerve injury.
    1. Abduction of the shoulder is impaired.
  c. **Diagnosis**
  i. Anteroposterior (AP) and axillary shoulder x-ray films should be obtained.
    1. X-ray reveals the humeral head displaced inferiorly and medially with an anterior dislocation (Fig. 4.1).

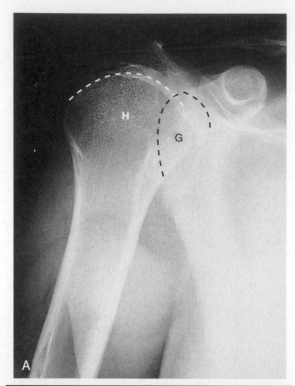

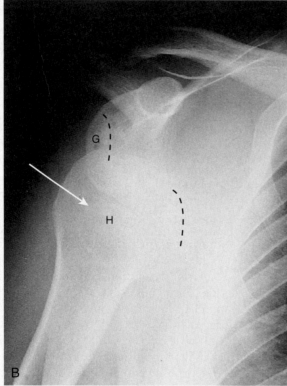

**Fig. 4.1** Shoulder dislocation. (A) AP view revealing that the humeral head *(H)* is located lateral to and overlapping the glenoid *(G)*. (B) Humeral head *(H)* is inferior and medial to the glenoid *(G)* *(arrows)*. *(From Mettler FA: Essentials of Radiology, 2nd ed. Philadelphia: Elsevier Saunders, 2005:287, Fig. 8-49.)*

2. Compression fracture of the posterior humeral head is evidence of an anterior dislocation.
3. Axillary view needed to diagnose posterior dislocation.
  ii. Magnetic resonance imaging (MRI) or arthrogram may be needed for diagnosis.
  **d. Treatment**
  i. Anterior dislocation should be reduced, and physical therapy (PT) begun to strengthen the rotator cuff muscles.
  ii. Surgery may be needed to correct recurrent dislocations.
  iii. Posterior dislocations should be seen by orthopedics.

**II. ROTATOR CUFF DISORDERS**
  **a. General**
  i. Rotator cuff is composed of four muscles.
   1. Supraspinatus.
   2. Infraspinatus.
   3. Subscapularis.
   4. Teres minor.
  ii. Disorders include rotator cuff tendinitis or tear.
  iii. Tendinitis is a common cause of shoulder pain in middle-aged patients.
   1. Etiology is loss of microvascular blood supply and repeated mechanical insult to the tendon.
  iv. Tear is more common in patients older than age 40.
   1. Etiology is acute injury, age-related degeneration, or altered blood supply to the tendon.
   2. Tears in young patients are secondary to physical activity or repeated trauma.
  **b. Clinical Manifestations**
  i. Tendinitis.
   1. Gradual onset of pain exacerbated by overhead activity.
   2. Night pain is common.
   3. Palpation over the greater tuberosity and subacromial bursa elicits tenderness and crepitus with shoulder motion.
  ii. Tear.
   1. Atrophy of muscles at the top and back of the shoulder may be noted.
   2. Recurrent shoulder pain with history of a specific injury triggering pain.
   3. Weakness, catching, and grating are noted when lifting arm overhead.
   4. Passive range of motion (ROM) is normal, but active ROM is limited.
   5. Difficulty holding arm elevated when lifted parallel to the floor.
    (a) A positive drop arm test is noted in severe tears.

### c. Diagnosis
  i. Tendinitis.
   1. X-ray of the shoulder is normal.
  ii. Tear.
   1. X-ray may reveal a high riding humerus.
   2. MRI is the test of choice to evaluate tear.
### d. Treatment
  i. Tendinitis.
   1. Rest from offending activity and nonsteroidal antiinflammatory drugs (NSAIDs).
   2. Steroid injection can be considered if rest and NSAIDs are not successful.
  ii. Tear.
   1. First treatment option is NSAIDs, sling, PT, and strengthening exercises.
   2. Steroid injection can provide short-term relief from pain and inflammation.
   3. Surgery is indicated only with significant symptoms and failed rehabilitation.

## III. SEPARATIONS
### a. General
  i. Result from direct trauma to the superior or lateral aspect of the shoulder with the arm adducted.
  ii. Three types.
   1. Type I.
    (a) Acromioclavicular (AC) joint ligaments are partially disrupted, but the coracoclavicular (CC) ligaments are non-tender.
    (b) Mild swelling with no deformity.
   2. Type II.
    (a) AC ligaments are torn; partial injury to the CC ligament.
    (b) Tenderness and swelling are noted.
   3. Type III.
    (a) AC and CC ligaments are completely disrupted, and clavicle is completely separated from the acromion.
    (b) Bruising is often present.
   4. Type IV.
    (a) Occurs with a forceful shoulder trauma with disruption of the AC and CC ligaments and displacement of clavicle into or through trapezius.
   5. Type V.
    (a) Significant disruption of the AC and CC ligaments and disruptions of the clavicle attachments.
### b. Clinical Manifestations
  i. Pain is noted over AC joint, and pain is noted on lifting the arm.
  ii. Patient supports arm in an adducted position, and any motion causes pain.

### c. Diagnosis
  i. AP x-ray film will confirm type II or type III separations.
   1. Weighted x-rays, with a 10-pound weight, may increase separation on the film.
### d. Treatment
  i. Type I and type II are each treated with a sling for a few days.
   1. Ice is helpful the first 48 hours along with pain medications.
  ii. Types III to V may require surgery.

## DISORDERS OF THE FOREARM/ WRIST/HAND

### I. DISLOCATIONS
### a. Elbow
  i. General
   1. Elbow dislocation results from a fall on an outstretched hand with the elbow extended or a twisting motion.
   2. Most are posterior and can be complete or perched.
   3. Concomitant fractures, of the radial head in adults or medial epicondyle in children, are common.
  ii. Clinical manifestations
   1. Present with severe pain, swelling, and inability to bend elbow.
   2. Must evaluate brachial artery, median nerve, and ulnar nerve for injury.
    (a) Weakness with wrist flexion and finger adduction with median nerve injury.
    (b) Weakness with finger abduction with ulnar nerve injury.
  iii. Diagnosis
   1. AP and lateral x-ray film assist in the diagnosis.
  iv. Treatment
   1. Reduction of the elbow should be performed as soon as possible.
   2. After reduction, the arm should be splinted.
   3. Elbow flexion and extension can begin in 3 to 5 weeks.
### b. Hand
  i. General
   1. Common injury due to hyperextension injury.
    (a) Involves complete tear of the volar capsule.
    (b) Proximal interphalangeal (PIP) joint is most affected.
  ii. Clinical manifestations
   1. Note joint deformity, pain, and swelling immediately after the injury.
   2. Joint instability is also noted.

iii. Diagnosis
   1. X-ray films are needed to rule out fracture.
iv. Treatment
   1. Closed reduction is required for PIP and distal interphalangeal (DIP) joint dislocations.
   2. Buddy taping to adjacent finger will stabilize joint.

## II. GAMEKEEPER'S THUMB
a. **General**
  i. Injury to ulnar collateral ligament of the thumb.
  ii. Due to a fall on thumb that forcibly deviates it radially.
    1. Frequently due to forced abduction of thumb against a ski pole (skier's thumb).
b. **Clinical Manifestations**
  i. Pain and swelling occurs shortly after the injury, pain worse with thumb extension or abduction.
  ii. Swelling is noted on the ulnar side of the thumb metacarpophalangeal (MCP) joint.
  iii. Note weakness with pinching the thumb and index finger.
c. **Diagnosis**
  i. Based on physical examination findings.
  ii. Check x-ray film to evaluate for an avulsion fracture.
d. **Treatment**
  i. Surgical treatment is required for complete tears.
  ii. Partial tears can be treated with thumb spica splint or cast.

## III. NURSEMAID'S ELBOW (SUBLUXATION OF THE RADIAL HEAD)
a. **General**
  i. Common elbow injury in children younger than age 5.
  ii. Due to increased ligament laxity.
  iii. Mechanism of injury is a pull on the forearm when the elbow is extended, and forearm is pronated.
  iv. Annular ligament slips proximally and becomes trapped between the radius and ulna.
b. **Clinical Manifestations**
  i. Pain noted immediately after injury.
  ii. Child then reluctant to use arm and extremity is held by the side with elbow slightly flexed and forearm pronated.
  iii. Tenderness noted over radial head.
c. **Diagnosis**
  i. X-ray film is normal.
  ii. Based on clinical findings.

d. **Treatment**
  i. Reduction is done by placing thumb over the radial head and supinating the forearm.
  ii. If successful, the child will begin using arm immediately.

## IV. SPRAINS (FINGERS)
a. **General**
  i. Typically a result of either radial or ulnar collateral ligament injury to the PIP or DIP joints.
  ii. Etiologies include sports, falls, work-related traumas, or direct blows.
  iii. Grades.
    1. Grade I.
     (a) Damage to the ligament, but no joint instability.
    2. Grade II.
     (a) Stretching and partial tearing of the ligament.
    3. Grade III.
     (a) Complete disruption of the ligament.
b. **Clinical Manifestations**
  i. Grade I.
    1. Swelling and tenderness on palpation, but no functional abnormality.
  ii. Grade II.
    1. Swelling with bruising is noted with some joint laxity.
  iii. Grade III.
    1. Joint is painful and feels unstable.
c. **Diagnosis**
  i. Based on clinical findings.
d. **Treatment**
  i. Grades I and II are treated by buddy taping injured finger to adjacent finger.
  ii. Grade III is buddy taped and referred for surgery.

## V. TENOSYNOVITIS
a. **Carpal Tunnel Syndrome**
  i. General
    1. Entrapment of the median nerve at the wrist.
    2. Common neuropathy of the upper extremity.
     (a) More common in middle-aged or pregnant women.
    3. Common precipitating causes include repetitive use trauma, tumors, pregnancy, hypothyroidism, rheumatoid arthritis, or diabetes.
  ii. Clinical manifestations
    1. Patients present with a vague ache that radiates into the thenar area.

2. Paresthesia and numbness are noted on the thumb and index, long, and radial half of the ring fingers.
3. May note frequently dropping items or inability to twist lids.
4. Often awakened at night with pain or numbness.
5. Thenar atrophy may occur.
6. Phalen test and Tinel sign are positive.
   (a) Phalen test is performed by placing wrists in flexion and noting aching or numbness in the median nerve distribution in 60 seconds.
   (b) Tinel sign is positive if tingling is noted in median nerve distribution with tapping over the median nerve.
iii. Diagnosis
1. Electromyograph and median nerve conduction velocity studies are abnormal.
iv. Treatment
1. Wrist splinting and NSAIDs are used in the treatment of mild cases.
   (a) Injection of steroids can be used if above fails.
2. Surgery is needed for patients with muscle atrophy, weak thenar muscles, or decreased sensation.

b. **de Quervain's Tenosynovitis**
i. General
1. Inflammation of the sheath around the abductor pollicis longus and extensor pollicis brevis tendons at the styloid process of the radius.
2. Repetitive use of the thumb involving pinching of the thumb while moving the wrist.
3. Common in females aged 30 to 50 years.
ii. Clinical manifestations
1. Note pain, swelling, and a locking of the tendon with movement of the thumb.
2. Patients note pain and swelling over the radial styloid, made worse with movement of the thumb.
3. Finkelstein test is positive.
   (a) Pain with full flexion of the thumb into the palm followed by ulnar deviation of the wrist.
iii. Diagnosis
1. Based on clinical findings.
iv. Treatment
1. Thumb spica splint or dorsal hand splint to immobilize thumb and wrist, ice, and use of NSAIDs are initial treatments.
2. Steroid injection can be used if splint, ice, and NSAID treatment fails.
3. If no improvement, surgery may be needed.

c. **Epicondylitis**
i. General
1. Lateral (tennis elbow).
   (a) Pain and tenderness at the site of origin of the extensor carpi radialis brevis muscle, lateral epicondyle of the humerus.
   (b) Typical patient is between ages 35 and 50.
2. Medial (golfer's elbow).
   (a) Pain and tenderness at the site of origin of the flexor and pronator muscles, just distal to the medial epicondyle.
ii. Clinical manifestations
1. Lateral.
   (a) Note gradual onset of pain in lateral elbow and forearm during activities involving wrist extension (turning a screwdriver or backhand in tennis).
   (b) On examination, tenderness is noted 1 cm distal to the lateral epicondyle.
   (c) Pain noted along the common extensor tendon when the long finger is extended against resistance and the elbow is held straight.
   (d) No numbness or tingling is noted.
   (e) Patients note pain with lifting with the palm down.
2. Medial.
   (a) Pain noted with active wrist flexion and forearm pronation (taking a golf swing, pitching a baseball, or swimming).
   (b) Area of tenderness is distal to the medial epicondyle.
   (c) Pain produced with bending of wrist with resistance when patient's forearm resting on table and hand supinated.
   (d) Patients note pain when lifting with the palm up.
iii. Diagnosis
1. Based on clinical findings.
iv. Treatment
1. Modification or elimination of the activity causing symptoms.
2. NSAIDs and PT may be helpful.
3. Tennis elbow wrap worn two finger widths below the lateral epicondyle may be helpful.

# DISORDERS OF THE BACK/SPINE

## I. ANKYLOSING SPONDYLITIS
a. **General**
i. A systemic, seronegative spondyloarthropathy.
ii. Affects the sacroiliac (SI) joint, spine, and hips.

1. SI joint involvement is necessary to make diagnosis.
  iii. More common in males between the ages of 20 and 40, and there is a direct relationship with presence of HLA-B27.
    2. Positive HLA-B27 noted in 90% of patients.

**b. Clinical Manifestations**
  i. Early symptoms include morning stiffness and general back pain.
    1. Pain is improved with bending forward.
  ii. As disease progresses, spinal ROM is lost.
    1. Positive Schober test.
  iii. Spinal fragility increases, and minor trauma may lead to significant neurologic deficit.
  iv. Physical examination will reveal SI joint tenderness and decreased chest expansion.
    1. Acute anterior uveitis may be noted.

**c. Diagnosis**
  i. Spine x-ray film reveals a bamboo spine (Fig. 4.2).
  ii. Laboratory tests reveal mild anemia, elevated erythrocyte sedimentation rate (ESR), and elevated creatine phosphokinase (CPK).

**d. Treatment**
  i. Antiinflammatory medications, such as NSAIDS and sulfasalazine, for pain relief and PT to maintain mobility of the spine.

## II. BACK STRAIN/SPRAIN
**a. General**
  i. Strain refers to damage to a muscle; sprain refers to damage to a ligament.
  ii. Due to injury to the paravertebral spinal muscles, ligamentous injuries of the facet joints, or anulus fibrosis.
  iii. Precipitated by repeated lifting and twisting.
  iv. Risk factors include poor fitness, smoking, and hypochondriasis.

**b. Clinical Manifestations**
  i. Symptoms are typically of limited duration.
  ii. Pain radiates into the buttocks and posterior thigh.
  iii. Patient may have trouble standing erect.
  iv. Physical examination reveals diffuse tenderness in the lower back or SI region.
  v. ROM is decreased, especially flexion.
  vi. Sensory examination and deep tendon reflexes are normal.

**c. Diagnosis**
  i. X-rays only needed if atypical symptoms present.
    1. Include pain at rest, pain at night, or significant trauma.

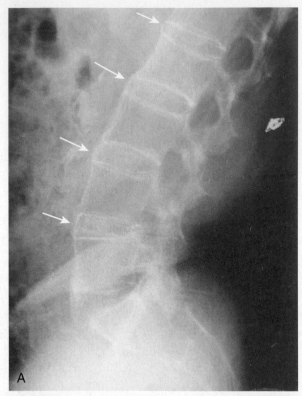
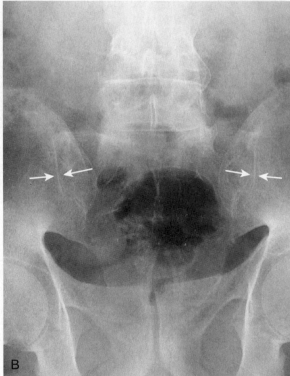

**Fig. 4.2** Ankylosing spondylitis. (A) Note "bamboo spine" appearance *(arrows)*. (B) Fusion of both SI joints is noted *(arrows)*. *(From Mettler FA: Essentials of Radiology, 2nd ed. Philadelphia: Elsevier Saunders, 2005:282, Fig. 8-39A.)*

### d. Treatment

i. Short period of bed rest (1 to 2 days).

ii. Cold therapy is started first, followed by heat therapy after 48 to 72 hours.

iii. Pain medications with NSAIDs or other non-narcotics.

iv. Muscle relaxants may be helpful first 3 to 5 days.

v. After pain has resolved, strengthening and conditioning should be started.

## III. CAUDA EQUINA SYNDROME

### a. General

i. Distal end of the spinal cord, conus medullaris, ends at the L1 to L2 level.

1. L2 to L5 area is filled with nerve roots, the cauda equina.

ii. Cauda equina syndrome is due to reduction in volume of lumbar spinal canal, causing compression and paralysis.

iii. Etiologies include central disk herniation, epidural abscess, hematoma, spinal stenosis, or fracture.

### b. Clinical Manifestations

i. Radicular pain and numbness involving both legs.

ii. Leg weakness is present.

iii. Difficulty with urinary and anal sphincter control.

iv. Physical examination may reveal difficulty walking, inability to walk on toes or heels, and loss of sensory function (perianal numbness).

### c. Diagnosis

i. Myelogram or MRI is diagnostic.

### d. Treatment

i. Requires emergency surgery for nerve decompression.

ii. Corticosteroids and analgesics may be needed..

## IV. HERNIATED DISK PULPOSUS

### a. General

i. Due to herniation of the nucleus pulposus into the lumbar spinal canal.

ii. Most commonly occurs at L4 to L5 or L5 to S1 levels with irritation of the L5 or S1 nerve root.

### b. Clinical Manifestations

i. Abrupt onset of symptoms.

1. Pain is severe and exaggerated by sitting, walking, standing, or coughing.

2. Pain radiates from the buttock down the posterior or posterolateral leg to the ankle or foot.

ii. Low back pain is accompanied by unilateral radicular leg pain.

iii. Physical examination reveals a positive straight leg raise, tenderness in the sciatic notch, and limited ROM.

iv. Neurologic symptoms vary with location of nerve impingement.

1. Table 4.1 summarizes neurologic findings.

### c. Diagnosis

i. MRI is very useful in diagnosing herniation.

### d. Treatment

i. NSAIDs are used in the acute phase with 1 to 3 days of bed rest.

1. Muscle relaxants, narcotics, or both may be helpful.

ii. Oral steroids or epidural injection may reduce pain.

iii. Muscle strengthening exercises are begun after acute attack is over.

iv. Surgery may be needed if no improvement.

1. Consider laminectomy, microscopic disk excision, or percutaneous disk excision.

## V. KYPHOSIS/SCOLIOSIS

### a. Kyphosis

i. General

1. Also called "round back."

2. Two major types of kyphosis.

(a) Congenital.

(i) Due to failure of formation or a failure of segmentation of the spine.

(ii) Can lead to paralysis.

(b) Scheuermann's.

(i) Idiopathic nonflexible kyphosis.

(ii) Have end-plate abnormalities and wedging of three or more vertebral bodies noted on lateral spine x-ray film.

**TABLE 4.1**

| Examination Findings of Cervical and Lumbar Radiculopathies | | | |
|---|---|---|---|
| Nerve Root | Motor Weakness | Decreased Reflex | Decreased Sensation |
| C5 | Deltoid, biceps | Biceps | Deltoid region |
| C6 | Biceps, wrist extensors | Biceps, brachioradialis | Dorsolateral aspect thumb and index finger |
| C7 | Triceps, finger extensors | Triceps | Index, long fingers, dorsum of hand |
| L4 | Anterior tibialis | Patellar tendon | Shin |
| L5 | Extensor hallucis longus | None | Top of foot, first web space |
| S1 | Hamstrings | Achilles tendon | Lateral foot |

ii. Clinical manifestations
1. Kyphosis greater than 40 degrees is abnormal.
iii. Diagnosis
1. Based on physical examination and x-ray findings.
iv. Treatment
1. Bracing is indicated if kyphosis measures more than 45 degrees.

**b. Scoliosis**
i. General
1. Lateral curvature of the spine.
2. May be structural or functional in nature.
(a) Structural.
(i) Have vertebral body rotation.
(ii) Caused by congenital malformation, degenerative or metabolic conditions, or idiopathy.
(b) Functional.
(i) Lateral curvature with no structural change or vertebral rotation.
(ii) Secondary to inequality in leg length, local inflammation, or nerve root irritation.
ii. Clinical manifestations
1. Typically diagnosed during adolescence.
2. Shoulder, pelvis, and waist asymmetry are noted on examination.
3. Scapular prominence may also be noted.
iii. Diagnosis
1. Screen for scoliosis with the Adams forward bend test.
(a) Confirmed by standing AP spinal x-ray.
2. Degree of curvature measured by the Cobb method.
iv. Treatment
1. Treatment varies with degree of curvature.
(a) Observation for curvature between 20 and 40 degrees, unless disease progressing, then brace.
(b) Surgical intervention for curvature greater than 40 degrees.
(c) Bracing is used for curvatures between 30 and 40 degrees.

**VI. LOW BACK PAIN**
**a. Etiologies**
i. Originating from the spine.
1. Mechanical.
(a) Make up over 95% of cases.
(b) Causes include the following:
(i) Lumbar spondylosis.
(ii) Disk herniation.
(iii) Spondylolisthesis.
(iv) Spinal stenosis.

(v) Fractures.
(vi) Idiopathic.
2. Neoplastic.
(a) Unusual cause of low back pain.
(b) Metastatic cancer from prostate, lung, breast, and thyroid are common.
3. Infectious.
(a) Includes vertebral osteomyelitis, epidural abscess, and septic diskitis.
(i) Diskitis is an infection of the disk space typically due to *Staphylococcus aureus*. Patient will maintain a straight spine. ESR will be elevated.
(ii) Epidural abscess is common in those with substance abuse disorders who use IV drugs. Patients present with fever and neck or back pain. Leukocytosis is common. Typically, due to *S. aureus*.
4. Inflammatory.
(a) Includes the spondyloarthropathies.
5. Metabolic.
(a) Includes compression fracture from osteoporosis.
ii. Originating from viscera.
1. Includes abdominal aortic aneurysm, pyelonephritis, kidney stones, chronic prostatitis, endometriosis, ovarian cysts, and inflammatory bowel disease.

**VII. SPINAL STENOSIS**
**a. General**
i. Narrowing of the lumbar spinal canal with compression of the nerve roots.
ii. Etiologies.
1. Congenital.
2. Acquired.
(a) Due to degenerative changes; more common in patients older than age 60.
(b) Obesity may be a predisposing factor.
3. Iatrogenic.
4. Other.
(a) Paget's disease.
(i) Disorder of bone metabolism.
(ii) More common in people over age 55.
(iii) Most frequently involves the skull, pelvis, lumbar spine, and femur.
(iv) Patients present with bone pain, fractures, deafness, and enlargement of bone.
(v) Laboratory testing reveals an elevated alkaline phosphatase.
(vi) Treatment consists of calcitonin and bisphosphonates.
(b) Acromegaly.

b. **Clinical Manifestations**
   i. Symptoms may develop following minor trauma or may be indolent.
   ii. Patients present with low back pain and stiffness.
   iii. Neurogenic claudication causing radicular complaints in one or both lower extremities.
      1. Symptoms progress from proximal to distal direction.
   iv. Note fatigue or weakness of the legs with walking or prolonged standing.
   v. May note short-term relief of discomfort with leaning forward.
   vi. See Table 4.2 for comparison of neurologic and vascular claudication.
   vii. Physical examination reveals muscle weakness in the legs, impaired proprioception, decreased reflexes, and possible decrease in urinary and anal sphincter tone.

c. **Diagnosis**
   i. Computed tomography (CT) scan, MRI, or myelogram is used to evaluate for stenosis.

d. **Treatment**
   i. NSAIDs, PT, and activity modification are initial treatment.
   ii. Surgery may be required.

## VIII. THORACIC OUTLET SYNDROME

a. **General**
   i. Due to compression of the lower trunk of brachial plexus and subclavian vessels.
      1. Caused by cervical rib, abnormal first thoracic rib, abnormal scalene muscle, or malunion clavicle fracture.
   ii. More common in women between the ages of 35 and 55.

b. **Clinical Manifestations**
   i. Pain and paresthesia begin in neck and shoulder and then extend to arm and hand.
   ii. Mild to moderate sensory impairment in C8 to T1 distribution.

c. **Diagnosis**
   i. Based on symptoms.
   ii. Electrodiagnostic and MRI may be needed.

d. **Treatment**
   i. Physical therapy, NSAIDs, and tricyclic antidepressants.
   ii. Surgery indicated for severe or progressive disease.

## IX. TORTICOLLIS

a. **Congenital**
   i. Head becomes tilted at or soon after birth. Most common cause is neck injury during delivery.
   ii. Imaging may be needed to exclude bony etiologies that may require stabilization.
   iii. Treatment includes passive stretching or botulinum toxin injection.

b. **Spasmatic (Cervical dystonia)**
   i. Contraction of neck muscles.
      1. Two forms.
         (a) Caput—involves most proximal cervical vertebrae.
         (b) Collis—involves lower cervical vertebrae.
   ii. Usually idiopathic in nature.
   iii. Noted between ages 20 to 60 years.
   iv. Major symptom is painful tonic contractions or spasms of the sternocleidomastoid, trapezius, or other neck muscles.
   v. Treatment includes physical therapy, massage, botulinum toxin, and anti-spasmodic drugs.

# DISORDERS OF THE HIP

## I. ASEPTIC NECROSIS (OSTEONECROSIS)

a. **General**
   i. Result of bone tissue death in the femoral head.
   ii. Etiologies include trauma to vascular supply or decrease in circulation.
      1. Risk factors include hip trauma/fracture, steroid use, alcoholism, sickle cell disease, rheumatoid arthritis (RA), and systemic lupus erythematosus (SLE).
   iii. Increased incidence in patients aged 30 to 50.

b. **Clinical Manifestations**
   i. Present with acute onset of dull or throbbing pain in groin, buttock, or lateral hip and a limp.
   ii. On physical examination, pain with internal or external rotation of the hip and decreased ROM are noted.

c. **Diagnosis**
   i. X-ray (AP and frog leg lateral views) of the hip reveals a flattened femoral head with joint space narrowing.

**TABLE 4.2**

| Comparison of Neurogenic and Vascular Claudication | | |
|---|---|---|
| **Feature** | **Neurogenic** | **Vascular** |
| Claudication distance | Varies | Fixed |
| Relief of pain | Sitting | Standing |
| Walking up hill | No discomfort | Discomfort |
| Type of pain | Numbness, ache | Tightness |
| Pulses | Present | Absent |
| Skin | Normal | Loss of hair |
| Weakness | Occasional | Rare |
| Back pain | Common | Uncommon |

ii. MRI and bone scan may reveal early changes.

iii. MRI is the gold standard.

d. **Treatment**

i. Protective weight bearing should be started until definitive treatment is established.

ii. Referral for surgery is indicated in most cases.

1. If collapse has occurred, hip arthroplasty is indicated.

## II. DISLOCATIONS

a. **General**

i. Occur when femoral head is displaced from the acetabulum.

ii. Typically occur due to high-energy trauma, such as a motor vehicle accident.

iii. Two types.

1. Posterior (the most common).

2. Anterior.

b. **Clinical Manifestations**

i. Posterior.

1. Hip is short and fixed in flexion, adduction, and internal rotation position.

2. Sciatic nerve injuries are common.

ii. Anterior.

1. Hip is in mild flexion, abduction, and external rotation position.

2. Femoral artery and obturator nerve injury may be present.

c. **Diagnosis**

i. X-ray film of a posterior dislocation reveals the affected femoral head appearing smaller than the opposite side.

1. Fractures of the posterior acetabular wall are common.

ii. X-ray film of an anterior dislocation reveals the affected femoral head appearing larger than the opposite side.

d. **Treatment**

i. Avascular necrosis can occur due to vascular compromise.

1. More common in posterior dislocations.

ii. After a fracture has been ruled out, reduction should occur as soon as possible.

iii. After reduction, crutch-assisted ambulation with limited weight bearing until pain-free.

# DISORDERS OF THE KNEE

## I. BURSITIS

a. **General**

i. Bursae lie between skin and bony prominences or between tendons, ligaments, and bone.

ii. Chronic pressure of friction leads to thickening of the lining, excess fluid formation, swelling, and pain.

iii. Prepatellar bursitis.

1. Lies between the skin and bony patella.

2. Most common bursitis of the knee.

3. Develops secondary to chronic kneeling (housemaid's knee).

b. **Clinical Manifestations**

i. Prepatellar bursitis presents with dome-shaped swelling over the anterior aspect of the knee.

1. Early in disease course, note pain with activity or direct pressure.

2. Movement of the knee does not increase pain.

c. **Diagnosis**

i. Aspiration of the bursa will assist in separating inflammatory, hemorrhagic, or septic bursitis.

1. Inflammatory bursitis presents with slightly yellow fluid.

2. Hemorrhagic bursitis presents with bloody fluid.

3. Septic bursitis presents with cloudy fluid.

d. **Treatment**

i. Nonoperative treatment includes NSAIDs, ice, and activity modifications.

ii. Aspiration may be therapeutic.

iii. Steroid injection may be needed.

iv. Septic bursitis treated with antibiotics to cover *S. aureus*.

## II. DISLOCATIONS

a. **General**

i. Severe injury resulting from violent trauma.

ii. Typically have three to four major ligaments injured with dislocation.

1. Vascular and nerve injuries are common.

iii. Classification based on direction of dislocation: anterior, posterior, lateral, medial, and rotatory.

1. Anterior dislocation is due to hyperextension of the knee.

2. Posterior dislocation is due to a direct blow to the anterior tibia with the knee flexed 90 degrees.

iv. Patella dislocation is due to a twisting injury on an extended knee.

1. More common in females.

b. **Clinical Manifestations**

i. Obvious deformity may be noted, including hemarthrosis and ecchymosis.

1. Dimple sign on the anteromedial surface is noted in posterolateral dislocation.

ii. Neurovascular complications are common, and status must be evaluated in all patients.

1. Complications involve popliteal artery and peroneal nerve.

iii. Patella dislocation presents with the patella displaced laterally over the lateral condyle.

c. **Diagnosis**
   i. X-ray film is required to determine the direction of the dislocation and presence of any fracture.

d. **Treatment**
   i. Reduction should be undertaken immediately.
      1. After reduction, the knee should be immobilized.
   ii. If reduction is not possible or vascular injury is present, immediate surgical intervention is required.
   iii. Flexing the hip, hyperextending the knee, and sliding the patella back into place reduce patella dislocation.
      1. Have immediate relief of pain.

## III. MENISCAL INJURIES

a. **General**
   i. Menisci are fibrocartilage pads that function as shock absorbers between the femur and tibia.
   ii. Mechanism of injury is a significant twisting knee injury, with the foot planted.

b. **Clinical Manifestations**
   i. After acute injury, patient can typically ambulate, and knee swelling, and stiffness develop over the next 2 to 3 days.
   ii. Patients note pain on the medial or lateral side of the knee.
      1. Locking or catching of the knee joint may occur.
      2. Climbing stairs brings about more pain than descending stairs.
   iii. On physical examination, note tenderness over the medial or lateral joint line.
      1. Large effusion or hemarthrosis may be present.
      2. ROM is limited due to presence of effusion.
   iv. Thessaly test, McMurray test, and Apley's compression tests are positive.

c. **Diagnosis**
   i. MRI is very sensitive for evaluation of meniscal injury.

d. **Treatment**
   i. Initial treatment is RICE (**R**est, **I**ce, **C**ompression, and **E**levation).
   ii. Surgical débridement or repair may be indicated.

## IV. SPRAINS/STRAINS

a. **Medial Collateral Ligament Injury**
   i. General
      1. Mechanism of injury is direct blow to the lateral portion of the knee or with significant twisting and torque on the lower extremity.
   ii. Clinical manifestations
      1. Patients typically report hearing or feeling a pop over the medial knee.
      2. Medial knee pain and swelling are noted.
      3. On physical examination, the ligament is tender to palpation.
      4. Degree of injury is evaluated by applying valgus stress to the knee when fully extended and in 20 to 30 degrees of flexion.
   iii. Diagnosis
      1. Based on history and physical examination.
      2. MRI used to diagnose severe tears.
   iv. Treatment
      1. Conservative therapy with RICE.
      2. Bracing may be helpful.

b. **Lateral Collateral Ligament Injury**
   i. General
      1. Mechanism of injury is a direct blow to the medial knee or anteromedial tibia with the knee flexed and foot planted.
   ii. Clinical manifestations
      1. Pain, stiffness, and localized swelling are noted.
      2. Varus stressing of the knee reveals increased laxity.
      3. If peroneal nerve damage is present, weakness of foot dorsiflexion and eversion is noted.
   iii. Diagnosis
      1. Based on history and physical examination.
   iv. Treatment
      1. Conservative therapy with RICE.
      2. Surgical repair is indicated.

c. **Anterior Cruciate Ligament (ACL) Injury**
   i. General
      1. Mechanism of injury is direct blow or indirect stress.
         (a) Requires a sudden change in direction of the weight-bearing knee.
   ii. Clinical manifestations
      1. Patient may note a pop in their knee at the time of injury.
      2. Note immediate swelling and pain after injury.
      3. Knee is very unstable and weight bearing is difficult.
      4. On physical examination, pain and tenderness is noted in the posterolateral area of the knee or near the tibial plateau.
      5. A positive anterior drawer, Lachman's test, or pivot shift test is noted.
   iii. Diagnosis
      1. Based on history and physical examination.
      2. MRI is highly sensitive and specific in the diagnosis of complete ACL tears.
   iv. Treatment

1. Conservative therapy with RICE.
2. Referral is needed for possible surgery.

**d. Posterior Cruciate Ligament Injury**
  i. General
   1. Mechanism of injury is hyperextending the knee or a direct blow to the anterior proximal tibia with the knee flexed and foot planted.
  ii. Clinical manifestations
   1. Patient may note a dull aching pain and stiffness.
    (a) Swelling is not typical.
   2. Physical examination may reveal only a mild effusion and posterior drawer test is positive.
  iii. Diagnosis
   1. Based on history and physical examination findings.
   2. MRI may be used to evaluate for possible ligament damage.
  iv. Treatment
   1. Conservative treatment and PT may be successful.
   2. Surgical intervention is the treatment of choice.

# DISORDERS OF THE ANKLE/FOOT

## I. DISLOCATIONS
**a. General**
  i. Can occur in one of four planes and are commonly associated with a fracture.
  ii. Posterior dislocation occurs when a backward force is applied when the foot is plantar flexed.
  iii. Anterior dislocation occurs when force is applied to anterior aspect of the tibia with the foot dorsiflexed.
**b. Clinical Manifestations**
  i. Pain, swelling, and deformity are noted at site of injury.
  ii. Patient is unable to bear weight, and ROM is decreased.
  iii. Neurovascular compromise can occur.
   1. Peroneal nerve is at risk.
**c. Diagnosis**
  i. X-ray film reveals widening of joint spaces.
**d. Treatment**
  i. All dislocations of the ankle should be referred.
  ii. Closed reduction should be performed immediately to limit risk of ischemia.
   1. Open reduction and fixation and posterior splint are typically required.

## II. SPRAINS/STRAINS
**a. General**
  i. Injury to the lateral ligaments is most common.
   1. Lateral ligaments include anterior talofibular, calcaneofibular, and posterior talofibular ligaments.
   2. Injury to the syndesmosis structures is less common and is called a high ankle sprain.
  ii. Mechanism of injury is increased rotational stress.
   1. Inversion injury is most common for lateral ankle sprain.
   2. Eversion injury leads to medial ankle sprain.
   3. Forceful external rotations lead to syndesmosis injury.
  iii. Grading of injury.
   1. Grade I.
    (a) Ligaments stretched, but no tear.
    (b) Ankle painful, but stable and has normal function.
   2. Grade II.
    (a) Some ligament tearing with moderate swelling and pain.
    (b) Some function limitations.
   3. Grade III.
    (a) Complete tear of the ligament with marked swelling, bruising, and joint instability.
**b. Clinical Manifestations**
  i. Pain, swelling, and loss of function are common.
  ii. On physical examination, note ecchymosis and swelling around the entire ankle.
  iii. Injury to the syndesmosis is noted by a positive squeeze test and external rotation test.
  iv. Lateral ankle sprain will have a positive anterior drawer test and talar tilt test.
   1. Anterior drawer evaluates the anterior talofibular ligament.
   2. Talar tilt test evaluates the calcaneofibular ligament.
**c. Diagnosis**
  i. AP, lateral, and mortise views required to rule out fracture.
**d. Treatment**
  i. Initial treatment is NSAIDs and RICE.
  ii. Brace to provide support and promote soft-tissue healing.

# FRACTURES

## I. GENERAL
**a. Definition**
  i. Fracture is a break in the continuity of bone or cartilage.
  ii. Pathologic fractures occur through abnormal bone.

iii. Greenstick fractures are incomplete angulated fractures of long bones in children.

iv. Table 4.3 summarizes common fractures.

b. **Descriptors**

i. Closed fracture: skin and soft tissue overlying the fracture are intact.

ii. Open fracture: fracture exposed to the outside environment.

iii. Types of fractures.

1. Transverse.

(a) Fracture occurs at a right angle to the long axis of the bone.

2. Oblique.

(a) Fracture runs oblique to the long axis of the bone.

3. Spiral.

(a) Fracture encircles the shaft of the bone in a spiral fashion.

4. Comminuted.

(a) Fracture has more than two fragments.

c. **Epiphyseal Fractures**

i. Salter-Harris classification.

1. Type I.

(a) Fracture extends through the epiphyseal plate, resulting in displacement.

2. Type II.

(a) As above, plus a triangular segment of metaphysis is fractured.

3. Type III.

(a) Fracture runs from the joint surface through epiphyseal plate and epiphysis.

4. Type IV.

(a) Fracture as in type III but also through the adjacent metaphysis.

5. Type V.

(a) Crush injury of the epiphysis.

6. See Fig. 4.3 for Salter-Harris classification.

d. **Accompanying Nerve Injuries**

i. Certain nerve injuries may accompany certain fractures.

ii. Table 4.4 summarizes nerve injuries that are associated with fractures.

## II. TYPES

a. **Ankle/Foot**

i. Ankle fractures involve the lateral, medial, or posterior malleolus.

1. Mechanism of injury is result of eversion or lateral rotation on the talus.

ii. Foot fractures involve the talus, calcaneus, metatarsal, and phalanges.

1. Talus fracture due to a twisting injury, fall, or high-energy impact.

**TABLE 4.3**

| Common Fractures | | |
| --- | --- | --- |
| **Fracture** | **Description** | **Mechanism** |
| Barton's | Intraarticular fracture dislocation of the wrist | High-velocity impact across radiocarpal joint with wrist in flexion or dorsiflexion |
| Bennett's | Oblique fracture through base of first metacarpal | Produced by direct force |
| Boxer's | Fracture neck of fourth and fifth metacarpal | Produced by striking clenched fist against an object |
| Galeazzi's | Fracture of shaft of radius with dislocation of distal radioulnar joint | Due to fall on outstretched hand with wrist in extension and forearm forcibly pronated |
| Hangman's | Fracture and dislocation of atlas and axis | Due to extreme hyperextension during abrupt deceleration |
| March | Stress fracture of the metatarsal | Due to repetitive trauma |
| Monteggia's | Fracture of the junction of the proximal and middle third of the ulna with anterior dislocation of the radial head | Due to fall on outstretched hand with forced pronation of forearm |
| Nightstick | Fracture of ulna, radius, or both | Due to direct trauma |
| Smith's | Extraarticular fracture of distal radius with volar displacement of distal fragment | Due to fall with force to back of hand |

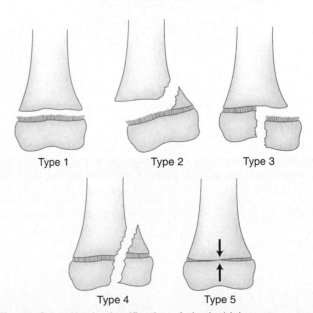

**Fig. 4.3** Salter-Harris classification of physical injury. *(From Green NE: Skeletal Trauma in Children, 3rd ed. Philadelphia: Elsevier Saunders 2003:21, Fig. 2-3.)*

Type 1   Type 2   Type 3   Type 4   Type 5

**TABLE 4.4**

| Nerve Injuries Associated with Fractures | |
| --- | --- |
| **Fracture** | **Nerve Injury** |
| Acetabulum | Sciatic |
| Femoral shaft | Peroneal |
| Humeral shaft | Radial |
| Lateral tibial plateau | Peroneal |
| Sacral | Cauda equina |

   2. Calcaneus fracture due to high-energy direct axial compression.
   3. Metatarsal fracture due to direct trauma or twisting force applied to a fixed forefoot.
   4. Phalangeal fracture due to direct trauma, such as dropping a heavy object or stubbing toes.
   iii. Deformity depends on extent of bone displacement.
   iv. Diagnosis made by x-ray.
      1. Standard AP and lateral views plus AP view 15 degrees internally rotated are needed to diagnosis ankle fracture.
      2. Foot fractures diagnosed by standard foot and ankle x-ray film.
      3. Ottawa Ankle Rules are used to determine if x-ray is needed for ankle or foot injuries.
         (a) Table 4.5 summarizes Ottawa Ankle Rules.
   v. Treatment.
      1. Elevation and ice to control swelling.
      2. Immobilization with splinting.
      3. Referral is indicated with severe displacement.
  **b. Forearm/Wrist/Hand**
      i. Boxer's.
         1. Mechanism of injury is direct blow of a closed fist against another object.

**TABLE 4.5**

| Ottawa Ankle Rules | |
| --- | --- |
| **Ankle X-Ray** | **Foot X-Ray** |
| Required if there is pain in the malleolar zone and the following: | Required if pain in midfoot zone and the following: |
| 1. Bone tenderness at posterior edge or tip of lateral malleolus or | 1. Bone tenderness at the base of the fifth metatarsal or |
| 2. Bone tenderness at posterior edge or tip of medial malleolus or | 2. Bone tenderness at the navicular bone or |
| 3. Inability to bear weight at time of injury and in ER | 3. Inability to bear weight at time of injury and in the ER |

   2. Fracture occurs at the distal end of the fifth metacarpal.
      (a) Fig. 4.4 shows boxer's fracture on x-ray film.
   3. Angulation of fracture greater than 30 degrees should be treated to limit deformity.
   4. Treatment is an ulnar gutter splint of the joint in flexion or percutaneous pinning.
  ii. Colles'.
   1. Mechanism of injury is due to fall on an outstretched hand.
   2. Transverse fracture of the distal radial metaphysis with dorsal displacement of the distal fragment.
      (a) Fracture is located within 2 cm of the articular surface.
      (b) Fig. 4.5 shows Colles' fracture on x-ray film.
      (c) Transverse facture of the distal radial metaphysis with volar displacement of the distal fragment is a reverse Colles' fracture or Smith's fracture.
   3. Physical examination reveals a "dinner fork" deformity of the wrist.
      (a) Due to dorsal displacement and angulation of the fracture.

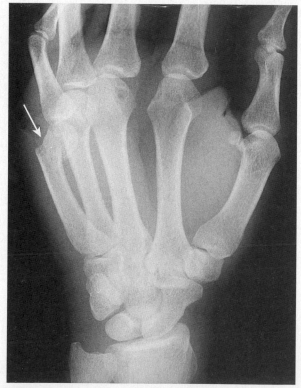

**Fig. 4.4** Boxer's fracture *(arrow)*. *(From Mettler FA: Essentials of Radiology, 2nd ed. Philadelphia: Elsevier Saunders, 2005:307, Fig. 8-78.)*

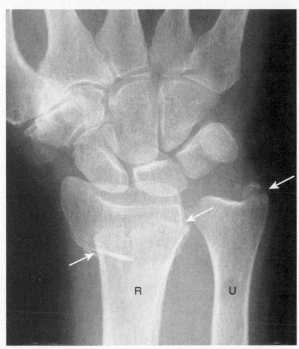

**Fig. 4.5** Colles' fracture *(arrows)*. *R*, Radius; *U*, ulna. *(From Mettler FA: Essentials of Radiology, 2nd ed. Philadelphia: Elsevier Saunders, 2005:300, Fig. 8-68A and B.)*

4. Posteroanterior (PA) and lateral x-ray films of the wrist reveal a fracture through the radial metaphysis.
5. Treatment is fracture reduction and reverse sugar-tong splinting with the wrist in flexion.

iii. Humeral.
  1. Humeral shaft fractures.
    (a) Mechanism of injury is due to direct trauma or severe twisting of the arm.
    (b) On physical examination, localized pain is noted with swelling.
        (i) The arm may be shortened or rotated.
    (c) Complications include radial nerve injury.
  2. Supracondylar fractures.
    (a) Fracture of the distal humerus proximal to the epicondyles.
    (b) Typically, an injury of the immature skeleton and due to a fall on the outstretched arm when the elbow is fully extended or hyperextended.
    (c) Patients present holding the upper extremity in extension to the side with swelling around the elbow.
  3. Epicondyle fracture.
    (a) Typically involves the medial epicondyle.

(b) Mechanism of injury is due to repetitive valgus stress.
  4. Treatment consists of simple immobilization with a splint, cast, sugar-tong, or sling and swathe splint.
    (a) If significant displacement is noted, a hanging cast may be required.
iv. Radial.
  1. Due to a fall on an outstretched hand.
  2. On physical examination, note localized tenderness over the radial head or pain with passive rotation of the forearm.
  3. X-ray film may be difficult to interpret.
    (a) Tenderness and a positive fat pad sign may be the only findings.
    (b) See Fig. 4.6 for radial fracture x-ray view.
  4. Treatment consists of long arm splint.
v. Scaphoid.
  1. Most common carpal bone fracture and most typically seen in young adults.
  2. Mechanism of injury is fall on an outstretched hand.
  3. Patient is tender in the anatomic snuffbox or with resisted supination and has limited ROM of the wrist and thumb.
  4. X-ray is often negative.
    (a) May require special scaphoid views or repeat x-ray 10 to 14 days after treatment.
  5. Treatment is thumb spica splint and referral.
    (a) Improper treatment may lead to avascular necrosis.

**c. Hip**
  i. General
    1. Incidence of hip fracture doubles each decade of life after age 50.
    2. Women affected more often than men.
    3. Mortality rate is high.
      (a) Deep vein thrombosis (DVT) and pulmonary embolism (PE) are serious complications.
  ii. Clinical manifestations
    1. Pain is the major feature, along with inability to bear weight.
    2. On physical examination, the affected leg is shortened and externally rotated.
  iii. Diagnosis
    1. X-ray film reveals fracture.
  iv. Treatment
    1. Surgical repair, hip arthroplasty, is indicated.

**d. Knee**
  i. General
    1. Result of significant trauma.
      (a) Patellar fracture due to direct blow.

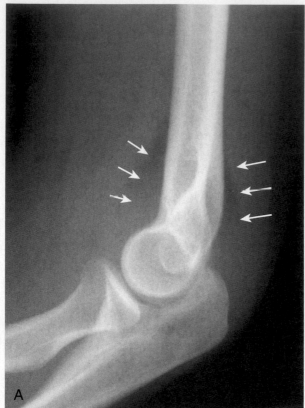

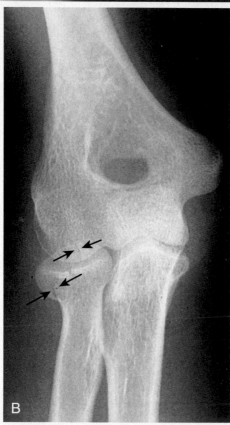

**Fig. 4.6** Positive fat pad in radial fracture. (A), Note anterior and posterior fat pads (arrows). (B) Note fracture line across humeral head *(arrows)*. *(From Mettler FA: Essentials of Radiology, 2nd ed. Philadelphia: Elsevier Saunders, 2005:294, Fig. 8-58.)*

(b) Tibial plateau fracture due to impact, direct axial load, or shearing force.

ii. Clinical manifestations
1. Patients present with knee pain and difficulty walking.
2. Physical examination reveals swelling and bruising.
3. Point tenderness over site of injury.

iii. Diagnosis
1. Patients present with large hemarthrosis with fat globules.
2. X-ray film reveals fracture.

iv. Treatment
1. Analgesics are required.
2. The extremity should be immobilized and made non–weight bearing.

e. **Shoulder**
i. Clavicle.
1. Very common fracture during childhood.
2. Mechanism of injury is typically direct force to lateral aspect of shoulder from a fall or sporting injury.
3. Patients present with pain over the fracture site, and the affected extremity is held close to the body.
4. Shoulder is typically slumped downward, forward, and inward.
5. Typically heals without difficulty.
(a) If displaced, may cause pressure on subclavian vessels or brachial plexus.
6. Treatment is immobilization with a figure-eight dressing.
7. Healing should be adequate in 6 weeks.

ii. Scapula.
1. Uncommon fracture noted primarily in men 30 to 40 years of age.
2. Mechanism of injury is typically violent direct trauma.
3. Typically, no displacement.
(a) May have associated injury to the ribs, chest wall, or shoulder girdle.
4. On examination, the shoulder is adducted, and the arm held close to the body.
(a) Increased pain with any movement.
5. Treatment is immobilization with a sling and swathe dressing.
(a) If significant displacement, the patient should be referred.

# INFECTIOUS DISEASES

I. **OSTEOMYELITIS**
a. **General**
i. Infection of the bone that may occur from a variety of methods.

1. Contiguous spread.
2. Hematogenous spread.
   ii. Organisms.
      1. *S. aureus.*
      2. *Escherichia coli.*
      3. *Pseudomonas aeruginosa.*
      4. *Salmonella.*
         (a) Common in children with sickle cell disease.
      5. Anaerobes.
   iii. Acute versus chronic.
      1. Acute disease evolves over days to weeks.
      2. Chronic disease evolves over weeks to months.

b. **Clinical Manifestations**
   i. Local pain and tenderness noted at site of infection.
      1. Most commonly affects long bones and vertebral bodies.
   ii. Signs of overlying infection may be present.
   iii. In chronic infection, sinus tracts may be present.
   iv. Fever may or may not be noted.
      1. Fever and chills more common in acute infection.

c. **Diagnosis**
   i. White blood cell (WBC) count is normal in chronic disease and elevated in acute disease; may note anemia of chronic disease.
      1. Sedimentation rate is elevated.
   ii. Diagnosis is made by x-ray.
      1. May be normal early, until substantial bone is lost.
      2. MRI/CT scan is more sensitive than plain x-rays.
   iii. Diagnosis and organism are confirmed by blood culture.

d. **Treatment**
   i. Treat with IV antibiotics or antifungals for 4 to 6 weeks.
      1. After IV treatment, oral antibiotics are used long term to decrease risk of flare up of disease.
      2. Table 4.6 summarizes treatment options for osteomyelitis.
   ii. Antibiotics are selected based on organism.
   iii. Monitor response to therapy by following sedimentation rate values.

## II. SEPTIC ARTHRITIS

a. **General**
   i. Arises due to hematogenous spread of bacteria to the synovial membrane lining a joint.
      1. Sources of infection include the following:
         (a) Urinary tract infection (UTI).
         (b) IV drugs in those with substance use disorder.

**TABLE 4.6**

| Treatment of Osteomyelitis | | |
| --- | --- | --- |
| **Organism** | **First Choice** | **Second Choice** |
| *Staphylococcus aureus* | Penicillin G | Second-generation cephalosporin Clindamycin Vancomycin |
| *Staphylococcus aureus*, penicillin-resistant | Nafcillin | Second-generation cephalosporin Clindamycin Vancomycin |
| *Staphylococcus aureus*, methicillin-resistant | Vancomycin | Teicoplanin |
| *Streptococcus* species | Penicillin G | Clindamycin Erythromycin Vancomycin |
| *Escherichia coli* | Quinolone | Third-generation cephalosporin |
| *Pseudomonas aeruginosa* | Piperacillin and gentamicin | Third-generation cephalosporin or quinolone |
| Anaerobes | Clindamycin | Ampicillin-sulbactam |
| Mixed | Ampicillin-sulbactam | Imipenem |

         (c) IV catheters.
         (d) Soft-tissue infections.
   ii. Common organisms include the following:
      1. *S. aureus.*
      2. *Neisseria gonorrhoeae.*
      3. Gram-negative bacilli.
      4. Parvovirus B19.
      5. Hepatitis B.

b. **Clinical Manifestations**
   i. Typical presentation includes swelling and pain in a single joint accompanied by fever.
   ii. Joint is warm to touch, and pain is noted with any movement.
   iii. Most affected joints in adults include the knee, hip, shoulder, wrist, ankle, and elbow.
   iv. In children, the most affected joint is the hip, followed by the knee.

c. **Diagnosis**
   i. Analysis of the synovial fluid is critical.
      1. WBC count is greater than $50,000/mm^3$ with a predominance of neutrophils.
      2. Gram stain and blood cultures may be positive.

d. **Treatment**
   i. Joint drainage is very important.
   ii. Systemic antibiotics are required for 3 to 4 weeks.
      1. Selection is based on most likely organism.

# NEOPLASTIC DISEASE

## I. BONE CYSTS
### a. General
  i. Common pseudotumor of the bone and most frequent cause of pathologic fractures in children.
  ii. Typical age of onset is 5 to 15 years and more common in boys than girls.
  iii. Most frequently noted in proximal humerus or upper femur.
### b. Clinical Manifestations
  i. Patients are typically asymptomatic unless pathologic fracture present.
### c. Diagnosis
  i. X-ray film reveals a solitary cyst located in the metaphyseal area with thinning of the adjacent cortical bone.
### d. Treatment
  i. Treatment depends on location of the cyst.
  ii. In weight-bearing bones, treatment should be aggressive.
  1. Consists of aspiration and injection of bone marrow.
  2. Curettage and bone grafting may be needed.

## II. BONE TUMORS
### a. General
  i. Benign disease is nonaggressive with very little tendency to metastasize.
  ii. Malignant disease is invasive, is destructive, and tends to metastasize.
  iii. Benign tumors include the following:
  1. Osteoid-forming tumors.
    (a) Osteoid osteoma.
    (b) Osteoblastoma.
  2. Chondroid-forming tumors.
    (a) Enchondroma.
    (b) Osteochondroma.
    (c) Chondroblastoma.
  iv. Malignant tumors include the following:
  1. Osteoid-forming tumors.
    (a) Osteosarcoma. (More information noted below.)
  2. Chondroid-forming sarcomas.
    (a) Primary chondrosarcoma.
    (b) Secondary chondrosarcoma.
  3. Ewing's family of tumors.
    (a) Ewing's sarcoma.
      (i) Found in patients between ages 5 and 25 years.
      (ii) Pelvis is most common location, followed by femur, tibia, and humerus.
      (iii) Present with localized pain or swelling for a few weeks to months.
      (iv) X-ray film of the tumor reveals a typical onion-skin appearance.
      (v) Treatment involves radiation therapy, chemotherapy, and surgery.
  v. Metastasis of primary malignancy to bone is common.
  1. Common primary sources include prostate, breast, kidney, thyroid, and lung.
  2. Common sites of bone metastasis in order of frequency: spine, pelvis, femur, ribs, proximal humerus, and skull.
### b. Clinical Manifestations
  i. Symptoms vary from being asymptomatic to dull, aching pain.
### c. Diagnosis
  i. Initial evaluations of bone tumors are plain x-rays.
### d. Treatment
  i. Varies from use of aspirin and NSAIDs to surgery for benign tumors.

## III. GANGLION CYSTS
### a. General
  i. Encapsulated, mobile mass found near a joint or tendon sheath.
  ii. Risk factors include repetitive movements or arthritic conditions.
### b. Clinical Manifestations
  i. Typically cause no clinical problem unless impinging nearby tissue.
  ii. Appear spontaneously and are more common on dorsum or palmar aspect of the wrist.
### c. Diagnosis
  i. Based on history and clinical findings.
### d. Treatment
  i. Cysts can be manually reduced, or aspiration can be performed.
  ii. Surgical excision is also an option.
  iii. Ganglion can recur.

## IV. OSTEOSARCOMA
### a. Diagnosis
  i. One of the most common primary malignant tumors of bone.
  ii. Typically noted in ages 10 to 30 years; more common in males.
  iii. Typically found in the metaphyseal areas of long bones.
### b. Clinical Manifestations
  i. Patients present with pain.
### c. Diagnosis
  i. X-ray film reveals lytic destruction.
### d. Treatment

i. Consists of chemotherapy and surgical treatment.
   1. Chemotherapeutic agents include methotrexate, doxorubicin, cisplatin, cyclophosphamide, etoposide, gemcitabine, and ifosfamide.
   2. Surgical treatment consists of limb-sparing surgery.

# OSTEOARTHRITIS

## I. GENERAL
a. **Most common rheumatic disease**
b. **Incidence increases with age (greater than 40 years old), obesity, and joint wear and tear**
c. **Classified as primary or secondary**
   i. Primary.
      1. No underlying etiologic factor.
   ii. Secondary.
      1. Have presence of underlying etiologic factor.
         (a) Previous trauma.
         (b) Congenital hip dysplasia.
         (c) Avascular necrosis.
         (d) Metabolic disorders.

## II. CLINICAL MANIFESTATIONS
a. **History of deep pain of gradual onset that worsens with activity and is relieved by rest**
b. **Morning stiffness lasts less than 30 minutes**
c. **On examination, note pain with ROM, tenderness, crepitus, and deformity of the following joints:**
   i. Hand deformities.
      1. Heberden's nodes.
         (a) Enlarged DIP joints.
      2. Bouchard's nodes.
         (a) Enlarged PIP joints.
   ii. Knee.
      1. Genu valgus or varus.
   iii. Hip.
      1. Loss of internal rotation and extension.
   iv. Foot.
      1. Affects first metatarsophalangeal joint.
   v. Spine.
      1. Commonly affects L3 to L4 intervertebral disk space.

## III. DIAGNOSIS
a. **Laboratory Results**
   i. ESR is normal and rheumatoid factor (RF) is negative.
   ii. Synovial fluid examination reveals mild inflammation, good mucin clot formation, and no crystals.
   iii. X-ray films reveal joint space narrowing, osteophytes, and subchondral cysts.

## IV. TREATMENT
a. **Weight reduction, PT, and support devices are used for joint preservation**
b. **NSAIDs are very beneficial for pain and inflammation control**
c. **Systemic steroids are typically not indicated**
   i. Intraarticular steroid injections are used for acute flare-ups.
d. **In severe disease, joint replacement may be needed**

# OSTEOPOROSIS

## I. GENERAL
a. **Characterized by decreased bone mass with normal bone structure, with associated reduced bone strength and increased risk for fracture**
b. **Disease is predominantly noted in White females**
c. **Estrogen is protective**
d. **Etiologies**
   i. Primary.
      1. Postmenopausal.
      2. Senile.
      3. Idiopathic.
   ii. Secondary.
      1. Endocrine.
         (a) Diabetes mellitus type 1, Addison's disease, thyroid disease.
      2. Neoplasia.
         (a) Multiple myeloma.
      3. Gastrointestinal.
         (a) Malabsorption.
      4. Rheumatologic.
      5. Drugs.
         (a) Steroids, anticonvulsants, anticoagulants, lithium, antidepressants.

## II. CLINICAL MANIFESTATIONS
a. **Vertebral compression and femur fractures are common**
b. **Low back pain may be the only symptom**

## III. DIAGNOSIS
a. **X-ray film reveals decreased bone density**
b. **X-ray film of spine may reveal wedge-shaped deformities with compression fractures**
c. **Bone density testing reveals decreased bone density**
   i. Table 4.7 interprets bone density testing.

**TABLE 4.7**

| Bone Density Test Interpretation | |
|---|---|
| **Classification** | **Density Results** |
| Normal | Less than –1 SD below normal |
| Osteopenia | Greater than –1 SD, but less than –2.5 SD below normal |
| Osteoporosis | Greater than –2.5 SD below normal |
| Severe | Greater than –2.5 SD below normal; osteoporosis and presence of a fracture |

*SD*, Standard deviation.

## IV. TREATMENT

a. **Estrogen replacement therapy can prevent or slow rate of osteoporosis**
   i. Contraindicated in women with high risk of endometrial cancer or breast cancer.
b. **Calcium supplements and vitamin D are important to maintain bone mass and slow or prevent disease**
c. **Bisphosphonates (alendronate and risedronate) increase bone density and prevent bone loss**
d. **Calcitonin inhibits osteoclastic bone resorption**
e. **Weight bearing and active lifestyle may help prevent osteoporosis**

## V. SCREENING

a. **U.S. Preventive Services Task Force (USP-STF) recommends screening in females aged 65 years and older and younger females whose facture risk is equal to or greater than that of a 65-year-old White female who has no additional risk factors**
b. **Screening not recommended in males**

# COMPARTMENT SYNDROME

## I. GENERAL

a. **Occurs when increased pressure in a compartment compromises blood flow and function of the tissue in that compartment**
b. **May occur acutely or chronically; acute syndrome is a surgical emergency**

## II. DEVELOPS AFTER THE FOLLOWING:

a. **Trauma, particularly long bone fractures**
b. **Open reduction and internal fixation of fractures**
c. **Crush injuries**
d. **Burns**
e. **Ischemia-reperfusion injury**

## III. CLINICAL MANIFESTATIONS

a. **Clinical signs vary based on compartment involved**
b. **Symptoms**
   i. Pain out of proportion to injury.
   ii. Deep ache or burning pain.
   iii. Paresthesias—suggests ischemic nerve injury.
c. **Physical Examination**
   i. Pain with passive stretch.
   ii. Tense compartment.
   iii. Pallor, decreased sensation, weakness, or paralysis.

## IV. DIAGNOSIS

a. **Based on clinical findings and measurement of compartment pressure**

## V. TREATMENT

a. **Immediate surgical consult and release of the compartment pressure via fasciotomy**

# RHEUMATOLOGIC CONDITIONS

## I. FIBROMYALGIA

a. **General**
   i. May coexist with SLE or RA.
   ii. Etiology of pain is unknown.
   iii. More common in females aged 20 to 55.
b. **Clinical Manifestations**
   i. Present with widespread pain for greater than 3 months and with fatigue.
      1. Light touch or breeze may be unpleasant.
   ii. Morning stiffness may be prominent.
   iii. Poor sleep is almost always present.
   iv. Pain is elicited by manual pressure at 11 or more defined tender points out of 18.
   v. Laboratory testing typically reveals no abnormal findings.
c. **Diagnosis**
   i. Based on clinical criteria including generalized pain for three months, fatigue, sleep disturbances, widespread tenderness, no joint swelling, and normal laboratory testing.
d. **Treatment**
   i. Nonpharmacologic.
      1. Exercise, cognitive-behavioral therapy, and non-opioid analgesics.
   ii. Pharmacologic.
      1. Treatment of chronic pain includes the following:
         (a) Tricyclic antidepressants.
            (i) May be combined with selective serotonin reuptake inhibitors or central-acting muscle relaxant.

(b) Gabapentin.

(c) Anxiolytics.

2. Tricyclic antidepressants, gabapentin, and anxiolytics can also be used to treat associated depression and improve sleep.

## II. GOUT/PSEUDOGOUT

### a. Gout

i. General

1. Secondary to purine metabolism disorders.

2. Most commonly affects middle-aged men.

3. Etiologies.

(a) Underexcretion of uric acid.

(i) Makes up 90% of cases.

(ii) Typically, a result of the following:

(1) Renal disease secondary to volume depletion.

(2) Drugs, such as aspirin, that decrease uric acid secretion.

(b) Overproduction of uric acid.

(i) Typically a result of the following:

(1) Purine metabolism enzyme deficiency.

(2) Increased nucleic acid turnover.

ii. Clinical manifestations

1. Two clinical stages.

(a) Asymptomatic.

(i) Increased serum uric acid in asymptomatic patient.

(b) Acute gouty arthritis.

(i) Lower extremity, monoarticular arthritis.

(1) Typically affects first metatarsophalangeal joint.

(ii) Joint tender, erythematous, warm, and swollen.

2. Acute attacks may be triggered by trauma, alcohol, stress, and acute illness.

iii. Diagnosis

1. Laboratory tests reveal a mild leukocytosis and elevated ESR.

2. Elevated serum uric acid.

3. Synovial fluid examination reveals monosodium urate crystals.

(a) Crystals are needle-shaped, negatively birefringent in polarized light.

iv. Treatment

1. Acute treatment.

(a) NSAIDs (indomethacin or naproxen) are useful in relieving pain.

(i) Aspirin should be avoided owing to decreasing uric acid secretion.

(b) Colchicine is used in acute attacks.

(c) If no relief with NSAIDs or colchicine, consider glucocorticoids.

2. Prophylaxis.

(a) Uricosuric drugs.

(i) Decreased tubular uric acid reabsorption.

(ii) Examples include probenecid and sulfinpyrazone.

(b) Allopurinol.

(i) Xanthine oxidase inhibitor lowers serum uric acid levels.

(ii) Side effects include leukocytosis and decreased renal function.

(c) Febuxostat.

(i) Xanthine oxidase inhibitor.

(ii) Side effects include elevated liver function tests, nausea, and arthralgias.

3. Complications of gout include acute obstructive uropathy leading to acute renal failure.

### b. Pseudogout

i. General

1. Also known as calcium pyrophosphate dihydrate (CPPD) deposition disease.

2. Typically noted in patients over 70 years of age.

3. Etiologies include the following:

(a) Hereditary.

(i) Autosomal dominant.

(b) Idiopathic.

4. Associated with other metabolic diseases.

(a) Hyperparathyroidism.

ii. Clinical manifestations

1. Acute attacks present with warmth, erythema, swelling, and tenderness.

(a) Typically affects the knee and first metatarsophalangeal joint.

2. Attacks last for days and are typically self-limiting.

iii. Diagnosis

1. CPPD crystals are noted in the synovial fluid.

2. X-ray films reveal chondrocalcinosis.

(a) Calcific deposits in the tendons, ligaments, and cartilage.

iv. Treatment

1. NSAIDs and intraarticular steroids are useful in acute attacks.

2. Colchicine used for prophylaxis.

## III. POLYARTERITIS NODOSA

### a. General

i. Vasculitis involving medium-sized arteries.

ii. Primarily affects middle-aged men.

iii. Commonly affects the skin, joints, nerves, and kidneys. Lungs are typically spared.

b. **Clinical Manifestations**
   i. Systemic symptoms include fever, malaise, and weight loss.
   ii. Renal involvement and peripheral neuropathy are common.
   iii. Examination of the skin reveals palpable purpura.
   iv. Nondeforming arthritis, involving any joint, may be noted.

c. **Diagnosis**
   i. Laboratory tests reveal elevated ESR, leukocytosis, anemia, and thrombocytosis.
   ii. Urinalysis is positive for protein and blood if kidneys are involved.
   iii. Diagnosed by tissue biopsy.

d. **Treatment**
   i. Consists of steroid and immunosuppressive (cyclophosphamide, methotrexate, or azathioprine) therapy.
   ii. May develop aneurysms and areas of occlusion.

## IV. POLYMYOSITIS/DERMATOMYOSITIS

a. **General**
   i. An idiopathic, inflammatory myopathy.
   ii. Peak prevalence ages 7 to 15 and 40 to 50 years.

b. **Clinical Manifestations**
   i. Patients present with symmetric, proximal muscle weakness.
      1. Patients will have difficulty arising from chairs, reaching overhead, or combing hair.
   ii. Dermatomyositis presents with skin changes.
      1. Gottron's papules: erythematous to violaceous papules on the extensor surface of the MCP and IP joints.
      2. Shawl sign: hyperpigmentation on upper back and V of the neck/upper chest.
      3. Pink-violet, erythema lesions, with or without edema, on the periorbital tissue.
   iii. Systemic symptoms include fatigue, arthralgias, weight loss, and muscle pain.

c. **Diagnosis**
   i. Laboratory results reveal elevated CPK, aldolase, and lactate dehydrogenase (LDH).
      1. Antinuclear antibody (ANA) is negative.
   ii. Evidence of chronic inflammation noted on muscle biopsy.
   iii. Electromyogram (EMG) results show the following patterns:
      1. Short duration, low amplitude.
      2. Fibrillation, even at rest.
      3. Bizarre, high-frequency discharges.

d. **Treatment**
   i. Center of treatment is the decreasing of inflammation with steroids, topical calcineurin inhibitors, methotrexate, or cyclophosphamide.
   ii. PT is important to maintain ROM and avoid contractures.

## V. POLYMYALGIA RHEUMATICA

a. **General**
   i. Cause of polymyalgia rheumatica (PMR) is unknown.
   ii. Inflammation of the synovial lining of the bursa and joints is noted.
   iii. Most affected areas are neck, shoulders, and hips.
   iv. Women are twice as likely as men to have PMR.
   v. Associated with the same HLA genes as RA.
   vi. Associated with giant cell arteritis.

b. **Clinical Manifestations**
   i. Note pain and stiffness in the neck, shoulders, and hip-girdle area that is worse in the morning.
   ii. On physical examination, note only decreased active or passive ROM.
   iii. MRI or ultrasound of the shoulders or hips reveals inflammation of the bursa.
   iv. Laboratory testing reveals an elevated ESR, elevated C-reactive protein (CRP), and anemia.

c. **Diagnosis**
   i. Diagnostic criteria include the following:
      1. Age older than 50.
      2. Aching and stiffness for longer than 1 month.
      3. Affects at least two of three areas: shoulders, neck, or pelvic girdle.
      4. Morning stiffness lasting longer than 1 hour.
      5. ESR greater than 40 mm/hour.
      6. Exclusion of other diseases
      7. Rapid response to treatment with steroids.

d. **Treatment**
   i. NSAIDs and prednisone are cornerstones of therapy.

## VI. REITER'S SYNDROME

a. **General**
   i. Also known as reactive arthritis.
   ii. Occurs secondary to chlamydial urethritis or gastrointestinal (GI) infections caused by *Shigella, Salmonella, Yersinia, Clostridium,* and *Campylobacter.*
   iii. Most prevalent in young adulthood.
   iv. Linked to HLA-B27.

b. **Clinical Manifestations**
   i. Signs and symptoms noted 1 to 4 weeks after initial infection.

ii. Acute disease presents with asymmetric arthritis in knees and ankles.
   1. Three typical features include the following:
      (a) Diffuse swelling of fingers and toes (sausage digits).
      (b) Tenderness of the Achilles tendon.
      (c) Low back pain with sacroiliitis.
iii. Conjunctivitis.
   1. Many will develop a mild, noninfectious conjunctivitis.
iv. Mucocutaneous lesions.
   1. May note small, shallow, painless ulcers on glans penis.

**c. Diagnosis**
   i. Laboratory tests reveal a leukocytosis and elevated ESR.
   ii. Synovial fluid reveals an increase in WBCs, mainly neutrophils.

**d. Treatment**
   i. NSAIDs and steroids are the primary treatments.
   ii. Sulfasalazine and methotrexate are second-line therapies.
   iii. Antibiotics are of no use in treating the arthritis but may be needed to treat the initial infection.

## VII. RHEUMATOID ARTHRITIS

**a. General**
   i. A chronic, systemic inflammatory disease.
   ii. More common in women of childbearing years.
   iii. Etiology is immune complex formation leading to an immune reaction.
   iv. Inflammation leads to destruction and deformity of cartilage, ligaments, and bone.

**b. Clinical Manifestations**
   i. Systemic symptoms include fatigue, malaise, and pain.
   ii. Patients note prolonged morning stiffness (greater than 60 minutes), and symptoms are made worse by movement.
   iii. Joints of the hands, wrists, elbows, shoulders, and feet are commonly affected.
      1. Joints affected include MCP and PIP.
      2. Findings include the following:
         (a) Ulnar deviation of fingers.
         (b) Palmar subluxation of PIP joints.
         (c) Hyperextension of PIP and flexion of DIP (swan-neck deformities).
         (d) Flexion of PIP and extension of DIP (boutonnière deformities).
   iv. Other physical findings include the following:
      1. Decreased dorsiflexion of the wrist.
      2. Atrophy of the thenar eminence.

3. Neck stiffness and pain.
4. Subluxation of metatarsal heads.

**c. Diagnosis**
   i. Laboratory findings include anemia of chronic disease, thrombocytosis, elevated ESR, and positive for rheumatoid factor (RF) and anti-cyclic citrullinated peptide (CCP).
   ii. Synovial fluid analysis reveals increased WBCs and poor mucin clot formation.
   iii. X-ray film shows evidence of joint deformity, presence of cysts, loss of cartilage, and erosive changes.
      1. Fig. 4.7 shows x-ray findings in RA.

**d. Treatment**
   i. First-line treatment includes exercise, rest, and NSAIDs.
   ii. Disease-modifying antirheumatic drugs (DMARDs).
      1. Hydroxychloroquine, sulfasalazine, and methotrexate may be needed for unremitting disease.
      2. Table 4.8 lists DMARDs.
   iii. Corticosteroid injections are used for flare-ups.

## VIII. SYSTEMIC LUPUS ERYTHEMATOSUS

**a. General**
   i. Most common in women of reproductive age.
   ii. Acute and chronic inflammatory process with multiple organ involvement.
      1. Linked to HLA-DR2 and HLA-DR3.

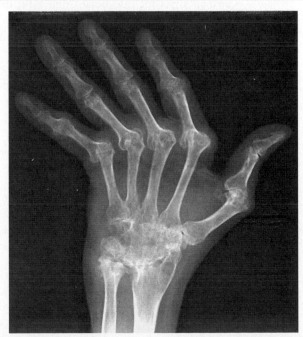

**Fig. 4.7** X-ray findings in rheumatoid arthritis. *(From Harris ED: Kelly's Textbook of Rheumatology, 7th ed. Philadelphia: Elsevier Saunders 2005:745, Fig. 51-6.)*

**TABLE 4.8**

### List of Disease-Modifying Antirheumatic Drugs

| Drug | Indication | Toxicity | Monitoring |
|------|-----------|----------|-----------|
| Hydroxychloroquine | Mild disease | Nausea, rash, retinal damage | Eye exam |
| Sulfasalazine | Mild disease | Nausea, hepatitis, G-6-PD anemia, myelosuppression | LFT and CBC |
| Methotrexate | First-line DMARD | Stomatitis, nausea, diarrhea, hepatitis, myelosuppression, teratogenic | CBC, LFTs, creatinine |
| Etanercept | TNF inhibitor | Avoid in patients with active or chronic infections, multiple sclerosis | Baseline PPD |
| Infliximab | TNF inhibitor | Avoid in patients with active or chronic infections, multiple sclerosis | Baseline PPD |
| Abatacept | Inhibitor of T-cell activation | Avoid in patients with active or chronic infections, pulmonary effects in COPD | Baseline PPD, no live vaccines |
| Rituximab | Inhibitor of T-cell activation | Avoid in patients with active or chronic infections, infusion reaction, hepatitis B reactivation | Effective contraception |

*CBC*, Complete blood count; *DMARD*, disease-modifying antirheumatic drug; *LFT*, liver function tests; *PPD*, purified protein derivative; *TNF*, tumor necrosis factor.

iii. May be drug induced, secondary to hydralazine and procainamide.

**b. Clinical Manifestations**

  i. Systemic symptoms include fatigue, weight loss, myalgias, and fever.

  ii. Affects multiple organ systems.

    1. Skin signs include facial butterfly rash and photosensitivity.

      (a) See Color Plate 1 for photo of typical facial rash noted in SLE.

    2. Nervous system signs include seizures and psychoses.

    3. Cardiac signs include pericardial effusions and myocarditis.

    4. Pulmonary signs include pleural effusions and pneumonitis.

    5. Renal signs include glomerulonephropathy.

    6. Musculoskeletal signs include symmetrical peripheral arthralgias/arthritis.

    7. Eye signs include keratoconjunctivitis sicca.

**c. Diagnosis**

  i. Laboratory tests reveal anemia, lymphopenia, and thrombocytopenia.

  ii. ANA is positive.

    1. Antibodies to double-stranded DNA and anti-Sm are specific for SLE.

    2. Antihistone is positive in drug-induced SLE.

  iii. False-positive VDRL may occur.

**d. Treatment**

  i. NSAIDs are useful for treatment of fever and joint pain.

  ii. Steroids are useful in cutaneous manifestations and multiple organ symptoms.

  iii. Hydroxychloroquine and chloroquine are used for the skin disease and mild systemic disease.

iv. Severe disease may require mycophenolate, cyclophosphamide, or azathioprine.

## IX. SYSTEMIC SCLEROSIS

**a. General**

  i. Multisystem disorder characterized by fibrosis of the skin, blood vessels, and visceral organs.

    1. Mechanism is overproduction and accumulation of collagen.

  ii. Two major subtypes.

    1. Diffuse cutaneous.

      (a) Skin changes noted on extremities, face, and trunk.

      (b) Risk of visceral disease is increased early in disease.

    2. Limited cutaneous.

      (a) Skin changes limited to distal extremities and face.

  iii. Typical age of onset is 20 to 40 years.

**b. Clinical Manifestations**

  i. Raynaud's phenomenon.

    1. Due to vasoconstriction of small arteries in the fingers, toes, nose, and earlobes.

  ii. Skin changes.

    1. Skin becomes thick, firm, and tightly bound to underlying subcutaneous tissue.

    2. Taut skin may lead to development of contractures.

  iii. Systemic features.

    1. Musculoskeletal.

      (a) May develop carpal tunnel syndrome.

    2. Gastrointestinal.

      (a) Dysphagia.

    3. Pulmonary.

      (a) Linear densities or honeycombing noted on chest x-ray film.

4. Cardiac.
    (a) Pericarditis and arrhythmias.
5. Renal.
    (a) Renal failure.
iv. Systemic symptoms include fatigue, stiff joints, weakness, and pain.

c. **Diagnosis**
    i. Laboratory tests reveal an elevated ESR, anemia, and positive ANA.
        1. ANA results.
            (a) Antitopoisomerase (Scl-70) positive in diffuse cutaneous disease.
            (b) Anticentromere positive in limited cutaneous disease.

d. **Treatment**
    i. Medications to control skin changes include D-penicillamine, azathioprine, and steroids.
    ii. Raynaud's can be managed by dressing warmly, discontinuing smoking, and use of calcium-channel blockers.

## X. SJÖGREN'S SYNDROME
a. **General**
    i. Inflammation and destruction of the salivary and lacrimal glands.
    ii. Etiologies.
        1. Primary.

2. Secondary.
    (a) Associated with RA or SLE.
iii. Typically affects women in their 50s and strongly associated with lymphoma.

b. **Clinical Manifestations**
    i. Patients have dry eyes with a foreign body sensation.
    ii. Dry mouth with an increase in dental caries, difficulty chewing or swallowing.
    iii. May develop constipation and pancreatic insufficiency.

c. **Diagnosis**
    i. Laboratory results reveal anemia of chronic disease, leukopenia, and mild eosinophilia.
    ii. ANA and RF tests are positive.
        1. Anti-La and Anti-Ro antibodies are positive.
    iii. Salivary gland biopsy will confirm the diagnosis.

d. **Treatment**
    i. Artificial tears and saliva are needed.
    ii. Systemic cyclophosphamide, tumor necrosis factor (TNF) inhibitors, and steroids are required in severe disease.
        1. Topical steroids in eye should be avoided owing to corneal thinning.

## XI. TABLE 4.9 SUMMARIES SEROLOGY TESTING USED IN RHEUMATIC DISEASE.

**TABLE 4.9**

| Summary of Serology Tests Used in Rheumatic Diseases | | |
|---|---|---|
| **Autoantibody** | **Diseases** | **Comments** |
| ANA | SLE | (+) in 95% of SLE<br>(+) in 10%–20% of healthy young females |
| Anti-histone | Drug-induced lupus | |
| Anti-ds DNA | SLE | (+) in 70% of SLE<br>More specific for SLE than ANA |
| Anti-Smith (Sm) | SLE | (+) in 20%–30% of SLE<br>More specific for SLE than ANA |
| Anti-RNP | SLE<br>Mixed connective tissue disease | |
| Anti-Ro/La | SLE<br>Sjögren's syndrome<br>Neonatal lupus | |
| Anti-Scl 70 | Diffuse scleroderma | (+) in 40% of patients with scleroderma |
| Anticentromere | CREST syndrome | (+) in >50% of patients with CREST |

*ANA*, Antinuclear antibody; *CREST*, **C**alcinosis, **R**aynaud's syndrome, **E**sophageal dysmotility, **S**clerodactyly, **T**elangiectasis; *(+)*, positive; *RNP*, ribonucleoprotein; *SLE*, systemic lupus erythematosus.

## QUESTIONS

### QUESTION 1
The Lachman's test is used to determine if an injury has occurred to which of the following structures?
A  Medial collateral
B  Posterior cruciate
C  Lateral collateral
D  Anterior cruciate
E  Medial meniscus

### QUESTION 2
A 45-year-old male presents with pain in his left great toe for the past 5 days. Physical examination of the foot reveals a red, tender, swollen great toe. Examination of the joint fluid reveals needle-shaped, negatively birefringent crystals. Which of the following is the most likely type of crystal in the fluid?
A  Calcium pyrophosphate
B  Monosodium urate
C  Cholesterol
D  Tyrosine
E  Cystine

### QUESTION 3
A 35-year-old female presents with symmetric skin thickening of the proximal extremities, face, and trunk. The ANA is positive for anti-topoisomerase. Which of the following is the most likely diagnosis?
A  Dermatomyositis
B  CREST syndrome
C  Mixed connective tissue disease
D  Diffuse cutaneous scleroderma
E  Systemic lupus erythematosus

### QUESTION 4
Which of the following is the initial therapy for medial epicondylitis?
A  Surgery
B  Antibiotics
C  Short arm splint
D  Intraarticular steroids
E  Nonsteroidal antiinflammatory drugs

### QUESTION 5
Which of the following is the mechanism of action of allopurinol (Zyloprim)?
A  Inhibits renal reabsorption of uric acid
B  Alkalinizes the urine
C  Inhibits xanthine oxidase
D  Activates dihydrofolate reductase
E  Activates macrophage enzymes

### QUESTION 6
Osteoporosis is most commonly noted in which of the following female populations?
A  Black
B  Asian
C  Hispanic
D  White
E  Indigenous Americans

### QUESTION 7
Which of the following is the most common type of malignant lesion to arise from bone cells?
A  Ewing's sarcoma
B  Chondrosarcoma
C  Osteosarcoma
D  Osteoid osteoma
E  Osteomalacia

### QUESTION 8
Which of the following physical examination findings is most commonly noted in patients with gamekeeper's thumb?
A  Inability to actively oppose thumb
B  Sensory loss ulnar nerve region
C  Positive Allen's test
D  Positive Finkelstein test
E  Positive Phalen test

### QUESTION 9
Which of the following are the most common widespread symptoms of fibromyalgia?
A  Vision loss and jaw claudication
B  Headache and nuchal rigidity
C  Diarrhea and abdominal pain
D  Depression and fatigue
E  Pain and stiffness

### QUESTION 10
A 2-year-old patient presents with right elbow pain. The patient holds the arm motionless at her side in slight flexion and pronation. Which of the following is the most likely diagnosis?
A  Subluxation of the annular ligament
B  Osteochondritis dissecans
C  Ruptured biceps tendon
D  Dislocation of the elbow
E  Olecranon bursitis

# ANSWERS

**1. D**

EXPLANATION: The Lachman's or anterior drawer test are used to evaluate for possible anterior cruciate ligament injuries. *Topic: Disorders of the Knee: Sprains/Strains*

☐ Correct ☐ Incorrect

**2. B**

EXPLANATION: Gout most commonly affects middle-aged men who present with a tender, red, swollen, and warm first metatarsophalangeal joint. Examination of the synovial fluid reveals needle-shaped, negatively birefringent monosodium urate crystals. *Topic: Gout*

☐ Correct ☐ Incorrect

**3. D**

EXPLANATION: Scleroderma is most commonly noted in patients aged 20 to 40 years, and patients present with thick, firm skin and Raynaud's phenomenon. Laboratory testing reveals a positive antitopoisomerase on ANA testing. *Topic: Systemic Sclerosis*

☐ Correct ☐ Incorrect

**4. E**

EXPLANATION: Medial epicondylitis presents with pain and point tenderness. Treatment consists of elimination of the activity causing symptoms, undertaking of PT, and use of NSAIDs. *Topic: Tenosynovitis*

☐ Correct ☐ Incorrect

**5. C**

EXPLANATION: Allopurinol (Zyloprim) is used in the treatment of gout and lowers serum uric acid levels by inhibiting xanthine oxidase. Side effects include decreasing renal function and leukocytosis. *Topic: Gout*

☐ Correct ☐ Incorrect

**6. D**

EXPLANATION: Osteoporosis is most commonly noted in White females. *Topic: Osteoporosis*

☐ Correct ☐ Incorrect

**7. C**

EXPLANATION: Osteosarcoma is the most common primary malignant tumor arising from bone. It is more commonly noted in males aged 10 to 30 years and is typically found in the metaphyseal areas of long bone. *Topic: Osteosarcoma*

☐ Correct ☐ Incorrect

**8. A**

EXPLANATION: People with gamekeeper's thumb, weakness of the ulnar collateral ligament, present with inability to oppose thumb, with weakness with pinch, and with recurrent effusions of the MCP joint. *Topic: Gamekeeper's thumb*

☐ Correct ☐ Incorrect

**9. E**

EXPLANATION: Fibromyalgia presents most commonly with widespread pain and stiffness. Other symptoms include fatigue, disrupted sleep, difficulties with memory, and psychological distress. *Topic: Fibromyalgia*

☐ Correct ☐ Incorrect

**10. A**

EXPLANATION: With subluxation of the annular ligament (nursemaid's elbow), the patient holds the arm motionless at their side in slight flexion and pronation. Reduction is accomplished by supinating and flexing the forearm while applying pressure over the radial head. *Topic: Nursemaid's elbow*

☐ Correct ☐ Incorrect

# CHAPTER 5
# ENDOCRINE SYSTEM

## EXAMINATION BLUEPRINT TOPICS

**ENDOCRINE BACKGROUND**
Information
Hypothalamic function
Feedback loops

**ADRENAL DISORDERS**
General function
Cushing's syndrome
Chronic corticoadrenal insufficiency
Acute corticoadrenal insufficiency
Glucocorticoids
Primary hyperaldosteronism

**DIABETES MELLITUS**
General

Type 1
Type 2
Compares Diabetes Mellitus Type 1 With Type 2
Hypoglycemia
Hypogondanism
Neoplasms

**PARATHYROID DISORDERS**
Hyperparathyroidism
Hypoparathyroidism

**PITUITARY DISORDERS**
General
Acromegaly/gigantism

Short stature and dwarfism
Syndrome of inappropriate antidiuretic hormone secretion (SIADH)
Diabetes insipidus
Hyperprolactinemia

**THYROID DISORDERS**
Hyperthyroidism
Hypothyroidism
Thyroiditis
Neoplastic disease

## ENDOCRINE BACKGROUND

### I. INFORMATION
   a. If there is excess hormone, order a suppression test
   b. If there are decreased levels of hormone, order a stimulation test
   c. Primary disease means malfunction of the target organ
   d. Secondary disease means malfunction of the pituitary gland
   e. Tertiary disease means malfunction of the hypothalamus

### II. HYPOTHALAMIC FUNCTION
   a. There are a number of releasing factors from the hypothalamus
      i. Gonadotropin-releasing hormone (GnRH) stimulates release of follicle-stimulating hormone (FSH) and luteinizing hormone (LH) from the anterior pituitary.
      ii. Thyrotropin-releasing hormone (TRH) stimulates release of thyroid-stimulating hormone (TSH) from the anterior pituitary.
      iii. Corticotropin-releasing hormone (CRH) stimulates release of adrenocorticotropic hormone (ACTH) from the anterior pituitary.
      iv. Growth hormone–releasing hormone (GHRH) stimulates release of growth hormone from the anterior pituitary.
      v. Exceptions:
         1. Oxytocin is produced in the hypothalamus and secreted by the posterior pituitary.
         2. Antidiuretic hormone (ADH) is produced in the hypothalamus and secreted by the posterior pituitary.

### III. FEEDBACK LOOPS
   a. Central basis of endocrine system
   b. With positive feedback, production of a hormone causes increased release of the hormone through stimulation of the hypothalamus and pituitary
   c. With negative feedback, production of a hormone causes decreased release of the hormone through down-regulation of the hypothalamus and pituitary (Fig. 5.1)

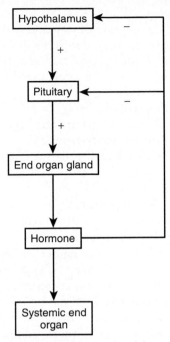

**Fig. 5.1** Negative feedback loop.

# ADRENAL DISORDERS

## I. GENERAL FUNCTION
### a. Location/Function
  i. Located on top of the kidneys bilaterally.
  ii. Each gland is composed of an outer cortex and an inner medulla.
    1. Cortex.
      (a) Composed of three zones that produce different steroid hormones (Table 5.1).
    2. Medulla.
      (a) A sympathetic ganglion that produces catecholamines.
### b. Tests of Adrenocortical Function
  i. Urine-free cortisol.
    1. Used with suspected adrenal hyperfunctioning.
  ii. Plasma cortisol.
    1. There is a diurnal variation in cortisol levels making it difficult to use as a screening test.
    2. Normal range is 5 to 20 μg/dL.

3. Typically, levels rise in the morning and decrease through the remainder of the day and overnight.
  iii. Plasma ACTH levels.
    1. Used to differentiate primary versus secondary adrenal dysfunction.
    2. Normal range is up to 100 pg/mL.
  iv. Provocative tests.
    1. ACTH stimulation test.
      (a) Screening test for adrenal hypofunction.
    2. CRH.
      (a) Used to separate ACTH-dependent from ACTH-independent hypercortisolism.
    3. Dexamethasone suppression test.
      (a) Used to screen for adrenal hyperfunction.

## II. CUSHING'S SYNDROME
### a. General
  i. Caused by glucocorticoid (cortisol) excess.
  ii. Causes of Cushing's syndrome.
    1. ACTH dependent.
      (a) ACTH-secreting benign pituitary adenoma (Cushing's disease).
        (i) Most common cause.
      (b) Nonpituitary ACTH-secreting neoplasm.
        (i) Small cell carcinoma of the lung (paraneoplastic syndrome).
        (ii) Endocrine tumors of foregut origin.
    2. ACTH independent.
      (a) Adrenal adenoma.
      (b) Adrenal carcinoma.
      (c) Glucocorticoid administration.
### b. Clinical Manifestations
  i. Patients classically present with the following:
    1. Weight gain.
      (a) Mainly centripetal with deposits in the dorsocervical fat pad (buffalo hump) and supraclavicular fossa.
    2. Plethora.
      (a) Present with a ruddy complexion.
    3. Striae.
      (a) Violaceous and occurring in thin skin.

**TABLE 5.1**

| Adrenal Gland Cortex | | | |
| --- | --- | --- | --- |
| Zone | Hormone Produced | Hormone Function | Hormone Controlling Release |
| Zona glomerulosa | Aldosterone | Regulates sodium balance | Renin |
| Zona fasciculata | Cortisol | Maintains physiologic integrity | ACTH |
| Zona reticularis | Androgen and estrogen precursors | Production of androgens and estrogens | Androgen-stimulating hormone |

4. Hypertension.
5. Proximal muscle weakness and wasting.
   (a) Test patient's ability to rise unassisted from a squatting position.
6. Oligomenorrhea or amenorrhea.
7. Moon facies.
   (a) Rounded face secondary to increased fatty deposits in the cheeks.

ii. Laboratory findings.
1. May see associated hyperglycemia, hypokalemia, and leukocytosis.

c. **Diagnosis**
i. Laboratory tests reveal an elevated cortisol level.
1. Initial screening of urine-free cortisol level is best.
ii. If urine-free cortisol levels are elevated, follow with a dexamethasone suppression test.
1. Dexamethasone suppression test: dexamethasone given at night with cortisol measured in the morning.
   (a) Positive results: elevated morning cortisol levels.
      (i) Low morning cortisol level excludes Cushing's syndrome as dexamethasone has properly suppressed cortisol secretion.
iii. If a dexamethasone suppression test reveals elevated morning cortisol, follow with a CRH stimulation test to separate ACTH-dependent from ACTH-independent disease.
1. CRH administration followed by measurement of ACTH levels.
   (a) ACTH >10 pg/dL is noted in ACTH-dependent disease.
      (i) Increased ACTH from pituitary macroadenoma (Cushing's disease) is the most common cause.
   (b) ACTH <10 pg/dL is noted in ACTH-independent disease.
      (i) Indicating an adrenal source as cause of excess cortisol secretion. ACTH is reduced in an unsuccessful attempt to suppress further cortisol secretion.

d. **Treatment**
i. If an adenoma or tumor is the cause, surgical removal of tumor is indicated, followed by hormone replacement therapy.
ii. Adrenal inhibitors include metyrapone and ketoconazole but are not indicated as sole therapy.

## III. CHRONIC CORTICOADRENAL INSUFFICIENCY
a. **General**
i. Caused by destruction or dysfunction of the adrenal cortex.

ii. Etiology.
1. Autoimmune destruction is the most common etiology (Addison's disease).
   (a) Called primary adrenal insufficiency as dysfunction occurs at the target organ (adrenal gland).
2. Tuberculosis.
3. Bilateral adrenal hemorrhage.
4. Adrenoleukodystrophy.
   (a) X-linked disorder with accumulation of long-chain fatty acids in adrenal cortex, testes, and brain.

b. **Clinical Manifestations**
i. Symptoms include weakness, fatigability, weight loss, myalgias, arthralgias, fever, anorexia, anxiety, and nausea and vomiting.
ii. On physical examination, hypotension with orthostatics and in primary disease only (disease of the adrenal gland) hyperpigmentation is noted.
1. Pigmentation is noted over the knuckles, elbows, posterior neck, and palmar creases.
2. The skin in pressure areas, belt line, also darkens.
iii. Laboratory findings include the following:
1. Eosinophilia.
2. Hyponatremia.
3. Hyperkalemia.
4. Hypoglycemia.

c. **Diagnosis**
i. A low morning serum cortisol level with an elevated ACTH level is diagnostic of primary disease.
1. Secondary disease has a low morning serum cortisol level with a low ACTH level, indicating pituitary involvement.
ii. Computed tomography (CT) scan of the adrenals may be needed to evaluate for tuberculosis of the adrenal glands.

d. **Treatment**
i. Drug of choice is hydrocortisone.
ii. If not resulting in adequate salt-retaining effect, fludrocortisone may be added.

## IV. ACUTE CORTICOADRENAL INSUFFICIENCY (ADRENAL CRISIS)
a. **General**
i. Due to insufficient cortisol.
ii. Most commonly seen in patients with primary adrenal insufficiency (Addison's disease).
iii. Adrenal crisis may occur after the following:
1. Stress such as trauma, surgery, or infection.
2. Sudden withdrawal of adrenocortical hormones.
3. Bilateral adrenalectomy.
4. Injury to both adrenals.

b. **Clinical Manifestations**
  i. Patients complain of headache, nausea and vomiting, abdominal pain, and diarrhea.
    1. Shock may be noted in adrenal crisis.
  ii. Confusion or coma may be present.
  iii. On physical examination, note the patient is hypotensive and has signs of cyanosis and dehydration.
  iv. Laboratory results reveal the following:
    1. Eosinophilia.
    2. Hyponatremia.
    3. Hyperkalemia.
    4. Hypoglycemia.

c. **Diagnosis**
  i. Evaluate patient for possible causes, such as infection.
  ii. Serum cortisol is low.
  iii. Plasma ACTH levels will be elevated if the patient has primary adrenal disease.
  iv. Diagnosis made by simplified cosyntropin stimulation test.
    1. A cortisol level below 20 μg/dL is a positive test.

d. **Treatment**
  i. Adrenal crisis.
    1. Management of underlying cause.
    2. Antibiotics for possible bacterial infection if suspected.
    3. IV saline and hydrocortisone or dexamethasone must be given immediately to avoid hypotensive emergency.
  ii. Convalescent.
    1. Continue with hydrocortisone and, as dosage decreases, may need to add mineralocorticoid to the treatment.

V. **GLUCOCORTICOIDS**
a. **General**
  i. Antiseizure medications enhance metabolism of glucocorticoids, making them less potent.
b. **Side Effects**
  i. Prolonged therapy or high doses may lead to a variety of side effects (Table 5.2).
    1. Decrease risk of side effects when:

**TABLE 5.2**

| Side Effects of Glucocorticoids | |
|---|---|
| Amenorrhea | Muscle weakness |
| Aseptic necrosis of bone | Osteoporosis |
| Diabetes | Personality change |
| Infection | Polyuria |
| Insomnia | Sex hormone suppression |
| Kidney stones | Weight gain |

(a) Dose equal to or less than the normal daily production.
(b) Duration of therapy less than 3 weeks.
(c) Administered as a single morning dose.

VI. **PRIMARY HYPERALDOSTERONISM**
a. **General**
  i. Due to unilateral adrenocortical adenoma (Conn's syndrome) or bilateral cortical hyperplasia.
  ii. More common in women than in men.
b. **Clinical Manifestations**
  i. Symptoms include muscle weakness, paresthesias, headache, polyuria, and polydipsia.
  ii. On physical examination, hypertension is noted.
  iii. Laboratory tests reveal hypokalemia.
c. **Diagnosis**
  i. All antihypertensive medications must be stopped before testing, and patients must have a high sodium intake during testing.
  ii. Diagnosis is made with noting a low plasma renin activity and an elevated 24-hour urine aldosterone level.
  iii. CT scan of the adrenal gland should be completed to evaluate for adrenal tumors.
d. **Treatment**
  i. Conn's syndrome is treated with adrenalectomy or lifelong spironolactone therapy.
  ii. Bilateral adrenal hyperplasia is treated with spironolactone.
  iii. Complications seen are those noted with chronic hypertension.

# DIABETES MELLITUS

I. **GENERAL**
a. **Leading cause of blindness, end-stage renal disease, and nontraumatic limb amputation in the United States**
b. **Increases risk for cardiovascular, cerebral, and peripheral vascular disease**
c. **Major factor in neonatal morbidity and mortality**
d. **Long-term complications including end organ damage are noted in type 1 and type 2 diabetes**
  i. Microvascular disease is more common in type 1.
  ii. Macrovascular disease is more common in type 2.
  iii. Table 5.3 summarizes primary complications noted in diabetes mellitus.

II. **TYPE 1**
a. **General**
  i. Previously known as insulin-dependent diabetes or juvenile diabetes.

**TABLE 5.3**

| Complications of Diabetes Mellitus |
| --- |
| **Eyes** |
| Diabetic retinopathy |
| Cataracts |
| **Renal** |
| Glomerulosclerosis |
| Renal tubular necrosis |
| Pyelonephritis |
| **Neurologic** |
| Peripheral neuropathy |
| Autonomic neuropathy (gastroparesis, erectile dysfunction, postural hypotension) |
| **Cardiovascular** |
| Heart disease (myocardial infarction, cardiomyopathy) |
| **Skin** |
| Lower extremity ulcers |
| **Infectious** |
| Malignant otitis externa |

ii. Patients have little or no insulin secretion capacity.
iii. Autoimmune disease.
  1. Associated with a specific HLA gene and the presence of autoantibodies to islet cells of the pancreas.
  2. Causes destruction of the pancreatic beta cells resulting in decreased/absent insulin production.

b. **Clinical Manifestations**
  i. At time of presentation, patients appear very ill.
  ii. Symptoms appear abruptly and include polyuria, polydipsia, polyphagia, and weight loss.
    1. May also present with ketoacidosis with or without coma.
  iii. Laboratory findings include:
    1. Glycosuria.
    2. Elevated serum glucose.
    3. Elevated glycosylated hemoglobin (hemoglobin A1c; HbA1c).
      (a) Reflects state of glycemia over the preceding 10 to 12 weeks.
    4. Ketonuria.
      (a) May also be noted in starvation, high-fat and low carbohydrate diets, alcoholic ketoacidosis, and fever.
    5. Proteinuria.
    6. Microalbuminuria.
      (a) Presence of microalbumin is an early predictor of diabetic nephropathy.

c. **Diagnosis**
  i. Requires one of the following:
    1. Hemoglobin A1c of 6.5% or higher.
    2. Symptoms of diabetes (polyuria, polydipsia, unexplained weight loss) plus random plasma glucose greater than 200 mg/dL.
    3. Fasting (at least 8 hours) plasma glucose greater than 126 mg/dL.
    4. A 2-hour (post-standard 75-g glucose tolerance test) plasma glucose greater than 200 mg/dL.

d. **Treatment**
  i. Prevention of long-term complications is vital.
  ii. Diet.
    1. Balance caloric intake with energy expenditure.
    2. Must match carbohydrate intake with insulin dosing.
    3. The American Dietetic Association (ADA) does not make specific dietary recommendations for percentages of macronutrients. A balanced diet, with moderate protein intake and low saturated fat and sodium intake is encouraged.
  iii. Insulin
    1. Insulin replacement along with lifestyle changes is required.
    2. Many different insulin regimens; each should be tailored to the individual patient.
    3. Frequent monitoring of plasma glucose levels is required to assist patient in maintaining adequate control of blood glucose.
    4. Basal insulin should cover baseline insulin requirements.
    5. Bolus insulin should cover insulin required for carbohydrate intake as well as correction of glucose.
    6. Table 5.4 summarizes insulin preparations.
  iv. Complications.
    1. Diabetic ketoacidosis.
      (a) Due to increased lipolysis, decreased glucose uptake, and increased proteolysis.
        (i) Results in hyperglycemia, ketonuria, and acidosis.
      (b) Precipitating factors include infections, inadequate insulin treatment, and myocardial ischemia/infarction.
      (c) Clinical signs include abdominal pain, nausea/vomiting, tachycardia, dehydration, and fruity breath odor.
      (d) Laboratory results reveal hyperglycemia (typically 250–500 mg/dL), presence of ketones in blood and urine, elevated anion gap metabolic acidosis (bicarbonate

**TABLE 5.4**

| Summary of Insulin Preparations | | | | |
| --- | --- | --- | --- | --- |
| **Class** | **Type** | **Onset** | **Peak** | **Duration** |
| Rapid-acting | Lispro or aspart | <15 minutes | 30–90 min | 3–4 hours |
| Short-acting | Regular | 30–60 min | 2–3 hours | 5–8 hours |
| Intermediate-acting | NPH | 1–2 hours | 5–10 hours | 18–24 hours |
| Long-acting | Glargine | 1–2 hours | no peak | 24–36 hours |

*NPH*, Neutral protamine Hagedorn.

<18 mEq/L and pH <7.30), and electrolyte abnormalities.
    (e) Treatment consists of IV fluids, IV regular insulin, correction of electrolyte abnormalities, and treatment of underlying cause.

## III. TYPE 2
  a. **General**
    i. Accounts for approximately 90% of all cases of clinical diabetes.
    ii. Patients retain some endogenous insulin secretion ability, but levels are low relative to glucose levels and level of insulin resistance.
    iii. High rate of genetic influence, not related to HLA genes, and also associated with metabolic syndrome, high-fat diets, obesity, and decreased physical activity.
    iv. Previously considered "adult-onset" but incidence in childhood is rising.
  b. **Clinical Manifestations**
    i. Insidious onset of symptoms and may be mild or symptomatic.
      1. May be an incidental finding on routine labs.
    ii. Symptoms include polyuria, polydipsia, blurry vision, fatigue, weakness, and dizziness.
      1. May present with symptoms of chronic complications such as vascular or neurologic disease.
    iii. Laboratory findings include the following:
      1. Glycosuria.
      2. Elevated serum glucose.
      3. Elevated glycosylated hemoglobin.
        (a) Reflects state of glycemia over the preceding 10 to 12 weeks.
      4. Proteinuria.
      5. Microalbuminuria.
        (a) Presence of microalbumin is an early predictor of diabetic nephropathy.

  c. **Diagnosis**
    i. Type 2 diabetes diagnosis requires one of the following:
      1. Symptoms of diabetes (polyuria, polydipsia) plus random plasma glucose greater than 200 mg/dL.
      2. Fasting (at least 8 hours) plasma glucose greater than 126 mg/dL.
      3. A 2-hour (post-standard 75 g glucose tolerance test) plasma glucose greater than 200 mg/dL.
    ii. Prediabetes diagnosis requires one of the following:
      1. Hemoglobin A1c of 5.7% to 6.4%.
      2. Fasting plasma glucose of 100 mg/dL to 125 mg/dL.
      3. 2-hour plasma glucose of 140 mg/dL to 199 mg/dL.
  d. **Treatment**
    i. Diet.
      1. Even modest weight loss in the obese patient will improve glycemic control.
      2. The ADA does not make specific dietary recommendations for percentages of macronutrients. A balanced diet, with moderate protein intake and low saturated fat and sodium intake is encouraged.
    ii. Oral antidiabetic medications.
      1. Indicated in patients who fail treatment with diet and exercise.
      2. Metformin is considered first-line therapy.
      3. Table 5.5 summarizes oral antidiabetic medications.
    iii. Monitoring.
      1. Regular self-monitoring allows patients to maintain tight control of blood sugar levels.
    iv. Complications.
      1. Hyperosmolar hyperglycemic state.
        (a) Most commonly noted in the elderly with diabetes mellitus type 2.
        (b) Etiology not fully understood, but patients have severe dehydration with hyperglycemia.
        (c) Symptoms include severe dehydration and alterations in mental status.
        (d) Laboratory results reveal severe hyperosmolarity (>350 mOsm/L) and hyperglycemia (typically >600 mg/dL).
          (i) Severe acidosis and ketosis are rare.
        (e) Treatment consists of IV fluids, IV regular insulin, correction of electrolyte abnormalities, and treatment of the underlying cause.
        (f) Table 5.6 compares insulin shock, diabetic ketoacidosis (DKA), and hyperosmolar shock.

**TABLE 5.5**

| Oral Antidiabetic Medications | | | | | |
|---|---|---|---|---|---|
| Drug | Classification | Mechanism of Action | Site of Metabolism | Duration of Action (Hours) | Side Effects |
| Glimepiride | Second-generation sulfonylurea | Increase pancreas insulin secretion | Liver | 24 | Hypoglycemia Weight gain |
| Glipizide | Second-generation sulfonylurea | Increase pancreas insulin secretion | Liver | 12–24 | Hypoglycemia Weight gain |
| Glyburide | Second-generation sulfonylurea | Increase pancreas insulin secretion | Liver | ≤24 | Hypoglycemia Weight gain |
| Repaglinide | Meglitinide analogue | Increase pancreas insulin secretion | Liver | <4 | Hypoglycemia Weight gain |
| Metformin | Biguanide | Decrease hepatic glucose production | Kidney | ≤24 | Abdominal pain Nausea Diarrhea Lactic acidosis |
| Pioglitazone | Thiazolidinedione | Decrease peripheral insulin resistance | Liver | 24 | Fluid retention Weight gain CHF |
| Rosiglitazone | Thiazolidinedione | Decrease peripheral insulin resistance | Liver | Up to 24 | Fluid retention Weight gain CHF |
| Acarbose | Alpha-glucosidase inhibitor | Decrease postprandial digestion of glucose | Gut | Local effect | Abdominal pain Nausea Diarrhea |
| Miglitol | Alpha-glucosidase inhibitor | Decrease postprandial digestion of glucose | Kidney | Local effect | Abdominal pain Nausea Diarrhea |

*CHF*, Congestive heart failure.

**TABLE 5.6**

| Comparison of Acute Complications of Diabetes Mellitus | | | |
|---|---|---|---|
| Feature | Insulin Shock | Diabetic Ketoacidosis | Hyperosmolar Shock |
| Insulin | Excessive | Insufficient | Normal or increased |
| Onset | Rapid | Gradual (days) | Gradual (days) |
| Skin | Cold sweats, pale | Dry, flushed | Dry, flushed |
| Respirations | Normal or shallow | Slow and deep | Typically normal |
| Heart rate | Rapid | Rapid | Typically normal |
| Blood pressure | Normal | Low | Normal |
| Blood glucose | Very low | High | Very high |
| pH | Normal | Low | Normal |
| Acetone | Absent | Positive | Absent |

**IV. TABLE 5.7 COMPARES DIABETES MELLITUS TYPE 1 WITH TYPE 2**

**V. HYPOGLYCEMIA**

    **a. General**
        i. There are two types.
            1. Fasting.
            2. Postprandial.
        ii. Etiologies (Table 5.8).

    **b. Clinical Manifestations**
        i. Symptoms typically begin when blood sugar level is less than 60 mg/dL.

            1. Impaired brain function when blood sugar is less than 50 mg/dL.
        ii. Symptoms include sweating, palpitations, hunger, tremor, weakness, headache, light-headedness, confusion, seizures, and coma.
        iii. In a patient with insulinoma, note the following:
            1. Symptoms develop in early morning or after missing a meal.
            2. Symptoms include blurry vision, headache, slurred speech, and weakness.

**TABLE 5.7**

| Comparison of Diabetes Mellitus Types 1 and 2 | | |
|---|---|---|
| | Diabetes Mellitus Type 1 | Diabetes Mellitus Type 2 |
| Body weight | Normal or lean | Overweight |
| C-peptide | Low or undetectable | Detectable or elevated |
| Family history | Weak family history | Strong family history |
| Insulin sensitivity | Normal | Very reduced |
| Islet cell antibodies | 80% are positive | Absent |
| Other autoimmune diseases | Present | Absent |
| Response to oral agents | Nonresponsive | Responsive |

**TABLE 5.8**

| Etiologies of Hypoglycemia |
|---|
| Fasting hypoglycemia |
| Endocrine disorders |
| Addison's disease |
| Myxedema |
| Hypopituitarism |
| Liver failure |
| Renal failure |
| Pancreatic B-cell tumor |
| Administration of insulin or sulfonylureas |
| Postprandial hypoglycemia |
| Postgastrectomy |
| Functional |
| Alcohol-related hypoglycemia |
| Autoimmune |
| Antibodies to insulin or insulin receptors |

c. **Diagnosis**
   i. The most dependable means of making the diagnosis is prolonged fasting in the hospital until hypoglycemia is noted.
   ii. Diagnosis of insulinoma is based on noting elevated insulin levels during a time of hypoglycemia.

d. **Treatment**
   i. Dextrose is used in the treatment of the patient with hypoglycemia due to administration of excess insulin.
   ii. Treatment of the patient with an insulinoma is surgical resection of the tumor, frequent feedings, and the use of diazoxide

## VI. HYPOGONADISM
a. **General**
   i. Umbrella term referring to decreased testosterone production from the testes.
   ii. Primary disease is due to a decrease in testicular function, resulting in decreased testosterone and spermatogenesis.
   iii. Secondary disease is due to decreased pituitary function resulting in decreased stimulation of the testes, which also causes decreased testosterone and spermatogenesis.

b. **Clinical Manifestations**
   i. Varied based on age of onset, primary versus secondary disease, and severity of disease.
   ii. Onset prior to puberty results in decreased muscle mass, lack of facial hair, lack of testicular growth.
   iii. Onset in adulthood results in decreased libido, mood changes, decreased muscle mass, and gynecomastia.

c. **Diagnosis**
   i. Primary disease: low serum testosterone and decreased sperm count with elevated serum LH and FSH.
   ii. Secondary disease: low serum testosterone and decreased sperm count with decreased LH and FSH.

d. **Management**
   i. Primary disease: testosterone replacement.
   ii. Secondary disease: GnRH analogues.

## I. NEOPLASMS
a. **Pheochromocytoma**
   i. General
      1. Catecholamine-secreting tumor that arises from the chromaffin cells of the adrenal medulla and the sympathetic ganglia.
      2. Rare cause of secondary hypertension.
   ii. Clinical
      1. Classic triad includes hypertension, sweating, and tachycardia.
      2. Other symptoms include palpitations, tremor, dyspnea, and weakness.
   iii. Diagnosis
      1. Must differentiate from panic attack and myocardial infarction.
      2. Elevated urinary and plasma metanephrines and catecholamines.
      3. Clonidine suppression test is positive.
         (a) Positive test: failure to suppress norepinephrine and epinephrine <500 pg/nL following administration of clonidine.
      4. CT scan to locate tumor.
   iv. Treatment
      1. Alpha blockage (phenoxybenzamine) followed by beta blockage (propranolol).
         (a) Beta blockage without alpha blockage can lead to worsening of hypertension.
      2. Surgical removal of tumor through an adrenalectomy.

b. **Multiple endocrine neoplasia (MEN)**
  i. General
    1. Rare, inherited disorder causing tumors on multiple endocrine glands, the small intestine, and stomach.
      (a) MEN 1 is autosomal dominant.
    2. Multiple types of multiple endocrine neoplasia (MEN) syndromes.
    3. Tumors are typically benign.
  ii. Clinical manifestations
    1. Symptoms vary based on the glands and organs affected.
    2. MEN 1 most commonly affects the parathyroid gland, pituitary gland, and pancreas.
    3. MEN 2a most commonly affects the parathyroid gland and thyroid gland and causes pheochromocytoma.
    4. MEN 2b most commonly affects the thyroid gland and causes pheochromocytoma and marfanoid habitus.
      (a) Nearly all patients with MEN 2b will develop medullary thyroid cancer, and prophylactic thyroidectomy is often indicated.
  iii. Diagnosis
    1. A combination of imaging (MRI, CT, PET, US) to determine location of tumors.
    2. Genetic testing for gene mutation.
  vi. Treatment
    1. Surgical removal of tumor and/or affected glands.

# PARATHYROID DISORDERS

## I. HYPERPARATHYROIDISM
  a. **General**
    i. More common in females than males and more common in patients older than age 50.
    ii. Caused by hypersecretion of parathyroid hormone.
      1. Due to parathyroid adenoma (most common), hyperplasia, or carcinoma.
    iii. Results in hypercalcemia
      1. Parathyroid hormone increases calcium levels through increased osteoclast activity in the bone (increased bone resorption) and increased renal tubular reabsorption of calcium in the kidney.
    iv. Primary hyperparathyroidism is due to excessive parathyroid hormone or multiple endocrine neoplasia (types 1 and 2a).
    v. Secondary hyperparathyroidism is due to renal failure, metastatic bone disease, osteomalacia, or multiple myeloma.

  b. **Clinical Manifestations**
    i. Most patients are asymptomatic; symptoms vary based on calcium level.
    ii. If symptomatic, have "bones, stones, abdominal moans, psychic groans, and fatigue overtones."
      1. Skeletal changes include loss of cortical bone and gain of trabecular bone, bone pain, and arthralgias.
      2. Urinary complaints include polyuria, polydipsia, and nephrolithiasis.
      3. Hypercalcemia may cause constipation, fatigue, anemia, weight loss, and hypertension in mild cases and increased thirst, anorexia, nausea, and vomiting in severe cases.
  c. **Diagnosis**
    i. Laboratory results reveal elevated parathyroid hormone, hypercalcemia, low phosphate in primary disease and elevated phosphate in secondary disease, and increased alkaline phosphatase (if bone disease is present).
      1. Diagnosis confirmed with presence of elevated levels of parathyroid hormone.
    ii. Skull x-ray may show "salt and pepper sign" consisting of multiple small areas of lucency secondary to increased trabecular bone resorption.
    iii. Must rule out other causes of hypercalcemia including malignant tumors, multiple myeloma, and sarcoidosis.
  d. **Treatment**
    i. Parathyroidectomy is recommended in patients with symptomatic disease.
      1. Postsurgical complications include hypocalcemia, paresthesias, and possibly tetany.
    ii. Medical treatment for hypercalcemia includes large fluid intake, bisphosphonates, and furosemide.
    iii. Complications include pathologic fractures, urinary tract infections, nephrolithiasis, and renal failure.

## II. HYPOPARATHYROIDISM
  a. **General**
    i. Most commonly noted after thyroidectomy; after surgical removal of parathyroid adenoma; or autoimmune, congenital, familial causes.
    ii. Pseudohypoparathyroidism is due to renal resistance to parathyroid hormone.
      1. Results in hypocalcemia, hyperphosphatemia, and increased serum parathyroid hormone.
  b. **Clinical Manifestations**
    i. Presentation varies with severity of hypocalcemia.
    ii. Acute disease causes circumoral tingling, tetany, muscle cramps, irritability, and seizures.

iii. Chronic disease symptoms include lethargy, personality changes, blurry vision, and mental retardation.
iv. Chvostek's sign and Trousseau's sign are present.
v. Nails may be brittle and skin may be dry.
vi. Deep tendon reflexes may be hyperactive.

**c. Diagnosis**
i. Laboratory tests reveal serum hypocalcemia and hyperphosphatemia with low-urine calcium and normal alkaline phosphatase.
ii. Low parathyroid hormone levels are necessary for diagnosis.
iii. EKG: prolonged QT interval.

**d. Treatment**
i. Treatment of acute attack includes intravenous (IV) calcium gluconate, vitamin D supplement, and magnesium supplement if levels are low.
ii. Maintenance therapy includes calcium and vitamin D supplements.
 1. Monitor serum calcium every 3 months.

# PITUITARY DISORDERS

## I. GENERAL
a. Table 5.9 summarizes pituitary hormones

## II. ACROMEGALY/GIGANTISM
**a. General**
i. Due to excessive growth hormone.
 1. It is called "gigantism" if it occurs before closure of epiphyses.

2. It is called "acromegaly" if it occurs after closure of epiphyses.
 (a) Acromegaly is almost always caused by pituitary adenoma.

**b. Clinical Manifestations**
i. Physical findings include large, doughy hands; wide feet; coarse facial features; prominent mandible; and wide tooth spacing.
ii. Hypertension and cardiomegaly are common.
iii. Increased risk of developing diabetes mellitus.
iv. Headaches are common, and bitemporal hemianopsia (loss of lateral visual field bilaterally) may develop secondary to impingement of optic chiasm.

**c. Diagnosis**
i. Initial screening reveals elevated serum insulin-like growth factor 1 (IGF-1).
ii. Once elevated IGF-1 is noted, an oral glucose suppression test is performed.
 1. Oral glucose is administered and an elevated growth hormone level is a positive result for acromegaly.
iii. Magnetic resonance imaging (MRI) may reveal a pituitary tumor.

**d. Treatment**
i. Pituitary adenomas are removed by transnasal-transsphenoidal resection surgery.
ii. Dopamine agonists can be used to shrink tumors.
iii. Somatostatin analogues (octreotide and lanreotide) can be used to treat patients with acromegaly despite surgery.
 1. Inhibit growth hormone (GH) secretion.

**TABLE 5.9**

| Pituitary Hormones | | |
| --- | --- | --- |
| **Anterior Hormone** | **Releasing/Inhibiting Agent** | **Function** |
| Adrenocorticotropic hormone (ACTH) | Corticotropin-releasing hormone (CRH) | Causes adrenal cortex to secrete adrenocortical hormone |
| Follicle-stimulating hormone (FSH) | Gonadotropin-releasing hormone (GnRH) | Causes growth of follicles in the ovaries prior to ovulation; also promotes formation of sperm in the testes |
| Growth hormone | Growth hormone–releasing hormone (GHRH) | Causes growth of almost all cells and tissues |
| Luteinizing hormone (LH) | Gonadotropin-releasing hormone (GnRH) | Plays a role in causing ovulation and causes secretion of female sex hormones by the ovaries and testosterone by the testes |
| Prolactin | Prolactin inhibitory hormone (PIH) | Promotes development of the breasts and secretion of milk |
| Thyroid-stimulating hormone (TSH) | Thyrotropin-releasing hormone (TRH) | Causes thyroid to release thyroid hormone |
| **Posterior Hormone** | **Stimulus** | **Function** |
| Antidiuretic hormone (ADH) | Increase in blood osmolality | Causes the kidneys to retain water |
| Oxytocin | Breast stimulation and contraction of uterus during parturition | Causes contraction of the uterus during birthing process and stimulates expression of milk from breasts |

## III. SHORT STATURE AND DWARFISM

a. **Short Stature**
  i. General
    1. Table 5.10 shows etiologies.
  ii. Clinical manifestations
    1. Familial short stature.
      (a) Establish growth curves at or below the fifth percentile by age 2.
      (b) Otherwise healthy with a normal physical examination.
      (c) Have normal bone age, and puberty occurs at the expected time.
    2. Constitutional delay.
      (a) Children grow or develop at or below the fifth percentile at normal growth velocity.
          (i) Growth curve parallel to the fifth percentile.
      (b) Have delay in puberty and skeletal maturation.
      (c) Child will likely mature to expected height for their family.
    3. Growth hormone deficiency.
      (a) Due to deficiency in growth hormone–releasing factor from the hypothalamus or deficiency in human growth hormone from the anterior pituitary.
      (b) Children grow at a diminished velocity.
    4. Primary hypothyroidism.
      (a) Diagnose with an elevated TSH and low thyroid hormone.
    5. Chronic diseases.
      (a) Due to lack of caloric intake or absorption.
      (b) Seen in children with cystic fibrosis, diabetes mellitus, chronic renal failure, inflammatory bowel disease, and celiac disease.
    6. Chromosomal abnormalities.
      (a) Turner's syndrome.
      (b) Trisomy 21.
    7. Medications.
      (a) Chronic use of medications (such as steroids, dextroamphetamine, and methylphenidate) may result in poor growth.

b. **Dwarfism**
  i. General
    1. Prototype is achondroplasia.
    2. Majority of cases result from new gene mutations.
  ii. Clinical manifestations
    1. Physical examination reveals short limbs, long narrow trunk, large head with midface hypoplasia, and prominent brows.
    2. Patients have delayed developmental milestones and have normal intelligence.
  iii. Diagnosis
    1. Genetic testing: mutation in the FGFR3 gene.
  iv. Treatment
    1. Complications include neurologic complications, bowing of legs, obesity, dental problems, and frequent ear infections.
    2. Surgery utilized to correct orthopedic problems.
    3. Use of growth hormone is controversial.

## IV. SYNDROME OF INAPPROPRIATE ANTIDIURETIC HORMONE SECRETION (SIADH)

a. **General**
  i. Inability to suppress antidiuretic hormone (ADH) secretion from the posterior pituitary gland.
  ii. Multiple possible causes including cancer (commonly small cell lung), pulmonary infection (such as pneumonia or tuberculosis), CNS disturbances (such as subarachnoid hemorrhage, head trauma, or meningitis), drug use (such as AVP analogues, SSRIs, and antipsychotics), or may be idiopathic.

b. **Clinical Manifestations**
  i. A small amount of very concentrated urine (oliguria, increased urine osmolality).
  ii. Polydipsia.

c. **Diagnosis**
  i. Euvolemic hyponatremia, serum hypoosmolality, high urine sodium, high urine osmolality.
  ii. Exclude other possible causes of euvolemic hyponatremia.

**TABLE 5.10**

| **Causes of Short Stature** | | |
| --- | --- | --- |
| **Normal Causes** | **Pathologic Disproportionate** | **Pathologic Proportionate** |
| Familial (genetic) | Rickets | Prenatal |
| Constitutional | Achondroplasia | Intrauterine growth restriction |
| | | Placental dysfunction |
| | | Intrauterine infections |
| | | Teratogens |
| | | Chromosomal abnormalities (Turner's syndrome or trisomy 21) |
| | | Postnatal |
| | | Malnutrition |
| | | Chronic disease |
| | | Drugs |
| | | Growth hormone deficiency |
| | | Glucocorticoid excess |

d. **Management**
   i. Targeted at managing the underlying cause.
   ii. Cautious fluid restriction.
   ii. Vasopressin receptor antagonists.

## V. DIABETES INSIPIDUS

a. **General**
   i. Due to deficiency of or resistance to antidiuretic hormone (ADH; vasopressin).
   ii. Etiologies.
      1. Central diabetes insipidus: deficiency of ADH from the posterior pituitary.
         (a) Primary.
            (i) May be familial with no sign of organic lesion.
         (b) Secondary.
            (i) Due to damage to the hypothalamus.
      2. Nephrogenic diabetes insipidus.
         (a) Due to defects in kidney tubules that interfere with response to ADH and water reabsorption.

b. **Clinical Manifestations**
   i. Symptoms include intense thirst (craving for ice water) and polyuria.
      1. Volume of ingested fluid varies from 2 to 20 L, and equally large volumes of urine are produced.
   ii. May present with hypernatremia and dehydration.
   iii. Urine specific gravity typically less than 1.005.

c. **Diagnosis**
   i. Diagnosis based on clinical picture with polyuria and dehydration.
      1. There is no single laboratory test for diagnosis of diabetes insipidus.
   ii. Central diabetes insipidus (CDI): vasopressin challenge test.
      1. Positive test: administration of nasal vasopressin results in transient decrease in symptoms.
   iii. Nephrogenic diabetes insipidus (NDI): water deprivation test.
      1. Monitoring urine volume and serum and urine osmolality after three to six hours of water deprivation.
      2. Positive test: low urine osmolality (<300 mOsm/kg)
      3. Can further differentiate central and nephrogenic causes by administration of exogenous vasopressin and measuring urine osmolality 2 hours after.
         (a) CDI: rise in urine osmolality by 50% to 100%.
         (b) NDI: minimal rise (<50 mOsm/kg) in urine osmolality.

d. **Treatment**
   i. CDI: desmopressin acetate.
      1. Given intranasally as needed for thirst and polyuria.
   ii. Central and nephrogenic diabetes insipidus may respond to hydrochlorothiazide.
      1. Nephrogenic disease urine output can be lowered with low-salt, low-protein diet.
   iii. Avoid thioridazine and lithium as they may worsen polyuria.

## VI. HYPERPROLACTINEMIA

a. **General**
   i. Main role of prolactin is in lactation.
   ii. Prolactin plus the effects of estrogen and progesterone allow breast development to take place.
   iii. The control of the secretion of prolactin is under inhibitory control.
      1. Prolactin inhibitory factor (PIF) is dopamine.
   iv. Etiologies are in the following three groups:
      1. Physiologic: exercise, pregnancy, stress, and suckling.
      2. Pharmacologic: estrogens, cimetidine, ranitidine, methyldopa, metoclopramide, phenothiazine, protease inhibitors, risperidone, selective serotonin reuptake inhibitors (SSRIs), and tricyclic antidepressants.
      3. Pathologic: acromegaly, chronic chest wall stimulation, cirrhosis, hypothyroidism, prolactin-secreting tumors, renal failure, and systemic lupus erythematosus (SLE).

b. **Clinical Manifestations**
   i. More common in females and sporadic in nature.
   ii. Increased levels may result in hypogonadotropic hypogonadism.
      1. Men may have erectile dysfunction, gynecomastia, and decreased libido.
      2. Women may have oligomenorrhea or amenorrhea and galactorrhea (typically bilateral).
         (a) Unilateral galactorrhea is suspicious for breast disorder and malignancy must be ruled out.
   iii. Large tumors may cause headaches and visual deficits.

c. **Diagnosis**
   i. Rule out conditions known to cause hyperprolactinemia.
      1. Liver function tests for cirrhosis.
      2. Beta–human chorionic gonadotropin (beta-hCG) for pregnancy.
      3. TSH for hypothyroidism.

4. Blood urea nitrogen (BUN) and creatinine for renal failure.
   ii. MRI of the pituitary to evaluate for tumor.
d. **Treatment**
   i. Stop all medications known to increase prolactin levels if possible.
   ii. Dopamine agonists.
      1. Initial treatment of choice for patients with large tumors or for those desiring normal sexual function and fertility.
         (a) Cabergoline.
         (b) Bromocriptine.
      2. Side effects include fatigue, nausea, dizziness, and orthostatic hypotension.
   iii. Surgery.
      1. Reserved for large tumors causing visual symptoms.
   iv. Radiation therapy.
      1. Used to prevent regrowth of tumor after surgery.

## THYROID DISORDERS

### I. HYPERTHYROIDISM
a. **General**
   i. Etiologies include the following:
      1. Graves' disease.
         (a) Most common cause of hyperthyroidism.
         (b) Autoimmune so patients may have a history of other autoimmune conditions.
         (c) More common in females.
      2. Toxic nodules of the thyroid.
         (a) Typically noted in the elderly.
      3. Subacute thyroiditis.
      4. Pregnancy/trophoblastic tumors.
      5. Use of amiodarone (hypothyroidism more common).
b. **Graves' Disease**
   i. General
      1. The most common cause of hyperthyroidism.
      2. Has diffuse enlargement and hyperactivity of the thyroid gland and presence of antibodies against the gland.
         (a) Have formation of autoantibodies to TSH receptors that stimulates the gland to hyperfunction.
      3. More common in females and onset typically between ages 20 and 40.
      4. Associated with other autoimmune diseases.
   ii. Clinical manifestations

1. Patients present with signs and symptoms of hyperthyroidism (Table 5.11).
2. For Graves' disease: physical examination presents with pretibial myxedema, exophthalmos, lid lag, and hyperreflexia.
3. Goiter, often with a bruit, is noted.
4. Patients may present with atrial fibrillation.
   iii. Diagnosis
      1. Primary hyperthyroidism: Serum triiodothyronine ($T_3$), thyroxine ($T_4$), and free $T_4$ are increased with a decreased TSH.
      2. Secondary hyperthyroidism: Serum triiodothyronine ($T_3$), thyroxine ($T_4$), and free $T_4$ are increased with an increased TSH.
      3. Elevated thyroid-stimulating antibody.
   iv. Treatment
      1. Propranolol is used for treatment of symptoms until hyperthyroidism is resolved.
         (a) Symptoms include tachycardia, tremor, diaphoresis, anxiety, and palpitations.
      2. Thiourea drugs—methimazole and propylthiouracil (PTU)—are used to inhibit thyroid hormone synthesis.
         (a) PTU is safer in pregnancy.
      3. Radioactive iodine is used to destroy an overactive thyroid.
         (a) Avoid in pregnant patients.
         (b) Monitor for hypothyroidism
      4. Thyroid surgery, although not used widely, is usually preferred for pregnant patients.
c. **Thyroid Storm**
   i. General
      1. Rare, severe form of thyrotoxicosis.
      2. May occur with stressful illness, thyroid surgery, or radioactive iodine.
      3. Very high mortality rate.
   ii. Clinical manifestations
      1. Present with marked delirium, severe tachycardia, vomiting, diarrhea, dehydration, and high fever.
   iii. Diagnosis
      1. Elevated free $T_4$ and decreased TSH.

**TABLE 5.11**

| Signs and Symptoms of Hyperthyroidism | |
|---|---|
| Appetite change | Menstrual disturbances |
| Diarrhea | Nervousness |
| Exertional shortness of breath | Palpitations |
| Fatigue | Sleep disturbances |
| Headache | Sweating |
| Heat intolerance | Tremor |
| Hyperactivity | Weakness |
| Irritability | Weight loss |

iv. Treatment
1. Treatment consists of thiourea drug, iodide, propranolol, and steroids.
   (a) Avoid propranolol in patients with heart failure.
2. Avoid aspirin, as it will raise free $T_4$ levels by displacement of thyroid hormone from carrier proteins.
3. Treatment with radioactive iodide or surgery is undertaken when patient is euthyroid.

## II. HYPOTHYROIDISM
### a. General
i. Etiologies include the following:
1. Autoimmune (Hashimoto's) thyroiditis.
   (a) Most common cause of hypothyroidism.
   (b) More common in females.
2. Post-ablative hypothyroidism.
3. Drug-induced: lithium, sulfonamides, amiodarone.
4. Iodine deficiency.
   (a) Not common in the United States due to fortification of table salt with iodine.
ii. Myxedema coma.
1. Hypothyroidism precipitated by an acute illness or trauma.
   (a) Very high mortality rate.
2. Patients present with signs and symptoms of hypothyroidism, hypothermia, and impaired mentation.
3. Laboratory results include decreased T3 and T4, elevated TSH, hyponatremia, and hypoglycemia.
4. Treatment is IV levothyroxine.

### b. Clinical Manifestations
i. Signs and symptoms of hypothyroidism (Table 5.12).
ii. Physical examination reveals dry, coarse skin; thin, brittle nails; thinning hair and lateral half of eyebrows; bradycardia; and delayed return of deep tendon reflexes.

### c. Diagnosis
i. Primary hypothyroidism: Serum triiodothyronine ($T_3$), thyroxine ($T_4$), and free $T_4$ are decreased with an increased TSH.
ii. Secondary hypothyroidism: Serum triiodothyronine ($T_3$), thyroxine ($T_4$), and free $T_4$ are decreased with a decreased TSH.
iii. Patients with Hashimoto's thyroiditis have high titers for antibodies to thyroid peroxidase and thyroglobulin.
iv. Table 5.13 interprets thyroid function tests.

### d. Treatment
i. Thyroid supplement with levothyroxine.
1. Smaller initial doses with slow titration should be started in the elderly and in patients with coronary artery disease.
2. Recheck thyroid hormone and TSH levels in 4 to 6 weeks.

## III. THYROIDITIS
### a. General
i. Classified as follows:
1. Lymphocytic thyroiditis.
   (a) More common in postpartum females.
2. Subacute thyroiditis.
   (a) More common in young and middle-aged females.
   (b) Viral infection suggested as the cause.
3. Infectious thyroiditis.
   (a) Bacterial infection caused by infection with *Staphylococcus* and *Streptococcus*.

### b. Clinical Manifestations
i. Lymphocytic thyroiditis presents with fatigue; weight loss; anxiety; and a nontender, modestly enlarged thyroid.
ii. Subacute thyroiditis presents with a painful, "woody," and enlarged thyroid.
iii. Infectious thyroiditis presents with a very painful, tender, red thyroid gland and with fever.

**TABLE 5.12**

| Signs and Symptoms of Hypothyroidism | |
|---|---|
| Arthralgias | Fatigue |
| Cold intolerance | Lethargy |
| Constipation | Menstrual disturbances |
| Decreased appetite | Muscle cramps |
| Decreased memory | Paresthesias |
| Decreased perspiration | Sleepiness |
| Depression | Weight gain |
| Dry skin | |

**TABLE 5.13**

| Thyroid Function Test Interpretation | | |
|---|---|---|
| | Thyroid-Stimulating Hormone Level | Thyroid Hormone Level |
| Overt hyperthyroidism | Low or undetectable | Elevated FT$_4$ or FT$_3$ |
| Subclinical hyperthyroidism | Low or undetectable | Normal FT$_4$ or FT$_3$ |
| Overt hypothyroidism | elevated (>5 mIU/L) | Low FT$_4$ |
| Subclinical hypothyroidism | elevated (>5 mIU/L) | Normal FT$_4$ |

*FT$_4$*, Free thyroxine; *FT$_3$*, free triiodothyronine.

c. **Diagnosis**
   i. Thyroid antibodies present in chronic lymphocytic (Hashimoto's) thyroiditis.
   ii. Radioactive iodide uptake is low in subacute thyroiditis.

d. **Treatment**
   i. Lymphocytic thyroiditis: observation and beta-blockers for symptom reduction.
   ii. Subacute thyroiditis: aspirin or NSAIDs for pain and inflammation.
   iii. Infectious thyroiditis: antibiotics and surgical drainage if needed.

## VI. NEOPLASTIC DISEASE

a. **General**
   i. Almost always manifests as a palpable thyroid nodule.
   ii. Cause of thyroid cancer is unknown.
   iii. Risk factors include radiation to the head and neck, as well as genetic causes.
   iv. Twice as common in females than males, but males have a worse prognosis.
   v. Papillary carcinoma is the most common type and is the least aggressive.
   vi. Other types include medullary, follicular, and anaplastic.
      1. Medullary thyroid cancer is very common in MEN 2a and 2b and has close to 100% penetrance with MEN 2b.

b. **Clinical Manifestations**
   i. May present with dysphagia or hoarseness (secondary to compression of the left recurrent laryngeal nerve).
   ii. May be asymptomatic with a single, hard nodule that is showing rapid, painless growth.
      1. Cancer more likely etiology of a thyroid nodule in a child or in a patient older than age 60.

c. **Diagnosis**
   i. Thyroid hormone levels are typically normal.
   ii. An iodine-123 ($^{123}$I) scan will reveal a thyroid nodule that is cold.
   iii. Diagnosis is based on cytology findings of a fine-needle aspiration of the thyroid.
   iv. Thyroid ultrasound can also be helpful to determine if nodule is cystic or fluid filled.

d. **Treatment**
   i. Thyroid surgery—a lobectomy or near-total thyroidectomy—is indicated.
   ii. $^{123}$I ablation is used in patients who have undergone a near-total thyroidectomy to destroy the remainder of the thyroid gland.
   iii. Thyroid replacement hormone (levothyroxine) is needed after thyroidectomy.

# QUESTIONS

## QUESTION 1
Which of the following presents with truncal fat distribution, moon facies, and hypertension?
A Hypoparathyroidism
B Cushing's disease
C Graves' disease
D Pheochromocytoma
E Diabetes mellitus type 2

## QUESTION 2
A 45-year-old patient presents with a history of weakness, orthostatic hypotension, and hyperpigmentation. Which of the following laboratory tests would assist in making the correct diagnosis?
A 24-hour urine test for catecholamines
B Glucose tolerance test
C ACTH level
D GH level
E TSH

## QUESTION 3
A 35-year-old female presents for evaluation of headache, vision changes, and delayed menses. On physical examination, bitemporal homonymous hemianopsia by confrontation is noted along with nipple discharge. Her pelvic examination is normal. Which of the following is the most likely diagnosis?
A Ovarian failure
B Hypothyroidism
C Addison's disease
D Pituitary adenoma
E Panhypopituitarism

# QUESTIONS—cont'd

## QUESTION 4

A 55-year-old patient presents with severe palpitations and fever. Thyroid studies reveal an elevated free $T_4$ and a TSH level that is undetectable. Which of the following is the most appropriate management of this patient pending further evaluation?

A Aspirin

B Synthroid

C Propranolol (Inderal)

D Cardiac pacing

E No treatment is indicated

## QUESTION 5

A 50-year-old female presents with a change in mental status and agitation. Physical examination reveals a temperature of 104.5° F and a heart rate of 130/minute, and a tremor is noted. Which of the following treatment options would be most helpful to this patient?

A Levodopa

B Lamotrigine

C Bromocriptine

D Propylthiouracil

E Fluoroquinolone

## QUESTION 6

In a patient with diabetes, the daily protein intake should be limited to what percent of total calories?

A 5% to 10%

B 10% to 20%

C 20% to 30%

D 30% to 40%

E 40% to 50%

## QUESTION 7

Which of the following inhibits ACTH secretion?

A Aldosterone

B Cortisol

C Glucose

D Calcium

E Dopamine

## QUESTION 8

Which of the following clinical features is noted in Cushing's syndrome?

A Hypopigmentation

B Diaphoresis

C Weight loss

D Thick skin

E Striae

## QUESTION 9

A 24-year-old female presents with short stature, round face, and obesity. Physical examination reveals shortening of the fourth and fifth digits on both hands, shortening of the fourth toes on each foot, and hypogonadism. Which of the following is the most likely diagnosis?

A Albright's osteodystrophy

B Cushing's disease

C Carcinoid syndrome

D Fanconi's syndrome

E Achondroplasia

# ANSWERS

**1. B**

EXPLANATION: Cushing's disease or syndrome typically presents with centripetal weight gain, moon facies, striae, hypertension, and proximal muscle weakness. ***Topic: Cushing's syndrome***

☐ Correct   ☐ Incorrect

**2. C**

EXPLANATION: Patients with Addison's disease (acute corticoadrenal insufficiency) present with headache and abdominal pain. On physical examination, orthostatic hypotension and hyperpigmentation are noted. Plasma ACTH levels are elevated in primary disease, and diagnosis can be made by cosyntropin stimulation test. ***Topic: Acute corticoadrenal insufficiency***

☐ Correct   ☐ Incorrect

**3. D**

EXPLANATION: Large pituitary adenomas present with headache and visual changes. Production of increased amounts of prolactin will lead to nipple discharge. ***Topic: Hyperprolactinemia***

☐ Correct   ☐ Incorrect

**4. C**

EXPLANATION: Hyperthyroidism presents with palpitations, diarrhea, fever, and other signs of increased metabolism. Laboratory testing reveals an elevated $T_4$ and decreased TSH. Early treatment consists of symptomatic control, such as beta-blockers (propranolol) for control of palpitations. Aspirin is contraindicated because it causes increased release of thyroid hormone. ***Topic: Hyperthyroidism***

☐ Correct   ☐ Incorrect

*Continued*

## ANSWERS—cont'd

**5.  D**

EXPLANATION: Thyroid storm symptoms include high fever, tachycardia, restlessness, agitation, tremor, and change in mental status. Treatment consists of propylthiouracil (PTU) or sodium iodide to inhibit thyroid hormone formation, propranolol for sympathetic blockage, hydrocortisone, and supportive therapy with IV fluids and oxygen. Must also treat the precipitating event. *Topic: Hyperthyroidism: thyroid storm*
☐ Correct    ☐ Incorrect

**6.  B**

EXPLANATION: Dietary management is important in the management of the diabetic patient. Cholesterol should be limited to 300 mg/day, protein limited to 10% to 20% of total calories, saturated fats restricted to 10% of total calories, and sodium restricted to less than 2.4 g/day. *Topic: Diabetes mellitus*
☐ Correct    ☐ Incorrect

**7.  B**

EXPLANATION: ACTH is released by the anterior pituitary and leads to the release of cortisol. Release is suppressed by negative feedback of cortisol. *Topic: Adrenal disorders*
☐ Correct    ☐ Incorrect

**8.  E**

EXPLANATION: Patients with Cushing's syndrome present with central obesity with a "moon face," thin extremities, muscle wasting, thinning of the skin, hirsutism, and purple striae. *Topic: Adrenal disorders*
☐ Correct    ☐ Incorrect

**9.  A**

EXPLANATION: Albright's osteodystrophy is a form of hypoparathyroidism that presents with obesity, short stature, round face, and short neck. Metacarpal and metatarsal shortening is also noted. *Topic: Hypoparathyroidism*
☐ Correct    ☐ Incorrect

# CHAPTER 6
# Eyes, Ears, Nose, and Throat System

## EXAMINATION BLUEPRINT TOPICS

**EYE DISORDERS**

**CONJUNCTIVAL DISORDERS**

Conjunctivitis

**CORNEAL DISORDERS**

Cataract

Corneal ulcer

Infectious

Keratitis

Pterygium

**LACRIMAL DISORDERS**

Dacryoadenitis/Dacryocystitis

**LID DISORDERS**

Blepharitis

Chalazion

Ectropion

Entropion

Hordeolum (stye)

**NEURO-OPHTHALMOLOGIC DISORDERS**

Nystagmus

Optic neuritis

Papilledema

**ORBITAL DISORDERS**

Orbital cellulitis

**RETINAL DISORDERS**

Macular degeneration

Retinal detachment

Retinopathy

**TRAUMATIC DISORDERS**

Blowout fracture

Foreign body

Corneal abrasion

Globe rupture

Hyphema

**VASCULAR DISORDERS**

Retinal vascular occlusion

**VISION ABNORMALITIES**

Amaurosis fugax

Amblyopia

Glaucoma

Scleritis

Strabismus

**EAR DISORDERS**

**EXTERNAL EAR**

Cerumen impaction

Otitis externa

Trauma

**INNER EAR**

Acoustic neuroma

Barotrauma

Dysfunction of eustachian tube

Labyrinthitis

Vertigo

**MIDDLE EAR**

Cholesteatoma

Otitis media

Tympanic membrane perforation

**HEARING IMPAIRMENT**

**OTHER ABNORMALITIES OF THE EAR**

Mastoiditis

Ménière's disease

Tinnitus

Foreign body: Ear

**NOSE/SINUS DISORDERS**

Epistaxis

Nasal polyps

Rhinitis

Acute sinusitis

Chronic sinusitis

Trauma

Foreign body: Nose

**OROPHARYNGEAL DISORDERS**

**DISEASES OF THE TEETH/GUMS**

Dental abscess

Gingivitis

**INFECTIOUS/INFLAMMATORY DISORDERS**

Aphthous ulcers

Oral candidiasis

Deep neck infection

Epiglottitis

Herpes simplex

Laryngitis

Peritonsillar abscess

Pharyngitis

**SALIVARY DISORDERS**

Sialadenitis

Parotitis

**TRAUMA**

Tooth Avulsion

**OTHER OROPHARYNGEAL DISORDERS**

Leukoplakia

**NEOPLASMS**

Oral cancer

# EYE DISORDERS

## CONJUNCTIVAL DISORDERS

### I. CONJUNCTIVITIS
  a. **General**
  i. Inflammation of the conjunctiva.
  ii. Etiologies.
  1. Bacterial.
   (a) *Streptococcus pneumoniae.*
   (b) *Haemophilus influenzae.*
   (c) *Staphylococcus aureus.*
   (d) *Moraxella catarrhalis.*
   (e) *Neisseria gonorrhoeae.*
   (f) *Chlamydia trachomatis.*
  2. Viral.
   (a) Adenovirus most common.
   (b) Herpes simplex virus types 1 and 2.
  3. Allergic.
  4. Chemical.
  5. Irritative.
  b. **Clinical Manifestations**
  i. Symptoms include foreign body sensation, a scratching or burning sensation, itching, and photophobia.
  ii. On physical examination, note hyperemia, tearing, exudate with eyelid mattering, and pseudoptosis.
  iii. Vision is normal.
  1. Examination findings vary depending on etiology.
   (a) Table 6.1 compares signs and symptoms of conjunctivitis.
   (b) Table 6.2 compares etiologies of the red eye.
  c. **Treatment**
  i. Bacterial.
  1. Typically self-limiting, lasting 7 to 10 days.
   (a) If treated, will last 1 to 3 days.
  2. Topical broad-spectrum antibiotics (e.g., erythromycin ointment, trimethoprim-polymyxin B, or fluoroquinolones).

  3. For contact lens wearers, cover for *Pseudomonas* (e.g., topical ciprofloxacin or ofloxacin).
  4. *N. gonorrhoeae* can treat with intramuscular (IM) ceftriaxone.
  5. *Chlamydia trachomatis* can treat with oral tetracycline, doxycycline, erythromycin, and/or azithromycin. Topical tetracycline can be used.
  iii. Viral.
  1. No specific treatment.
  2. Herpes conjunctivitis should be treated with antivirals (acyclovir) to prevent corneal involvement.
  iv. Allergic.
  1. Topical antihistamines (e.g., Olopatadine, Pheniramine-Naphazoline)
  2. A short course of topical or oral steroids may be indicated.

## CORNEAL DISORDERS

### I. CATARACT
  a. **General**
  i. Any opacity in the lens, with aging being the most common cause.
  1. Other causes include trauma (foreign body or blunt force), systemic disease (diabetes), smoking, congenital, and drugs (steroids).
  2. Most common in patients 60 years and older.
  ii. Due to protein that aggregates in the lens, scattering light and reducing transparency.
  1. A yellow-brown color may be noted due to these proteins.
  b. **Clinical Manifestations**
  i. Patients present with the following:
  1. Painless blurry vision or vision loss.
  2. Glare.
  3. Myopia.
  4. Monocular double vision.
  5. Absent red reflex.
  6. Leukocoria.

**TABLE 6.1**

| Signs and Symptoms of Conjunctivitis | | | | |
| --- | --- | --- | --- | --- |
| **Signs and Symptoms** | **Bacterial** | **Viral** | **Chlamydial** | **Allergic** |
| Itching | Minimal | Minimal | Minimal | Severe |
| Hyperemia | Generalized: bright red | Generalized | Generalized | Generalized: milky |
| Tearing | Moderate | Profuse | Moderate | Moderate |
| Discharge | Profuse/Purulent | Minimal/Watery | Profuse | Minimal/Watery |
| Preauricular adenopathy | Uncommon | Common | Varies | None |
| Sore throat and fever | Occasionally | Occasionally | Never | Never |

**TABLE 6.2**

**Etiologies of the Red Eye**

| Factor | Allergic Conjunctivitis | Bacterial Conjunctivitis | Viral Conjunctivitis | Corneal Ulcer | Anterior Uveitis | Acute Glaucoma | Anterior Scleritis |
|---|---|---|---|---|---|---|---|
| Symptoms/ Signs | Bilateral, itchy eyes | No itching or adenopathy | Itching, preauricular adenopathy | Irregular corneal light reflex | Photophobia, ciliary flush | Headache, nausea, vomiting | Pain, worse at night |
| Vision | Normal | Normal | May be impaired | Impaired | Slightly blurred | Decreased | Normal |
| Discharge | Watery | Mucopurulent | Watery | None | Tearing | Tearing | None |
| Pain | None | Minimal | Minimal | Present | Photophobia | Severe | Severe |
| Pupil size | Normal | Normal | Normal | Normal | Miotic | Mid-dilated | Normal |
| Pupillary response | Normal | Normal | Normal | Normal | Nonreactive | Nonreactive | Normal |
| Redness | Diffuse | Diffuse | Segmental or diffuse | Localized or diffuse | Ciliary flush | Diffuse with ciliary flush | Local or diffuse |
| Management | Topical antihistamines | Topical antibiotics | Supportive | Topical cycloplegics Topical antibiotics | Topical steroids | Laser Surgical iridectomy | Steroids NSAIDs |

c. **Diagnosis**
  i. Measure visual acuity to determine impairment of vision.
  ii. Slit-lamp examination needed.
d. **Treatment**
  i. Surgical treatment, with or without lens implant, is the definitive treatment.

## II. CORNEAL ULCER
a. **General**
  i. Cornea ulceration as a result of direct injury to the eye, or from a bacterial, fungal, or viral infection.
  ii. Risk factors include contact lens use, dry eyes, inability to close the eye, immunocompromised.
b. **Clinical Manifestations**
  i. Patients may present with eye redness, eye pain, excessive tearing, sensation of a foreign body in the eye, and worsening or blurry vision.
  ii. Table 6.2 compares etiologies of the red eye.
c. **Diagnosis**
  i. Ciliary injection (limbal flush), erythema, corneal opacification.
  ii. Examine with slit lamp; increased fluorescein uptake.
d. **Treatment**
  i. Vision-threatening eye emergency; send to ophthalmologist immediately.
  ii. Do not need to patch the eye.

## III. INFECTIOUS
a. **General**
  i. Corneal ulceration or inflammation caused by bacterial or viral infections.
  ii. More common with contact lens wear.
  iii. Recent outbreak of shingles, chickenpox, or cold sores.
b. **Clinical Manifestations**
  i. Patients may present with eye redness, eye pain, excessive tearing, sensation of a foreign body in the eye, and worsening or blurry vision.
c. **Diagnosis**
  i. Ciliary injection (limbal flush), erythema, corneal opacification.
  ii. Fluorescein staining to evaluate for epithelial defect.
  iii. Obtain cultures if possible.
d. **Treatment**
  i. Vision-threatening eye emergency; send to ophthalmologist immediately.
  ii. Topical fluoroquinolones for bacterial source.
  iii. Topical antivirals (acyclovir or ganciclovir ointment) or oral antivirals (acyclovir, valacyclovir) for viral cause.
  iii. Do not patch the eye.

## IV. KERATITIS
a. **General**
  i. Characterized by inflammation of the cornea.
  ii. May or may not be associated with infectious cause.

1. Causes include minor injury, contact lens overuse, foreign body.
2. Infectious causes include bacteria, viruses, fungi, and parasites.

b. **Clinical Manifestations**
   i. Eye redness, eye pain, excess tears, discharge, blurred or decreased vision, photophobia, foreign body sensation.
   ii. May progress to corneal ulcer if untreated.

c. **Diagnosis**
   i. Test visual acuity.
   ii. Fluorescein staining needed to evaluate for epithelial defect.
      1. Dendritic branching seen in reactivation of herpes simplex virus.
   iii. Corneal cultures.

d. **Treatment**
   i. Noninfectious causes, treat symptomatically.
   ii. Topical fluoroquinolones for bacterial source.
   iii. Topical antivirals (acyclovir or ganciclovir ointment) or oral antivirals (acyclovir, valacyclovir) for viral cause.

### V. PTERYGIUM

a. **General**
   i. A fleshy, triangular encroachment onto the cornea.
   ii. Typically bilateral and on the nasal side.
   iii. Due to irritation secondary to ultraviolet light, drying, and wind.

b. **Clinical Manifestations**
   i. On physical examination, note triangular lesion on the nasal side of the cornea.

c. **Treatment**
   i. If large, may be removed surgically.

## LACRIMAL DISORDERS

### I. DACRYOADENITIS/DACRYOCYSTITIS

a. **General**
   i. Dacryoadenitis is acute inflammation of the lacrimal gland.
      1. Rare condition seen in children (as a complication of mumps, measles, or influenza) or in adults (associated with gonorrhea).
   ii. Dacryocystitis is infection of the lacrimal sac.
      1. Occurs more commonly in infants and older females.
      2. Is unilateral and due to obstruction of the nasolacrimal duct.
      3. Common infectious agents include *H. influenzae*, *S. aureus*, and beta-hemolytic *Streptococcus*.

b. **Clinical Manifestations**
   i. Dacryoadenitis presents with severe pain, swelling, and injection over the temporal aspect of the upper eyelid.
   ii. Dacryocystitis presents with tearing and discharge. Inflammation, pain, swelling, and tenderness are noted in medial side of the lower lid.

c. **Treatment**
   i. Dacryoadenitis is observed, treated with antibiotics if needed.
      1. Surgery is rarely needed.
   ii. Dacryocystitis is treated with oral antibiotics and warm compresses.

## LID DISORDERS

### I. BLEPHARITIS

a. **General**
   i. Inflammation of the eyelid margin.
   ii. Anterior blepharitis is a chronic bilateral inflammation of the base of the eyelids.
      1. Two types.
         (a) Infectious.
            (i) Due to *S. aureus* or *S. epidermidis*.
         (b) Seborrheic.
   iii. Posterior blepharitis is inflammation of the eyelids secondary to dysfunction of the meibomian glands.
      1. More common than anterior blepharitis.
      2. A bilateral chronic condition.

b. **Clinical Manifestations**
   i. Major symptoms include irritation, burning, tearing, and itching of the eyelids.
   ii. The eyes are red-rimmed, and many scales are noted on the upper and lower lashes.
      1. In staphylococcal, the scales are dry and the lids red.
      2. In seborrheic, the scales are greasy and lid margins less red.

c. **Treatment**
   i. Eyelids and lid margins should be kept clean.
   ii. Staphylococcal infection is treated with antistaphylococcal antibiotics or sulfonamide eye ointment.
   iii. Posterior blepharitis is typically treated with systemic antibiotics, doxycycline or erythromycin, and a weak topical steroid.

### II. CHALAZION

a. **General**
   i. Idiopathic, sterile chronic granulomatous inflammation of the meibomian gland.

b. **Clinical Manifestations**
   i. Painless, localized, rubbery nodule that develops over a week.
      1. Swelling points to the conjunctival surface.
   ii. No acute inflammatory signs.
c. **Treatment**
   i. Small lesions resolve without intervention.
   ii. Intralesional steroid injections may be used in small lesions.
   iii. Surgical excision with removal of the material may be needed if refractory.

### III. ECTROPION
a. **General**
   i. Sagging and eversion (turn outward) of the lower lid.
   ii. Typically bilateral and noted in the elderly.
   iii. Caused by relaxation of the orbicularis oculi muscle.
b. **Clinical Manifestations**
   i. Symptoms include tearing and irritation.
   ii. On examination, note sagging and eversion of the lid.
c. **Treatment**
   i. Lubricating drops for symptomatic relief.
   ii. Treated surgically with horizontal shortening of the lid.

### IV. ENTROPION
a. **General**
   i. Turning inward of the lower lid due to laxity of the lower lid muscles.
b. **Clinical Manifestations**
   i. Lower lid is inverted inward.
   ii. Eyelashes may impinge on cornea and cause ulcerations.
c. **Treatment**
   i. Lubricating drops for symptomatic relief.
   ii. Treated surgically to evert the lid.

### V. HORDEOLUM (STYE)
a. **General**
   i. Infection of the glands of the eyelid.
   ii. Most are caused by infection with staphylococcal species.
b. **Clinical Manifestations**
   i. Symptoms include pain, redness, and swelling.
   ii. Internal hordeolum may point toward the skin or conjunctiva.
   iii. External hordeolum always points toward the skin.
c. **Treatment**
   i. Warm compressions to area three to four times a day.

   ii. If no improvement in 48 hours, incision and drainage may be needed.
   iii. Antibiotic ointment may be helpful.

## NEURO-OPHTHALMOLOGIC DISORDERS

### I. NYSTAGMUS
a. **General**
   i. Is the rhythmic regular oscillation of the eyes.
   ii. Major symptoms include vertigo, oscillopsia, and blurred vision.
b. **Clinical Manifestations**
   i. Pathologic nystagmus.
      1. Central nystagmus noted with lesions of the cerebellum. Vestibular organs are normal.
      2. Peripheral nystagmus noted in disease related to vestibular organs.
c. **Etiologies**
   i. Disease such as brain tumors, head trauma, multiple sclerosis, benign paroxysmal positional vertigo, and Ménière's disease.
   ii. Toxins such as alcohol, benzodiazepines, lithium, phenytoin, and salicylates.
d. **Treatment**
   i. Treat underlying cause.

### II. OPTIC NEURITIS
a. **General**
   i. An inflammatory, demyelinating disease of optic nerve that causes acute vision loss.
   ii. Typically monocular.
   iii. Highly associated with multiple sclerosis.
b. **Clinical Manifestations**
   i. Vision loss, visual field defects, or decrease in color vision develops over days to weeks.
   ii. Eye pain, worse with eye movement.
   iii. Afferent pupillary defect (Marcus-Gunn pupil).
c. **Treatment**
   i. Treat underlying cause. MRI to confirm diagnosis and assess for multiple sclerosis.
   ii. IV corticosteroids.

### III. PAPILLEDEMA
a. **General**
   i. Optic nerve swelling due to increased intracranial pressure.
b. **Etiologies**
   i. Intracranial mass lesions.
   ii. Cerebral edema.
   iii. Increased cerebrospinal fluid (CSF) production.
   iv. Decreased CSF absorption.
   v. Obstructive hydrocephalus.
   vi. Pseudotumor cerebri.

c. **Clinical**
  i. Optic disk is elevated, and cup may be obliterated.
  ii. Disk margins become obscured.
  iii. Other symptoms, such as headache, are noted as causes of papilledema.
d. **Treatment**
  i. Treat underlying cause.
  ii. Acetazolamide decreases production of aqueous humor and CSF.

# ORBITAL DISORDERS

## I. ORBITAL CELLULITIS
a. **General**
  i. Occurs most commonly in children.
  ii. May be the result of trauma or extension of sinusitis through the ethmoid sinus to the orbit.
  iii. Most common organisms are *S. aureus*, streptococci and *H. influenzae*.
  iv. Infection of the content of the orbit.
b. **Clinical Manifestations**
  i. Children may present with proptosis.
  ii. Present with edema, erythema, hyperemia, and pain.
    1. Infection may spread rapidly.
  iii. Physical examination in post septal reveals chemosis, limited eye movements, reduction of vision, and erythema.
    1. Preseptal cellulitis presents with swelling and pain (not worse with eye movements), and normal visual acuity.
  iv. Laboratory testing reveals leukocytosis.
c. **Diagnosis**
  i. CT scan or MRI needed to separate preseptal from postseptal involvement.
d. **Treatment**
  i. IV antibiotics are required for post-septal cellulitis. Include vancomycin plus ceftriaxone, cefotaxime, ampicillin-sulbactam, or piperacillin-tazobactam.
    1. Surgical drainage is indicated if optic nerve function worsens even with antibiotics.
  ii. Oral antibiotics for preseptal cellulitis: Trimethoprim-sulfamethoxazole or clindamycin plus amoxicillin, amoxicillin-clavulanic, or cefdinir.

# RETINAL DISORDERS

## I. MACULAR DEGENERATION
a. **General**
  i. Age-related macular degeneration is the leading cause of permanent blindness in the elderly.
  ii. Causes central vision loss.
  iii. Two types.
    1. Atrophic (dry): most common, progresses over decades.
    2. Exudative (wet): choroidal neovascularization that leaks blood and fluid into macula; more aggressive (progresses over months).
b. **Clinical Manifestations**
  i. In atrophic (dry) degeneration, drusen are noted in an ophthalmoscopic examination.
    1. Drusen are discrete, round, yellow-white deposits beneath the pigment epithelium and scattered throughout the macula.
    2. Visual impairment is variable.
      1. Metamorphopsia: straight lines appear bent.
  ii. In exudative (wet) degeneration vision loss is severe.
    1. Neovascularization may be noted on ophthalmoscopic examination.
c. **Treatment**
  i. Atrophic degeneration.
    1. Monitor for loss of central vision with Amsler grid.
    2. Antioxidants and vitamins with zinc may slow progression.
  ii. Exudative degeneration.
    1. Intravitreous injection of a vascular endothelial growth factor inhibitor (e.g., bevacizumab).
    2. Laser photocoagulation is needed if neovascularization is present.

## II. RETINAL DETACHMENT
a. **General**
  i. Separation of the sensory retina from the underlying pigmented epithelium.
    1. Unilateral vision changes.
  ii. Caused by trauma or can be spontaneous.
  iii. Most commonly in people over age 50 with severe myopia or history of cataract surgery.
b. **Clinical Manifestations**
  i. Patient may state that a curtain came down over their eye.
  ii. Flashes and floaters may be noted, vision is blurry and progressively worsens.
  iii. On funduscopic examination, the retina is noted hanging in the vitreous fluid.
    1. Shafer's sign: brown-colored pigment clumps of vitreous cells in anterior vitreous humor.
c. **Treatment**
  i. Ophthalmologic emergency, immediate referral needed.
  ii. Keep patient supine with head turned to side of detachment so that gravity helps the portion of the retina fall back into place.

iii. Photocoagulation or cryotherapy may be needed to correct the tear.

## III. RETINOPATHY
a. **Diabetic**
   i. General
      1. Changes in retinal vessels lead to microaneurysms, neovascularization, hemorrhages, and edema.
      2. Occurs faster in diabetes type 2 than type 1.
      3. Classified as either proliferative or nonproliferative.
   ii. Clinical manifestations
      1. Varies with classification.
         (a) Proliferative.
            (i) Neovascularization.
            (ii) Hemorrhage in the vitreous body.
            (iii) May lead to retinal detachment.
         (b) Nonproliferative.
            (i) Venous dilation.
            (ii) Microaneurysms.
            (iii) Retinal hemorrhages.
            (iv) Edema.
            (v) Hard exudates.
      2. See Color Plate 2 for funduscopic view in diabetic retinopathy.
   iii. Diagnosis
      1. Based on history and funduscopic examination.
   iv. Treatment
      1. Management of blood sugar and blood pressure is vital.
      2. Yearly ophthalmoscopic examination is needed for patients with diabetes.
      3. Neovascularization is treated with laser photocoagulation.
      4. Laser surgery for macular edema.
b. **Hypertensive**
   i. General
      1. Due to systemic hypertension.
   ii. Clinical manifestations
      1. Vision is impaired.
      2. On funduscopic examination, note the following:
         (a) Silver or copper wiring.
         (b) Arteriovenous (AV) nicking.
         (c) Flame-shaped hemorrhages.
         (d) Cotton-wool spots.
         (e) Retinal edema.
         (f) Retinal pigmentation.
   iii. Diagnosis
      1. Based on history and physical examination findings.
   iv. Treatment
      1. Will have improvement with blood pressure control.

## TRAUMATIC DISORDERS

### I. BLOWOUT FRACTURE
a. **General**
   i. Occurs with blunt force to the globe or orbit rim.
   ii. Inferior "floor" blowout fractures are the most common.
b. **Clinical Manifestations**
   i. Infraorbital anesthesia is common.
      1. Anesthesia of the maxillary teeth and upper lip is common.
   ii. Diplopia is common.
      1. If noted on upward gaze the inferior rectus muscle is entrapped.
   iii. A step-off deformity may be palpated over the intraorbital ridge.
   iv. Enophthalmos is rare.
c. **Diagnosis**
   i. Plain x-ray films may note hanging teardrop sign (herniation of orbital fat into the maxillary sinus) or bone fragments in the sinus.
   ii. Computed tomography (CT) scan of the orbit is needed to confirm diagnosis and to determine extent of damage.
d. **Treatment**
   i. Nasal decongestants and corticosteroids to reduce pain and swelling, antibiotics. Avoid nose blowing or sneezing.
   ii. Surgical repair is required if present with enophthalmos or persistent diplopia.

### II. FOREIGN BODY
a. **Clinical Manifestations**
   i. Surface foreign bodies present with pain and irritation that are noted with eye movement.
   ii. Intraocular foreign bodies present with discomfort or blurry vision.
      1. A history of striking metal, explosion, or projectile injury is typically present.
b. **Diagnosis**
   i. Visual acuity should be determined on all patients.
   ii. With intraocular foreign bodies, a slit lamp should be used to locate site of entry.
      1. CT scan or plain film x-ray should be done to identify radiopaque particles.
      2. Magnetic resonance imaging (MRI) is contraindicated.
c. **Treatment**
   i. For removal of the surface foreign body, a topical anesthetic and a swab or fine-gauge needle are used to remove the foreign body.
      1. Topical anesthetic should not be used long term.
      2. Steroids should also be avoided.

ii. Intraocular foreign bodies should be removed by an ophthalmologist whenever possible.

iii. Metallic rings surrounding copper or iron fragments can be removed with a drill that has a burr tip.

iv. After removal, antibiotic (erythromycin) ointment should be applied and the eye pressure patched.

v. All patients should be seen within 48 hours by an ophthalmologist.

## III. CORNEAL ABRASION

a. **General**

   i. Traumatic erosion of the corneal surface.

   ii. Secondary to trauma or contact lens wear.

b. **Clinical Manifestations**

   i. Patients present with pain, tearing, and photophobia.

   ii. A foreign body sensation is typically noted.

c. **Diagnosis**

   i. Must test visual acuity.

      1. May need topical anesthetic to facilitate visual acuity testing.

   ii. Fluorescein staining needed to evaluate for epithelial defect.

d. **Treatment**

   i. Most heal spontaneously within 48 hours.

   ii. Pain control with a cycloplegic, such as cyclopentolate or scopolamine, and oral analgesic.

   iii. Erythromycin ointment, sulfacetamide, polymyxin/trimethoprim, or ciprofloxacin may be needed.

      1. Abrasions from organic material or soft contact lenses should not be patched.

      2. Soft contact wearers are at risk of infection with *Pseudomonas* and should be treated with fluoroquinolone or tobramycin.

   iv. Follow up in 48 hours and avoid contact lenses for 1 week after healing.

## IV. GLOBE RUPTURE

a. **General**

   i. Occurs when the outer membranes of the eye are penetrated by trauma.

b. **Clinical Manifestations**

   i. Reduced vision.

c. **Diagnosis**

   i. Physical examination:

      1. Enophthalmos or exophthalmos.

      2. May have severe conjunctival hemorrhage.

      3. Teardrop or irregularly shaped pupil.

   ii. Fluorescein staining: positive Seidel's test (fluorescein dye parted by clear stream of aqueous humor).

d. **Treatment**

   i. Leave impaled objects, protect with rigid eye shield.

   ii. Emergency ophthalmology consult.

   iii. IV antibiotics. Avoid topical eye solutions. May need tetanus prophylaxis.

## V. HYPHEMA

a. **General**

   i. Traumatic forces tear vessels, which bleed into the aqueous humor.

   ii. Rule out globe rupture.

b. **Clinical Manifestations**

   i. Blood may settle out into a visible layer.

   ii. Vision loss, photophobia, and eye pain may be noted.

   iii. Increased intraocular pressure.

c. **Treatment**

   i. Eye shield and bed rest.

   ii. Will resolve by spontaneous absorption. Elevate head of bed to 30 degrees to reduce staining of the cornea.

   iii. Topical glucocorticoids reduce risk of bleeding. Topical tetracaine may help with pain.

   iv. Can lead to permanent vision loss.

   v. Admit if large hyphemia (50% or more of anterior chamber) or patients with bleeding or clotting disorders.

# VASCULAR DISORDERS

## I. RETINAL VASCULAR OCCLUSION

a. **General**

   i. Typically presents with painless monocular vision loss.

   ii. Central artery occlusion is noted in patients older than 50 years of age and is associated with atherosclerotic disease.

b. **Clinical Manifestations**

   i. Patients with central retinal artery occlusion present with painless monocular vision loss.

      1. Most commonly caused by carotid artery emboli.

      2. On funduscopic examination, a cherry-red spot is noted on the macula, boxcar appearance of the retinal vessels.

   ii. Central retinal vein occlusion presents with sudden painless monocular vision loss.

      1. Funduscopic examination varies from small retinal hemorrhages to cotton-wool spots to deep and superficial retinal hemorrhages.

c. **Treatment**

   i. Referral to an ophthalmologist is required.

   ii. In central retinal vein occlusion, intravitreal anti-vascular endothelial growth factor used to decrease macular edema, as well as laser photocoagulation.

iii. Central artery occlusion is treated with revascularization techniques and ocular massage.

    1. Treatment should be attempted but poor prognosis.

# VISION ABNORMALITIES

## I. AMAUROSIS FUGAX

### a. General

i. Transient monocular vision loss with complete recovery.

    1. Often lasts minutes.

ii. Caused by etiologies affecting the eye or optic nerve.

    1. Retinal emboli or ischemia.

    2. Transient ischemic attack, giant cell arteritis, migraine, SLE, central retinal artery occlusion.

### b. Clinical Manifestations

i. Descending vision loss, "curtain or shade" coming down. Resolves within an hour.

### c. Diagnosis

i. Determine cause via history, physical, ophthalmologic exam, MRI, or EEG.

### d. Treatment

i. Treat underlying cause.

## II. AMBLYOPIA

### a. General

i. Clear vision fails to develop in one or both eyes in childhood or infancy.

    1. When the development of vision in one eye is affected, the brain cannot effectively combine the two images and it suppresses one of them, leading to the development of amblyopia in that eye.

      (a) Refractive amblyopia: asymmetric refractive error (anisometropia).

      (b) Strabismic amblyopia: constant eye turn in one eye.

      (a) Deprivation amblyopia: impaired vision in one eye.

### b. Clinical Manifestations

i. Poor depth perception.

ii. Squinting or shutting an eye.

iii. Eye strain.

### c. Diagnosis

i. Visual acuity difference of two or more lines between eyes or poor visual acuity.

ii. Corneal light reflex testing: may show asymmetric alignment.

iii. Eye preference testing (asymmetry of vision).

iv. Red reflex may be abnormal.

### d. Treatment

i. Children with suspected amblyopia should be referred to an ophthalmologist.

ii. Treatment may include prescription glasses for amblyopic eye and patching the non-amblyopic eye with an eye patch.

## III. GLAUCOMA

### a. General

i. Due to increased intraocular pressure causing optic nerve damage.

    1. Increased intraocular pressure due to impaired outflow of aqueous humor or impaired access of aqueous humor to the drainage system.

ii. Leading cause of preventable blindness in the United States.

iii. Classification.

    1. Primary.

      (a) Open-angle.

        (i) Most common type of glaucoma.

        (ii) Due to inadequate drainage of aqueous humor.

      (b) Angle-closure.

        (i) Restricted flow of aqueous humor.

        (ii) Acute angle-closure glaucoma is an ophthalmic emergency.

    2. Congenital.

    3. Secondary: steroid induced, uveitis, diabetic retinopathy, and ocular trauma.

### b. Clinical Manifestations

i. Primary angle-closure glaucoma presents with sudden onset of eye pain, headache, blurred vision and halos, nausea and vomiting, fixed and dilated pupil, and hyperemia.

ii. Open-angle glaucoma is asymptomatic early with gradual loss of peripheral vision and halos around lights.

iii. Table 6.2 compares etiologies of the red eye.

### c. Diagnosis

i. Increased intraocular pressure measured by tonometry (greater than 21 mmHg).

ii. Gonioscopy.

    1. Determines if anterior chamber angle is wide (open), narrow, or closed.

iii. Optic disk assessment.

    1. Will note enlargement of optic disk, disk pallor, and increased cup–disk ratio.

iv. Visual field defects.

    1. Involves mainly the peripheral field.

v. Conjunctival erythema, mid-dilated fixed pupil (with poor reaction to light), cloudy cornea.

### d. Treatment

i. Combination therapy to reduce intraocular pressure.

1. Topical agents to reduce intraocular pressure (e.g., timolol, apraclonidine).
2. Cholinergic to reduce miosis (e.g., pilocarpine).
3. Systemic agents to help reduce intraocular pressure (e.g., mannitol or acetazolamide).

   ii. Surgical treatment is definitive.
1. Includes peripheral iridotomy, laser trabeculoplasty, and trabeculectomy.

## IV. SCLERITIS
a. **General**
   i. Scleral inflammation (scleritis).
1. Can occur in one or both eyes.
   ii. Often related to underlying cause: autoimmune disease (rheumatoid arthritis, other vascular/connective tissue diseases).
b. **Clinical Manifestations**
   i. Eye pain is the hallmark, worse at night.
1. Tenderness may radiate to other parts of the head.
   ii. Photophobia and tearing.
   iii. Red eye.
   iv. Table 6.2 compares etiologies of the red eye.
c. **Diagnosis**
   i. Laboratory testing for other underlying causes (based on history and physical).
d. **Treatment**
   i. Treat underlying cause.
1. May include corticosteroids, nonsteroidal anti-inflammatory drugs (NSAIDs), immunosuppressives, and biologics.

## V. STRABISMUS
a. **General**
   i. Defined as any deviation from perfect ocular alignment.
   ii. Misalignment may be in any direction.
1. Esotropia is convergent strabismus (crossed eyes).
      (a) The most common type of strabismus.
2. Exotropia is divergent strabismus (directed outward).
   iii. Present in 4% to 5% of children.
1. Stable ocular alignment not present until age 2 to 3 months.
b. **Clinical Manifestations**
   i. Children present with diplopia, scotoma, and amblyopia.
   ii. On physical examination, the strabismus may be noted (asymmetric corneal reflex).
   iii. Convergence testing is used to test for disjunctive movements.
c. **Diagnosis**
   i. Angle of strabismus determined by the cover-uncover test.

ii. Hirschberg corneal light reflex test is used to determine eye position by evaluating for centering of light reflection in both eyes.
d. **Treatment**
   i. Treatment should be started as soon as possible.
   ii. Nonsurgical treatment.
1. Occlusion therapy is used to treat amblyopia.
      (a) The sound eye is covered to stimulate the amblyopic eye.
2. Spectacles are used to treat strabismus, and prisms are used to treat diplopia.
   iii. Surgical treatment.
1. Resection and recession are used to strengthen and weaken the appropriate muscles.

# EAR DISORDERS

## EXTERNAL EAR

## I. CERUMEN IMPACTION
a. **General**
   i. Precipitated by use of cotton-tipped applicators to clean ears.
   ii. Foreign bodies in the external ear canal may also be present.
b. **Clinical Manifestations**
   i. Present with decreased hearing (conduction type), pressure or fullness in the ear, dizziness, tinnitus, or pain.
   ii. On physical examination the tympanic membrane (TM) may not be visualized and the external auditory canal may be occluded with cerumen.
c. **Treatment**
   i. Cerumen softeners are used and then a cerumen spoon or loop is used to remove the cerumen.
   ii. Softening of the cerumen can occur with half-strength hydrogen peroxide, mineral oil, or over-the-counter preparations.
   iii. Irrigation of the ear may also be needed (only if TM intact).

## II. OTITIS EXTERNA
a. **General**
   i. Defined as infection and inflammation of the external auditory canal.
   ii. Four different categories.
1. Acute localized.
2. Acute diffuse (swimmer's ear).
3. Chronic.
4. Malignant (necrotizing external otitis).

iii. Etiology includes the following:
    1. *Pseudomonas aeruginosa* (most common).
    2. *S. aureus.*
    3. Group A *Streptococcus.*
    4. *Aspergillus.*

**b. Clinical Manifestations**
  i. Acute localized infection presents with pain and tenderness.
    1. On physical examination, the canal is erythematous and tenderness is noted over the tragus.
    2. Preauricular lymphadenopathy may be noted.
  ii. Acute diffuse disease presents with pain and itching.
    1. On physical examination, the canal is seen to be erythematous, swollen, and hemorrhagic.
  iii. Patients with chronic disease present with drainage and itching.
  iv. Patients with malignant disease present with a severe, necrotizing infection.
    1. Associated with elderly diabetic patients and infection due to *P. aeruginosa.*

**c. Diagnosis**
  i. Based on history and physical examination.

**d. Treatment**
  i. Gentle cleaning with saline or alcohol and acetic acid mixture, remove debris and cerumen.
  ii. Topical antibiotics also started (cover for *Pseudomonas* and *Staphylococcus*) with or without glucocorticoid for inflammation.
  iii. IV antipseudomonal antibiotics, such as ceftazidime or piperacillin, plus aminoglycosides or fluoroquinolones, are required for the treatment of malignant otitis externa.

## III. TRAUMA

**a. General**
  i. Results from blunt trauma to auricle during sports (wrestling, rugby, boxing).

**b. Clinical Manifestations**
  i. Presents as a tender, tense, fluctuant collection of blood on the anterior aspect of the pinna.
  ii. Skin is erythematous or ecchymotic.
  iii. Cauliflower ear is a chronic, bulbous deformity of the pinna in the former area of the hematoma.

**c. Treatment**
  i. Drain as soon as possible after injury.
  ii. If hematoma older than 7 days, refer to ear, nose, and throat (ENT) physician.
  iii. Complications include bleeding, infection, and cauliflower ear.

# INNER EAR

## I. ACOUSTIC NEUROMA

**a. General**
  i. Schwannomas are Schwann cell–derived tumors that develop in the cerebellopontine angle and compress cranial nerve VIII.
  ii. Median age at diagnosis is 50.
  iii. Most tumors are unilateral.

**b. Clinical Manifestations**
  i. Progressive sensorineural hearing loss and tinnitus are noted.
  ii. Unsteadiness while walking.
  iii. Facial numbness (CN V) and/or facial paresis (CN VII).

**c. Diagnosis**
  i. MRI is the test of choice: enhancing lesion in middle ear, extension into the cerebellopontine angle.

**d. Treatment**
  a. Surgical removal of tumor or focused radiation treatment.

## II. BAROTRAUMA

**a. General**
  i. Injury caused by barometric pressure change.
  ii. Usually results from water diving, ascending into the atmosphere, or mechanical respiratory support.
  iii. Injury can occur in the ears, sinuses, or lungs.

**b. Clinical Manifestations**
  i. External ear barotrauma.
    1. Patients experience pain and bloody discharge.
    2. May note petechiae, hemorrhagic blebs, or rupture of the TM on physical examination.
  ii. Middle ear barotrauma.
    1. Due to impaired eustachian tube functioning, secondary to upper respiratory infection (URI), allergy, or trauma.
    2. Noted in patients with URI and flying in a plane.
     (a) Pain and fullness noted on descent if patient fails to "pop" ears.
  iii. Decompression sickness ("the bends").
    1. Occurs most often after divers descend and remain deeper than 10 meters.
    2. Due to nitrogen becoming insoluble and forming bubbles in the blood and tissue.
    3. Present with steady, throbbing pain in the joints, pruritus, headache, seizures, hemiplegia, and visual disturbances.
    4. Pulmonary effects include substernal pain, dyspnea, and cough.

c. **Treatment**

    i. Treatment of ear barotrauma consists of keeping ear dry, pain control, decongestants, or antihistamines.

       1. Prevent with use of decongestants prior to flying.

       2. Auto-insufflation (e.g., yawning, swallowing, chewing gum).

    ii. Treatment of decompression sickness consists of recompression therapy in a compression chamber.

## III. DYSFUNCTION OF EUSTACHIAN TUBE

a. **General**

    i. Defined as failure of the functional valve of the eustachian tube to open and/or close properly.

    ii. Eustachian tube has the following three functions:

       1. Equalization of pressure.

       2. Protection of the middle ear from infection.

       3. Clearance of ear secretions.

b. **Etiologies**

    i. Dilatory dysfunction due to infection, allergies, smoking, gastroesophageal reflux disease (GERD), and anatomic abnormalities.

c. **Clinical Manifestations**

    i. Ear fullness or pressure, hearing loss, and tinnitus are noted.

    ii. Physical examination varies with etiology.

d. **Treatment**

    i. Treat the underlying cause. Decongestants for congestive symptoms.

    ii. Auto-insufflation (e.g., yawning, swallowing, chewing gum).

## IV. LABYRINTHITIS

a. **General**

    i. Acute unilateral infection or inflammation of the vestibular and cochlear system of CN VIII.

    1. Typically due to viral infection.

    2. A history of recent URI.

    ii. May last 7 to 10 days and typically is self-limited.

b. **Clinical Manifestations**

    i. Present with continuous vertigo, nystagmus, nausea, and vomiting.

       1. Nystagmus is horizontal and rotatory away from affected side.

       2. Tinnitus or hearing loss.

    ii. On physical examination, the vertigo is noted to remain whether the patient opens or closes the eyes.

    iii. Gait instability may be noted.

c. **Diagnosis**

    i. Clinical diagnosis.

    ii. Neuroimaging scan may be needed to rule out central causes of dizziness.

d. **Treatment**

    i. Typically self-limiting and may require symptomatic treatment.

       1. Glucocorticoids first-line.

       2. Antihistamines or anticholinergics.

       3. Benzodiazepines.

    ii. Complications are uncommon.

## V. VERTIGO

a. **General**

    i. Vertigo described as a dizziness, spinning, imbalance, lightheadedness, or sensation of ground moving.

    ii. Due to a disturbance in the vestibular system.

    iii. Physiologic vertigo.

       1. Etiologies include the following:

          (a) Due to mismatch in sensory systems.

          (b) Patient subjected to unfamiliar head movements.

          (c) Unusual head or neck positions.

          (d) Spinning.

    iv. Pathologic vertigo.

       1. Etiologies include the following:

          (a) Peripheral.

             (i) Severe vertigo with sudden onset.

             (ii) Nystagmus is horizontal or rotatory and fatigable.

             (iii) Other symptoms include tinnitus, hearing loss, nausea, and vomiting.

             (iv) Etiologies include the following:

                (1) Benign paroxysmal positional vertigo (BPPV).

                (2) Labyrinthitis.

                (3) Ménière's disease.

                (4) Vestibular neuritis.

          (b) Central.

             (i) Less severe and vague vertigo. Ear symptoms rarely present.

             (ii) Nystagmus is vertical and continuous.

             (iii) Etiologies include the following:

                (1) Multiple sclerosis.

                (2) Vertebrobasilar insufficiency.

          (c) Table 6.3 compares peripheral and central vertigo.

b. **Diagnosis**

    i. Dix-Hallpike maneuver is used to assist in the diagnosis of BPPV.

    ii. Electronystagmography (calorics), warm and cold, to test vestibular function.

c. **Treatment**

    i. Treatment of acute vertigo consists of bed rest and medications to manage nausea and vomiting.

**TABLE 6.3**

| Peripheral and Central Vertigo | | |
| --- | --- | --- |
| Signs/Symptoms | Peripheral | Central |
| Severity of vertigo | Marked, spontaneous | Mild, gradual |
| Tinnitus/Deafness | Often present | Usually absent |
| Vertical nystagmus | Never | Occasionally |
| Horizontal nystagmus | Uncommon | Common |
| Duration | Finite, intermittent | Variable, chronic |
| Central nervous system signs | None | Common |
| Etiologies | Infection Ménière's trauma Toxin | Vascular Neoplasm |

1. Medications include the following:
   (a) Antihistamines/anticholinergics such as meclizine and dimenhydrinate.
   (b) Dopamine blockers such as promethazine and prochlorperazine.
   (c) Benzodiazepines such as diazepam and lorazepam.
   (d) Serotonin antagonists such as ondansetron.
2. Epley maneuver for canalith repositioning in BPPV.

# MIDDLE EAR

## I. CHOLESTEATOMA
### a. General
   i. Keratinized, desquamated epithelial collection in the middle ear or mastoid.
   ii. Primary disease occurs most commonly due to eustachian tube dysfunction.
   iii. Secondary disease occurs due to TM perforation.
### b. Clinical Manifestations
   i. Hearing loss, dizziness, and otorrhea are noted.
   ii. Patients may be asymptomatic.
   iii. Physical examination.
      1. Otoscopic examination reveals cellular debris on the TM and possible perforation of the TM.
### c. Treatment
   i. Treatment of choice is surgical removal of debris.

## II. OTITIS MEDIA
### a. General
   i. Due to inflammation that results in fluid collection in the middle ear.

   ii. Risk factors include the following:
      1. Day-care attendance.
      2. Sibling with acute otitis media.
      3. Parental smoking.
      4. Drinking from a bottle while lying flat.
   iii. Etiology
      1. Most cases are viral (respiratory syncytial virus, rhinovirus, influenza, and enterovirus).
      2. Bacterial causes include the following:
         (a) *S. pneumoniae.*
         (b) *H. influenzae.*
         (c) *M. catarrhalis.*
         (d) Group A *Streptococcus.*
   iv. Chronic otitis media: complication of acute otitis media.
### b. Clinical Manifestations
   i. Children present with fever, irritability, crying, lethargy, and pulling at their ears.
   ii. Older children and adults present with earache and ear drainage.
   iii. Physical examination reveals an erythematous tympanic membrane (TM).
      1. TM may be bulging, retracted, or perforated.
      2. An air-fluid level may be noted behind the TM, and mobility of the TM is diminished.
      3. Hearing may be decreased.
   iv. Chronic otitis media may present with persistent or recurrent purulent otorrhea with TM perforation, some degree of conductive hearing loss.
      1. May have developed a cholesteatoma.
### c. Diagnosis
   i. Based on history and physical examination.
   ii. Culture, via tympanocentesis, is rarely done, unless patient appears toxic or has recurrent infection.
### d. Treatment
   i. Symptomatic treatment, mainly pain control with acetaminophen or ibuprofen, is required.
   ii. Antibiotic treatment includes the following:
      1. Amoxicillin.
      2. Erythromycin/Sulfisoxazole.
      3. Amoxicillin/Clavulanate.
      4. Cefpodoxime.
      5. Trimethoprim-sulfamethoxazole.
   iii. Most patients start to respond in 48 to 72 hours.
   iv. Complications include chronic otitis media, mastoiditis, and intracranial extension.
      1. Recurrent disease may require placement of tympanostomy tubes or tonsillectomy/adenoidectomy.
      2. Chronic otitis media may require systemic antibiotics and tympanic membrane repair.

### III. TYMPANIC MEMBRANE PERFORATION

a. **General**
   i. Occurs as a result of penetrating or noise trauma.
   ii. Occurs typically in the pars tensa, anteriorly or inferiorly.

b. **Clinical Manifestations**
   i. Present with acute onset of pain, hearing loss, and with or without bloody otorrhea.
   ii. May also have tinnitus and vertigo.

c. **Diagnosis**
   i. Perforation is noted on otoscopic examination.

d. **Treatment**
   i. Most perforated TMs will heal spontaneously.
   ii. A follow-up hearing test is needed to confirm that hearing has returned to baseline.
   iii. Avoid water and topical aminoglycosides (ototoxic) with TM rupture.

# HEARING IMPAIRMENT

a. **General**
   i. Almost 10% of the adult population has some hearing loss.
   ii. Two types of hearing loss.
      1. Conductive.
         (a) Lesion in the auricle, external auditory canal, or middle ear.
      2. Sensorineural.
         (a) Lesion in the inner ear or cranial nerve VIII.

b. **Etiologies**
   i. Conductive.
      1. Obstruction of external auditory canal due to cerumen (most common), foreign body, swelling, neoplasm, or TM perforation.
      2. Cholesteatoma.
      3. Otosclerosis.
         (a) Due to fixation of the ossicular bones and results in a low-frequency conductive hearing loss.
         (b) Schwartz sign is positive in otosclerosis.
   ii. Sensorineural.
      1. Presbycusis.
         (a) Most common cause of sensorineural hearing loss and is age-associated.
         (b) High-frequency hearing loss.
      2. Ménière's disease.
      3. Central nervous system (CNS) lesion (e.g., acoustic neuroma).
      4. Drug induced.
         (a) Mechanism is damage to hair cells in the organ of Corti.
         (b) Common medications include salicylates, quinine, aminoglycosides, cisplatin, and loop diuretics.

c. **Diagnosis**
   i. Differentiate conductive and sensorineural hearing losses with the Weber and Rinne tests.
      1. Weber.
         (a) Vibrating tuning fork placed on the head in the midline.
         (b) With unilateral conductive hearing loss, the tone is perceived in the affected ear.
         (c) With unilateral sensorineural hearing loss the tone is perceived in the unaffected ear.
      2. Rinne.
         (a) Vibrating tuning fork placed near opening of auditory canal (air conduction) and then placed on mastoid process (bone conduction).
         (b) Normally and with sensorineural hearing loss, air conduction is greater than bone conduction.
         (c) With conductive hearing loss, bone conduction is greater than air conduction.
   ii. Audiologic assessment.
      1. Used to determine level of hearing loss.

d. **Treatment**
   i. Conductive hearing loss can be treated with surgical intervention and correction.
   ii. Sensorineural hearing loss is permanent and corrected with hearing aids.

# OTHER ABNORMALITIES OF THE EAR

### I. MASTOIDITIS

a. **General**
   i. A rare complication of otitis media.
      1. Caused by same microorganisms as otitis media.
   ii. Infection of the mastoid air cells.

b. **Clinical Manifestations**
   i. Present with pain (worse at night), fever, swelling, tenderness, and redness behind the ear in the area of the mastoid bone.
   ii. On physical examination, the mastoid area is red and tender and the pinna may be displaced.

c. **Diagnosis**
   i. CT with contrast first-line.

d. **Treatment**
   i. IV antibiotics and drainage (myringotomy). May also need tympanostomy tube.
   ii. Mastoidectomy may be needed in severe or refractory disease.
   iii. Complications include brain abscess and septic lateral sinus thrombosis.

## II. MÉNIÈRE'S DISEASE

a. **General**

    i. Results from malfunction of the endolymphatic sac in the inner ear.

b. **Clinical Manifestations**

    i. Present with debilitating vertigo, progressive sensorineural hearing loss, and tinnitus.

        1. Onset of vertigo is sudden and lasts minutes to hours.

            (a) Rarely lasts longer than 24 to 48 hours.

    ii. May also note a fullness or pressure in the affected ear.

    iii. Horizontal nystagmus.

c. **Diagnosis**

    i. Based on history and physical examination.

    ii. Electronystagmography with warm and cold calorics can be used to differentiate central from peripheral causes of vertigo.

d. **Treatment**

    i. Dietary modifications: sodium restriction, eliminate caffeine, nicotine, alcohol, and chocolate.

    ii. Pharmacologic treatment to reduce endolymphatic pressure consists of the following:

        1. Benzodiazepines for acute disease.

        2. Anticholinergics (e.g., scopolamine).

        3. Antihistamines (e.g., meclizine and dimenhydrinate).

        4. Diuretics (e.g. hydrochlorothiazide).

    iii. Surgical drainage of the endolymphatic system or ablation of cranial nerve VIII, or labyrinth may be needed in severe cases.

## III. TINNITUS

a. **General**

    i. Perception of sound in proximity to the head in the absence of an external source.

    ii. Most often a buzzing, ringing, or hissing sound.

b. **Etiologies**

    i. Vascular disorders: arteriovenous (AV) shunts and arterial bruits.

    ii. Neurologic disorders.

    iii. Eustachian tube dysfunction.

    iv. Ototoxic drugs such as salicylates, cisplatin, and loop diuretics.

    v. Presbycusis.

    vi. Otosclerosis.

c. **Diagnosis**

    i. Special testing, such as angiography and audiometric tests, may be needed.

    ii. Refer to ENT.

d. **Treatment**

    i. Treat underlying cause.

    ii. Discontinue toxic medications.

## IV. FOREIGN BODY: EAR

a. **Foreign Body External Auditory Canal**

    i. General

        1. Most common in children under age 6.

        2. Most common objects include beads, pebbles, small toys, popcorn, and insects.

    ii. Clinical manifestations

        1. May be asymptomatic or present with decreased hearing, ear pain, or drainage.

    ii. Treatment

        1. Removal of foreign body.

# NOSE/SINUS DISORDERS

## I. EPISTAXIS

a. **General**

    i. Common etiologies of epistaxis.

        1. Infection.

        2. Trauma.

        3. Allergic rhinitis.

        4. Atrophic rhinitis.

        5. Hypertension.

        6. Tumors.

    ii. Divided into two groups.

        1. Anterior.

            (a) Makes up 90% of nosebleeds, and most originate from Kiesselbach plexus.

        2. Posterior.

            (a) More common in the elderly and due to arteriosclerosis.

b. **Clinical Manifestations**

    i. Anterior bleeds are typically unilateral and without sensation of blood in the posterior pharynx.

    ii. Posterior bleeds are typically profuse, and blood is noted draining down posterior pharynx.

c. **Treatment**

    i. Anterior nosebleeds are treated with the following:

        1. Direct pressure.

            (a) Compress elastic area of nose for 10 to 15 minutes.

        2. Vasoconstrictive agents.

            (a) Agents include phenylephrine, oxymetazoline, or epinephrine.

        3. Nasal packing.

            (a) Perform when direct pressure or vasoconstrictors are not successful.

            (b) Consider prophylactic treatment against toxic shock syndrome.

               (i) Includes cephalexin, clindamycin, or amoxicillin/clavulanate.

        4. Cautery.

            (a) Done with silver nitrate or electrocautery.

    ii. Posterior nosebleeds are treated with the following:
1. Posterior nasal packing.
   (a) Carries a significant morbidity, includes difficulty swallowing, otitis media, sinusitis, and hypoxia.
2. Embolization.
3. Ligation.

## II. NASAL POLYPS
### a. General
    i. Two types.
1. Eosinophilic.
   (a) Most common type.
   (b) Associated with intrinsic asthma and aspirin sensitivity.
2. Neutrophilic.
   (a) Associated with cystic fibrosis, sinusitis, and immune deficiency.

### b. Clinical Manifestations
    i. May cause severe obstruction and anosmia.
    ii. Type of nasal secretion varies with type of polyp.
1. Eosinophilic type presents with seromucous secretion.
2. Neutrophilic type presents with purulent secretions.
    iii. On physical examination, polyps will be noted.
    iv. Nasal cytology reveals increased eosinophils, with or without increased number of basophils, in eosinophilic type and increased neutrophils, with or without bacteria, in neutrophilic type.

### c. Treatment
    i. Eosinophilic type treated with intranasal or oral corticosteroids.
    ii. Neutrophilic type treated with antibiotics.
    iii. Surgical removal may be necessary if medical therapy unsuccessful.

## III. RHINITIS
### a. General
    i. Several types:
1. Allergic is most common type.
2. Infectious due to common cold (rhinovirus).
3. Vasomotor dilation due to temperature change, humidity, potent smells.
    ii. Allergic type is type I hypersensitivity reaction mediating the allergic response.
1. Onset at any age, greatest incidence during adolescence and peak prevalence 20 to 30 years.
2. Involves the excess production of immune globulin E (IgE).

3. Two phases:
   (a) Early phase.
      (i) Due to degranulation of mast cells, evokes an inflammatory response and release of histamine, leukotrienes, cytokines, and prostaglandins.
      (ii) Occurs within 10 to 15 minutes of exposure.
      (iii) Symptoms include sneezing, rhinorrhea, itching, and increased vascular permeability.
   (b) Late phase.
      (i) Release of cytokines and leukotrienes causes an influx of inflammatory cells (eosinophils).
      (ii) Can begin 4 to 6 hours after initial exposure.
      (iii) Symptoms include nasal congestion and postnasal drip.
4. Etiologies.
   (a) Seasonal: occurs during certain seasons and typically due to tree pollen in the spring, grasses in the late spring and summer, and weeds in the fall.
   (a) Perennial: symptoms are usually constant and typically due to indoor allergens, such as dust mites, animal dander, cockroaches, and mold spores.

### b. Clinical Manifestations
    i. Seasonal allergic rhinitis presents with sneezing; watery rhinorrhea; itching of the nose, eyes, and throat; red and watery eyes; and nasal congestion.
1. Symptoms are worse in the morning and aggravated by dry, windy conditions.
2. Physical examination of the nose reveals blue, pale, boggy turbinates; wet, swollen mucosa; and nasal congestion.
    ii. Perennial allergic rhinitis presents with nasal congestion and postnasal drip.
1. Physical examination may be normal or may reveal only nasal congestion.
    iii. In children, may note allergic shiners, mouth breathing, and the nasal salute.

### c. Diagnosis
    i. Allergy testing is done to establish the presence of atopic disease.

### d. Treatment
    i. Three major options for allergic rhinitis.
1. Avoidance and environmental control.
   (a) Consists of avoiding outdoor allergens, keeping windows closed, using air conditioning, decreasing home humidity, removing carpets and pets from often-used

living areas, encasing items in hypoallergenic coverings, and using air purifiers.

2. Pharmacotherapy.
   (a) Done through a variety of medications.
   (b) Antihistamines are most effective on early-phase symptoms and have little effect on nasal congestion.
   (c) Intranasal corticosteroids are the most effective medications for overall control of allergic rhinitis.
       (i) May take 1 to 2 weeks for maximum effect.
       (ii) They act on the late-phase symptoms.
       (iii) No systemic side effects compared with oral corticosteroids.
   (d) Decongestants improve nasal congestion, but have no effect on sneezing, rhinorrhea, or pruritus.
   (e) Anticholinergics control only rhinorrhea.
   (f) Intranasal cromolyn must be used prior to onset of symptoms.
   (g) Table 6.4 lists medications used in allergic rhinitis.

3. Immunotherapy.
   (a) Attempts to increase the threshold level for the appearance of symptoms.
   (b) Done through the gradual increase in dose of antigen until a reaction occurs.

## IV. ACUTE SINUSITIS
### a. General
   i. Defined as acute sinusitis when less than 4 weeks duration.
   ii. Typically occurs as a result of a preceding viral upper respiratory tract infection.
   iii. Mechanism includes obstruction of the sinus ostia or impaired ciliary clearance.
   iv. Etiologies include allergic rhinitis, barotrauma, chemical irritants, and infections.
      1. Infectious agents include bacterial, viral, and fungal.
         (a) Bacterial.
            (i) *S. pneumoniae.*
            (ii) *H. influenzae* (nontypable).
            (iii) *M. catarrhalis.*
            (iv) Anaerobes.
            (v) *P. aeruginosa.*
            (vi) *S. aureus.*

**TABLE 6.4**

**Medications for Allergic Rhinitis**

| Class | Medication | Mechanism of Action | Side Effects |
|---|---|---|---|
| Antihistamines | **First generation** Diphenhydramine Hydroxyzine Chlorpheniramine **Second generation** Fexofenadine Loratadine Cetirizine Azelastine | Antagonize the H1 receptor–mediated effects of histamine | First-generation side effects include sedation and anticholinergic effects. Second-generation side effects have little sedation and no anticholinergic effects. |
| Decongestants | Oxymetazoline | Act on alpha-adrenergic receptors of the mucosa of the respiratory tract | May have rebound nasal congestion |
| Corticosteroids (intranasal and oral) | **Nasal** Triamcinolone Budesonide Fluticasone Mometasone **Oral** Prednisone | Act at a wide variety of steps, cell types, and mediators, suppressing inflammatory response | Nasal corticosteroids have no systemic side effects. Oral corticosteroids may suppress the HPA axis. |
| Mast-cell stabilizers | Cromolyn | Inhibit the release of mediators, such as histamine, from mast cells | Nasal irritation |
| Anticholinergic agents | Ipratropium bromide | Antagonize the action of acetylcholine at muscarinic receptors | Blurry vision Dizziness Dry mouth Headache Palpitations |
| Leukotriene modifiers | Montelukast | Antagonize the action of leukotriene receptors or inhibit the formation of leukotrienes | Headache |

*HPA,* Hypothalamic–pituitary–adrenal.

(b) Viral.
  (i) Rhinovirus.
  (ii) Parainfluenza.
  (iii) Influenza.
(c) Fungal.
  (i) *Rhizopus.*
  (ii) *Rhizomucor.*
  (iii) *Mucor.*
  (iv) *Aspergillus.*

**b. Clinical Manifestations**

i. Patients present with fever, nasal drainage and congestion, facial pain or pressure, and headache.
  1. Upper molar tooth pain and halitosis are associated with bacterial sinusitis.
ii. Sinus pressure or pain is localized over infected sinus.
  1. Maxillary sinus is most frequently infected, followed by ethmoid, frontal, and sphenoid.
  2. Pain or pressure worse with bending forward.
iii. On physical examination, tenderness with palpation is noted over the infected sinus.
  1. Decreased transillumination may be noted.
iv. Laboratory testing reveals a leukocytosis.

**c. Diagnosis**

i. Clinical diagnosis. Signs and symptoms should be present for more than 10 days.
ii. CT scan (test of choice) or sinus x-ray may reveal air–fluid levels, opacification, and mucosal thickening.
  1. Fig. 6.1 shows common x-ray findings of a sinus infection.

**d. Treatment**

i. For symptoms present for less than 10 days, decongestants, analgesics, and nasal saline lavage may be helpful.
ii. For symptoms present longer than 10 days or more severe symptoms, antibiotics are indicated.
  1. Amoxicillin-clavulanate, doxycycline, and levofloxacin are indicated.

## V. CHRONIC SINUSITIS

**a. General**

i. Defined by signs and symptoms lasting longer than 12 weeks.
ii. Associated with infection by bacteria or fungi.
  1. *S. aureus* is the most common bacterial cause.
  2. *Aspergillus* is the most common fungal cause.
iii. Mechanism is based on impaired mucociliary clearance from repeated infections.
  1. Certain conditions, such as cystic fibrosis, can predispose patients to chronic bacterial sinusitis.

**b. Clinical Manifestations**

i. Present with headaches, fatigue, irritability, low-grade fever, facial pressure, and postnasal discharge.

**c. Diagnosis**

i. Biopsy or histology to identify the organism.

**d. Treatment**

i. Includes repeated courses of antibiotics or antifungals, intranasal glucocorticoids, and irrigation of the sinus.

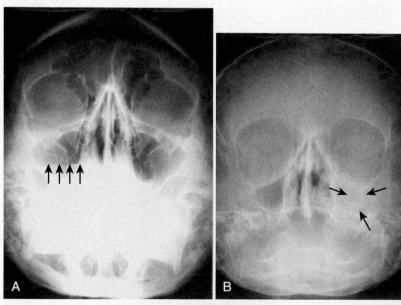

**Fig. 6.1** Sinus infection x-ray. **(A)** Water's view showing air–fluid level *(arrows)* in acute sinusitis. **(B)** Opacification of the left maxillary sinus *(arrows)*. *(From Mettler FA: Essentials of Radiology, 2nd ed. Philadelphia: Elsevier Saunders, 2005:37, Fig. 2-27A.)*

ii. Surgery may be needed to remove impacted mucus.

## VI. TRAUMA
a. **General**
   i. Direct blows to the nose can cause serious nasal injuries:
      1. Simple linear fracture.
      2. Naso-orbito-ethmoid fractures.
      3. Septal fractures or dislocation.
b. **Clinical Manifestations**
   i. Nasal deformity, tenderness, periorbital swelling or ecchymoses, trouble breathing through nose, and epistaxis.
c. **Diagnosis**
   i. CT scan of maxillofacial bones, orbits and base of skull if any of the following are suspected: naso-orbito-ethmoid fracture, frontal sinus fracture, instability of the palate, cerebrospinal fluid leak.
d. **Treatment**
   i. Pain management, control of epistaxis, and management of open wounds.
   ii. Emergency otolaryngology consultation for patients with septal hematoma or abscess, concern for associated orbital or frontal sinus fracture, septal cartilage injury, or for closed reduction.

## VII. FOREIGN BODY: NOSE
a. **General**
   i. Occur most commonly in young children.
   ii. Objects include beads, toys, and organic material.
b. **Clinical Manifestations**
   i. May have no symptoms.
   ii. May note mucopurulent discharge, foul odor, and epistaxis.
c. **Diagnosis**
   i. Otoscopic or endoscopy may be needed.
   ii. Plain radiographs not indicated.
d. **Treatment**
   i. Positive pressure technique or via instrumentation.

# OROPHARYNGEAL DISORDERS

## DISEASES OF THE TEETH/GUMS

### I. DENTAL ABSCESS
a. **General**
   i. Periodontal abscess may be focal or diffuse.
   ii. Due to entrapment of plaque and debris in the periodontal pocket.
   iii. Periodontal disease is the most common cause of tooth loss.

b. **Clinical manifestations**
   i. Present with a painful, red, fluctuant swelling of the gingiva.
   ii. Gingiva is very tender to palpation.
   iii. Pus can be expelled from the periodontal pocket after probing of the pocket.
c. **Treatment**
   i. Small abscesses can be treated with warm saline rinses and oral antibiotics (penicillin or erythromycin).
   ii. Large abscesses require incision and drainage.

### II. GINGIVITIS
a. **General**
   i. Inflammatory process with gingival redness, swelling, and bleeding provoked by brushing or flossing.
   ii. Is a precursor to periodontitis.
b. **Etiology**
   i. Associated with plaque buildup.
   ii. Non–plaque-induced disease.
      1. Pregnancy gingivitis.
      2. Linear gingival erythema: seen in HIV.
      3. Drug induced: phenytoin, calcium channel blockers, and cyclosporine.
c. **Treatment**
   i. Oral rinses with chlorhexidine.
   ii. If oral antibiotics are needed, use penicillin plus metronidazole or clindamycin.

# INFECTIOUS/INFLAMMATORY DISORDERS

### I. APHTHOUS ULCERS
a. **General**
   i. One of the most common oral lesions.
   ii. Etiology is unknown, but may be linked to human herpesvirus 6.
      1. Linked to celiac disease and inflammatory bowel disease.
   iii. Three factors known to predispose to ulcer formations.
      1. Immune imbalance.
      2. Defect in mucosal barrier.
      3. Allergic response.
   iv. Involve the nonkeratinized epithelium and begin as an erythematous macule that ulcerates and forms a central fibropurulent eschar.
b. **Clinical Manifestations**
   i. Present with multiple, painful, shallow (yellow, white, or gray) ulcers that measure from 2 to 3 mm to several cm in diameter.
   ii. Mainly involve the labial or buccal mucosa.
   iii. Disease may be more severe in immunocompromised patients.

**c. Treatment**
  i. Treatment consists of topical corticosteroids, such as dexamethasone or fluocinonide.
  ii. Topical analgesics.

## II. ORAL CANDIDIASIS
**a. General**
  i. Most cases due to infection with the fungal organism *Candida albicans*, which can infect any mucosal surface in the body.
  ii. *Candida* is normal flora in many areas of the body and only causes disease when normal host defenses are altered.
     1. Risk factors include immunocompromised states, use of inhaled corticosteroids without a spacer, recent antibiotic use, dentures, or xerostomia.
**b. Clinical Manifestations**
  i. Patients present with multiple white patches on the tongue, palate, and other areas of the oral mucosa.
  ii. The patches are easily removed by scraping with a tongue blade to reveal a red, irritated mucosa.
**c. Diagnosis**
  i. Budding yeast and hyphae can be seen on KOH preparation of scraping.
**d. Treatment**
  i. Topical antifungal agents, such as nystatin or clotrimazole, are effective.
  ii. If systemic treatment is required, fluconazole or itraconazole are effective.
  iii. Dentures must be removed and properly cleaned.

## III. DEEP NECK INFECTION
**a. General**
  i. Infection of the deep neck space behind the posterior pharyngeal wall.
     1. Most common in children; adults more commonly caused by penetrating trauma or dental infections.
  ii. Often polymicrobial.
**b. Clinical Manifestations**
  i. Torticollis, neck stiffness.
  ii. Fever, sore throat, dysphagia, muffled voice, drooling.
**c. Diagnosis**
  i. Physical exam may reveal pharyngeal wall edema, cervical lymphadenopathy, lateral neck swelling.
  ii. CT with contrast image of choice.
**d. Treatment**
  i. Surgical incision and drainage with antibiotics for large abscesses.
  ii. Smaller abscesses (less than 2.5 cm) may be observed with systemic antibiotics.

  iii. IV ampicillin-sulbactam or clindamycin.

## IV. EPIGLOTTITIS
**a. General**
  i. Due to inflammation (cellulitis) of the epiglottis and adjacent supraglottic structures.
  ii. More common in children.
  iii. Caused by the following:
     1. *H. influenzae* type b.
     2. *S. pneumoniae.*
     3. *S. pyogenes.*
     4. *S. aureus.*
  iv. A respiratory emergency.
**b. Clinical Manifestations**
  i. Present with a short, rapidly progressive febrile illness.
  ii. Also have sore throat, pain with swallowing, and shortness of breath.
  iii. On physical examination, the patient appears toxic, assumes a forward-leaning, neck-extended position, and with drooling of secretions.
     1. A child may also present with stridor and tachypnea.
  iv. Indirect laryngoscopy demonstrates a cherry-red epiglottis.
  v. Examination of the pharynx with tongue depressor may result in loss of the airway.
**c. Diagnosis**
  i. Laboratory tests reveal a leukocytosis, and blood cultures are typically positive.
  ii. X-ray of the neck shows an enlarged edematous epiglottis (thumbprint sign) and normal subglottic space (Fig. 6.2).
**c. Treatment**
  i. Maintaining a patent airway is most important.
  ii. Antibiotic treatment consists of the following:
     1. Cefotaxime.
     2. Ceftriaxone.
     3. Ampicillin/sulbactam.
  iii. Secondary attacks can be decreased with the prophylactic use of rifampin.
  iv. Incidence of disease has decreased with mass vaccination for *H. influenzae* type b.

## V. HERPES SIMPLEX
**a. General**
  i. Typically due to herpes simplex type 1 (HSV-1), but herpes simplex type 2 can also cause infection.
  ii. Present with an acute infection, the virus lies dormant and is then reactivated to cause latent infections.
     1. Reactivation may occur secondary to menses, trauma, fever, stress, or exposure to ultraviolet light.

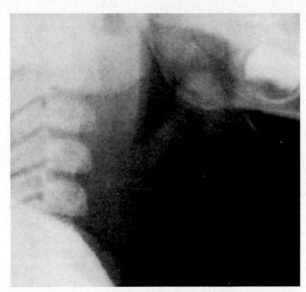

**Fig. 6.2** Soft-tissue x-ray of the lateral neck showing an edematous epiglottis space (thumbprint sign). *(From Behrman RE: Nelson's Textbook of Pediatrics, 17th ed. Philadelphia: Elsevier Saunders 2004:1406, Fig. 371-2.)*

b. **Clinical Manifestations**
  i. Appear as a group or single vesicular lesion that becomes pustular to form single or multiple ulcers.
  ii. May present with a burning pain prior to vesicle formation.
  iii. Lesions are very painful and last 5 to 10 days.
  iv. Fever and lymphadenopathy may also be noted and may occur prior to the appearance of the vesicles.
c. **Diagnosis**
  i. Giemsa stain may reveal giant multinucleated cells (Tzanck smear).
  ii. Immunofluorescence or antigen detection testing can be used in oral herpes infections to assist in diagnosis.
  iii. Viral culture can be used.
d. **Treatment**
  i. Treatment consists of the antivirals acyclovir, valacyclovir, or famciclovir.
    1. Can be given orally or used topically.
  ii. Avoiding contact with infected patients can reduce the risk of transmission.
  iii. Suppression therapy with antivirals can be used if history of frequent recurrences.

## VI. LARYNGITIS
a. **General**
  i. Defined as inflammation of the larynx caused by a variety of infectious agents.
    1. Most frequent noninfectious cause is voice abuse.

  ii. Most commonly due to viral agents, such as rhinovirus, influenza, adenovirus, respiratory syncytial virus, or parainfluenza.
    1. Bacterial cause less common and typically due to *S. pyogenes* or *M. catarrhalis*.
b. **Clinical Manifestations**
  i. Symptoms include hoarseness, aphonia, rhinitis, and pharyngitis.
  ii. On physical examination, the larynx is noted to be hyperemic, edematous, and with or without ulcerations.
c. **Treatment**
  i. Treatment is typically supportive with voice rest, warm saline gargles, and increased humidity.

## VII. PERITONSILLAR ABSCESS
a. **General**
  i. A complication of adenotonsillitis and typically due to infection with a mixture of aerobic and anaerobic bacterial organisms.
  ii. Develops when a bacterial infection extends beyond the tonsillar capsule and into surrounding tissues.
    1. Abscess develops between the capsule wall and the pharyngeal muscles.
b. **Clinical Manifestations**
  i. Present with severe odynophagia, fever, muffled "hot potato" voice, and drooling.
  ii. On physical examination, it is noted that the infected tonsil is displaced to the midline or beyond (uvula deviation to contralateral side).
c. **Diagnosis**
  i. Typically a clinical diagnosis.
  ii. CT scan is preferred imaging test.
d. **Treatment**
  i. Needle aspiration or incision and drainage may be required.
  ii. Systemic antibiotics, such as amoxicillin-clavulanic acid, ampicillin-sulbactam or clindamycin, are required.

## VIII. PHARYNGITIS
a. **General**
  i. Acute infection of the pharyngeal mucosa.
  ii. Etiologies include the following:
    1. *Streptococcus pyogenes* most common bacterial cause.
    2. Viral most common cause overall:
      (a) Adenovirus.
      (b) Rhinovirus.
      (c) Enterovirus.
      (d) Influenza A and B.
      (e) Epstein-Barr virus.
      (f) Respiratory syncytial virus.

b. **Clinical Manifestations**
   i. Presents with mild sore throat to severe pain with swallowing or talking, with or without fever.
   ii. On physical examination, the pharynx is erythematous with or without exudates and cervical lymphadenopathy is noted.
   iii. Symptoms and physical examination findings vary with etiology.
      1. Rhinorrhea suggests viral etiology.
      2. Pharyngeal exudates suggest streptococcal infection or Epstein-Barr virus.
      3. Vesicles or ulcers suggest herpes simplex.
      4. Conjunctival congestion suggests adenovirus.

c. **Diagnosis**
   i. Diagnosis of *S. pyogenes* can be made with rapid streptococcus screen or throat culture.
   ii. Testing for suspected influenza or mononucleosis.

d. **Treatment**
   i. Complications of *S. pyogenes* infection include rheumatic fever and acute glomerulonephritis.
   ii. If bacterial, treatment consists of penicillin, amoxicillin, erythromycin, clarithromycin, or azithromycin.
   iii. Symptomatic treatment consists of fluids, warm saline gargles, and NSAIDs.

# SALIVARY DISORDERS

## I. SIALADENITIS
a. **General**
   i. Inflammation resulting from decreased saliva production or alterations in saliva flow.
      1. May be due to virus (mumps), bacteria (*S. aureus*), Sjögren's syndrome, or sarcoidosis.
   ii. There may or may not be an obstruction.
      1. A sialolithiasis (stone in the salivary duct) may be the cause.
   iii. Typically noted only in adults.

b. **Clinical Manifestations**
   i. Present with painful swelling and erythema of the salivary gland, especially with eating.
   ii. If a stone is present, it may be palpated.

c. **Diagnosis**
   i. CT scan may be needed to rule out a malignant tumor or abscess.
   ii. Sialography or ultrasound may be helpful in finding an obstruction.

d. **Treatment**
   i. Conservative therapy and antistaphylococcal antibiotics are the most successful treatments.
      1. Conservative treatment consists of oral hygiene, increased hydration, massage of affected gland, and use of sialagogues.

## II. PAROTITIS
a. **General**
   i. Acute infection of the parotid gland.
   ii. Most commonly caused by *S. aureus* or mixed aerobes and/or anaerobes.
   iii. Occurs in settings of dehydration or poor oral hygiene.

b. **Clinical Manifestations**
   i. Sudden onset of firm, erythematous swelling of the preauricular and postauricular areas that extend to the angle of the mandible.
   ii. Also note local pain and tenderness with trismus and dysphagia.
   iii. On physical examination, purulent material may be noted from Stensen's duct.

c. **Diagnosis**
   i. CT scan or ultrasound may be needed to aid in diagnosis.
   ii. Amylase is elevated.

d. **Treatment**
   i. Antibiotics including nafcillin plus metronidazole or clindamycin are needed.

# TRAUMA

## I. TOOTH AVULSION
a. **General**
   i. An avulsed tooth is a medical emergency and should be replaced immediately (within 15 minutes to an hour).
      1. Primary teeth should not be reimplanted.
      2. Avulsed permanent teeth should be reimplanted immediately by the first capable person.

b. **Diagnosis**
   i. Dental radiographs should be taken to assess the severity of displacement or the occurrence of a root fracture, bony fracture, or permanent tooth bud displacement.

c. **Treatment**
   i. Remove debris by gentle rinsing with saline or tap water.
   ii. Tooth should be placed back in the socket ideally within 15 minutes to an hour (or longer if stored in cold milk, culture media, or patient's saliva).
   iii. Refer to dentist.

# OTHER OROPHARYNGEAL DISORDERS

## I. LEUKOPLAKIA
a. **General**
   i. Leukoplakia appears as white patches in the oral cavity that cannot be removed with scraping.
      1. Noted in smokers and smokeless tobacco users; thought to be premalignant.

ii. Oral hairy leukoplakia is a white lesion found on the sides of the tongue or soft palate.
    1. Not malignant or premalignant.
    2. May be noted in patients with human immunodeficiency virus (HIV), post transplantation, or on chronic steroids.
  b. **Clinical Manifestations**
    i. Appear as painless, well-defined, white patches that cannot be removed with scraping.
  c. **Diagnosis**
    i. Biopsy is required to evaluate for malignant conditions.
  d. **Treatment**
    i. Cryotherapy, laser ablation, or surgical excision if at risk for malignancy or malignant.

# NEOPLASMS

## I. ORAL CANCER
  a. **General**
    i. Most common type is squamous cell carcinoma.

ii. Alcohol and tobacco use account for up to 80% of cases of squamous cell carcinoma of the head and neck.
iii. Leukoplakia is benign but can progress to carcinoma.
  b. **Clinical Manifestations**
    i. Persistent papules, erosions, ulcers, or plaques in the mouth.
    ii. Mouth or tongue pain, trouble swallowing or speaking.
  c. **Diagnosis**
    i. Biopsy to confirm.
  d. **Treatment**
    i. Based on extent of locoregional disease (tumor size, depth of invasion, involvement of regional lymph nodes, and metastases). Treatment may involve surgery, radiation therapy, or chemotherapy.

# QUESTIONS

### QUESTION 1
Which of the following is a clinical finding of bacterial conjunctivitis?
A  Conjunctival itching
B  Fever
C  Profuse discharge
D  Severe pruritus
E  Periauricular adenopathy

### QUESTION 2
Which of the following is the first step in the evaluation of the patient with a foreign body in the eye?
A  Visual acuity
B  Schiøtz tonometry
C  Fluorescein staining
D  MRI scanning
E  Upper lid eversion

### QUESTION 3
A patient presents with vertigo after a recent URI. The patient denies tinnitus or hearing loss. On physical examination, it is noted that the vertigo is present with the patient's eyes open or closed. Which of the following is the most likely diagnosis?
A  Benign paroxysmal positional vertigo
B  Vestibular neuronitis
C  Ménière's disease
D  Acoustic neuroma
E  Multiple sclerosis

### QUESTION 4
A 75-year-old female presents with epistaxis. The bleeding is brisk, and blood is noted in the posterior pharynx. Which of the following is the most appropriate intervention?
A  Posterior nasal packing
B  Silver nitrate
C  Vasoconstrictors
D  Embolization
E  Protamine sulfate

### QUESTION 5
A 30-year-old patient presents with odynophagia. On physical examination, the uvula is noted to be to the left of midline. Which of the following is the treatment of choice?
A  Erythromycin
B  Cefazolin
C  Vancomycin
D  Clindamycin
E  Fluconazole

### QUESTION 6
Which of the following is a risk factor for malignant otitis externa?
A  Smoking
B  Diabetes
C  Neomycin use
D  Perforated TM
E  Chronic sinusitis

*Continued*

## QUESTIONS—cont'd

### QUESTION 7
Which of the following types of hypersensitivity immune response is noted in allergic rhinitis?
A  Type I
B  Type II
C  Type III
D  Type IV

### QUESTION 8
At what age should ocular alignment be stable?
A  2 to 3 months
B  4 to 5 months
C  6 to 7 months
D  8 to 9 months
E  10 to 11 months

### QUESTION 9
Which of the following is the pathophysiologic mechanism in the development of cataracts?
A  Epithelial keratitis
B  Protein aggregates
C  Retinal ganglion cell apoptosis
D  Degeneration of retinal pigment epithelium
E  Immune complex formation on the optic nerve

### QUESTION 10
A 25-year-old patient presents with a complaint of gradual hearing loss. Physical examination reveals a normal otoscopic examination and a positive Schwartze test. Audiogram reveals an air–bone gap. Which of the following is the most likely diagnosis?
A  Otosclerosis
B  Presbyacusia
C  Cholesteatoma
D  Acoustic neuroma
E  Cerumen impaction

## ANSWERS

**1.  C**
EXPLANATION: Bacterial conjunctivitis presents with bright red hyperemia, moderate tearing, and profuse discharge. Preauricular adenopathy is more common in viral conjunctivitis. *Topic: Conjunctivitis*
☐ Correct   ☐ Incorrect

**2.  A**
EXPLANATION: Visual acuity should be determined before the evaluation of any patient with possible ocular foreign body. *Topic: Foreign body: Eye*
☐ Correct   ☐ Incorrect

**3.  B**
EXPLANATION: Vestibular neuronitis (labyrinthitis) typically develops after a viral infection and presents with vertigo (present with eyes open or closed), nystagmus, nausea, and vomiting. No tinnitus or hearing loss is noted. *Topic: Labyrinthitis*
☐ Correct   ☐ Incorrect

**4.  A**
EXPLANATION: Posterior epistaxis typically presents with profuse bleeding down the posterior pharynx and is most commonly treated with posterior nasal packing and possibly embolization or ligation. *Topic: Epistaxis*
☐ Correct   ☐ Incorrect

**5.  D**
EXPLANATION: Odynophagia and displacement of the uvula or tonsil past midline is the typical presentation of peritonsillar abscess. Peritonsillar abscess is typically treated with systemic antibiotics such as ampicillin-sulbactam or clindamycin. *Topic: Peritonsillar abscess*
☐ Correct   ☐ Incorrect

**6.  B**
EXPLANATION: Malignant otitis externa is most commonly noted in elderly diabetic patients and typically is due to infection with *P. aeruginosa*. *Topic: Otitis externa*
☐ Correct   ☐ Incorrect

**7.  A**
EXPLANATION: Type I hypersensitivity reaction, with increased production of IgE, mediates the immune response in allergic rhinitis. *Topic: Allergic rhinitis*
☐ Correct   ☐ Incorrect

**8.  A**
EXPLANATION: Ocular alignment should be stable by 2 to 3 months. If alignment is not stable, the patient should be evaluated by an ophthalmologist. *Topic: Strabismus*
☐ Correct   ☐ Incorrect

## ANSWERS—cont'd

**9. B**
EXPLANATION: The pathophysiologic mechanism of cataracts is the development of protein aggregates that scatter light rays and reduce transparency. *Topic: Cataracts*
☐ Correct ☐ Incorrect

**10. A**
EXPLANATION: Patients with otosclerosis typically present between the ages of 20 and 30 with progressive hearing loss. Otoscopic examination is normal and the Schwartz sign positive. Presbyacusia is hearing loss of advancing age. Acoustic neuroma presents with hearing loss and vertigo. Cerumen impaction would present with an abnormal otoscopic examination. Cholesteatoma presents with hearing loss, but cellular debris is noted in the auditory canal. *Topic: Hearing impairment*
☐ Correct ☐ Incorrect

# CHAPTER 7
# NEUROLOGIC SYSTEM

## EXAMINATION BLUEPRINT TOPICS

**CLOSED HEAD INJURIES**

Concussion

**CRANIAL NERVE PALSIES**

Bell's palsy

**ENCEPHALOPATHIC DISORDERS**

Wernicke's encephalopathy

**HEADACHES**

Cluster headache

Migraine

Tension headache

**INFECTIOUS DISORDERS**

Encephalitis

Meningitis: bacterial

**MOVEMENT DISORDERS**

Amyotrophic lateral sclerosis

Essential tremor

Huntington's disease

Parkinson's disease

Tourette's syndrome

**NEOPLASMS**

Benign

Malignant

**NEUROCOGNITIVE DISORDERS**

Delirium/altered level of consciousness

**ALZHEIMER'S DISEASE**

General

Clinical manifestations

Diagnosis

Treatment

**NEUROMUSCULAR DISORDERS**

Cerebral palsy

Multiple sclerosis

Myasthenia gravis

**PERIPHERAL NERVE DISORDERS**

Carpal tunnel syndrome

Guillain-Barré syndrome

Diabetic peripheral neuropathy

**SEIZURE DISORDERS**

Seizure disorders

Status epilepticus

**VASCULAR DISORDERS**

Arteriovenous malformation

Cerebral aneurysm

Normal-pressure hydrocephalus

Subarachnoid hemorrhage

Stroke

Syncope

Complex regional pain syndrome

## CLOSED HEAD INJURIES

### I. CONCUSSION
  a. **General**
    i. Transient loss or change of consciousness followed by complete recovery.
    ii. Caused by direct blow to head, face, or neck.
  b. **Clinical**
    i. Hallmark symptoms are confusion and amnesia.
    ii. Other symptoms include headache, dizziness, and nausea/vomiting.
    iii. No focal neurologic symptoms are typically present.
  c. **Grading system**
    i. See Table 7.1.
  d. **Treatment**
    i. Patients can typically return to activity when they are symptom free during rest and exertion and when neuropsychological tests are normal.

  e. **Complications**
    i. Post-concussive syndrome.
      1. Common sequela of traumatic brain injury (TBI).
      2. Patients have concussion symptoms that persist for months after injury.
      3. Risk factors include female sex and increasing age.
  f. **Clinical**
    i. Symptoms include headache, dizziness, fatigue, anxiety, insomnia, and loss of concentration and memory.
  g. **Treatment**
    i. Symptomatic therapy.

## CRANIAL NERVE PALSIES

### I. BELL'S PALSY
  a. **General**
    i. Unilateral facial paralysis (cranial nerve VII) of unknown etiology.

**TABLE 7.1**

**Concussion Grading Scale**

| | Grade I | Grade II | Grade III |
|---|---|---|---|
| Colorado Medical Society Guidelines | Confusion<br>No loss of consciousness | Confusion<br>Posttraumatic amnesia<br>No loss of consciousness | Any loss of consciousness |
| American Academy of Neurology Guidelines | Confusion<br>Symptoms last <15 minutes<br>No loss of consciousness | Symptoms last >15 minutes<br>No loss of consciousness | Loss of consciousness<br>IIIa lasts seconds<br>IIIb lasts minutes |

**TABLE 7.2**

**Summary of Cranial Nerve Dysfunction**

| Cranial Nerve | Name | Symptoms of Dysfunction | Possible cause(s) |
|---|---|---|---|
| I | Olfactory | Anosmia | Trauma, Neoplasm |
| II | Optic | Visual field defects, decreased visual acuity | Trauma, neoplasm, multiple sclerosis |
| III | Oculomotor | Fixed and dilated pupil, ptosis | Increased intracranial pressure, microvascular damage (diabetes mellitus), trauma |
| IV | Trochlear | Diplopia | Trauma (whiplash, concussion) |
| V | Trigeminal | Sensory: deficit on clinical exam<br>Motor: Mandibular paralysis | Trauma, idiopathic, HTN |
| VI | Abducens | Inability to gaze laterally | Multiple sclerosis, CVA |
| VII | Facial | Facial weakness or paralysis | Bell's palsy, CVA |
| VIII | Vestibulocochlear | Deafness | Acoustic neuroma, excessive exposure to loud noise |
| IX | Glossopharyngeal | Impaired gag reflex | Trauma |
| X | Vagus | Uvula deviation to unaffected side | Trauma, brainstem lesion |
| XI | Accessory | Weakness of shoulder shrug | CVA |
| XII | Hypoglossal | Protruded tongue deviates to the affected side | Brainstem lesion, trauma |

CVA, Cerebrovascular accident; HTN, hypertension.

1. Possible link to herpes simplex virus.
   b. Table of symptoms of cranial nerve dysfunction can be found in Table 7.2.
b. **Clinical Manifestations**
   i. Typically note facial paralysis upon waking.
   ii. Patients will have trouble closing their eye on the affected side.
   iii. Paralysis may be preceded by pain behind the ear.
   iv. On physical examination, note cranial nerve VII palsy, loss of taste on the anterior two-thirds of the tongue, and hyperacusis.
   v. Inability to wrinkle the forehead can help differentiate Bell's palsy from an upper motor neuron lesion.
c. **Diagnosis**
   i. One of exclusion.
   ii. Rule out herpes zoster oticus (Ramsay Hunt syndrome).
      1. May note herpetic lesions in the external auditory canal.
   iii. Rule out cerebrovascular accident (CVA).

d. **Treatment**
   i. Most cases resolve without treatment, however varying degrees of facial paralysis may persist.
   ii. Eye protection should be used to prevent the eye from drying.
   iii. Oral corticosteroids should be used early to reduce the risk of permanent sequelae.

# ENCEPHALOPATHIC DISORDERS

## WERNICKE'S ENCEPHALOPATHY
a. **General**
   i. An acute condition caused by thiamine deficiency (vitamin B1).
   ii. Affects the peripheral and central nervous systems.
   iii. It is commonly associated with alcohol use disorder but many also be secondary to dietary deficiencies, eating disorders, or chemotherapy.

b. **Clinical Manifestations**
    i. Classic triad of symptoms: confusion, ataxia, and nystagmus.
c. **Diagnosis**
    i. A clinical diagnosis that requires ruling out of other possible causes of neurologic dysfunction.
        1. A patient history of chronic vomiting, insufficient dietary intake, or alcohol use disorder may be present.
    ii. Laboratory testing will confirm decreased thiamine levels.
    iii. CSF analysis, brain CT and MRI, and EEG will all be normal.
d. **Treatment**
    i. IV or IM thiamine replacement, typically given for 3 to 7 days.
        1. Parenteral thiamine is used for acute treatment as intestinal absorption may be impaired.

# HEADACHES

## I. CLUSTER HEADACHE
a. **General**
    i. Recurrent episodes of frequent headaches separated by periods of being headache free.
    ii. The cause is unknown.
    iii. More common in males than females by a 4:1 ratio.
    iv. Headaches may cease during pregnancy.
b. **Clinical Manifestations**
    i. History of recurrent episodes of unilateral, orbital, supraorbital, or temporal pain.
    ii. Accompanied by conjunctival injection, lacrimation, rhinorrhea, nasal congestion, or ptosis.
    iii. Attacks typically last 15–30 minutes but may last up to 3 hours and can occur from every other day to up to eight times per day.
c. **Diagnosis**
    i. Based on history and physical exam.
    ii. Other causes of headache must be ruled out.
d. **Treatment**
    i. High-flow oxygen can serve as an effective abortive therapy.
    ii. Classic treatment is ergotamine tartrate.
    iii. Other options include sumatriptan.
    iv. Preventive therapy includes verapamil, steroids, lithium, and topiramate.

## II. MIGRAINE
a. **General**
    i. Affects females more than males, primarily between ages 25 and 45 years.

**TABLE 7.3**

| Migraine Headache Triggers |
| --- |
| Alcohol |
| Glare |
| Lack of sleep/Fatigue |
| Menses |
| Oral contraceptives |
| Physical exertion |
| Stress |
| Weather changes |

    ii. Increased risk for migraine in patients with relatives with migraines.
    iii. May be brought on by certain triggers (Table 7.3).
b. **Clinical Manifestations**
    i. May have prodrome symptoms 24 to 48 hours before headache attack.
        1. Symptoms include hyperactivity, mild euphoria, lethargy, depression, and craving for certain foods.
    ii. Migraines may or may not have an aura.
        1. Aura includes homonymous visual disturbances (scotoma), unilateral numbness, unilateral weakness, or ataxia.
    iii. Headache lasts 4 to 72 hours and is described as unilateral throbbing or pulsatile pain that is moderate to severe in intensity.
    iv. Associated symptoms include nausea and vomiting, photophobia, and phonophobia.
        1. Patients report lying flat in a quiet, dark room to relieve symptoms.
    v. Headache is intensified with physical activity.
c. **Diagnosis**
    i. Diagnosis is based on history and physical examination.
    ii. Diagnostic testing is used to rule out other causes of headache.
d. **Treatment**
    i. Acute treatment.
        1. Nonpharmacologic therapy includes behavior modification, biofeedback, hypnosis, and meditation.
        2. Abortive pharmacologic therapy includes the following:
        (a) Mild attacks.
            (i) Acetaminophen.
            (ii) Nonsteroidal antiinflammatory drugs (NSAIDs).
        (b) Moderate to severe attacks.
            (i) Butalbital with caffeine and aspirin.
            (ii) Dihydroergotamine.
            (iii) 5-HT receptor agonists (sumatriptan)
                (1) Vasoconstrictive agents, such as 5-HT receptor agonists,

should be avoided in patients with uncontrolled hypertension or coronary artery disease.

(iv) Ergotamine.

ii. Preventive treatment.

1. Recommended if headache limits normal daily activities 3 or more days per month, if headaches are severe, or if headaches are associated with a complication.

2. Treatment options include the following:

(a) β-Adrenergic blockers.

(b) NSAIDs.

(c) Tricyclic antidepressants.

(d) Calcium channel antagonists.

(e) Anticonvulsants.

## III. TENSION HEADACHE

a. **General**

i. Most common type of primary headache disorder.

ii. More common in females than males and typically begins in the second decade of life.

iii. Symptoms may worsen in times of stress.

b. **Clinical Manifestations**

i. Patients have recurrent attacks of diffuse, tight, bandlike or "vise grip," bilateral, mild to moderate pain.

ii. Pain may last from minutes to days.

iii. Pain does not worsen with physical exertion, and there is no associated nausea, vomiting, or photophobia.

c. **Diagnosis**

i. Based on history and physical examination and ruling out other causes.

d. **Treatment**

i. Typically responds to acetaminophen and NSAIDs.

1. Frequent use of pain medications can lead to an increase in the number of headaches.

ii. Chronic tension headaches may require prophylactic treatment with tricyclic antidepressants.

## IV. TABLE 7.4 SUMMARIZES VARIOUS TYPES OF HEADACHES

# INFECTIOUS DISORDERS

## I. ENCEPHALITIS

a. **General**

i. Encephalitis is an infection of the brain parenchyma.

ii. Etiology is typically viral and includes the following:

1. Enterovirus.

2. Arboviruses.

**TABLE 7.4**

| Summary of Various Types of Headaches | | | |
|---|---|---|---|
| **Characteristic** | **Migraine Headache** | **Tension Headache** | **Cluster Headache** |
| Onset | Female > males (+) Family history Peak in adolescence | Females > males Variable age of onset | Male > females Age 20–50 |
| Frequency | 1–2 per month | 5–20 per day | Daily with periods free of headache |
| Triggers | Stress Hormonal changes Caffeine Red wine Chocolate Aged cheese Nitrates, MSG | Fatigue Stress | Alcohol |
| Location | Unilateral > bilateral Bifrontal in 40% | Bilateral Neck or occipital | Unilateral Temporal or orbital |
| Pain | Pulsating Moderate to severe | Pressure or squeezing Waxing severity | Quick onset Excruciating pain Deep and continuous |
| Duration | 4–72 hours | Minutes to days | 30–180 minutes |
| Associated symptoms | Nausea, vomiting Photophobia Phonophobia Aura | None | Ptosis, miosis, lacrimation, conjunctival injection Rhinorrhea, nasal congestion |

*MSG*, Monosodium glutamate.

(a) Transmitted by mosquitoes and ticks.

(b) Cause the following:

(i) California encephalitis.

(ii) Eastern and western equine encephalitis.

(iii) St. Louis encephalitis.

(iv) West Nile encephalitis.

3. Herpes simplex virus.

4. CMV.

5. Rubella.

6. Measles.

iii. Incidence peaks in the late summer.

b. **Clinical Manifestations**

i. Patients present with fever, malaise, myalgias, gastrointestinal symptoms, respiratory symptoms, and rash.

ii. Signs of meningeal irritation, such as headache, photophobia, and stiff neck.

iii. May also develop seizures and a decreased level of consciousness.

iv. Presence of altered mental status, motor or sensory deficits, and altered behavior are noted in encephalitis but not in meningitis.

c. **Diagnosis**

i. Computed tomography (CT) scan of the head should be performed first if viral encephalitis is suspected.

ii. Cerebrospinal fluid (CSF) testing is essential.

1. Gram stain is negative for bacteria.

2. Cell count reveals a white blood cell (WBC) count typically between 50 and 250/mm$^3$, with a majority of the cells being mononuclear leukocytes.

3. Glucose values are typically normal or slightly decreased.

4. Protein is typically greater than 100 mg/dL.

5. C-reactive protein is normal.

iii. Polymerase chain reaction (PCR) testing for herpes simplex virus.

d. **Treatment**

i. Treatment is directed at symptomatic control.

1. Acetaminophen is the drug of choice for controlling fever and headache.

2. Anticonvulsants are not routinely indicated.

ii. Encephalitis caused by herpes simplex virus should be treated with antivirals, such as acyclovir.

iii. Prognosis with encephalitis varies with the cause.

1. Eastern equine encephalitis has a high mortality rate, whereas California encephalitis has a low mortality rate.

2. Complications include difficulty concentrating, behavioral and speech disorders, and memory loss.

## II. MENINGITIS: BACTERIAL

a. **General**

i. Inflammation of the arachnoid, pia mater, and CSF.

ii. Bacterial meningitis is a medical emergency, requiring immediate diagnosis and antibiotic treatment.

iii. Etiology.

1. Table 7.5 lists etiologies by age group.

iv. Clinical settings.

1. Meningococcal meningitis noted in areas of crowded conditions such as classrooms, military settings, prison systems, or dormitories.

(a) Meningococcal meningitis is the only type that occurs in outbreaks.

2. Pneumococcal meningitis is noted in patients with acute otitis media and pneumonia.

3. *Staphylococcus aureus* meningitis noted as a complication of a neurosurgical procedure, trauma, or secondary to endocarditis.

b. **Clinical Manifestations**

i. Present with acute onset of fever, headache, vomiting, and stiff neck.

ii. On physical examination, there is evidence of the following:

1. Meningeal irritation noted by drowsiness, obtundation, stiff neck, and positive Kernig's and Brudzinski's signs.

(a) With patient supine and hip and knee flexed to 90 degrees, further extension of the knee causes pain in the neck or hamstring. This is a positive Kernig's sign.

(b) Flexing the neck of a supine patient resulting in flexion of the hip and knee is a positive Brudzinski's sign.

2. Petechial or purpuric rash that is non-blanching may be noted in meningococcal infection.

3. Neurologic findings include the following:

(a) Cranial nerve abnormalities.

**TABLE 7.5**

**Etiology of Meningitis Based on Age Group**

| Neonates | Children (Age <15 years) | Adults (Age >15 Years) |
|---|---|---|
| Streptococci group B Gram-negative bacilli (Escherichia coli) Listeria monocytogenes | *Streptococcus pneumoniae* *Neisseria meningitidis* *Haemophilus influenzae* | *Streptococcus pneumoniae* *Listeria monocytogenes* *Staphylococcus aureus* Gram-negative bacilli *Neisseria meningitidis* |

**TABLE 7.6**

**Laboratory Findings in Meningitis**

| Agent | Opening Pressure (mm H$_2$O) | WBC Count (mm$^3$) | Neutrophil (%) | Lymphocyte (%) | Protein | Glucose |
|---|---|---|---|---|---|---|
| Normal | <200 | <5 | None | 100 | <50 mg/dL | >50 mg/dL |
| Bacterial | High | >100 | >80 | <20 | >100 mg/dL | <40 mg/dL |
| Viral | High | >50 | <50 | >50 | >50 mg/dL | >50 mg/dL |
| Fungal | High | >50 | <50 | >50 | >50 mg/dL | <40 mg/dL |

**TABLE 7.7**

**Antibiotic Choices for Selective Bacteria in Meningitis**

| Organism | First Choices | Second Choices | Duration of Therapy (Days) |
|---|---|---|---|
| Streptococcus pneumoniae | Penicillin G, ampicillin, or ceftriaxone | Vancomycin or chloramphenicol | 10–14 |
| Neisseria meningitidis | Penicillin G or ampicillin | Ceftriaxone | 7 |
| Haemophilus influenzae | Ampicillin or ceftriaxone | Third-generation cephalosporin or chloramphenicol | 10 |
| Listeria monocytogenes | Ampicillin or penicillin G | Trimethoprim-sulfamethoxazole | 14–21 |
| Staphylococcus aureus | Nafcillin | Vancomycin | 14 |
| Gram-negative bacilli | Cefotaxime or ceftazidime | Meropenem or aztreonam | 21 |
| Pseudomonas aeruginosa | Cefepime or ceftazidime plus tobramycin | Meropenem plus aminoglycoside | 21 |
| Streptococcus agalactiae | Penicillin G or ampicillin | Ceftriaxone or cefotaxime | 14–21 |

(i) Typically cranial nerves III, IV, VI, and VII.
(b) Seizures.
(c) Focal cerebral signs such as hemiparesis, dysphagia, and visual field defects.
(d) Papilledema is rare.

**c. Diagnosis**
i. CSF should be obtained and examined.
1. Gram stain should be evaluated for white blood cells (WBCs) and bacteria.
2. Rapid antigen testing can be used to test for *Haemophilus influenzae*, *Streptococcus pneumoniae*, Group B *Streptococcus*, *Neisseria meningitidis*, and *Escherichia coli*.
3. Cell count reveals a WBC count typically greater than 100/mm$^3$, with a majority of the cells being polymorphonuclear leukocytes.
4. Glucose values typically less than 40 mg/dL.
5. Protein typically greater than 100 mg/dL.
6. Lactic acid levels are elevated in bacterial meningitis and low/normal in viral meningitis.
ii. Initial CT of the head is not indicated unless signs of mass effect of focal neurologic deficit on physical examination.

iii. Table 7.6 shows laboratory results of the various etiologies of meningitis.

**d. Treatment**
i. Bactericidal agents should be used whenever possible.
1. Certain antibiotics should be avoided, such as first- and second-generation cephalosporins and clindamycin, because adequate levels cannot be achieved in the CSF.
2. Table 7.7 lists antibiotic choices for selective bacteria causing meningitis.
ii. Initial therapy for bacterial meningitis of unknown cause varies based on age group (Table 7.8).
iii. Chemoprophylaxis of close contacts of patients with meningococcal meningitis is needed.
1. Oral rifampin is the drug of choice.
(a) May result in reddish-orange dissociation of sweat, saliva, urine, and tears.
(b) Avoid use in pregnant patients.
2. Oral ciprofloxacin, ofloxacin, or ceftriaxone can be used as alternatives.
iv. Dexamethasone is given to lower risk of complications.
1. Complications include hydrocephalus, deafness, seizures, and cranial nerve palsies.

**TABLE 7.8**

| Initial Therapy for Bacterial Meningitis of Unknown Cause | | |
|---|---|---|
| **Age Group** | **First Choice** | **Second Choice** |
| Neonate | Ampicillin plus cefotaxime | Ampicillin plus gentamicin |
| Children | Cefotaxime or ceftriaxone plus vancomycin | Ampicillin plus chloramphenicol or meropenem |
| Adults | Cefotaxime or ceftriaxone plus vancomycin | Meropenem |
| Elderly | Cefotaxime or ceftriaxone plus ampicillin plus vancomycin | Cefotaxime plus vancomycin plus trimethoprim-sulfamethoxazole |

# MOVEMENT DISORDERS

## I. AMYOTROPHIC LATERAL SCLEROSIS (LOU GEHRIG'S DISEASE)

### a. General

i. Upper and lower motor neuron disorder of unknown cause that presents with progressive weakness.

ii. Most common motor neuron disease that typically affects patients older than 40 years and more males than females.

### b. Clinical Manifestations

i. The first sign is muscle weakness and atrophy in the hands.

  a. Patients may complain of a weakened grip or difficulty opening jars or buttoning shirts.

ii. May also note fasciculations (including the tongue), spasticity, dysarthria, and dysphagia.

iii. Sensory systems, voluntary eye muscles, and urinary sphincter are spared from the disease.

iv. May note signs of both upper and lower motor neuron disease (Table 7.9).

### c. Diagnosis

i. Based on history and physical examination.

ii. EMG may show changes of chronic partial denervation and reinnervation with spontaneous

**TABLE 7.9**

| Signs of Upper and Lower Motor Neuron Disease | |
|---|---|
| **Upper Motor Neuron Disease** | **Lower Motor Neuron Disease** |
| Spasticity | Flaccid paralysis |
| Hyperreflexia | Areflexia or hyporeflexia |
| No fasciculations | Fasciculations |
| Upward Babinski reflex | Downward Babinski reflex |
| Little or no muscle atrophy | Loss of muscle tone and atrophy |

abnormal activity in resting muscle in at least three limbs.

### d. Treatment

i. Riluzole may reduce progression of the disease and may extend life expectancy by 3 to 6 months.

ii. Edaravone is given IV and has been shown to reduce daily functioning declines.

iii. Supportive care.

iv. Life expectancy is typically 3 to 5 years.

## II. ESSENTIAL TREMOR

### a. General

i. The cause is unknown, but it can be inherited in an autosomal dominant pattern.

### b. Clinical Manifestations

i. May begin at any age and is enhanced by emotional stress.

ii. Typically involves the hands or head.

iii. Physical examination is normal except for the intention tremor.

  a. Tremor will worsen when performing actions that require refined hand movements such as buttoning a shirt.

  b. Patients may report an improvement in symptoms with alcohol consumption.

iv. Patients lack the hypokinetic features and rigidity of Parkinson's disease.

### c. Treatment

i. Many patients do not require treatment.

ii. Beta-blockers (propranolol) are the most effective treatments.

  1. If not effective, can utilize primidone.

iii. Modest doses of alcohol may improve the tremor, but are not a recommended therapy.

## III. HUNTINGTON'S DISEASE

### a. General

i. A genetic disorder characterized by choreiform movements, mental status decline, and personality changes.

  1. Located on chromosome 4 (CAG trinucleotide repeat).

  2. Autosomal dominant pattern of inheritance with 100% disease penetrance.

ii. Onset of symptoms is typically from age 30 to 50 years.

### b. Clinical Manifestations

i. Patients present with insidious onset of clumsiness and random, brief, fidgety movements.

ii. Involuntary choreic, "dance-like," movements.

  1. Worse with voluntary movements, increased by emotional stress, and disappear with sleep.

  2. Gait is irregular, unsteady, and dancelike.

iii. Dementia.

  1. Includes memory loss and apathy.

iv. Personality changes.
  1. Include agitation, psychosis, irritability, and antisocial behavior.
v. On physical examination, the reflexes are brisk, and the patient is not able to maintain tongue protrusion.
vi. Laboratory and CSF studies are normal.
vii. CT or MRI of the brain reveals cerebral atrophy.

#### c. Diagnosis
i. Based on history, especially family history, and physical examination.
ii. Confirm diagnosis with genetic testing.

#### d. Treatment
i. There is no cure for the disease.
  1. Genetic counseling, physical and occupational therapies, and nutritional counseling are important.
ii. Initially, the movement disorder can be controlled with tetrabenazine, deutetrabenazine, risperidone, or haloperidol.
iii. Death typically occurs about 15 years after onset of symptoms.

## IV. PARKINSON'S DISEASE

#### a. General
i. A progressive, degenerative disease resulting from loss of dopaminergic neurons in the substantia nigra, in the basal ganglia.
ii. A very common disorder, affecting males more than females.
iii. The mean age of onset is 60 years.
  a. Young onset Parkinson's disease is onset before the age of 50 years.
  b. Juvenile Parkinsonism has disease onset before the age of 21 years.
iv. Drug-induced parkinsonism can be noted with dopamine receptor antagonists, such as antiemetics, antipsychotics, and reserpine.

#### b. Clinical Manifestations
i. The classic triad of Parkinson's disease includes the following:
  1. Tremor: a resting, pill-rolling tremor that decreases with movement.
  2. Cogwheel rigidity.
  3. Bradykinesia.
    (a) Accounts for slowing of movements, lack of facial expression (masked facies), staring expression from decreased blinking, impaired swallowing, monotone speech, and micrographia.
ii. Also note postural instability.
iii. Gait is shuffling with short steps and decreased arm swing.
iv. Depression and dementia are common.

#### c. Diagnosis
i. History and physical examination are typically diagnostic.
ii. CT scan of the brain is often done to rule out other pathology.

#### d. Treatment
i. A progressive disorder without a cure.
ii. Treatment is lifelong and must include psychological support for the patient and family.
iii. Medications.
  1. Levodopa plus carbidopa.
    (a) Levodopa is metabolized to dopamine.
    (b) Carbidopa inactivates enzymes that metabolize levodopa allowing a smaller dose to be used and reducing side effects.
    (c) Levodopa can suppress tremor, but it is more useful in controlling bradykinesia and rigidity.
    (d) Over time, patients lose their response to levodopa.
    (e) Side effects include nausea and vomiting, hypotension, dyskinesias, and confusion.
  2. Dopamine agonist.
    (a) Bromocriptine and pergolide.
      (i) Side effects include anorexia, nausea, vomiting, and postural hypotension.
      (ii) Avoid in patients with mental illness or recent myocardial infarction.
    (b) Pramipexole and ropinirole.
      (i) Side effects include fatigue, nausea, edema, confusion, and postural hypotension.
      (ii) May also note excessive sleepiness.
  3. Anticholinergics.
    (a) More helpful with tremor and rigidity.
    (b) Drugs include benztropine mesylate, procyclidine, and trihexyphenidyl.
    (c) Side effects include dry mouth, nausea, constipation, palpitations, urinary retention, agitation, confusion, and increased intraocular pressure.
    (d) Contraindicated in patients with narrow-angle glaucoma and prostatic hypertrophy.
  4. Amantadine.
    (a) Mode of action is unknown but appears to improve all the features of Parkinson's disease.
    (b) Side effects are rare at the normal dose.
  5. Selegiline.
    (a) A monoamine oxidase B inhibitor that inhibits the breakdown of dopamine.

(b) It is not neuroprotective, but may delay the need for levodopa.

6. Catechol-O-methyl transferase (COMT) inhibitors.

(a) Options include tolcapone or entacapone.

(b) Prolong and potentiate effects of levodopa.

(c) Not used as a single agent.

iv. Surgery.

1. Deep brain stimulation may be effective for relieving symptoms.

2. Stereotactic thalamotomy is done in cases of disabling tremor.

## V. TOURETTE'S SYNDROME

a. **General**

i. Neurological disorder manifested by motor and phonic tics with onset during childhood.

1. Most common cause of tics.

ii. Inherited in autosomal dominant pattern.

iii. Likely due to a disturbance in the striatal-thalamic-cortical spinal system, which leads to disinhibition of the motor and limbic system.

b. **Clinical**

i. Tics are the clinical hallmark.

1. Tics are sudden, brief, intermittent movements or utterances.

2. Can be simple (eye blinking, facial grimacing, head jerking) and complex (bizarre gait, kicking, body gyrations).

3. Involuntary utterances range from simple noises to obscene words, repetition of words, and repetition of a phrase.

ii. Onset typically between 2 and 15 years of age.

1. Tics resolve by age 18 in half of the patients.

iii. Physical examination is typically normal except for the presence of tics.

c. **Diagnosis**

i. Based on clinical features.

d. **Treatment**

i. Dopamine antagonists such as fluphenazine or pimozide for tics.

ii. Habit reversal training may be effective in improving tics and controlling symptoms.

## NEOPLASMS

### I. BENIGN

a. **General**

i. There are many types of benign neoplasms. Two common forms are discussed in this section.

1. Meningiomas: Most common type of primary brain tumor. Arises in the brain or spinal cord.

2. Acoustic neuromas: Benign Schwann cell tumors arising from the vestibular segment of CNXIII. Often associated with neurofibromatosis I.

iii. Pituitary adenomas are discussed in Chapter 5 Endocrine System.

b. **Clinical Manifestations**

i. Meningiomas: Symptoms vary based on size and location. Include visual changes, headaches, memory loss, loss of smell, and seizures.

ii. Acoustic neuromas: unilateral sensorineural hearing loss, tinnitus, and imbalance.

c. **Diagnosis**

i. Meningiomas: CT scan.

ii. Acoustic neuromas: CT scan.

d. **Treatment**

i. Meningiomas: Surgical removal.

ii. Acoustic neuromas: Surgical removal.

### II. MALIGNANT

a. **General**

i. Primary brain tumors are most commonly glioblastomas.

ii. Primary lung and breast cancer and melanoma most commonly metastasize to the brain.

b. **Clinical Manifestations**

i. Red flag symptoms include new onset headaches that become more frequent and severe, focal neuro deficits, visual disturbances, and new onset seizures.

c. **Diagnosis**

i. MRI with biopsy.

d. **Treatment**

i. Surgical removal if possible.

ii. Radiation and chemotherapy are often used.

## NEUROCOGNITIVE DISORDERS

### I. DELIRIUM/ALTERED LEVEL OF CONSCIOUSNESS

a. **General**

i. Delirium and confused states are very common.

ii. Delirium has the following four key factors:

1. Reduced ability to focus or sustain attention.

2. Perceptual disturbance.

3. Short course with fluctuations.

(a) Verses dementia, which is progressive.

4. Due to a medical condition, substance, or medication.

b. **Etiologies**

i. See Table 7.10 for common causes of delirium and confusional states.

**TABLE 7.10**

| Common Causes of Delirium and Confusional States | |
|---|---|
| Drugs/Toxins | Prescription medications: opioids, sedatives<br>Nonprescription medications: antihistamines<br>Drugs of abuse: ethanol, hallucinogens<br>Withdrawal states: ethanol, benzodiazepines<br>Drug side effects |
| Infections | Sepsis<br>Systemic infections |
| Metabolic abnor-malities | Hyponatremia/Hypernatremia<br>Hypocalcemia/Hypercalcemia<br>Hypothyroidism/Hyperthyroidism<br>Hypoglycemia/Hyperglycemia<br>Hypoosmolar/Hyperosmolar states<br>Hypoxemia<br>Wernicke's encephalopathy |
| Brain disorders | Central nervous system infections<br>Epileptic seizures<br>Hypertensive encephalopathy |
| Systemic failure | Cardiac failure<br>Liver failure<br>Renal failure |
| Physical disorders | Burns<br>Hypothermia/Hyperthermia<br>Trauma |

**TABLE 7.11**

| Degenerative Dementias | | |
|---|---|---|
| **Neurodegenerative** | **Traumatic** | **Infectious** |
| Alzheimer's disease<br>Lewy body disease<br>Huntington's disease<br>Parkinson's disease<br>Pick's disease (fronto-temporal) | Dementia pugilistica ("punch drunk") | AIDS, encephalopathy<br>Progressive multifocal leukoencephalopathy<br>Creutzfeldt-Jakob disease |

    e. Table 7.11 shows various etiologies of degenerative dementias

## II. CLINICAL MANIFESTATIONS

    a. **Patient is typically older than 65 years and presents with the following:**
        i. Early stage.
            1. Memory loss.
                (a) The patient has difficulty learning new material (anterograde amnesia) and has impaired recent memory.
            2. Word-finding problems.
                (a) Word-finding pauses with diminished verbal fluency.
            3. Visuospatial disturbances.
                (a) Decline in drawing and driving abilities.
        ii. Intermediate stage.
            1. Develops aphasia, apraxia, and behavioral disturbances.
            2. Sleep-wake cycle disturbances.
            3. Decline in activities of daily living.
            4. May wander, get lost, and is at an increased risk for falls.
        iii. Terminal stage.
            1. Further cognitive decline, motor abnormalities, and both urinary and fecal incontinence.
            2. Recent and remote memories are lost.
            3. May be unable to swallow and eat.

## III. DIAGNOSIS

    a. **Definitive diagnosis can be proven only at autopsy with the demonstration of neurofibrillary tangles and senile plaques**
    b. **Evaluate each patient to exclude other possible causes of dementia**
        i. This includes evaluating serum chemistries, vitamin $B_{12}$, thyroid-stimulating hormone (TSH), and CSF studies.

## IV. TREATMENT

    a. **There is no cure. Treatment is palliative only**
    b. **Education, counseling, and support groups for family and caregivers are essential**

    c. **Evaluation**
        i. Electrolytes, renal function, glucose, calcium, complete blood count (CBC), and urinalysis should be obtained.
        ii. In elderly patients who present with delirium, there should be high suspicion for urinary tract infection (UTI) (urosepsis) as the source of infection.
        iii. Obtain drug levels for current medication and toxicology.
        iv. CT scan and possible spinal tap.
    d. **Treatment**
        i. Avoid factors that trigger or aggravate delirium.
        ii. Treat the underlying cause.
        iii. Provide supportive care.

# ALZHEIMER'S DISEASE

## I. GENERAL

    a. **A progressive dementia with insidious onset and characterized by atrophy of the cerebral cortex**
    b. **A very common cause of dementia**
    c. **Genetic mutations have been implicated**
        i. Increased risk if there is history of a first-degree relative being affected by the disease.
    d. **A mean of 10 years passes from onset of disease to death**

c. **Medications for specific behavioral problems may be indicated**
   i. Delusions.
      1. Risperidone, olanzapine, or quetiapine can be used.
      2. Haloperidol should be avoided because of side effects including tardive dyskinesia and prolonged QT interval.
   ii. Agitation.
      1. Trazodone, divalproex, or carbamazepine can be used.
      2. Anticholinergic agents are contraindicated because of possible worsening of dementia.
d. **Medications for Alzheimer's disease**
   i. Amyloid beta-directed monoclonal antibody reduces amyloid beta build up.
      1. Aducanumab
   ii. Acetylcholinesterase inhibitors will improve cognition, activities of daily living, and apathy.
      1. Donepezil.
      2. Rivastigmine.
      3. Galantamine.
      4. Side effects of the acetylcholinesterase inhibitors include nausea, vomiting, diarrhea, and muscle cramps.
   iii. *N*-methyl-D-aspartate receptor antagonist.
      1. Memantine.
      2. Is neuroprotective.

# NEUROMUSCULAR DISORDERS

## I. CEREBRAL PALSY
a. **General**
   i. Group of congenital, permanent, nonprogressive motor disabilities.
   ii. Risk factors include prematurity, multiple gestation, low birth weight, and abnormal prenatal or perinatal history.
b. **Clinical Manifestations**
   i. Nonprogressive, but clinical presentation may vary over time.
   ii. Subtypes include spastic, dyskinetic, and ataxic.
   iii. Excessive irritability, decreased interaction, weakness, difficulty feeding, rigid body positions, or hypotonia.
   iv. Findings vary based on the location of the brain affected.
c. **Diagnosis**
   i. Relies on historical information and physical exam findings.
   ii. MRI, cranial US in neonates, and EEG (if seizures) can help rule out other possible causes.

d. **Treatment**
   i. There is no cure and management is directed at relieving symptoms.
      1. Multiple specialists are necessary to coordinate care.
   ii. Pain and spasticity can be managed with botulinum toxin and benzodiazepines.
   iii. Surgical management options include baclofen pump, tendon release, spinal fusion, and deep brain stimulation.

## I. MULTIPLE SCLEROSIS
a. **General**
   i. Cause is unknown, but mediated by immune-initiated inflammatory demyelination and axonal injury.
   ii. More common in the temperate zones of the world and decreases in incidence toward the equator.
   ii. Females are affected more often than males, and symptoms typically begin between the ages of 15 and 45 years.
b. **Clinical Manifestations**
   i. Common presenting symptoms include weakness, numbness, tingling, and unsteadiness in a limb.
      1. Heat may worsen the symptoms.
   ii. Visual symptoms are common and include diplopia, monocular vision loss, and blurry vision (optic neuritis).
      1. Optic neuritis is the most common visual symptom and it affects approximately half of all patients with MS at some stage of the illness.
   iii. Spasticity is common and consists of increased muscle tone, hyperreflexia, limb spasms, weakness, and loss of dexterity.
      1. Typically affects the upper more than the lower extremities.
   iv. Lhermitte's sign is positive with the sensation of electricity down the back with passive flexion of the neck.
   v. The pattern of disease varies from relapsing-remitting, secondary and primary progressive, and progressive-relapsing.
c. **Diagnosis**
   i. Based on clinical features and laboratory results.
   ii. Laboratory tests reveal the following:
      1. CSF.
         (a) Increased CSF immunoglobulin levels.
            (i) Discrete oligoclonal bands.
         (b) CSF protein is normal or mildly elevated.
         (c) CSF cell count is less than 50 mononuclear cells/mm$^3$.
         (d) Increased levels of myelin basic protein.

2. Sensory evoked potentials.
   (a) Loss of myelin slows conduction velocity and possible conduction blocks.
   (b) Visual evoked potentials are prolonged in multiple sclerosis.
3. MRI scanning.
   (a) Reveals multifocal, hyperintense lesions in the periventricular cerebral white matter, cerebellum, brain stem, and/or spinal cord.
   (b) MRI is the test of choice.

**d. Treatment**
  i. Treatment of common symptoms.
    1. Spasticity treated with baclofen or diazepam.
     (a) Dystonic spasms (brief, painful posturing of the extremities) are treated with carbamazepine or phenytoin.
    2. Fatigue treated with amantadine.
    3. Depression treated with serotonin reuptake inhibitors.
  ii. Treatment of multiple sclerosis.
    1. A brief course of IV corticosteroids can be helpful in an acute relapse.
    2. Immunomodulatory therapy, interferon beta-1b (Betaseron), reduces the frequency and severity of relapses, slows the progression of the disease, and reduces the number of brain lesions.
    3. Plasma exchange.

**e. Prognosis**
  i. There are various disease patterns.
    1. Clinically isolated syndrome.
    2. Relapsing-remitting.
     (a) The most common form, affecting approximately 80% to 90% of patients with MS.
    3. Secondary progressive.
    4. Primary progressive.

## II. MYASTHENIA GRAVIS
**a. General**
  i. An acquired autoimmune disorder that causes a decrease in acetylcholine receptors at the motor end plate.
  ii. Fluctuating weakness of commonly used voluntary muscles that results in increased weakness with activity of affected muscles.
  iii. Occurs at all ages, with females primarily affected in their 20s and males in their 50s or 60s.
  iv. Approximately 50% of patients with a thymoma will have symptoms of myasthenia gravis (MSG) throughout the course of their disease.

**b. Clinical Manifestations**
  i. In early stages, the disease often affects the eye muscles, causing ptosis and diplopia.
    1. Other facial muscles may be affected, resulting in loss of facial expression, jaw drop, and choking on food.
  ii. Limb muscle involvement leads to abnormal fatigability.
    1. Patients will have trouble combing hair, climbing stairs, or lifting objects repeatedly.
  iii. Deep tendon reflexes remain normal.

**c. Diagnosis**
  i. Based on history and physical examination findings.
  ii. Anticholinesterase challenge test in which intravenous (IV) edrophonium or intramuscular (IM) neostigmine results in improved strength within seconds to minutes.
  iii. EMG reveals a decrease in action potentials amplitude over a number of muscle contractions.
  iv. Serology testing may reveal presence of antibodies to acetylcholine receptor binding sites.

**d. Treatment**
  i. Anticholinesterase drugs such as pyridostigmine bromide and neostigmine bromide are the cornerstones of treatment.
  ii. Other treatment options include alternate-day prednisone treatment, thymectomy, azathioprine, plasmapheresis, and IV immunoglobulin.
  iii. Aminoglycosides, telithromycin, and magnesium sulfate may exacerbate the disease and should be avoided.

# PERIPHERAL NERVE DISORDERS

## I. CARPAL TUNNEL SYNDROME
**a. General**
  i. Common condition that occurs with compression of the medial nerve.
  ii. Risk factors include pregnancy, wrist fracture, hand deformity, diabetes, and rheumatoid arthritis.
  ii. Significantly more common in males than females.

**b. Clinical Manifestations**
  i. Grip weakness, pain or numbness in the fingers following median nerve distribution (thumb, index, and middle finger).
  ii. The patient may wake up in the middle of the night with symptoms.

**c. Diagnosis**
  i. Clinical presentation:

1. Phalen test: flexing the wrist to 90 degrees for one minute elicits symptoms.
2. Tinel test: symptoms are elicited by tapping over the median nerve.

ii. Electromyography (EMG) showing nerve conduction delay.

### d. Treatment

i. Splinting the wrist in a neutral position, including overnight.
ii. Oral or local injections of corticosteroids.
iii. Carpal tunnel release: surgical incision in the carpal ligament to relieve median nerve pressure.

## IV. GUILLAIN-BARRÉ SYNDROME

### a. General

i. An acute or subacute polyradiculoneuropathy most likely due to an immune-mediated mechanism.
ii. Due to lymphocytic infiltration and macrophage-mediated demyelination and axonal degeneration.
iii. Typically follows some type of infection such as *Campylobacter*, Epstein-Barr virus, and cytomegalovirus (CMV).

### b. Clinical Manifestations

i. Initial symptoms include ataxia and tingling or a pins-and-needles sensation in the feet.
ii. Weakness then develops, typically involving the legs.
iii. On physical examination, the deep tendon reflexes are lost early, and weakness is noted in a bilateral and ascending pattern.

### c. Diagnosis

i. Diagnosis based on history and physical examination of progressive bilateral weakness and areflexia.
ii. Spinal fluid studies may reveal an elevated total protein and normal cell count.
iii. Electromyogram (EMG) results are consistent with demyelination and decreased nerve conduction studies.

### d. Treatment

i. Typically requires hospitalization because of the risk for respiratory muscle involvement and the need for ventilatory support.
ii. Treatment options include plasmapheresis and high doses of human immunoglobulin.

## III. DIABETIC PERIPHERAL NEUROPATHY

### a. General

i. Symptomatic, possibly disabling neuropathy seen in nearly one half of patients with diabetes.
ii. Can have peripheral and/or autonomic neuropathy.

### b. Clinical Manifestations

i. Focal neuropathy.
1. Begins suddenly and patients present with pain.
2. Self-limited, typically lasting 6 to 8 weeks.
3. Treatment is aimed at pain control.

ii. Sensorimotor polyneuropathy.
1. Most common neurologic syndrome seen in diabetes.
2. Affects distal sensorimotor nerves of the hands and feet.
3. Patients report numbness or tingling in a "stocking-glove pattern."
4. Pain is common and may be described as burning, gnawing, numbness, and/or tingling.
5. Physical examination findings include loss of vibratory sensation, light touch, two-point discrimination, and thermal sensitivity.

iii. Autonomic.
1. May affect many different organ systems.
   (a) Cardiac symptoms include resting tachycardia, decreased heart rate variability, and prolonged QTc.
   (b) Vascular symptoms include postural hypotension.
   (c) Gastrointestinal symptoms include constipation and gastroparesis.
   (d) Genitourinary symptoms include bladder hypotonia, incontinence, and erectile dysfunction.

### c. Diagnosis

i. A complete history and physical examination are needed.
1. Neurologic examination must include a detailed sensory examination.
ii. Nerve conduction studies and electromyography may be needed.

### d. Treatment

i. Tight glycemic control is the best early treatment.
ii. Treatment of autonomic symptoms.
1. Gastroparesis treated with metoclopramide or domperidone.
   (a) Ondansetron can be used to mitigate associated nausea.
2. Genitourinary complaints treated with bethanechol or alpha-blockers.
3. Erectile dysfunction can be treated with sildenafil.
   (a) Sildenafil should be avoided in patients with heart disease.
iii. Neuropathic pain control.
1. Tricyclic antidepressants such as amitriptyline and desipramine.

2. Anticonvulsants such as carbamazepine and gabapentin.
3. Topical therapy such as capsaicin.
4. Long-term opiate use and pain specialist management may be needed in refractory cases.

# SEIZURE DISORDERS

I. **SEIZURE DISORDERS EXHIBIT SUDDEN, EXCESSIVE, AND DISORDERLY DISCHARGE OF CEREBRAL NEURONS THAT RESULT IN ABNORMAL MOVEMENTS OR PERCEPTIONS THAT ARE OF SHORT DURATION BUT TEND TO RECUR**
   a. **Classification**
      i. Focal/Partial:
         1. Simple.
            (a) Confined to a single locus in the brain.
            (b) Patients often have abnormal activity of a single limb and do not lose consciousness.
            (c) Seizures may be followed by a transient neurologic deficit (Todd's paralysis).
            (d) Can occur at any age.
         2. Complex.
            (a) Patients have complex sensory hallucinations, mental distortion, and loss of consciousness.
            (b) Motor dysfunction includes automatisms.
      ii. Generalized.
         1. Tonic-clonic.
            (a) Have loss of consciousness, followed by tonic (stiffening) then clonic (rhythmic jerking) phases.
            (b) Urinary incontinence is common.
            (c) Followed by a postictal period.
         2. Absence.
            (a) Have brief, abrupt, and self-limiting loss of consciousness.
            (b) Patients typically stare and then exhibit rapid eye blinking that lasts 3 to 5 seconds.
               (i) Often reported as periods of "daydreaming."
            (c) No postictal period.
         3. Myoclonic.
            (a) Have short periods of muscle contraction that may reoccur for several minutes.
            (b) No loss of consciousness.
         4. Atonic
            (a) Sudden loss of control of muscles, mainly in the legs.

            (b) Often referred to as "drop seizures" as patients suddenly collapse to the floor.
         iii. Febrile.
            1. Consist of generalized tonic-clonic seizures of short duration, accompanied by high fever.
            2. Occur most often between 6 months and 4 years of age.
   b. **Clinical Manifestations**
      i. A detailed history is vital in making the diagnosis.
      ii. Physical examination is typically normal.
      iii. Evaluate for head trauma.
   c. **Diagnosis**
      i. Electroencephalography (EEG) is the most important test in diagnosing seizures.
         1. Note epileptiform abnormalities on the EEG.
      ii. MRI should be obtained on all adults with new-onset seizures to rule out other abnormalities.
   d. **Treatment**
      i. No treatment can cure epilepsy, but it can control frequency of seizures.
      ii. Drug levels monitored to minimize side effects.
      iii. About 70% of patients will achieve a 5-year remission of seizures.
      iv. Driving precautions must be taken in patients with seizure disorders.
      v. Table 7.12 shows antiepileptic agent selections.
      vi. Table 7.13 summarizes antiepileptic medications.

II. **STATUS EPILEPTICUS**
   a. **General**
      i. A single seizure lasting longer than 5 minutes or multiple seizures that occur without the

**TABLE 7.12**

| Antiepileptic Agent Selection | | |
| --- | --- | --- |
| **Type of Epilepsy** | **Preferred Agent** | **Alternative Agent** |
| **Partial** | | |
| Simple | Phenytoin Carbamazepine | Phenobarbital |
| Complex | Phenytoin Carbamazepine | Phenobarbital |
| **Generalized** | | |
| Tonic-clonic | Valproic acid Lamotrigine | Phenobarbital Carbamazepine |
| Absence | Ethosuximide | Valproic acid |
| Myoclonic | Clonazepam | Lamotrigine Valproic acid |

**TABLE 7.13**

## Summary of Antiepileptic Medications

| Drug | Mechanism of Action | Side Effects | Notes |
|---|---|---|---|
| Carbamazepine | Blocks sodium channels, reducing abnormal impulses | Aplastic anemia<br>Drowsiness<br>Nausea/Vomiting<br>Respiratory depression<br>Stupor or coma<br>Vertigo/Ataxia | |
| Ethosuximide | Reduces propagation of abnormal electrical activity | Agitation<br>Dizziness<br>Drowsiness<br>Nausea/Vomiting | Stevens-Johnson syndrome may occur.<br>Aplastic anemia |
| Gabapentin | Unknown | Ataxia<br>Dizziness<br>Fatigue<br>Somnolence | Typically used as an add-on agent |
| Lamotrigine | Blocks sodium channels and prevents repeat firing | Ataxia<br>Diplopia<br>Drowsiness<br>Rash | Increase dose slowly to avoid potential for severe rash |
| Phenytoin | Stabilize neuronal cells by decreasing flux of sodium ions | Ataxia<br>Gingival hyperplasia<br>Nausea/Vomiting<br>Nystagmus | Teratogenic: cleft lip and palate, and congenital heart disease |
| Phenobarbital | Unknown | Nausea/Vomiting<br>Nystagmus<br>Rash<br>Sedation<br>Vertigo/Ataxia | |
| Valproic acid | Enhances GABA action at inhibitory synapses, reducing abnormal discharge in the brain | Ataxia<br>Hepatic toxicity<br>Nausea/Vomiting<br>Sedation<br>Tremor | Monitor liver function tests.<br>May cause thrombocytopenia and bleeding |

*GABA,* γ-Aminobutyric acid.

patient regaining consciousness between episodes.

ii. The most common cause is a patient with known seizure disorder who has subtherapeutic levels of antiseizure medications.

b. **Clinical Manifestations**

i. Present most commonly with tonic-clonic seizures, but other types are possible.

c. **Diagnosis**

i. Must rule out potential causes such as alcohol withdrawal, metabolic abnormalities, febrile, tumor, anoxia, psychogenic, or trauma.

1. Drug screen, chemistry profile, lumbar puncture, and CT/MRI are typically indicated.

ii. Definitive diagnosis requires EEG.

d. **Treatment**

i. Treatment should be started immediately.

ii. Prognosis varies with etiology.

1. Death occurs in up to 10% of adults.

iii. Treatment protocol.

1. IV lorazepam or diazepam or IM midazolam should be started immediately.

2. The second phase includes phenytoin or fosphenytoin.

3. Thiamine and glucose.

4. Patients who fail to respond to benzodiazepine often require intubation and sedation. Intubation is most often indicated in patients seizures secondary to toxic or metabolic etiologies.

# VASCULAR DISORDERS

## I. ARTERIOVENOUS MALFORMATION

a. **General**

i. Malformations of arteries and veins that become tangled and form direct connections.

ii. Idiopathic and not considered hereditary.

iii. Often congenital.

b. **Clinical Manifestations**
   i. Symptoms vary based on location and severity.
   ii. AVMs in the brain may cause progressive neurological deficits, headaches, or seizures.
c. **Diagnosis**
   i. CT or MRI.
d. **Treatment**
   i. Ranges from observation to surgical removal.

## II. CEREBRAL ANEURYSM
a. **General**
   i. Thin-walled outpouchings that protrude from the arteries.
   ii. Different types.
      1. Saccular (berry).
         (a) Most common intracranial aneurysm.
         (b) Typically located on the circle of Willis or major branches.
      2. Fusiform.
         (a) Elongated dilations of large arteries.
         (b) Associated with atherosclerosis.
         (c) Typically develop in the basilar artery.
      3. Mycotic.
         (a) Due to an infected emboli.
         (b) Frequently multiple and found in the distal cerebral arteries.
b. **Clinical Manifestations**
   i. Signs and symptoms vary depending on the location of the aneurysm and the compression of surrounding structures.
c. **Diagnosis**
   i. CT scan, magnetic resonance arteriography, or angiography is commonly used to make diagnosis.
d. **Treatment**
   i. Saccular aneurysms treated by surgical clipping.
   ii. Fusiform aneurysms are treated with total occlusion.

## III. NORMAL-PRESSURE HYDROCEPHALUS
a. **General**
   i. Dilation of the cerebral ventricles and secondary to prior CNS insult.
      1. Insults include subarachnoid hemorrhage, trauma, infection, or tumors.
   ii. Typically seen in adults older than 60 years, and incidence higher in males than females.
b. **Clinical Manifestations**
   i. Present with wide-based, shuffling gait (apraxia), dementia, and urinary incontinence.
   ii. Also note weakness, malaise, and lethargy.
c. **Diagnosis**
   i. Based on history and physical examination.
   ii. Lumbar puncture reveals an elevated opening pressure.
   iii. CT scan or MRI shows enlarged ventricles.

d. **Treatment**
   i. Removal of CSF provides temporary relief.
   ii. Ventriculoperitoneal shunt is the treatment of choice.

## IV. SUBARACHNOID HEMORRHAGE
a. **General**
   i. Rupture of vessels on or near the surface of the brain or ventricles.
   ii. Mainly affects young adults; males and females are affected equally.
   iii. Trauma is the most common cause of subarachnoid hemorrhage.
      1. Rupture of an aneurysm is the most common nontraumatic cause.
      2. Arteriovenous malformation is another cause.
   iv. Risk factors include the following:
      1. Smoking.
      2. Binge drinking.
      3. Phenylpropanolamine or other sympathomimetics.
b. **Clinical Manifestations**
   i. Patients describe pain as the worst headache of their lives and or a rapid-onset "thunder-clap" headache.
   ii. Rapidly developing pain and stiff neck.
   iii. Blood pressure may be elevated, and there may be mental status changes.
   iv. On physical examination, focal neurologic deficit is not noted unless there is compression of surrounding brain structures.
   v. Funduscopic examination reveals well-circumscribed, bright red, preretinal hemorrhages.
c. **Diagnosis**
   i. Diagnosed by CT scan, which reveals an area of high attenuation consistent with bleeding.
   ii. If CT scan is negative and suspicion remains high, lumbar puncture is indicated.
      1. Will note a constant number of red blood cells in each tube.
         a. Conversely, in a traumatic tap, the number of red blood cells will decrease with each following tube.
      2. Opening pressure is elevated.
   iii. Cerebral angiography is the definitive study to identify the source of the bleed.
d. **Treatment**
   i. Maintain airway, breathing, and circulation.
   ii. Control blood pressure.
   iii. Surgery clipping or coiling may be needed depending on the cause.
   iv. Overall mortality is 45%, with 10% dying before reaching the hospital.

**TABLE 7.14**

**Comparison of Epidural, Subdural, and Subarachnoid Hematomas**

| Hematoma | Vessel | Mechanism | Presentation | CT Scan Findings |
|---|---|---|---|---|
| Epidural | Artery | Skull fracture | Spinal fluid rhinorrhea<br>Unconsciousness followed by resolution and then later unconsciousness (injury, unconsciousness, resolution, unconsciousness) | Convex (lentiform, lemon-shape) shaped<br>Typically beneath the temporal bone<br>Sharply demarcated |
| Subdural | Venous | Head injury | Symptoms develop later after injury with headache, confusion, coma, and hemiparesis (injury, latency period, unconsciousness) | Concave, crescent-shaped<br>Subdural = Banana shape |
| Subarachnoid | Artery | Aneurysm | Worst headache of life<br>Stiff neck and delirium | Hyperdense, amorphous appearance in the subarachnoid space |

    v. Medical complications include rebleeding, vasospasm, hydrocephalus, seizures, and hyponatremia.

  e. **Table 7.14 compares epidural, subdural, and subarachnoid hematomas.**

## V. STROKE

  a. **General**

    i. Multiple types of strokes.

      1. Ischemic.

        (a) Caused by insufficient blood flow to part or all the brain.

        (b) Neurologic deficit lasts longer than 24 hours.

          (i) If less than 24 hours, episodes are termed a "transient ischemic attack."

        (c) No extravasated blood into the brain.

        (d) Account for 60% to 65% of all strokes.

        (e) Two types of ischemic strokes.

          (i) Thrombosis.

            (1) Occlusion forms locally at the site.

          (ii) Embolic.

            (1) Due to a piece of clot breaking off from another location and traveling to the brain.

            (2) Sources include mural thrombi, valvular heart disease, and arrhythmias (atrial fibrillation).

      2. Hemorrhagic.

        (a) Extravasation of blood into the brain.

        (b) Account for 15% of all strokes.

      3. Small vessel (lacunar).

        (a) Caused by occlusion of small arterioles.

        (b) Account for 20% of all strokes.

        (c) Typically due to long-standing hypertension.

    ii. Risk factors for stroke include the following:

      1. Increasing age.

      2. Atrial fibrillation.

      3. Hypercoagulable states.

      4. Hypertension.

      5. Smoking.

      6. Diabetes.

      7. Elevated serum lipids.

      8. Recent myocardial infarction.

      9. Carotid stenosis.

     10. Transient ischemic attack (TIA).

        (a) Defined as a transient episode of neurologic dysfunction, without acute infarction.

        (b) The most common source is embolic from carotid or vertebrobasilar circulation.

        (c) Clinical presentation and work-up same as for cerebrovascular accident (CVA).

        (d) Treatment should be aggressive and include antiplatelet therapy and carotid endarterectomy or angioplasty.

  b. **Clinical Manifestations**

    i. Signs and symptoms depend on location within the brain that has been deprived of blood flow.

    ii. Table 7.15 summarizes clinical manifestations of stroke.

  c. **Diagnosis**

    i. Neurologic examination will suggest location and size of stroke.

    ii. Electrocardiogram (EKG) is indicated to rule out arrhythmia.

    iii. Carotid Doppler and echocardiogram indicated to rule out a possible embolic source.

    iv. A non-contrast CT scan is the standard initial study.

      1. Evaluate for possible hemorrhage.

    v. MRI is more sensitive for detecting early ischemia.

    vi. MRI angiography or CT angiography.

    vii. Digital subtraction angiography (DSA) is the gold standard for carotid artery stenosis, vasculitis, cerebral aneurysms, and cerebrovascular malformations.

**TABLE 7.15**

| Clinical Manifestations of Stroke | |
|---|---|
| **Occluded Blood Vessel** | **Clinical Manifestations** |
| Anterior cerebral artery (rare) | Upper motor neuron weakness<br>Neglect of contralateral leg<br>Urinary incontinence<br>Transcortical motor aphasia |
| Basilar artery | Bilateral sensory abnormalities<br>Cerebellar dysfunction<br>Cranial nerve abnormalities<br>Paralysis/Weakness of all extremities<br>Impaired vision |
| Internal carotid artery | Ipsilateral blindness |
| Middle cerebral artery (common) | Contralateral weakness<br>Sensory loss in the face and arm<br>Expressive aphasia (if dominant side)<br>Anosognosia and spatial disorientation (if nondominant side) |
| Posterior cerebral artery | Highly variable<br>Difficulty reading and performing calculations<br>Memory impairment |
| Vertebral artery | Vertigo<br>Nausea/Vomiting<br>Nystagmus<br>Ipsilateral cerebellar ataxia |

   **d. Treatment**
     i. Modify risk factors.
       1. Carotid endarterectomy for carotid stenosis.
         a. Typically indicated in patients with 70%+ of blockage.
         b. Perioperative mortality is between 1% and 2%.
       2. Aspirin or anticoagulation for patients with atrial fibrillation or hypercoagulable states.
       3. Control hypertension.
     ii. Thrombolytic therapy is the only effective method for the acute treatment of ischemic stroke.
       1. Must be started within 3 hours from onset of stroke.
       2. CT scan must be obtained to rule out hemorrhage.
       3. Blood pressure must be less than 185 mm Hg systolic or 110 mm Hg diastolic.
        (a) If elevated, must lower before starting thrombolytic therapy.
       4. Contraindications include the following:
        (a) Significant head trauma or prior stroke in the past 3 months.
        (b) Current symptoms or prior history of intracranial hemorrhage.
        (c) Active internal bleeding, platelet count <100,000/mm$^3$.
        (d) CT indicating multilobar infarct.
        (e) Blood glucose <50mg/dL.

        (f) Current use of anticoagulation with INR >1.7 or PT >15 seconds, direct thrombin inhibitors or direct factor Xa inhibitors with elevated laboratory tests, or heparin use in the past 48 hours with abnormally elevated aPTT.
       2. Relative contraindications include:
        (a) Minor or quickly improving stroke symptoms.
        (b) Pregnancy.
        (c) Seizure at onset of symptoms.
        (d) Major surgery or trauma in the past 14 days.
        (e) GI or urinary hemorrhage in the past 21 days.
        (f) Myocardial infarction in the past 3 months.
     iii. Hemorrhagic stroke treated with mannitol, hyperventilation, and head elevation to decrease increased intracranial pressure.
     iv. Prophylactic heparin indicated, unless other contraindications, to decrease risk for pulmonary embolism or deep venous thrombosis.

**VI. SYNCOPE**
   **a. General**
     i. Defined as abrupt loss of consciousness and postural tone, followed by rapid and complete recovery.
     ii. May have presyncopal symptoms of dizziness without loss of postural tone.
   **b. Etiologies**
     i. Cardiac arrhythmias, such as ventricular tachycardia.
       1. Prodromal or presyncopal symptoms are typically absent.
     ii. Valvular heart disease, such as aortic stenosis and hypertrophic cardiomyopathy.
     iii. Orthostatic hypotension.
       1. Symptoms occur with transition from sitting or lying to standing.
     iv. Vasovagal.
       1. Seizures.
       2. Metabolic.
       3. Anaphylaxis.
   **c. Clinical**
     i. Symptoms include lightheadedness; sudden, brief loss of consciousness and decreased muscle tone; dizziness; and weakness.
     ii. Focal neurologic deficits suggest possible TIA or seizure disorder.
   **d. Diagnosis**
     i. Ambulatory EKG, echocardiogram, CT scan of the brain, and carotid ultrasound are needed to identify possible etiology.

1. Tilt table or electrophysiologic study needed in severe cases.
  e. **Treatment**
    i. Treat underlying etiology.

## II. COMPLEX REGIONAL PAIN SYNDROME
  a. **General**
    i. Disorder of a body region characterized by pain, swelling, limited range of motion, vasomotor instability, skin changes, and patchy bone demineralization.
    ii. Frequently follows an injury, surgery, or vascular event.
  b. **Clinical Manifestations**
    i. Occurs most commonly in upper and lower extremities.
    ii. Three stages.
      1. Stage 1: burning, throbbing pain, aching, sensitivity to touch or cold, and localized edema in a limb.
      2. Stage 2: note progression of soft tissue edema, thickening of skin, muscle wasting, and brawny skin.

3. Stage 3: note limitations of movement, contractures of the digits, and brittle ridged nails.
  c. **Diagnosis**
    i. Primarily a clinical diagnosis.
    ii. Elevated resting skin temperature and decreased sweat production.
    ii. Decreased perfusion of affected region on bone scintigraphy.
    iii. MRI may show characteristic findings and aid in excluding possible differential diagnoses.
  d. **Treatment**
    i. Multidisciplinary approach.
      1. Includes patient education, counseling, physical therapy (PT), occupational therapy (OT), and smoking cessation.
    ii. Medications include gabapentin, bisphosphonates, and glucocorticoids.
      i. Invasive therapies such as injections, nerve stimulations, nerve blocks, and sympathectomy are used.

# QUESTIONS

### QUESTION 1

Which of the following physical examination findings is typically noted in Parkinson's disease?

**A** Bilateral visual field defects

**B** Intermittent blank staring episodes

**C** Cogwheeling of an upper extremity

**D** Sensory loss over chest dermatomes

**E** Chorea-like movements of extremities

### QUESTION 2

A 65-year-old patient with a history of hypertension and chronic obstructive pulmonary disease (COPD) presents with left facial drooping and weakness on the right side of the body. Which of the following is the first best step in the evaluation of this patient?

**A** Chest x-ray

**B** Cerebral CT scan

**C** Carotid ultrasound

**D** Neurology consult

**E** Magnetic resonance angiography

### QUESTION 3

A 50-year-old female is brought into the emergency room after suffering a seizure while eating dinner. The patient developed convulsive jerking in the upper and lower extremities that lasted approximately 5 minutes. The patient also lost consciousness for 2 to 3 minutes. The patient has no prior history of seizures. Which of the following is the most likely diagnosis?

**A** Complex partial seizure

**B** Absence seizure

**C** Tonic-clonic seizure

**D** Myoclonic seizure

**E** Atonic seizure

## QUESTIONS—cont'd

### QUESTION 4

A 15-year-old male presents to the emergency room with a history of being hit on the side of the head with a baseball bat. He is a little slow to respond, but is not lethargic. He is otherwise in good health. Physical examination is completely normal with the exception of a small collection of blood posterior to the left ear, near the site of the impact. Which of the following is the next best step in the evaluation of this patient?

**A** Pneumoencephalography

**B** Cerebral angiography

**C** CT scan of the skull

**D** MRI of the brain

**E** Lumbar puncture

### QUESTION 5

A 70-year-old patient presents with neck stiffness and headache. Lumbar puncture laboratory testing reveals 500 WBCs with 100% neutrophils, total protein 230 mg/dL, and glucose 40 mg/dL. Which of the following is the best treatment option for this patient?

**A** Ceftriaxone (Rocephin)

**B** Ceftriaxone and ampicillin

**C** Acyclovir (Zovirax)

**D** Acyclovir and amphotericin B

**E** Ampicillin and amphotericin B

### QUESTION 6

A patient presents with a history of debilitating migraine headaches 4 to 5 days per month. Which of the following medications can be used as prophylactic treatment for migraine headaches?

**A** Sumatriptan (Imitrex)

**B** Ergotamine tartrate (Cafergot)

**C** Desipramine (Norpramin)

**D** Acetaminophen (Tylenol)

**E** Oxycodone (OxyContin)

### QUESTION 7

Which of the following is the vector involved with transmission of West Nile encephalitis?

**A** Bats

**B** Snails

**C** Wild birds

**D** Wild rodents

**E** White-tailed deer

### QUESTION 8

A 30-year-old female presents with weakness in the lower extremities. On physical examination, reflexes are decreased in the lower extremities. CSF studies reveal a normal cell count and elevated total protein. Which of the following is the most likely diagnosis?

**A** Viral meningitis

**B** Myasthenia gravis

**C** Guillain-Barré syndrome

**D** Huntington's disease

**E** Parkinson's disease

### QUESTION 9

Which of the following differentiates common migraine from classic migraine?

**A** Lack of neurologic prodrome

**B** Presence of phonophobia

**C** Presence of incontinence

**D** Presence of nausea

**E** Throbbing pain

### QUESTION 10

A patient presents with an aneurysm of the posterior communicating artery. Which of the following cranial nerves is most likely to be affected?

**A** II

**B** III

**C** IV

**D** V

**E** VI

# ANSWERS

**1. C**
EXPLANATION: Patients with Parkinson's disease classically present with the triad of tremor, bradykinesia, and cogwheel rigidity. *Topic: Parkinson's disease*
☐ Correct   ☐ Incorrect

**2. B**
EXPLANATION: Evaluation of the possible stroke patient begins with a CT scan to evaluate for possible hemorrhage. Carotid ultrasound may be needed later to evaluate for possible embolic source. *Topic: Stroke*
☐ Correct   ☐ Incorrect

**3. C**
EXPLANATION: Tonic-clonic seizures present with tonic (stiffening) and then clonic (rhythmic jerking) phases. Urinary incontinence and loss of consciousness are common. T*opic: Seizure disorders*
☐ Correct   ☐ Incorrect

**4. C**
EXPLANATION: Any patient with trauma to the head must have subarachnoid, epidural, or subdural hemorrhage ruled out. CT scan of the skull and brain are the test of choice in the evaluation of patients with head trauma. *Topic: Subarachnoid hemorrhage*
☐ Correct   ☐ Incorrect

**5. B**
EXPLANATION: Bacterial meningitis in the elderly may be caused by *S. pneumoniae*, *N. meningitidis*, and *Listeria monocytogenes*. Treatment in the elderly must include ceftriaxone and ampicillin to cover the most common organisms. *Topic: Meningitis*
☐ Correct   ☐ Incorrect

**6. C**
EXPLANATION: Preventive treatment is indicated if headaches limit normal daily activities three or more days per month, if headaches are severe, or if headaches are associated with complications. Treatment options include beta-blockers, NSAIDs, and tricyclic antidepressants. Sumatriptan, ergotamine, and acetaminophen are used for acute treatment. *Topic: Headaches*
☐ Correct   ☐ Incorrect

**7. C**
EXPLANATION: West Nile encephalitis is transmitted by mosquitoes and wild birds. *Topic: Encephalitis*
☐ Correct   ☐ Incorrect

**8. C**
EXPLANATION: Guillain-Barré syndrome typically follows an infection and presents with ascending weakness. Reflexes are diminished, and the CSF reveals a normal cell count and elevated total protein. Topic: Guillain-Barré syndrome
☐ Correct   ☐ Incorrect

**9. A**
EXPLANATION: Common migraine is a migraine without an aura or neurologic prodrome. Classic migraine includes an aura or neurologic prodrome. *Topic: Headaches*
☐ Correct   ☐ Incorrect

**10. B**
EXPLANATION: Cranial nerve III (oculomotor) is located adjacent to the posterior communicating artery and may be affected by an aneurysm. *Topic: Cerebral aneurysm*
☐ Correct   ☐ Incorrect

# CHAPTER 8

# REPRODUCTIVE SYSTEM

## EXAMINATION BLUEPRINT TOPICS

**BREAST DISORDERS**
Abscess
Carcinoma
Fibroadenoma
Fibrocystic disease
Galactorrhea
Gynecomastia
Mastitis

**CERVICAL DISORDERS**
Carcinoma
Cervicitis
Dysplasia
Incompetent cervix (cervical insufficiency)

**COMPLICATED PREGNANCY**
Abortion
Abruptio placentae
Cord prolapse
Dystocia: shoulder
Ectopic pregnancy
Fetal distress
Gestational diabetes
Gestational trophoblastic disease
Molar pregnancy (hydatidiform moles)
Multiple gestation
Placenta previa
Postpartum hemorrhage
Hypertension disorders in pregnancy

Premature rupture of membranes
Rh incompatibility

**CONTRACEPTIVE METHODS**
Natural methods
Barrier methods
Spermicides
Intrauterine devices (IUDs)
Hormonal
Sterilization
Emergency contraception pill

**INFERTILITY**
General
Male infertility
Female infertility

**MENOPAUSE**
General
Clinical manifestations
Diagnosis
Treatment

**MENSTRUAL CYCLE**
Menarche
Menstrual cycle

**MENSTRUAL DISORDERS**
Amenorrhea
Dysmenorrhea
Premenstrual syndrome (PMS)

**OVARIAN DISORDERS**
Cysts
Ovarian neoplasms
Ovarian torsion

**PELVIC INFLAMMATORY DISEASE (PID)**
General
Clinical manifestations
Diagnosis
Treatment
Complications

**UNCOMPLICATED PREGNANCY**
Prenatal diagnosis/care
Normal labor/delivery

**UTERINE DISORDERS**
Dysfunctional uterine bleeding (DUB)
Endometrial cancer
Endometriosis
Adenomyosis
Leiomyoma (uterine fibroids)
Metritis
Uterine prolapse

**VAGINAR/VULVAR DISORDERS**
Cystocele
Neoplasms
Rectocele
Vaginitis

## BREAST DISORDERS

### I. ABSCESS

**a. General**
   i. An acute inflammatory process that results in the formation of a collection of pus.
   ii. It may also develop in patients with acute mastitis.
   iii. Breast abscesses are categorized as lactational or nonlactational.

   a. Lactational breast abscess is typically due to *Staphylococcus aureus*.
   v. Subareolar breast abscess is typically due to a mixed infection, including anaerobes, staphylococci, and streptococci.

**b. Clinical Manifestations**
   i. May present with a painful, erythematous mass in the breast with occasional drainage through the skin or nipple duct.

c. **Diagnosis**
   i. Based on physical examination findings.
d. **Treatment**
   i. Incision and drainage or needle aspiration required.
   ii. Carcinoma should be excluded by performing a biopsy.
   iii. Antibiotics are needed.
      1. Lactational abscess can be treated with nafcillin, cefazolin, or vancomycin.
      2. Subareolar abscess requires broad-spectrum antibiotics with anaerobic coverage.
   iv. Complications.
      1. Fistula may develop in subareolar abscess.

## II. CARCINOMA
a. **General**
   i. Lifetime incidence of breast cancer for women in the US is about 13% (1 in 8).
      1. Most cases are diagnosed after age 40.
   ii. Risk factors.
      1. Increasing age.
      2. Family history of gynecologic malignancies.
      3. First-degree relative with breast cancer.
      4. Personal history of breast cancer.
      5. Exposure to ionizing radiation before age 30.
      6. Significant alcohol use.
      7. Presence of BRCA1 or BRCA2 gene.
      8. Nulliparity.
   iii. Prevention.
      1. Early pregnancy.
      2. Prolonged lactation.
      3. Chemical or surgical sterilization.
      4. Exercise.
      5. Low-fat diet.
b. **Clinical Manifestations**
   i. Present with masses, skin changes, nipple discharge, or symptoms of metastatic disease.
      1. Breast pain is rarely a presenting symptom of breast cancer.
   ii. The mass is most often detected by a patient on self-breast examination.
      1. Mass is typically nontender, irregular, firm, and immobile.
      2. Half occur in the upper outer quadrant of the breast.
   iii. Skin dimpling, tissue edema, "peau d'orange" appearance, and nipple retraction or discharge may be noted.
   iv. May also have nonspecific symptoms such as anorexia, weight loss, fatigue, dyspnea, and bone pain.
c. **Diagnosis**
   i. Mammogram is used to detect early lesions.

1. Screening guidelines.
   (a) U.S. Preventive Services Task Force (USPSTF) recommends a mammogram every 1 to 2 years between ages 50 and 74.
2. Findings suggestive of carcinoma include:
   (a) Spiculated mass.
   (b) Asymmetric local fibrosis.
   (c) Microcalcifications with a linear, branched pattern.
3. See Fig. 8.1 for example of a positive mammogram for breast cancer.
   ii. Ultrasound (US) is also used to separate fluid-filled cysts from solid masses.
      1. Also helpful for axillary masses.
   iii. Needle biopsy, fine-needle aspiration, or excisional biopsy is needed to diagnose.
      1. If fine-needle aspiration is negative, an excisional biopsy should be done.
   iv. Types of invasive breast cancer.
      1. Infiltrating ductal carcinoma.
      2. Invasive lobular carcinoma.
      3. Paget's disease of the nipple.
      4. Inflammatory breast carcinoma.

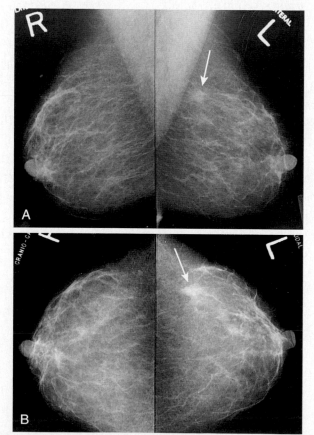

**Fig. 8.1 (A)** and **(B)** Mammogram of breast cancer reveals a mass *(arrows)* in the left breast. *(From Mettler FA: Essentials of Radiology, 2nd ed. Philadelphia: Elsevier Saunders, 2005:118, Fig. 4-2.)*

**TABLE 8.1**

| Types of Noninvasive Breast Cancer | | | | |
| --- | --- | --- | --- | --- |
| **Type** | **Age** | **Mammogram Results** | **Diagnosis** | **Treatment** |
| Ductal carcinoma in situ | 50s | Clustered microcalcifications | Needle or excisional biopsy | Surgical excision |
| Lobular carcinoma in situ | 40s | Not seen on mammogram | Diagnosed incidentally on biopsy for other condition | Local excision |

5. Table 8.1 summarizes noninvasive breast cancer.

d. **Treatment**
   i. Surgical treatment options.
      1. Wide local excision or lumpectomy.
         (a) This is a breast-conserving treatment option.
         (b) Can be used if tumor less than 4 cm and tumor is not fixed to underlying tissue.
         (c) Radiation therapy is also utilized.
      2. Simple mastectomy.
         (a) Includes removal of breast tissue, nipple-areolar complex, and skin.
         (b) There is no axillary node dissection.
      3. Modified radical mastectomy.
         (a) Includes removal of breast tissue, nipple-areolar complex, skin, pectoralis fascia, and axillary lymph nodes.
      4. Radical mastectomy.
         (a) Includes removal of breast tissue, nipple-areolar complex, skin, axillary lymph nodes, and pectoralis major and minor.
      5. Radiation therapy indicated in patients with high risk of local recurrence.
   ii. Medical treatment options.
      1. Include chemotherapy and hormone (anti-estrogen) therapy.
      2. Are used to control micrometastases.
      3. Are indicated in lymph node–positive patients or high-risk lymph node–negative patients.
      4. Chemotherapy typically includes cyclophosphamide, methotrexate, and 5-fluorouracil (CMF).
         (a) Monoclonal antibodies, such as trastuzumab, indicated with chemotherapy.
      5. The most common hormone therapy includes aromatic inhibitors (exemestane) or tamoxifen.
   iii. Prognosis
      1. Overall 5-year disease-free survival rate varies between 18% and 95%
         (a) Survival rate varies with stage of cancer.
      2. Patients with positive estrogen and progesterone receptors have a more favorable prognosis.

## III. FIBROADENOMA
a. **General**
   i. Benign tumors are most commonly noted in women younger than 40 years of age.
b. **Clinical Manifestations**
   i. On physical examination, palpated as round, well-circumscribed, rubbery, nontender, mobile firm lesion.
      1. Lesions may change during menstrual cycle or pregnancy.
   ii. Most are 1 to 5 cm in diameter.
   iii. No axillary involvement or nipple discharge.
c. **Diagnosis**
   i. Diagnosis based on physical examination and biopsy results.
d. **Treatment**
   i. If no family history of breast cancer and if the patient is stable, she can be followed clinically.
   ii. If suspicious for cancer, a fine-needle aspiration should be done.
   iii. Large fibroadenoma can be removed by excisional biopsy.

## IV. FIBROCYSTIC DISEASE
a. **General**
   i. Very common benign breast condition.
   ii. Common in women between the ages of 30 and 40.
   iii. Due to exaggerated stromal response to hormones.
b. **Clinical Manifestations**
   i. Present with breast swelling, pain, and tenderness.
   ii. Are typically multiple, well demarcated, and mobile.
   iii. May involve both breasts and vary in presentation through the menstrual cycle.
   iv. No axillary lymph node involvement or nipple discharge.
c. **Diagnosis**
   i. Biopsy is needed to diagnose possible carcinoma.

d. Treatment
   i. NSAIDs and oral contraceptive pills (OCPs) improve symptoms.
   ii. Decreasing intake of nicotine and caffeine may reduce symptoms.
   iii. If symptoms are severe, danazol, an androgen, can be used.

### V. GALACTORRHEA
a. General
   i. Milky nipple discharge that occurs unrelated to lactation.
   ii. Not a disease, but a sign of an underlying condition.
   iii. Unilateral nipple discharge is concerning for breast cancer.
b. Clinical Presentation
   i. Patients may have spontaneous leaking from one or both nipples
   ii. Menstrual cycles may be abnormal or absent.
   iii. If a pituitary adenoma is the cause, the patient may complain of headaches or visual disturbances.
c. Diagnosis
   i. Serum prolactin levels can rule out prolactin-secreting pituitary adenoma.
      1. Follow with MRI to rule out adenoma if elevated.
   ii. Thorough breast exam with possible mammography to rule out breast cancer.
   iii. Medication review: antidepressants, antipsychotics, and hypertensive medications can cause galactorrhea.
d. Treatment
   i. Targeted at underlying cause.

### VI. GYNECOMASTIA
a. **Benign proliferation of glandular tissue of the male breast**
b. **Etiology**
c. **Diagnosis made by physical examination**
   i. Check the testosterone level (typically low).
   ii. A mammogram is needed if cancer is suspected.
d. Treatment
   i. Treat the underlying cause.
   ii. Stop an offending drug if applicable.
   iii. Tamoxifen or testosterone therapy may be indicated.

### VII. MASTITIS
a. General
   i. Regional infection of the breast.
   ii. Typically seen in lactating women and caused by a patient's skin flora or oral flora of an infant.

iii. The organism enters through skin erosion or crack in the nipple.
b. Clinical Manifestations
   i. Present with fever, chills, and malaise.
   ii. On physical examination, the area is noted to be tender, red, and warm to the touch.
   iii. Laboratory tests may reveal an elevated white blood cell (WBC) count.
c. Diagnosis
   i. Diagnosis made based on physical examination findings.
d. Treatment
   i. Treated with oral dicloxacillin.
   ii. Complications include development of breast abscess.
   iii. Patients should be instructed to continue to breastfeed or to continue to use a breast pump to prevent accumulation of infected material.

## CERVICAL DISORDERS

### I. CARCINOMA
a. General
   i. Cervical cancer and premalignant cervical dysplasia are correlated with onset of sexual activity at an early age and with increased number of sexual partners.
   ii. Human papillomavirus (HPV) is the primary causative agent.
      1. Serotypes 16 and 18 are most commonly correlated with cervical cancer.
   iii. The most common cell type is squamous cell carcinoma followed by adenocarcinoma.
      1. Clear cell carcinoma, a type of adenocarcinoma, is linked to exposure in utero of diethylstilbestrol (DES).
         a. DES was banned in 1971 by the FDA.
b. Clinical Manifestations
   i. Classic presentation is postcoital bleeding.
      1. Other symptoms may include abnormal vaginal bleeding, watery vaginal discharge, or pelvic pain.
   ii. On bimanual examination, a mass within the cervix may be palpated.
c. Diagnosis
   i. Screen for disease with Pap smear.
      1. Per United States Preventive Services task Force (USPSTF) cervical cytology screening is recommended every 3 years between ages 21 and 29.
      2. For ages 30 to 65 years, cervical cytology screening alone every 3 years or every 5 years with high-risk human papillomavirus (hrHPV) in combination with cytology.

3. In women who have had adequate screening and not at high risk, stop screening at age 65.
   ii. With any abnormal Pap smear, consider cervical biopsy via colposcopy.

d. **Treatment**
   i. With microinvasion carcinoma, a cone biopsy should be performed if the patient wishes to maintain fertility.
   ii. With invasive cervical carcinoma, if it has not spread beyond the cervix, uterine corpus, and vagina, radical hysterectomy is indicated.
   iii. Curative or palliative radiation therapy can also be used.
   iv. Cisplatin-based chemotherapy with radiation therapy has been found to be effective against bulky stage disease.

## II. CERVICITIS

a. **General**
   i. General term referring to inflammation of the cervix; typically caused by infection.
   ii. Most common infectious agents include the following:
       1. *Chlamydia trachomatis.*
       2. *Neisseria gonorrhoeae.*
       3. Herpes simplex virus.
       4. *Trichomonas vaginalis.*

b. **Clinical Manifestations**
   i. Acute cervicitis.
      1. The primary symptom is purulent vaginal discharge.
         (a) Gonorrhea: thick and creamy discharge.
         (b) Chlamydia: purulent discharge.
         (c) *Trichomonas*: foamy and greenish-white discharge.
      2. Other symptoms include leukorrhea (caused by endocervical inflammation), infertility, pelvic discomfort, and dyspareunia.
      3. On physical examination, note acutely inflamed, edematous cervix with purulent discharge.
         a. A "strawberry cervix" is pathognomonic for trichomoniasis.
   ii. Chronic cervicitis.
      1. Leukorrhea is the major symptom.

c. **Diagnosis**
   i. Diagnosis made through various methods.
      1. Wet mount: motile flagellated *Trichomonas vaginalis* may be noted.
      2. Gram stain reveals gram-negative, intracellular diplococci in gonorrhea.
      3. Viral culture for viral causes.
      4. Polymerase chain reaction (PCR) testing for gonorrhea and chlamydia.

d. **Treatment**
   i. Treatment is based on the specific organism found.
      1. *T. vaginalis*: metronidazole.
      2. Gonorrhea: ceftriaxone.
      3. Chlamydia: doxycycline or azithromycin.
      4. Herpes: acyclovir.

## III. DYSPLASIA

a. **General**
   i. Thought to be a precursor to cervical cancer.
   ii. Cervical intraepithelial neoplasia (CIN) I takes approximately 7 years to become cervical cancer; it takes approximately 4 years for CIN II to become cervical cancer.

b. **Clinical Manifestations**
   i. No clinical signs or symptoms.

c. **Diagnosis**
   i. Diagnosis made by Pap smear and confirmed by biopsy.

d. **Treatment**
   i. CIN I followed with a colposcopy every 3 to 4 months. If persists, treat with loop electrosurgical excision procedure (LEEP).
   ii. CIN II or III treated with destruction or excision of the lesions.
      1. Cryotherapy or laser therapy can be used.
      2. LEEP is used to remove endocervical lesions.

## IV. INCOMPETENT CERVIX (CERVICAL INSUFFICIENCY)

a. **General**
   i. Painless dilation of the cervix, often in the second trimester.
   ii. Defined as the inability of the uterine cervix to retain a pregnancy in the absence of the signs and symptoms of clinical contractions, or labor, in the second trimester.
   ii. With an incompetent cervix, fetal membranes are exposed to vaginal flora and to risk of increased trauma.
   iii. Infection, vaginal discharge, and premature rupture of membranes are common in patients with incompetent cervix.
   iv. Increased risk of incompetent cervix with history of prior incompetent cervix, surgery, cervical trauma, DES exposure, or treatment for CIN.

b. **Clinical Manifestations**
   i. Patients present with painless dilation and effacement of the cervix, often during the second trimester of pregnancy.
   ii. May also note bleeding, vaginal discharge, or rupture of membranes.

c. **Diagnosis**
   i. Diagnosis is based on physical examination.

d. Treatment
  i. Strict bed rest.
  ii. High likelihood of fetal demise.
  ii. In future pregnancies, placement of a cerclage, a suture placed vaginally to close the cervix, can be used.

# COMPLICATED PREGNANCY

## I. ABORTION
  a. General
    i. Spontaneous abortion is a pregnancy that ends before week 20 of gestation.
      1. Between 60% and 80% of all spontaneous abortions occur during the first trimester.
    ii. Most first-trimester abortions are associated with abnormal chromosomes, while second-trimester abortions are associated with infection, uterus/cervix abnormalities, exposure to toxins, and trauma.
    iii. Many different types of abortions.
      1. Complete: complete expulsion of all products of conception before 20 weeks of gestation.
      2. Incomplete: partial expulsion of some but not all products of conception before 20 weeks of gestation.
      3. Inevitable: no expulsion of products, but bleeding and dilation of the cervix are evidence that a viable pregnancy is not likely.
      4. Threatened: any intrauterine bleeding before 20 weeks of gestation, without dilation or expulsion of products of conception.
      5. Missed: fetal demise before 20 weeks of gestation with complete retention of the products of conception; cervical os may be open or closed
  b. Diagnosis
    i. Present with vaginal bleeding, abdominal cramping, abdominal pain, and decreased symptoms of pregnancy.
    ii. Serial beta–human chorionic gonadotropin (hCG) levels should be obtained and doubling should occur every 48–72 hours early in pregnancy when pregnancy is viable.
      a. Elevated hCG may indicate multiple gestation or gestational trophoblastic disease.
    iii. Ultrasound should be obtained to detect fetal heart activity.
  c. Treatment
    i. Incomplete or missed abortions should be allowed to finish.
    ii. Dilation and evacuation may be required to remove all products of conception.

    iii. Patients with threatened abortions should be placed on pelvic rest and monitored for continued bleeding.
    iv. All Rh-negative patients should receive RhoGAM with any vaginal bleeding.

## II. ABRUPTIO PLACENTAE
  a. General
    i. The premature separation of the placenta from the uterine wall.
    ii. Most occur after 30 weeks of gestation and before the onset of labor.
    iii. May result in premature delivery, uterine tetany, disseminated intravascular coagulation (DIC), and shock.
    iv. Cause is unknown, but risk factors include maternal hypertension, prior history of abruptio placentae, maternal trauma (abuse, motor vehicle collisions), advanced age, multiparity, smoking, maternal cocaine use, and alcohol use.
  b. Clinical Manifestations
    i. Present with third-trimester vaginal bleeding and severe to moderate abdominal pain.
    ii. On physical examination, will note vaginal bleeding and a firm, tender uterus.
  c. Diagnosis
    i. Diagnosis based on clinical findings.
    ii. Confirmed by inspection of the placenta at time of delivery.
  d. Treatment
    i. The first step is to stabilize the patient and prepare for more hemorrhage.
    ii. Prepare for delivery and monitor for complications such as disseminated intravascular coagulation (DIC) and shock.

## III. CORD PROLAPSE
  a. General
    i. The umbilical cord passes through the cervical os prior to fetal delivery causing cord compression and fetal hypoxia.
  b. Clinical Manifestations
    i. Cord may be visualized on vaginal exam.
    ii. Irregular fetal heartbeat may occur.
    iii. Variable decelerations result from sudden drops in fetal heart rate and are associated with cord compression.
  c. Diagnosis
    i. Visualization or palpation of umbilical cord on pelvic exam.
    ii. Fetal bradycardia (<120 bpm) is may occur.
  d. Treatment
    i. Emergent delivery, typically by cesarean section.

1. Manual elevation of fetal presentation may be necessary until delivery can occur.

## IV. DYSTOCIA: SHOULDER
### a. General
  i. Impaction of the anterior shoulder against the pubic symphysis after delivery of the head.
  ii. The rate is 1 in 300 live births.
    1. Increased risk in newborns with macrosomia.
### b. Clinical Manifestations
  i. On examination, the fetal head may appear to retract toward the maternal perineum.
### c. Diagnosis
  i. Warning signs include prolonged second stages of labor and the use of forceps or vacuum with delivery.
### d. Treatment
  i. McRoberts maneuver used to disimpact the shoulder.
    1. Maternal thighs flexed onto the abdomen increases inlet diameter and removes sacral prominence as a possible obstruction.
    2. Suprapubic pressure can also be used with this maneuver to disimpact the shoulder.
  ii. Complications
    1. Maternal complications include soft-tissue injury.
    2. Fetal complications are more severe and include brachial plexus injury including Erb's palsy, clavicle fracture, and fetal hypoxia.

## V. ECTOPIC PREGNANCY
### a. General
  i. Implantation of the egg occurs outside of the uterus, most commonly in the fallopian tubes (98%).
  ii. Occurs in approximately 1 in 100 pregnancies.
  iii. Risk factors for ectopic pregnancy include history of STI or PID, prior ectopic pregnancy, previous abdominal or tubal surgery, endometriosis, or use of IUD.
### b. Clinical Manifestations
  i. Symptoms include unilateral pelvic pain and vaginal bleeding.
  ii. On physical examination, may note a tender adnexal mass, uterus small for gestational age, and cervical bleeding.
  iii. Laboratory results reveal beta-hCG levels low for gestational age and a level that does not double every 48–72 hours early in the pregnancy.
### c. Diagnosis
  i. Based on symptoms, physical examination, and laboratory findings.
  ii. Transvaginal ultrasound may reveal an adnexal mass or extrauterine pregnancy.
  iii. If no mass is noted on physical examination or ultrasound, the patient should be followed with serial beta-hCG levels to evaluate for possible ectopic pregnancy.
### d. Treatment
  i. The patient should be stabilized if the ectopic pregnancy has ruptured, and then an exploratory laparotomy should be performed.
  ii. Methotrexate can be used in uncomplicated, stable ectopic pregnancies and serial beta-hCG should be followed until it returns to the pre-pregnancy normal level.

## VI. FETAL DISTRESS
### a. Presence of signs that suggest that the fetus may not be well
### b. Etiologies
  i. Abnormal fetal presentation/position.
  ii. Multiple gestation.
  iii. Shoulder dystocia.
  iv. Umbilical cord prolapse.
  v. Nuchal cord.
  vi. Placental abruption.
  vii. Breathing problems.
### c. Clinical Manifestations
  i. Decreased fetal movements.
  ii. Meconium present in amniotic fluid.
### d. Evaluation
  i. Monitor fetal movements.
    1. Normal is at least 10 fetal movements per 12 hours of maternal activity or more than 2 hours when mother is at rest.
  ii. Monitor with stress tests.
    1. Nonstress test (NST).
      (a) Measures fetal heart rate for 20 minutes and also monitors fetal movement.
      (b) A reactive (normal) test shows fetal heart rate acceleration.
    2. Contraction stress test (CST).
      (a) Measures response of fetal heart rate to the stress of a uterine contraction.
      (b) A negative (normal) test shows no fetal heart rate deceleration.
  iii. Ultrasound
      (a) Measures fetal movement, muscle tone, breathing movement and amniotic fluid volume.

## VII. GESTATIONAL DIABETES
### a. General
  i. Impaired carbohydrate metabolism that first manifests during pregnancy.
  ii. Risk factors for the development of diabetes during pregnancy include age older than 25 years,

**TABLE 8.2**

| Complications of Diabetes During Pregnancy | |
|---|---|
| **Maternal** | **Fetal** |
| Infection | Shoulder dystocia |
| Miscarriage | Traumatic delivery |
| Neuropathy | Intrauterine growth retardation |
| Postpartum hemorrhage | Delayed organ maturity |
| Preeclampsia | Macrosomia |
| Vascular or end-organ involvement | Congenital abnormalities |

obesity, positive family history, history of macrosomia, and previous miscarriage.

   iii. Patients who develop gestational diabetes are at an increased risk of developing gestational diabetes in later pregnancies and overt diabetes within 5 years.

   iv. Complications of diabetes (Table 8.2).

**b. Clinical Manifestations**

   i. If a patient has one or more risk factors, screen for diabetes at the first prenatal visit.

   ii. Screening is typically done between 24–28 weeks.

   iii. Screening is done by measuring glucose 1 hour after a 50-g glucose load.

     1. Normal fasting glucose is less than 95 mg/dL, and normal 1-hour glucose post 50-g glucose load is less than 180 mg/dL.

**c. Diagnosis**

   i. Oral glucose tolerance testing (OGTT) is done if the screening test is positive.

   ii. OGTT involves a 100-g glucose dose and then measuring fasting, and 1-, 2-, 3-hour blood-glucose levels.

   iii. Gestational diabetes is diagnosed if two or more of the levels are elevated.

**d. Treatment**

   i. Strict glucose control is vital to the wellbeing of the mother and infant.

   ii. Diet control with an American Dietetic Association (ADA) diet is indicated.

   iii. Insulin may be needed if control with diet is inadequate.

   iv. Oral hypoglycemic agents are not indicated due to crossing the placenta and because of possible teratogenic effects.

     a. Glyburide can be used but with caution.

## VIII. GESTATIONAL TROPHOBLASTIC DISEASE

**a. General**

   i. Wide group of interrelated diseases resulting in abnormal proliferation of trophoblastic tissue.

   ii. Four major groups.

     1. Molar pregnancy: benign.

     2. Invasive mole.

      (a) A malignant disorder in which the molar villi and trophoblasts penetrate the myometrium.

     3. Choriocarcinoma: malignant.

     4. Placental site trophoblastic tumor: malignant.

**b. Clinical Manifestations**

   i. Irregular or heavy vaginal bleeding early in the pregnancy.

   ii. All are able to produce hCG.

**c. Diagnosis**

   i. hCG serves as a tumor marker for this disease.

   ii. Ultrasound can be used to aid in diagnosis.

**d. Treatment**

   i. Varies with type of disease.

   ii. Malignant types are very sensitive to chemotherapy.

## IX. MOLAR PREGNANCY (HYDATIDIFORM MOLES)

**a. General**

   i. Two types.

     1. Complete.

      (a) Results from fertilization of an empty ovum by a normal sperm.

      (b) Have trophoblastic development and the absence of fetal parts.

     2. Incomplete.

      (a) Results when two sperm fertilize a normal ovum at the same time.

   ii. Incidence 1 in 1000 pregnancies; occurs most commonly in women younger than age 20 or older than age 40.

**b. Clinical Manifestations**

   i. Present with painless, irregular, or heavy vaginal bleeding early in pregnancy.

   ii. May also note severe nausea and vomiting.

   iii. Physical examination may reveal molar clusters (grapelike) protruding into the vagina and blood in the cervical os in complete molar pregnancy.

     1. Physical examination is normal in incomplete molar pregnancy.

   iv. Laboratory results reveal a markedly elevated beta-hCG relative to that of a normal pregnancy.

   v. Ultrasound reveals no fetal heart tones.

**c. Diagnosis**

   i. Based on laboratory and ultrasound results.

     1. A "snowstorm" or "whiteout" appearance on pelvic US.

**d. Treatment**

   i. Immediate removal of uterine contents.

   ii. Monitor beta-hCG levels for 1 year to identify invasive moles.

   iii. Pregnancy should also be avoided during this 1-year follow-up.

## X. MULTIPLE GESTATION

**a. General**
   i. Monozygotic, or identical, twins result when a fertilized ovum divides into two separate ova.
   ii. Dizygotic, or nonidentical, twins result when two ova are released and fertilized.
   iii. Twins occur in approximately 1 in 80 pregnancies.
   iv. Triplets occur in approximately 1 in 8000 pregnancies.
      1. Increased risk with ovulation-enhancing drugs and IVF.

**b. Complications**
   i. Increased risk of preterm labor, umbilical cord prolapse, postpartum hemorrhage, gestational diabetes, preeclampsia, and placenta previa.

**c. Diagnosis**
   i. Possible diagnosis indicated by rapid uterine growth, excessive maternal weight gain, and elevated beta-hCG.
   ii. Diagnosed by ultrasound.

**d. Treatment**
   i. Because of increased risk of complications, multiple gestations should be managed as a high-risk pregnancy.

## XI. PLACENTA PREVIA

**a. General**
   i. Abnormal implantation of the placenta over the internal cervical os.
      1. Complete previa occurs when the placenta completely covers the internal os.
      2. Partial previa occurs when the placenta covers part of the internal os.
      3. Marginal previa occurs when the edge of the placenta reaches the margin of the os.
   ii. Major cause of painless antepartum bleeding.
   iii. Bleeding is due to disruptions in placental attachment during normal development and thinning of the cervix during the third trimester.
   iv. May be complicated by placenta accreta in which there is abnormal invasion of the placenta into the uterine wall.
      1. Placenta accreta does not allow the placenta to separate from the uterine wall after delivery.
      2. Results in severe hemorrhage and is treated with hysterectomy following cesarean delivery.

**b. Clinical Manifestations**
   i. Presents with sudden, profuse, painless vaginal bleeding after week 28 of gestation.
   ii. Vaginal examination is contraindicated in placenta previa.

**c. Diagnosis**
   i. Diagnosis is made by ultrasound.

**d. Treatment**
   i. If placenta previa is suspected, stabilize the patient, prepare for bleeding, and deliver via cesarean section.
   ii. If signs of fetal distress or severe hemorrhaging, emergency cesarean section is indicated.

## XII. POSTPARTUM HEMORRHAGE

**a. General**
   i. Defined as blood loss greater than 500 mL in a vaginal delivery and greater than 1000 mL in a cesarean section.
   ii. See Table 8.3 for etiologies of postpartum hemorrhage.

**b. Diagnosis**
   i. Uterine atony is the major cause of postpartum bleeding.
      1. On physical examination, note that the uterus will be soft, enlarged, and boggy.
      2. Treated with IV oxytocin and uterine massage.

**c. Treatment**
   i. Fluid resuscitation should be started and the patient should be monitored for signs of DIC.

## XIII. HYPERTENSION DISORDERS IN PREGNANCY

**a. General**
   i. In the obstetric patient, hypertension is defined as a blood pressure greater than 140/90 mm Hg.
   ii. There are four defined hypertensive states in pregnancy.
      1. Preeclampsia and eclampsia.
      2. Chronic hypertension.
      (a) Defined as hypertension present before conception, before 20 weeks of gestation, or continuing more than 6 weeks postpartum.
      3. Chronic hypertension with superimposed preeclampsia.
      (a) Defined as worsening hypertension or worsening proteinuria in the last half of pregnancy.

**TABLE 8.3**

| Causes of Postpartum Bleeding | |
| --- | --- |
| **Vaginal** | **Cesarean** |
| Vaginal and cervical lacerations | Uterine atony |
| Uterine atony | Surgery |
| Placenta accreta | Placenta accreta |
| Retained products of conception | Uterine rupture |
| Uterine inversion or rupture | |

4. Transient hypertension.
   (a) Hypertension that develops between midpregnancy and 48 hours after delivery.

b. **Preeclampsia**
   i. General
      1. Presence of edema, proteinuria, and hypertension.
         (a) May develop any time after 20 weeks of gestation, but typically seen in the third trimester.
      2. Involves generalized arteriolar vasoconstriction and intravascular depletion.
      3. Maternal complications are related to the arteriolar vasoconstriction and include renal failure, oliguria, edema, thrombocytopenia, and DIC.
      4. Fetal complications are related to prematurity and include intrauterine growth restriction, placental abruption, fetal distress, and stillbirth.
   ii. Clinical manifestations (Table 8.4).
   iii. Diagnosis
      1. Based on physical examination and laboratory findings.
   iv. Treatment
      1. Delivery is the ultimate treatment.
      2. Magnesium sulfate may be indicated to decrease risk of seizures.
      3. In severe disease, hydralazine can be used to control blood pressure.

c. **Eclampsia**
   i. General
      1. Defined as the development of seizures that are not attributed to any other cause in a patient with preeclampsia.
   ii. Clinical manifestations
      1. Seizures are tonic-clonic.
   iii. Diagnosis

1. Based on findings of elevated blood pressure, proteinuria, edema, and seizures.
   iv. Treatment
      1. Seizure control and prophylaxis with magnesium sulfate.
      2. Blood pressure control with IV hydralazine, IV labetalol, or oral nifedipine.
      3. Once the patient is stable, delivery should be started.

c. **HELLP Syndrome**
   i. General
      1. Subcategory of severe preeclampsia.
      2. Uncommon but has a high rate of stillbirth and neonatal death.
      3. Can occur postpartum in a patient with a history of preeclampsia.
   ii. Clinical manifestations
      1. Patients present with the following:
         (a) *H*emolytic anemia.
         (b) *E*levated *L*iver function tests.
         (c) *L*ow *P*latelets.
      2. Physical examination may reveal epigastric pain due to liver capsule distension and progressive nausea and vomiting.
   iii. Diagnosis
      1. Based on laboratory findings.
   iv. Treatment
      1. Delivery is the definitive treatment.
      2. Treat hypertension and seizure risk as for eclampsia.

**XIV. PREMATURE RUPTURE OF MEMBRANES**
   a. **General**
      i. Defined as rupture of membranes at least 1 hour before the onset of labor.
      ii. Preterm rupture of membranes is rupture that occurs before 37 weeks of gestation.
      iii. Prolonged premature rupture of membranes is rupture more than 18 hours before onset of labor.

**TABLE 8.4**

| Manifestations of Preeclampsia | | | | |
|---|---|---|---|---|
| **Severity** | **Blood Pressure (mm Hg)** | **Proteinuria** | **Edema** | **Other** |
| Mild | 140/90 to 160/110 or ≥30 increase in systolic BP ≥15 increase in diastolic BP | >300 mg/24 hr or 1–2+ on dipstick | Hands and/or face | |
| Severe | >160/110 | >5 g/24 hr or 3–4+ on dipstick | Hands and/or face | Altered consciousness Headache Abdominal pain Elevated liver function tests Oliguria Pulmonary edema Thrombocytopenia |

**b. Clinical Manifestations**
  i. Suspected with a history of amniotic fluid leaking from the vagina.
**c. Diagnosis**
  i. Nitrazine or fern test confirms diagnosis.
    1. Nitrazine test detects the pH of the fluid that is alkaline if amniotic fluid.
    2. Fern test detects crystallization of salts in the amniotic fluid.
**d. Treatment**
  i. Evaluate for signs of infection, chorioamnionitis.
  ii. Chorioamnionitis is an infection of the amniotic fluid.
    1. Commonly caused by group B *Streptococcus* and treated with IV antibiotics.

## XV. RH INCOMPATIBILITY
**a. General**
  i. If a woman is Rh-negative and the fetus is Rh-positive, the woman may become sensitized to Rh antigen and develop antibodies against the fetal blood.
  ii. Antibodies may cross the placenta and cause hemolysis of the fetal red blood cells.
**b. Diagnosis**
  i. In a patient who has a positive antibody screen for Rh, a titer should be checked and monitored throughout the pregnancy.
    1. If titer increases, amniocentesis should be performed and the amniotic fluid tested for bilirubin.
    2. Bilirubin levels are used to predict severity of disease.
    3. Ultrasound is used to evaluate for signs of fetal hydrops, and a fetal hemoglobin is obtained.
  ii. If placenta abruption or any antepartum bleeding occurs, a Kleihauer-Betke test is needed to determine the amount of fetal blood cells in the maternal circulation.
    1. RhoGAM dose may need to be increased based on test results.
**c. Treatment**
  i. If a patient is Rh-negative and has a negative antibody screen, the goal is to keep the patient from becoming sensitized.
    1. With any exposure to fetal blood, the patient should be given RhoGAM, anti-D immunoglobulin.
    2. RhoGAM is given at 28 weeks of gestation and then again postpartum if the neonate is Rh-positive.
  ii. In the sensitized Rh-negative patient with severe disease, fetal transfusion may be needed.

## CONTRACEPTIVE METHODS

## I. NATURAL METHODS
**a. Periodic Abstinence (Rhythm Method)**
  i. Method.
    1. Requires abstinence shortly before and after the predicted ovulation period.
    2. Ovulation assessment methods include taking basal temperature, tracking menstrual cycle, evaluation of cervical mucus, and monitoring for premenstrual or ovulatory symptoms.
  ii. Effectiveness.
    1. Failure rate is high at 20% to 30%.
  iii. Advantages/Disadvantages.
    1. No use of chemicals or barriers.
    2. May require long periods of abstinence.
    3. Must be motivated to monitor and use ovulation assessment methods.
**b. Coitus Interruptus**
  i. Method.
    1. Requires withdrawal of penis from vagina before ejaculation.
  ii. Effectiveness.
    1. Failure rate is high at 15% to 25%.
  iii. Advantages/Disadvantages.
    1. Must have sufficient self-control to withdraw before ejaculation.
    2. No use of chemicals or barriers.
**c. Lactational Amenorrhea**
  i. Method.
    1. After delivery, ovulation is delayed due to hypothalamic suppression of ovulation secondary to nursing and lactation.
    2. Should be used for a maximum of 6 months after delivery.
  ii. Effectiveness.
    1. Failure rate is high at 15% to 55%.
    2. Failure rate can be decreased to 2% if the method is not used for longer than 6 months and if breastfeeding is the only form of nutrition for the infant.
**d. Natural methods are physiologically based, do not use barriers, and are the least effective methods of contraception**

## II. BARRIER METHODS
**a. Male/Female Condom**
  i. Method.
    1. Male condom is placed over the penis and prevents the ejaculate from entering the female reproductive tract.
    2. Female condom has two flexible rings. One is placed into the vagina, and the other stays outside near the introitus.

ii. Effectiveness.
1. Male condom has a failure rate of 10% to 15%.
   (a) Decreases to 2% if used properly.
2. Female condom has a failure rate of 15% to 20%.

iii. Advantages/Disadvantages.
1. Male condoms are widely available and help prevent the transmission of STIs.
   (a) The only method of contraception that protects against human immunodeficiency virus (HIV).
2. Female condoms protect against STIs but are more costly than male condoms.

b. **Diaphragm**
   i. Method.
   1. A domed sheet of rubber or latex that is placed in the vagina so that it covers the cervix.
   2. Must be placed before intercourse and left in place for 6 to 8 hours after intercourse.
   3. Spermicide must also be used.
   ii. Effectiveness.
   1. Failure rate is 5% to 15%.
   iii. Advantages/Disadvantages.
   1. May lead to bladder irritation and cystitis.
   2. If diaphragm left in place too long, the patient could become colonized with *S. aureus* and develop toxic shock syndrome.
   3. Diaphragm must be fitted and replaced every 5 years or when a patient gains or loses more than 10 pounds.

c. **Cervical Cap**
   i. Method.
   1. Small, soft cap that fits over the cervix and is held in place by suction.
   ii. Effectiveness.
   1. Failure rate is 5% to 20%, primarily due to movement of the cap.
   iii. Advantages/Disadvantages.
   1. Can be left in place for 1 to 2 days.
   2. Must be fitted and requires use of spermicide.

## III. SPERMICIDES

a. **Method**
   i. Disrupt the cell membrane of sperm and act as a mechanical barrier to sperm in the cervical canal.
   ii. Must be placed in the vagina 30 minutes before intercourse.
   iii. May be used alone but is more effective if used with condoms, diaphragms, or cervical caps.

b. **Effectiveness**
   i. Failure rate is 10% to 30%.

c. **Advantages/Disadvantages**
   i. Widely available in a variety of forms including vaginal creams, jellies, suppositories, and foam.
   ii. Can cause vaginal irritation.

## IV. INTRAUTERINE DEVICES (IUDS)

a. **Method**
   i. Plastic or metal device that is placed in the endometrial cavity.
   ii. May elicit a spermicidal inflammatory response resulting in the sperm being destroyed.
   iii. Has no effect on ovulation.

b. **Effectiveness**
   i. Very low failure rate of <1%.

c. **Advantages/Disadvantages**
   i. Contraindications to use of IUD.
   1. Absolute.
      (a) Current pregnancy.
      (b) Abnormal vaginal bleeding.
      (c) Gynecologic cancer.
      (d) Acute cervical or uterine infection.
      (e) History of PID.
   2. Relative.
      (a) Nulliparity.
      (b) Prior ectopic pregnancy.
      (c) History of STI.
      (d) Moderate to severe dysmenorrhea.
   ii. Must be prescribed, inserted, and removed by a health-care provider.

## V. HORMONAL

a. **Oral Contraceptive/Contraceptive Patch**
   i. Method.
   1. Composed of progesterone alone or progesterone and estrogen.
   2. Interferes with the pulsatile release of follicle stimulating hormone (FSH) and luteinizing hormone (LH) and suppresses ovulation.
   3. Also changes the endometrium to not allow for implantation.
   ii. Effectiveness.
   1. Very effective, with a theoretic failure rate of less than 1%. The actual failure rate is about 3% due to human error (inconsistent use).
      (a) May have decreased effectiveness due to interaction with other medications.
         (i) Effectiveness decreased with concurrent use of many medications, including penicillins, tetracycline, sulfonamides, rifampin, phenytoin, and barbiturates.
   iii. Advantages/Disadvantages.

**TABLE 8.5**

| Contraindications to Use of Oral Contraceptive Pills | |
|---|---|
| **Absolute** | **Relative** |
| Thromboembolism | Uterine fibroids |
| Pulmonary embolism | Lactation |
| Myocardial infarction | Hypertension |
| Stroke | |
| Breast/Endometrial cancer | |
| Hepatic tumor or abnormal liver function | |

1. Complications include increased coagulability and increased risk of pulmonary embolism, thromboembolism, stroke, and myocardial infarction.
   (a) Increased risk with increased doses of estrogen.
2. Oral contraceptive pills are contraindicated in women older than 35 years of age who use tobacco.
   (a) Table 8.5 lists contraindications.
3. Oral contraceptive pills decrease risk of ovarian and endometrial cancer, ectopic pregnancy, anemia, and PID.

b. **Depo-Provera (Medroxyprogesterone acetate)**
   i. Method.
      1. Progestin that is injected intramuscularly (IM) and slowly released over 3 months.
      2. Mechanism of action is via suppression of ovulation, thickening cervical mucus, and making endometrium unsuitable for implantation.
   ii. Effectiveness.
      1. Very low failure rate of 0.3%.
   iii. Advantages/Disadvantages.
      1. May lead to irregular vaginal bleeding, depression, breast tenderness, and weight gain.
      2. Long-term use may lead to loss of bone mineral density, osteoporosis, and osteoporotic fracture.
      3. After discontinuing may have a significant delay, up to 18 months, in return of normal ovulation.

**VI. STERILIZATION**
   a. **Tubal Sterilization**
      i. Method.
         1. Pregnancy inhibited by surgically blocking both fallopian tubes and preventing sperm and ovum from meeting.
         2. Can be done by clipping, banding, or coagulation of the tubes.
         3. Performed under general anesthesia.

      ii. Effectiveness.
         1. Failure rate of only 0.2% to 0.4%.
      iii. Advantages/Disadvantages.
         1. Very low rate of ectopic pregnancy.
         2. May be reversed, but success rates vary from 40% to 80%.
   b. **Vasectomy**
      i. Method.
         1. Sterilization via ligation of vas deferens.
         2. Can be performed under local anesthesia.
         3. Due to the possibility of viable sperm being present in the proximal collecting system, another form of contraception should be used for 4 to 6 weeks until azoospermia can be confirmed through microscopic evaluation.
      ii. Effectiveness.
         1. Failure rate is less than 1%.
      iii. Advantages/Disadvantages.
         1. Complications are rare and include bleeding and infection after the procedure.
         2. Success rate of reanastomosis is 60% to 70%.

**VII. EMERGENCY CONTRACEPTION PILL**
   a. **Method**
      i. Thought to inhibit or delay in ovulation and cause insufficient corpus luteum function.
      ii. Products contain ethinyl estradiol and/or levonorgestrel.
   b. **Effectiveness**
      i. Failure rate of 15% to 25%.
      ii. Most effective when used within 72 hours of unprotected intercourse.
   c. **Advantages/Disadvantages**
      i. Should not be used in patients with a known or suspected pregnancy.
      ii. If pregnancy does occur, emergency contraception has no effect on fetal development.

# INFERTILITY

**I. GENERAL**
   a. **Infertility is defined as the inability to conceive after 1 year of unprotected intercourse**
   b. **Male factors are attributed to approximately 25% of cases of infertility, female factors to approximately 45%, and unidentifiable factors to approximately 30%**

**II. MALE INFERTILITY**
   a. **Etiology**
      i. May be due to endocrine causes, anatomic defects, abnormal sperm production or motility, and sexual dysfunction.

**TABLE 8.6**

| Etiologies of Male Infertility | | |
| --- | --- | --- |
| **Endocrine** | **Abnormal Spermatogenesis** | **Sexual Dysfunction** |
| Hypothalamic dysfunction | Varicocele | Impotence |
| Anabolic steroids | Cryptorchidism | |
| Thyroid disease | | |
| Hyperprolactinemia | | |

    ii. Risk factors include exposure to chemicals, radiation, and excessive heat. See Table 8.6 for etiologies.

  **b. Diagnosis**

    i. Review for history of previous pregnancies fathered by patient, for chemical or toxin exposure, and for history of STIs, mumps, or trauma to the genitals.

    ii. Physical examination should include signs of testosterone deficiency, varicocele, and patency of urethral meatus.

    iii. Laboratory evaluation includes semen analysis.

      1. Analysis includes sperm count, volume, motility, morphology, pH, and WBC count.

      2. If abnormal, evaluation should continue with thyroid testing and serum testosterone, prolactin, and FSH level.

  **c. Treatment**

    i. Avoid environmental exposures.

    ii. Reproductive techniques such as intracytoplasmic sperm injection.

      1. Sperm are retrieved, and a single sperm is injected directly into an egg and then implanted.

## III. FEMALE INFERTILITY

  **a. Etiology**

    i. May be due to ovulatory, cervical, uterine, tubal, or peritoneal causes.

    ii. Ovulatory factors disrupt the hypothalamic pituitary ovarian axis and lead to infertility by impairing follicle formation, ovulation, or endometrial development.

    iii. See Table 8.7.

  **b. Diagnosis**

    i. May require laparoscopic evaluation, evaluation for evidence of ovulation, endometrial biopsy, progestin challenge, FSH, LH, prolactin and thyroid function tests, and pelvic examination.

  **c. Treatment**

    i. Varies with etiology.

    ii. Ovulation can be induced with clomiphene citrate.

      1. Clomiphene stimulates release of GnRH, which stimulates FSH and LH release, as well as follicular development.

      2. A major side effect is multiple-gestation pregnancy.

    iii. Techniques such as intrauterine insemination (IUI), in vitro fertilization (IVF), and gamete intrafallopian transfer (GIFT) can also be used.

# MENOPAUSE

## I. GENERAL

  **a. Denotes the final menstruation and marks the end of reproductive capabilities**

  **b. In the United States, menopause typically occurs between the ages of 48 and 52**

    i. If menopause occurs before age 40, it is considered premature and is due to primary ovarian insufficiency.

  **c. Due to diminished estrogen production that leads to increased levels of FSH and LH**

  **d. With menopause, women lose the benefits of estrogen on lipid profile and vascular endothelium**

    i. Leads to increased risk of coronary artery disease.

    ii. Also includes loss of bone resorption that leads to osteopenia and osteoporosis.

## II. CLINICAL MANIFESTATIONS

  **a. Symptoms include vasomotor flushing, sweats, mood changes, and depression**

    i. Due to decrease in estradiol levels.

**TABLE 8.7**

| Causes of Female Infertility | | | | |
| --- | --- | --- | --- | --- |
| **Cervical** | **Uterine** | **Tubal** | **Peritoneal** | **Ovulatory** |
| Cervical stenosis | Malformations | Pelvic inflammatory disease | Adhesions | Pituitary insufficiency |
| Cervicitis | Leiomyoma | Tubal ligation | Endometriosis | Hyperprolactinemia |
| | Asherman's syndrome | Endometriosis | | Polycystic ovarian disease |
| | | | | Ovarian tumor |
| | | | | Thyroid disease |
| | | | | Obesity |

b. Physical examination may reveal decreasing breast size, as well as vaginal, urethral, and cervical atrophy

c. Laboratory tests reveal an elevated FSH

### III. DIAGNOSIS

a. Based on history and physical examination

### IV. TREATMENT

a. Hormone replacement therapy may be considered

i. Benefits include decreased number of hip fractures and improvement of symptoms noted during menopause.

ii. Risk factors include cholestatic hepatic dysfunction, increased incidence of estrogen-dependent neoplasm, increased risk of thromboembolic events, or undiagnosed vaginal bleeding.

iii. Progesterone is used in combination with estrogen therapy to decrease risk of endometrial hyperplasia and cancer that occur with unopposed estrogen use in post-menopausal women.

## MENSTRUAL CYCLE

### I. MENARCHE

a. The average age of onset is about 12 years, with the majority falling between 10–15 years

b. The menstrual cycle is typically irregular, due to anovulatory cycles, for the first 6 months to 1 year after menarche.

### II. MENSTRUAL CYCLE (FIG. 8.2)

a. Two phases: follicular and luteal

b. Follicular (Proliferative) Phase

i. Day 1 of menses through ovulation.

ii. Release of follicle-stimulating hormone (FSH) from the anterior pituitary results in development of a primary ovarian follicle.

ii. The ovarian follicle produces estrogen, which causes the uterine lining proliferation.

iii. At mid-cycle, typically about day 14, LH (from the anterior pituitary) spikes in response to the estrogen surge. This stimulates release of the ovum from the follicle (ovulation).

c. Luteal (Secretory) Phase

i. Begins after release of the ovum.

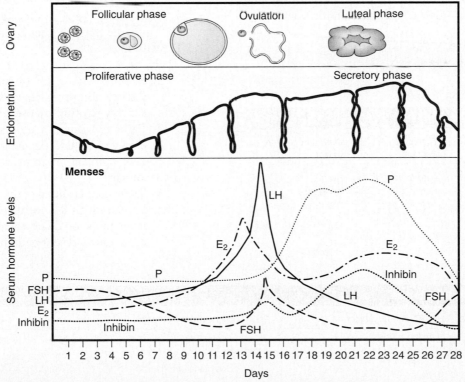

**Fig. 8.2** The normal menstrual cycle. $E_2$, Estradiol; *FSH*, follicle-stimulating hormone; *LH*, luteinizing hormone; *P*, progesterone. *(From Larsen PR: Williams Textbook of Endocrinology, 10th ed. Philadelphia: Elsevier Saunders 2003:607, Fig. 16-22.)*

ii. Follicle remnants in the ovary develop into the corpus luteum and secrete progesterone.
   1. Release of progesterone causes reduction in FSH and LH from the anterior pituitary through negative feedback.
iii. Progesterone maintains the uterine lining in preparation for implantation of the fertilized ovum.
   1. If fertilization occurs, the developing trophoblast synthesizes hCG that maintains the corpus luteum until the placenta develops.
iv. If there is no fertilization, the corpus luteum degenerates and progesterone levels fall.
v. Without progesterone, the endometrial lining is sloughed off (menstruation).
vi. The withdrawal of estrogen and progesterone leads to gradual increase in FSH from the anterior pituitary.
vii. Release of FSH results in development of primary ovarian follicles and the start of the follicular phase, continuing the cycle.

# MENSTRUAL DISORDERS

## I. AMENORRHEA
a. **General**
   i. Amenorrhea is the absence of menses.
      1. Primary amenorrhea is absence of menses in a woman who has not undergone menarche by age 16.
         (a) Table 8.8 lists etiologies of primary amenorrhea.
      2. Secondary amenorrhea is the absence of menses for 6 months in a woman who previously had normal menses.
         (a) The leading cause of secondary amenorrhea is pregnancy.
         (b) Table 8.9 lists etiologies of secondary amenorrhea.
b. **Clinical Manifestations**
   i. Primary.
      1. Workup based on phenotypic picture.
         (a) Based on presence or absence of uterus and breasts.
      2. Workup of a phenotypic female with absence of either uterus or breasts must include karyotype studies, testosterone level, and FSH level.
c. **Diagnosis**
   i. Table 8.10 shows diagnostic features of primary amenorrhea.
   ii. Diagnosis of secondary amenorrhea.
      1. Begins with a pregnancy test.
      2. Thyroid-stimulating hormone (TSH) and prolactin levels should be checked to evaluate for hypothyroidism and hyperprolactinemia.
      3. If prolactin is normal, a progesterone challenge test should be done.
         (a) The presence of withdrawal bleeding shows estrogen levels are adequate and the outflow tract is patent.
d. **Treatment**
   i. Primary.
      1. Patients with a functional uterus and congenital abnormalities can be treated with surgery to allow menses flow.
      2. Patients without a uterus are treated with estrogen replacement to promote breast development and to prevent osteoporosis.
   ii. Secondary.
      1. Treatment is aimed at the underlying cause.
      2. Patients with a positive progesterone challenge test should be treated with oral contraceptives to prevent endometrial hyperplasia.

**TABLE 8.8**

| Causes of Primary Amenorrhea | | |
| --- | --- | --- |
| **Outflow Obstruction** | **End-Organ Disease** | **Central Regulatory Disease** |
| Imperforate hymen | Ovarian failure | Hypothalamic disorder |
| Transverse vaginal septum | Gonadal agenesis | Pituitary disorder |
| Vaginal agenesis | | |
| Testicular feminization | | |

**TABLE 8.9**

| Causes of Secondary Amenorrhea | | | |
| --- | --- | --- | --- |
| **Anatomic** | **Ovarian Dysfunction** | **Hyperprolactinemia** | **Hypothalamic Disorders** |
| Syndrome | Premature ovarian failure | Primary hypothyroidism | Stress |
| Cervical stenosis | Polycystic ovarian disease | Medications | Anorexia nervosa |
| | | Dopamine antagonists | Weight loss |
| | | TCA | |
| | | MAO inhibitors | |
| | | Pituitary tumor | |

*MAO*, Monoamine oxidase; *TCA*, tricyclic antidepressants.

**TABLE 8.10**

| Diagnosis of Primary Amenorrhea | | |
|---|---|---|
| | **Uterus Present** | **Uterus Absent** |
| **Breasts Present** | Testicular feminization Müllerian agenesis | Congenital abnormalities |
| **Breasts Absent** | Gonadal agenesis Enzyme deficiency in testosterone synthesis | Gonadal failure/ agenesis Hypothalamic-pituitary axis dysfunction Hypothalamic, pituitary, or ovarian dysfunction |

## II. DYSMENORRHEA

a. **General**
   i. Pain and cramping during the menstrual cycle that interferes with normal daily activities.
   ii. Classified as primary or secondary.
   iii. Etiology.
      1. Primary dysmenorrhea has no obvious cause.
         (a) May be due to high levels of prostaglandins.
      2. Secondary dysmenorrhea is due to an identifiable underlying cause such as endometriosis, fibroids, cervical stenosis, or pelvic adhesions.

b. **Clinical Manifestations**
   i. Primary dysmenorrhea.
      1. Crampy pain typically occurs on the first or second day of menstruation.
      2. Associated symptoms may include headache, nausea, and vomiting.
      3. It is more common in the years following menarche and typically improves with age.
      4. On physical examination, no abnormalities are typically noted except generalized tenderness in the lower abdomen/pelvis.
   ii. Secondary dysmenorrhea.
      1. Patients with cervical stenosis present with scant menses and severe cramping pain that is relieved with increased menstrual flow.
         (a) Physical examination reveals scarring of the external os.
      2. Patients with pelvic adhesions typically have a history of pelvic infections or prior pelvic surgery.

c. **Diagnosis**
   i. Primary dysmenorrhea diagnosis is based on history and lack of organic cause.

d. **Treatment**
   i. Primary dysmenorrhea is treated with NSAIDs and oral contraceptive pills.
   ii. Treatment of secondary dysmenorrhea is based on the cause.

1. Endometriosis is treated with oral contraceptives, medroxyprogesterone, danazol, or surgery.
2. Cervical stenosis is treated with cervical dilation.
3. Pelvic adhesions are treated with NSAIDs and oral contraceptive pills. If no relief, surgery can be used to lyse the adhesions.

## III. PREMENSTRUAL SYNDROME (PMS)

a. **General**
   i. Occurs during the second half of the menstrual cycle and often during the first few days of menses.
   ii. Etiology is thought to be due to changes in gonadal steroids during the luteal phase.
   iii. Clinically significant disease occurs in 3% to 8% of women.

b. **Clinical Manifestations**
   i. Symptoms include somatic, emotional, and behavioral complaints.
      1. Somatic complaints include breast swelling and tenderness, abdominal bloating, headache, fatigue, and constipation.
      2. Emotional complaints include irritability, depression, anxiety, and libido changes.
      3. Behavioral complaints include mood swings, food cravings, poor concentration, and sensitivity to noise.

c. **Diagnosis**
   i. Based on history and physical examination.
   ii. To confirm diagnosis, the patient must have a symptom-free follicular phase for about 1 week.

d. **Treatment**
   i. NSAIDs and oral contraceptive pills bring symptomatic relief.
   ii. Selective serotonin reuptake inhibitors (SSRIs) may be needed in some patients who are experiencing more severe psychological symptoms.

# OVARIAN DISORDERS

## I. CYSTS

a. **General**
   i. Functional cysts result from normal physiologic functioning of the ovaries.
   ii. Two types of functional cysts: follicular and corpus luteum cysts.
   iii. Most commonly occur between puberty and menopause.
   iv. Smoking increases risk of functional cysts.

b. **Clinical Manifestations**
   i. Follicular cysts are typically asymptomatic and an incidental finding, but large cysts can cause

pelvic pain and dyspareunia and can lead to ovarian torsion.

1. Tend to be less than 8 cm in size.

ii. Theca lutein cysts may cause pelvic pain and amenorrhea or delayed menses.

1. Tend to be larger than follicular cysts and more firm or solid on palpation.

iii. Physical examination varies with the type of cyst.

iv. A torsed or ruptured cyst will cause pain on palpation, acute abdominal pain, and rebound tenderness.

v. Polycystic ovary disease (PCOS).

1. Present with anovulation, oligomenorrhea, amenorrhea, hirsutism, obesity, and enlarged ovaries.

a. **Patients may present with infertility.**

c. **Diagnosis**

i. Pelvic ultrasound is the test of choice for the workup of ovarian cysts.

ii. For PCOS, ultrasound may show a "string of pearls"—typically 12 or more follicles per ovary.

d. **Treatment**

i. Treatment varies with age and size of cyst.

1. Premenarchal and cyst greater than 2 cm: treat with exploratory laparotomy.

2. Reproductive age and cyst less than 6–8 cm: observe for 6 weeks.

3. Reproductive age and cyst greater than 8 cm: treat with exploratory laparotomy.

4. Postmenopausal age and palpable cyst: treat with exploratory laparotomy.

ii. Polycystic ovary syndrome.

1. Treatment depends on symptoms and desire for fertility.

(a) If fertility is desired, start clomiphene citrate.

(i) Clomiphene has an approximately 10% rate of multiple gestation.

(b) If fertility is not desired, start estrogen-progestin contraceptives.

## II. OVARIAN NEOPLASMS

a. **General**

i. Second most-common cancer of the female genital tract.

ii. Ovarian carcinoma spreads primarily by direct exfoliation of malignant cells.

iii. The cause is unknown but may be due to malignant transformation of ovarian tissue after a long period of chronic uninterrupted ovulation.

1. Increase risk of disease with presence of *BRCA1* gene or *BRCA2* gene.

iv. Increased risk with positive family history, with history of uninterrupted ovulation, and with breast cancer.

1. Oral contraceptives may have a protective effect.

v. Table 8.11 summarizes ovarian carcinoma.

b. **Clinical Manifestations**

i. Patients are often asymptomatic until the disease is advanced.

ii. May present with vague lower abdominal pain and abdominal enlargement.

iii. Physical examination reveals a solid, fixed pelvic mass and possible ascites.

1. Malignant tumors tend to be fixed, solid, bilateral, and nodular.

c. **Diagnosis**

i. Pelvic ultrasound is the test of choice.

1. Malignant masses tend to be greater than 8 cm in size, solid, multilocular, and bilateral.

ii. Tumor markers such as CA-125, alpha-fetoprotein (AFP), and hCG are present.

d. **Treatment**

i. Varies with cell type (see Table 8.11).

**TABLE 8.11**

### Summary of Ovarian Carcinoma

|  | Epithelial Tumors | Germ Cell | Sex Cord Stroma |
|---|---|---|---|
| Frequency | 65%–70% | 15%–20% | 5%–10% |
| Age group | 50s | 1–25 years | All ages |
| Clinical | Elevated CA-125 | Rapidly enlarging mass | Have hormone production |
| Treatment | Surgery<br>Cisplatin-based chemotherapy | Surgery<br>Multidrug chemotherapy | Surgery |
| Cell types | Serous<br>Mucinous<br>Endometrioid<br>Clear cell | Teratoma<br>Choriocarcinoma<br>Dysgerminoma | Sertoli-Leydig cell<br>Fibroma<br>Granulosa-theca cell |
| 5-year survival rate | <20% | 60%–85% | 90% |

## III. OVARIAN TORSION

a. **General**
   i. Occurs when the ovary, and typically the fallopian tube, twists on itself resulting in reduced blood supply to the ovary.
   ii. Occurs with ovarian instability typically secondary to ovarian cysts, neoplasia or polycystic ovary syndrome.

b. **Clinical Manifestations**
   i. Acute unilateral lower abdominal pain that radiates to the adnexal region.
   ii. Possible nausea and/or vomiting.

c. **Diagnosis**
   i. Doppler ultrasound reveals reduced blood supply to the ovary.

d. **Management**
   i. An obstetric emergency.
   ii. Prompt surgical detorsion of the ovary is needed. Oophorectomy may be indicated if ovarian necrosis has occurred.

# PELVIC INFLAMMATORY DISEASE (PID)

## I. GENERAL

a. **A serious complication of STIs**
   i. Infectious agents include *N. gonorrhoeae, C. trachomatis,* and anaerobic organisms.

b. **Increased risk of infertility and ectopic pregnancy with PID.**

c. **Incidence is highest in the 15- to 19-year-old age group.**

d. **Risk factors: non-White ethnicity, being unmarried, cigarette smoking, and use of IUDs.**

e. **Barrier contraceptives decrease the risk of PID**

## II. CLINICAL MANIFESTATIONS

a. **Major symptoms are abdominal or pelvic pain**
   i. Pain can be bilateral or unilateral and is described as a burning, cramping, or stabbing pain.

b. **May also note increased vaginal discharge, abnormal bleeding, dyspareunia, and gastrointestinal or urinary tract symptoms**

c. **Fever may be noted**

d. **On physical examination, note lower abdominal tenderness, cervical motion tenderness (Chandelier's sign), and purulent cervical discharge**

e. **Laboratory tests reveal an elevated WBC count**

## III. DIAGNOSIS

a. **Ultrasound is not helpful in making the diagnosis**

b. **Definitive diagnosis is made by laparoscopy**

c. **Cultures are obtained to identify the causative agent**

## IV. TREATMENT

a. **Patients often need to be hospitalized**

b. **Antibiotics include broad-spectrum cephalosporins, such as cefoxitin or cefotetan, and doxycycline**

c. **Clindamycin and gentamicin can be used if a patient is allergic to cephalosporins**

## V. COMPLICATIONS

a. **Perihepatitis (Fitz-Hugh–Curtis syndrome)**
   i. Infection of liver capsule and peritoneal surfaces.
   ii. Symptoms include severe right upper quadrant pain.
   iii. Visualized on laparoscopic exam and may be described as "violin strings."

# UNCOMPLICATED PREGNANCY

## I. PRENATAL DIAGNOSIS/CARE

a. **Pregnancy Diagnosis**
   i. In the patient with normal menstrual periods, a delay of more than a few days may suggest pregnancy.
   ii. Diagnosis can be made by serum or urine assay for beta-hCG.
   iii. Ultrasound can also be used to confirm or detect a pregnancy as early as 5 weeks of gestation by detecting the gestational sac or the fetal heart at 6 weeks of gestation.
   iv. Pregnancy dating.
      1. Nägele's rule.
         (a) Estimated date of confinement (EDC) is the first day of the last menstrual period minus 3 months plus 7 days.
      2. Ultrasound.
         (a) Uses fetal crown-to-rump length, at 7 to 10 weeks, to determine gestational age.
         (b) Can also use femur length.
      3. Other landmarks.
         (a) Fetal quickening (first fetal movements) at 16 to 20 weeks.
         (b) Fetal heart tones may be detected by Doppler ultrasound at 12 weeks of gestation.
   v. Signs and symptoms of pregnancy.
      1. Chadwick's sign.
         (a) Bluish discoloration of the vagina and the cervix.

2. Goodell's sign.
   (a) Softening and cyanosis of the cervix after 4 weeks.
3. Breast swelling and tenderness.
4. Development of the lines of nigra from the umbilicus to the pubis.
5. Palmar erythema.
6. Symptoms include amenorrhea, nausea and vomiting, breast pain, and quickening.

vi. Time frames.
   1. First trimester.
      (a) Lasts until 14 weeks of gestational age.
   2. Second trimester.
      (a) Lasts from 14 to 28 weeks of gestation.
   3. Third trimester.
      (a) Lasts from 28 weeks of gestation to delivery.

b. **Prenatal Care**
   i. Initial visit.
   1. Complete history, including history of prior pregnancies, and physical examination are required.
      (a) Examination with Pap smear and cultures for gonorrhea and chlamydia are required.
   2. Initial laboratory tests include complete blood count, blood type and antibody screen, rapid plasma reagin (RPR), chlamydia testing, rubella titer, varicella immunity, hepatitis B surface antigen, and urinalysis.
      (a) HIV counseling and testing should be offered.
   ii. Follow-up visits.
   1. With each return visit, the patient should have weight and blood pressure checked, urinalysis, measurement of fundal height, and evaluation of fetal heart tones.
      (a) Fundal height varies with gestational age.
         (i) 12 weeks: just above pubic symphysis.
         (ii) 14 to 16 weeks: midway between pubic symphysis and umbilicus.
         (iii) 20 to 22 weeks: level of umbilicus.
         (iv) 22 to 38 weeks: height equal to gestational age (weeks).
         (v) 38 to 40 weeks: 2 to 3 cm below xiphoid process.
   2. Genetic and congenital screening.
      (a) Typically occurs during the second trimester but may be done in the first trimester.
      (b) Between weeks 15 and 18, evaluate with the triple screen.
         (i) Tests include maternal serum AFP, beta-hCG, and estriol.
         (ii) Elevated AFP correlated with increased risk of neural tube defect and maternal AFP is decreased in Down syndrome.
         (iii) Decreased estriol indicates a risk of trisomy 21 or trisomy 18.
         (iv) Increased hCG is associated with trisomy 21, and decreased hCG is associated with trisomy 18.
      (c) Screening ultrasound.
         (i) Offered between weeks 18 and 20.
         (ii) Provides a fetal anatomic survey.
   3. Oral glucose tolerance testing (OGTT).
      (a) Completed during the second trimester (24 to 28 weeks) if screening tests are positive for hyperglycemia.
      (b) Fasting result greater than 95 mg/dL or 1-hour result greater than 180 mg/dL significant for gestational diabetes on OGTT.
   4. Group B *Streptococcus* screening.
      (a) Done at 35 to 37 weeks.

## II. NORMAL LABOR/DELIVERY

a. **General**
   i. Defined as contractions that cause change in cervical effacement or dilation.

b. **Examination**
   i. Obstetric.
   1. Includes determining fetal presentation and lie.
      (a) Determined by using the Leopold maneuvers that involve palpating the maternal abdomen.
      (b) Fetal lie evident if the infant is transverse or longitudinal in the uterus.
      (c) Fetal presentation is if the infant is breech or vertex.
   2. If the fetal position or lie is difficult to determine, an ultrasound can be used.
   ii. Cervical.
   1. Cervical examination assists with determining phase of labor and labor progression.
   2. Based on the following five items:
      (a) Dilation.
         (i) Determines how open the cervix is at the internal os.
         (ii) Ranges from closed to 10 cm.
      (b) Effacement.
         (i) Determines how thin the cervix is between internal and external os.
         (ii) Is typically 3 to 5 cm in length and is measured in percent effacement.

(c) Station.
- (i) Determined by the relationship of the fetal head to the ischial spines of the pelvis.
- (ii) Zero station is when the presenting part is at the level of the ischial spines.
- (iii) Ranges from –3 to +3 or –5 to +5, with negative stations being above the ischial spines and positive stations being below the ischial spines.

(d) Cervical position.
- (i) Determines if cervical position is posterior, mid, or anterior.

(e) Cervical consistency.
- (i) Determines if the cervix is firm, soft, or in between.

3. Bishop scoring system used to determine if the cervix is favorable to spontaneous delivery.
- (a) A score of greater than 8 is favorable.

c. **Induction and Augmentation**
   i. General.
   1. Induction of labor is an attempt to begin labor in a nonlaboring patient.
      (a) Indications for induction include post-term pregnancy, preeclampsia, premature rupture of membranes, fetal distress, or growth restriction.
   2. Augmentation of labor is the process of increasing already-present labor.
   ii. Induction preparation.
   1. Success of induction is related to Bishop score. A score of less than 5 leads to an increased number of failed inductions.
   2. Can prepare a patient for induction by use of prostaglandins to ripen the cervix.
      (a) Contraindications to the use of prostaglandins include maternal asthma or glaucoma, more than one prior cesarean section, or unstable fetal status.
   iii. Induction.
   1. Can be performed with amniotomy or Pitocin (oxytocin).
   2. Pitocin, given by continuous IV infusion, stimulates uterine contraction.
   3. Amniotomy is the rupture of the amniotic sac with the use of an amniotic hook.
   iv. Augmentation.
   1. Pitocin and amniotomy can also be used to augment labor in those with inadequate labor.

d. **Fetal Monitoring**
   i. Contraction monitoring.
   1. External tocometer is used to obtain a record of the contractions.
   2. It is used to monitor frequency of contractions and to compare to fetal heart monitoring records.
   ii. Fetal heart monitoring.
   1. Continuous monitoring is done after determining the baseline to monitor for fetal distress.
   2. Baseline fetal heart rate is between 110 and 160 beats/minute.
      (a) With rates above 160, the fetal distress may be secondary to infection, hypoxia, or anemia.
   3. Fetal heart tracing should show variability between heartbeats.
   4. Decelerations can be noted on fetal heart monitoring.
      (a) Early decelerations.
         (i) Begin and end at the same time as the contraction.
         (ii) A result of increased vagal tone due to head compression during the contraction.
      (b) Variable decelerations.
         (i) Occur at any time and drop more than early or late decelerations.
         (ii) A result of umbilical cord compression.
      (c) Late decelerations.
         (i) Begin at the peak of a contraction and slowly return to baseline after the contraction is complete.
         (ii) A result of uteroplacental compromise.
      (d) "VEAL CHOP"
         1. V = Variable/C = cord compression
         2. E = Early/H = head compression
         3. A = Accelerations/O = okay
         4. L = Late/P = placental insufficiency
   iii. Fetal scalp electrode.
   1. Used to sense depolarizations of the fetal heart.
   2. Used in the fetus with repetitive decelerations or difficult to monitor externally.
   3. Contraindications include fetal thrombocytopenia, maternal hepatitis, or HIV.
   iv. Fetal scalp pH.
   1. If fetal heart tracings are abnormal, fetal scalp pH can be obtained to evaluate for fetal hypoxia and acidosis.
   2. pH greater than 7.25 is normal, and pH less than 7.20 is abnormal.
   v. Intrauterine pressure catheter.
   1. Used to determine timing and strength of contractions.

2. Used in those patients difficult to monitor externally or when absolute values of contraction strength are needed.

e. **Labor Progression**
   i. Cardinal movements of labor.
      1. Engagement.
         (a) When the fetal presenting part enters the pelvis.
      2. Flexion.
         (a) Head flexes to allow the smallest diameter to present to the pelvis.
      3. Descent.
         (a) Passage of the head into the pelvis.
      4. Internal rotation.
         (a) Fetal vertex moves from occiput transverse position to a position where the sagittal suture is parallel to the anteroposterior diameter of the pelvis.
      5. Extension.
         (a) Vertex extends as it passes beneath the pubic symphysis.
      6. External rotation.
         (a) The fetus externally rotates after the head is delivered so that the shoulders can be delivered.
   ii. Stages of labor.
      1. Stage 1.
         (a) Begins with the onset of labor to complete dilation and effacement of the cervix.
         (b) Average duration is 10 to 12 hours in nulliparous and 6 to 8 hours in multiparous patients.
         (c) Divided into the following two phases:
            (i) Latent phase from onset of labor until 3 to 4 cm of dilation.
            (ii) Active phase ranges until greater than 9 cm of dilation.
         (d) Transit time is affected by three things.
            (i) Power: the strength and frequency of contractions.
            (ii) Passenger: size and position of the fetus.
            (iii) Pelvis: size and shape of the pelvis.
         (e) Dystocia: an abnormally slow or halted labor. Typically diagnosed during the first or second stages of labor. Often results in cesarean delivery.
      2. Stage 2.
         (a) From the time of full dilation and effacement to delivery of the infant.
         (b) Normal time frame is less than 2 hours in nulliparous and less than 1 hour in multiparous patients.
         (c) Once the fetal head is delivered, the mouth and upper airway should be suctioned.

         (d) If stage 2 is prolonged, an operative vaginal delivery may be needed.
            (i) Use of forceps or vacuum extraction.
         (e) Episiotomy may be needed to speed up delivery, minimize risk of laceration, or assist with shoulder dystocia.
            (i) Two common types: midline and mediolateral.
            (ii) Lacerations.
               (1) First-degree: involves mucosa and skin.
               (2) Second-degree: extends into perineal body but not the anal sphincter.
               (3) Third-degree: extends into or through the anal sphincter.
               (4) Fourth-degree: anal mucosa is entered.
      3. Stage 3.
         (a) From delivery of the infant to delivery of the placenta.
         (b) Normal time frame is less than 30 minutes.
         (c) Three signs of placental separation.
            (i) Cord lengthening.
            (ii) Rush of blood.
            (iii) Uterine fundal rebound.
         (d) Retained placenta.
            (i) Diagnosis made when placenta has not been delivered in 30 minutes.
            (ii) May be removed by manual extraction.

# UTERINE DISORDERS

## I. DYSFUNCTIONAL UTERINE BLEEDING (DUB)
   a. **General**
      i. Relies heavily on exclusion. If no pathologic cause of menorrhagia, metrorrhagia, or menometrorrhagia is found, the diagnosis of DUB is made.
      ii. May be secondary to anovulation with a disruption of the hypothalamic-pituitary-gonadal axis that causes continuous estrogen stimulation of the endometrium that overgrows and sloughs off at irregular times and in varying amounts rather than the predictable, physiologic cyclic pattern.
      iii. More often to occur near menarche and menopause. When this occurs in the months preceding menopause, it is called perimenopause.
   b. **Diagnosis**
      i. A careful workup including history and physical examination to rule out other causes before the diagnosis is made.

ii. Endometrial biopsy is the gold standard to determine the presence of a proliferative (normal with menstruation) endometrium versus a hyperplastic (abnormal) endometrium.

**c. Treatment**

i. Oral contraceptives are used to regulate the menstrual cycle if the patient is stable, not hemorrhaging, and pregnancy is not desired at this time.

ii. If excessive bleeding occurs, multiple pills each day (typically 3–4) can be used for one week.

iii. With ovulatory dysfunctional uterine bleeding, NSAIDs can decrease menstrual blood loss.

iv. If there is no response to medical therapy, surgical intervention may be necessary.

1. Endometrial ablation is the first treatment of choice.

2. Hysterectomy is the definitive treatment and is reserved for refractory cases.

v. Iron deficiency anemia is common and should be managed accordingly if present.

## II. ENDOMETRIAL CANCER

**a. General**

i. Most common gynecologic cancer in the United States.

1. Mean age at diagnosis is 60 years and diagnosis it is uncommon under age 45 years.

2. Occurs about 75% of the time in postmenopausal women, followed by perimenopausal women, and is much less common in women who are menstruating.

ii. The most common type is adenocarcinoma, followed by mucinous, clear cell, and squamous cell.

**b. Risk Factors**

i. Nulliparity.

ii. Late menopause.

iii. Diabetes mellitus.

iv. Obesity.

v. Unopposed estrogen therapy.

vi. Tamoxifen use.

vii. Lynch syndrome.

**c. Clinical Manifestations**

i. The most common symptom is post-menopausal irregular bleeding, including prolonged heavy bleeding or spotting.

ii. Patients typically will have a normal pelvic examination, but a pelvic mass may be noted.

**d. Diagnosis**

i. Endometrial biopsy is the gold standard for diagnosis.

ii. Pelvic ultrasound is needed to rule out fibroids, polyps, and endometrial hyperplasia.

**e. Treatment**

i. Depends on staging.

ii. Treatment includes surgical staging, total abdominal hysterectomy and bilateral salpingo-oophorectomy, and postoperative radiation therapy.

## III. ENDOMETRIOSIS

**a. General**

i. Presence of endometrial tissue outside of the endometrial cavity.

1. Most common sites are ovary, pelvic peritoneum, round ligament, fallopian tubes, and sigmoid colon.

ii. Found in women of reproductive age.

**b. Clinical Manifestations**

i. Patients report pain. Symptoms include dysmenorrhea, dyspareunia, infertility, abnormal bleeding, and chronic pelvic pain.

1. Symptoms and severity vary with area involved.

ii. Physical examination findings may be absent or subtle early in the disease.

1. When disease is more disseminated, a physical exam may show uterosacral nodularity or a fixed or retroverted uterus.

a. Note that up to approximately 25% of women have a physiologic retroverted uterus.

2. If an ovary is involved, a tender, fixed adnexal mass may be noted.

**c. Diagnosis**

i. Pelvic and/or transvaginal ultrasound is often used for screening.

j. Gold standard diagnosis requires a laparoscopic exam with direct visualization and biopsy of endometrial implants.

1. While invasive, this may also be therapeutic (see Treatment).

**d. Treatment**

i. Treatment aimed at suppression and atrophy of endometrial tissue.

ii. Options include the following:

1. Oral contraceptives or medroxyprogesterone.

(a) Suppresses ovulation and menstruation, avoiding dysmenorrhea.

2. Danazol, an androgen derivative, or gonadotropin-releasing hormone (GnRH) analogs.

(a) Suppress FSH and LH, which results in diminished estrogen production and a decrease in endometriosis.

(b) Side effects of danazol include acne, weight gain, edema, and hirsutism.

(c) Side effects of GnRH analogs include hot flashes and decreased bone density.

3. Surgical treatment.

(a) Conservation options include ablation, electrocauterization, or excision of visible endometrial implants.

(b) Definitive therapy includes abdominal hysterectomy and bilateral salpingo-oophorectomy, lysis of adhesions, and removal of endometrial implants.

## IV. ADENOMYOSIS

a. **General**
   i. Extension of endometrial glands and stroma into the uterine musculature (myometrium).
   ii. The cause is unknown.
   iii. Typically develops in parous women in their late 30s or early 40s.

b. **Clinical Manifestations**
   i. Patients may be asymptomatic.
   ii. Most common symptoms are secondary dysmenorrhea, menorrhagia, or both.
   iii. On physical examination, may note a tender, symmetrically enlarged globular uterus with a boggy, soft consistency.

c. **Diagnosis**
   i. Definitive diagnosis is made via hysterectomy.
   ii. Transvaginal ultrasound or magnetic resonance imaging (MRI) are possible screening tools.

d. **Treatment**
   i. Analgesics may be used in mild disease.
   ii. Hormonal manipulation (progestins, GnRH analogues, or aromatic inhibitors) may reduce menorrhagia and dysmenorrhea.
   iii. Total abdominal hysterectomy is the definitive treatment.

## V. LEIOMYOMA (UTERINE FIBROIDS)

a. **General**
   i. Due to local proliferation of smooth muscle cells of the uterus.
      1. Etiology is unknown.
   ii. Typically occur in women of childbearing age and regress during menopause.
   iii. More common in Black women.

b. **Clinical Manifestations**
   i. Most women have no clinical symptoms.
   ii. The most common symptom, when symptoms are present, is heavy or prolonged uterine bleeding.
   iii. Symptoms also include pressure-related symptoms (pelvic pressure, fullness, or heaviness), infertility, and first trimester spontaneous abortion.

iv. Physical examination may be normal or reveal masses noted on bimanual or abdominal examination.
   1. Uterus is enlarged, nontender, and irregularly shaped.

c. **Diagnosis**
   i. Transvaginal ultrasound reveals hypoechogenic areas of shadowing among normal myometrial material.

d. **Treatment**
   i. Treatment is typically not required.
   ii. If treatment is needed, it is aimed at decreasing uterine bleeding.
   iii. Treatment is needed if severe pain, infertility, or evidence of continued growth of fibroid is present.
      1. Medical treatment to shrink the fibroids includes medroxyprogesterone, danazol, and GnRH agonists.
      2. Surgical treatment includes myomectomy and hysterectomy.

## VI. METRITIS

a. **General**
   i. Endometritis is an infection of the uterine endometrium.
   ii. Endomyometritis is an infection invading into the myometrium.
   iii. Infection preceded by instrumentation or disruption of the intrauterine cavity.
      1. Most common after cesarean section, vaginal deliveries, dilation and evacuation or curettage, and IUD placement.

b. **Clinical Manifestations**
   i. Patients typically have fever ($\geq 38.0°C$).
   ii. Bimanual examination reveals uterine tenderness.
   iii. Laboratory tests reveal leukocytosis.

c. **Diagnosis**
   i. Based on clinical history and presence of uterine tenderness, fever, and elevated white blood cell (WBC) count.

d. **Treatment**
   i. Severe disease is treated with intravenous clindamycin plus gentamicin.
   ii. Mild disease is treated with a second-generation cephalosporin.
   iii. Chronic disease is treated with doxycycline.

## VII. UTERINE PROLAPSE

a. **General**
   i. Abnormal protrusion of the uterus through the pelvic-floor aperture.
   ii. Due to injury or stretching of the cardinal ligaments.

iii. Occurs most commonly in multiparous women.

iv. Most commonly secondary to childbirth injury, but also noted with pelvic tumors, sacral nerve disorders, systemic disorders (obesity and asthma), and local conditions (ascites).

v. Prolapse of the bladder into the anterior vaginal wall is called cystocele.

vi. Prolapse of the rectum into the posterior vaginal wall is called rectocele.

**b. Clinical Manifestations**

i. Symptoms include vaginal pressure, sensation of something "falling out," stress urinary incontinence, and constipation.

ii. Depending on the staging, patients present with a firm mass in the lower vagina, cervix projecting through the introitus, and vaginal inversion with cervix and uterus projecting between the legs.

iii. Physical examination reveals descent of the cervix according to the following staging:
stage 1: Into the vaginal canal.
stage 2: Equal with the introitus.
stage 3: Outside of the introitus.
stage 4: Uterus full outside the introitus.

**c. Diagnosis**

i. Based on physical examination findings.

**d. Treatment**

i. Kegel exercises (to strengthen the pelvic-floor muscle) can be used for prevention.

ii. Medical treatment includes a vaginal pessary and use of estrogens to improve tissue tone.

iii. Surgical treatment to improve vaginal support may be needed.

# VAGINAR/VULVAR DISORDERS

## I. CYSTOCELE

**a. General**

i. Descent of a portion of the posterior bladder wall and trigone into the vagina.

ii. Typically due to the trauma of parturition.

**b. Clinical Manifestations**

i. A small cystocele causes no significant symptoms.

ii. If a large cystocele, the patient may complain of vaginal pressure or a protruding mass.

iii. Symptoms are aggravated with prolonged standing, coughing, or straining.

iv. Urinary incontinence is also noted.

v. On physical examination, note a relaxed vaginal outlet with a thin-walled, smooth, bulging mass involving the anterior vaginal wall.

1. With straining, the mass may project through the vaginal introitus.

**c. Treatment**

i. Kegel exercises may assist in prevention.

ii. Medical measures include a vaginal pessary, Kegel exercises, or estrogens.

iii. Surgery is seldom indicated unless the cystocele is large or causing significant impairment in the patient's daily life.

1. Anterior vaginal colporrhaphy is most effective in patients with a large cystocele.

## II. NEOPLASMS

**a. Vaginal**

i. General

1. Peak incidence in women ages 60 to 70 years.

2. The most common type is squamous cell.

(a) It is rare in young females, but increased risk of clear cell adenocarcinoma of the vagina with exposure to DES.

ii. Clinical manifestations

1. Many are asymptomatic or may present with vaginal discharge, bleeding, and urinary symptoms.

iii. Diagnosis

1. Disease is screened for with the Pap smear and colposcopy.

2. Diagnosis is confirmed by biopsy.

iv. Treatment

1. Surgical resection and radiation therapy are used to treat vaginal carcinoma.

2. A 5-year survival rate varies with clinical stage.

**b. Vulva**

i. General

1. More common in older patients, with peak incidence in women in their 70s.

2. Risk factors include smoking, vulvar dystrophy, CIN, and human papillomavirus (HPV) infection.

3. Squamous cell most common histology.

ii. Clinical manifestations

1. Symptoms include vulvar pruritus and vulvodynia.

2. May also present with vulvar bleeding or mass.

3. A mass, ulcer, or plaque noted on the labia.

iii. Diagnosis

1. Confirmed with biopsy.

iv. Treatment

1. Wide local excision with regional lymphadenectomy is the treatment of choice.

2. If metastatic disease is noted, pelvic radiation is indicated.

## III. RECTOCELE
### a. General
i. Herniation of the rectum into the vaginal vault.

ii. Due to injury of the endopelvic fascia of the rectovaginal septum.

iii. Risk factors include chronic constipation, multiparity, and obesity.

### b. Clinical Manifestations
i. Small rectoceles are typically asymptomatic.

ii. With larger rectoceles, vaginal pressure, rectal fullness, and incomplete evacuation are noted.

iii. On physical examination, a soft, thin-walled rectovaginal septum projecting into the vagina is noted.

### c. Diagnosis
i. Based on history and physical examination findings.

### d. Treatment
i. Conservative management includes increasing fluid intake, stool softeners, pelvic floor exercises, and vaginal pessary use.

ii. Surgical measures include posterior colpoperineorrhaphy.

## IV. VAGINITIS
### a. Yeast Infection (Candida)
i. General

1. Most commonly caused by *Candida albicans*.

2. Predisposing factors include use of antibiotics, diabetes mellitus, increased estrogen levels, and decreased cellular immunity.

3. Make up 20% to 25% of all causes of vaginitis.

ii. Clinical manifestations

1. Symptoms include vulvar and vaginal pruritus, burning, dysuria, dyspareunia, and vaginal discharge.

2. On physical examination, there is vulvar edema and erythema with a thick white vaginal discharge.

iii. Diagnosis

1. Branching hyphae and spores noted on KOH test.

2. Gram stain and culture are also used in diagnosis.

3. See Fig. 8.3.

iv. Treatment

1. Consists of -azole agents (e.g., clotrimazole, miconazole) via topical application (vaginal suppository).

2. Oral fluconazole is also effective.

### b. *Trichomonas vaginalis (T. vaginalis)*
i. General

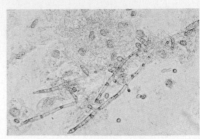

**Fig. 8.3** Yeast and mycelia. Saline preparation positive for yeast and mycelia. *(From Mandell G. Principles and Practice of Infectious Disease. Philadelphia: Elsevier Churchill Livingstone 2005:1364, Fig. 103-10.)*

1. A sexually transmitted infection (STI) caused by a unicellular flagellated protozoan.

2. Make up 15% to 20% of all causes of vaginitis. Can cause cervicitis as well.

ii. Clinical manifestations

1. Present with a profuse unpleasant-smelling discharge.

2. The discharge may be yellow or green in color and frothy in appearance.

3. May also note vulvar erythema, edema, and pruritus.

4. On physical examination, may note erythematous, punctate epithelial papillae, or a "strawberry" appearance of the cervix.

iii. Diagnosis

1. Wet prep reveals motile protozoan.

2. See Fig. 8.4.

iv. Treatment

1. Treatment consists of metronidazole for 7 days.

### c. *Gardnerella vaginalis*
i. General

1. Risk factors include low socioeconomic status, IUD usage, multiple sexual partners, and smoking.

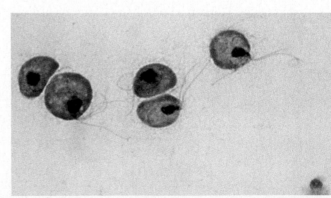

**Fig. 8.4** *Trichomonas vaginalis. (From Kumar V. In: Robbins and Cotran, eds.: Pathologic Basis of Disease, 7th ed. Philadelphia: Elsevier Saunders 2005:1064, Fig. 22-4.)*

2. Make up 40% to 50% of all causes of vaginitis.

ii. Clinical manifestations
1. Patients may be asymptomatic.
2. Symptomatic patients note a profuse nonirritating discharge with a "fishy odor."

iii. Diagnosis
1. On wet prep, note epithelial cells covered by bacteria (clue cells).
    (a) Clue cells are vaginal squamous epithelial cells covered with *G. vaginalis*, giving the cells a granular appearance.
    (b) See Fig. 8.5.
2. The "fishy" odor can be enhanced with addition of KOH to the vaginal prep (whiff test).
3. Vaginal pH is greater than 4.5.

iv. Treatment
1. Treatment consists of metronidazole or clindamycin.

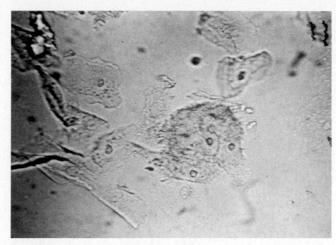

**Fig. 8.5** Clue cells seen in bacterial vaginosis. *(From Ferri FF: Ferri's Clinical Advisor: Instant Diagnosis and Treatment. Philadelphia: Elsevier Saunders 2005:876, Fig. 1-290.)*

# QUESTIONS

## QUESTION 1

Which of the following physical examination findings is typically seen in fibroadenoma of the breast?

**A** Rubbery mass
**B** Dimpling
**C** Retraction
**D** Nipple flattening
**E** Nipple discharge

## QUESTION 2

What is the average doubling time for beta-hCG during the first trimester of pregnancy?

**A** 2 days
**B** 4 days
**C** 6 days
**D** 8 days
**E** 10 days

## QUESTION 3

A 24-year-old pregnant patient presents with pelvic pain and brisk vaginal bleeding. Beta-hCG is elevated with a level consistent with 10 weeks of gestation. Pelvic ultrasound fails to demonstrate an intrauterine gestational sac. Which of the following is the most likely diagnosis?

**A** Endometriosis
**B** Ectopic pregnancy
**C** Pelvic inflammatory disease
**D** Threatened abortion
**E** Chorioamnionitis

## QUESTION 4

A 30-year-old female presents with a nontender mass in the right breast. No nipple discharge is noted. Which of the following is the next best step in the evaluation of this patient?

**A** Simple mastectomy
**B** Excisional biopsy
**C** Fine-needle aspiration
**D** Mammography
**E** Breast MRI

## QUESTION 5

Which of the following is the treatment of choice for *Trichomonas vaginalis*?

**A** Podophyllin
**B** Doxycycline
**C** Metronidazole
**D** Penicillin
**E** Nystatin

## QUESTION 6

Which of the following is a risk factor for the development of endometrial cancer?

**A** Anorexia
**B** Multiparity
**C** Early menopause
**D** Diabetes insipidus
**E** Chronic tamoxifen use

*Continued*

## QUESTIONS—cont'd

### QUESTION 7

Release of which of the following hormones results in development of the primary ovarian follicle?

A Estrogen

B Prolactin

C Progesterone

D FSH

E LH

### QUESTION 8

A 25-year-old primigravida at 42 weeks of gestation delivers after induction with oxytocin. The second stage of labor lasted 3 hours. Then 10 minutes after delivery, she has copious vaginal bleeding of about 500 mL over a 5-minute period. On examination, the fundus is noted to be soft and boggy. Which of the following is the most likely cause of the hemorrhage?

A Uterine atony

B Placenta previa

C Uterine inversion

D Cervical laceration

E Retained placental tissue

### QUESTION 9

Which of the following hormones is responsible for milk production in a lactating female?

A Oxytocin

B Prolactin

C DHEA

D FSH

E LH

### QUESTION 10

A 30-year-old female, in her 37th week of pregnancy, presents with a sudden onset of painless, profuse vaginal bleeding. Vitals are pulse 106/minute, respirations 20/minute, blood pressure 106/64 mm Hg, and temperature 98.6° F (37° C). Which of the following is the most likely diagnosis?

A Cervical laceration

B Abruptio placentae

C Uterine rupture

D Placenta previa

E Uterine atony

## ANSWERS

**1. A**

EXPLANATION: Dimpling, retraction, and nipple flattening or discharge are more commonly noted in breast cancer. Fibroadenoma presents with a well-circumscribed, rubbery, nontender, mobile, firm mass. *Topic: Fibroadenoma*

☐ Correct ☐ Incorrect

**2. A**

EXPLANATION: During the first trimester of a normal pregnancy, the beta-hCG will double every 2 days. In ectopic pregnancy, the beta-hCG does not double as expected in a normal pregnancy. *Topic: Uncomplicated pregnancy*

☐ Correct ☐ Incorrect

**3. B**

EXPLANATION: Ectopic pregnancy presents classically with amenorrhea, vaginal bleeding, and lower abdominal pain. Appropriate beta-hCG levels and transvaginal ultrasound that reveals no intrauterine gestational sac are consistent with the diagnosis of ectopic pregnancy. *Topic: Ectopic pregnancy*

☐ Correct ☐ Incorrect

**4. C**

EXPLANATION: The evaluation of the patient with a breast mass includes a fine-needle aspiration followed by excisional biopsy if aspirate is negative. *Topic: Breast: carcinoma*

☐ Correct ☐ Incorrect

**5. C**

EXPLANATION: *Trichomonas vaginalis* is noted with a foul-smelling, green vaginal discharge and is treated with metronidazole (Flagyl). *Topic: Vaginitis*

☐ Correct ☐ Incorrect

**6. E**

EXPLANATION: Risk factors for endometrial cancer include obesity, nulliparity, late menopause, diabetes mellitus, breast or ovarian cancer, chronic unopposed estrogen stimulation, and chronic tamoxifen use. However, studies that support diabetes mellitus as a risk factor for endometrial cancer do not adjust for obesity, which is a risk factor for type 2 diabetes. *Topic: Endometrial cancer*

☐ Correct ☐ Incorrect

**7. D**

EXPLANATION: Release of FSH from the anterior pituitary gland results in development of primary ovarian follicles. The ovarian follicle produces estrogen, which causes the uterine lining to proliferate. *Topic: Menstrual cycle*

☐ Correct ☐ Incorrect

## ANSWERS—cont'd

**8.  A**

EXPLANATION: Uterine atony, failure of the uterus to contract after placental separation, is a common cause of hemorrhage. Predisposing factors include oxytocic augmentation of labor, prolonged labor, and multiple gestations. On examination, the uterus will be soft and boggy. *Topic: Complicated pregnancy*

☐ **Correct**   ☐ **Incorrect**

**9.  B**

EXPLANATION: Prolactin is secreted by the anterior pituitary and is responsible for lactation. Oxytocin is secreted by the posterior pituitary and is responsible for uterine contraction and milk ejection. LH and FSH are involved in ovulation. *Topic: Breast*

☐ **Correct**   ☐ **Incorrect**

**10.  D**

EXPLANATION: Patients with placenta previa, a major cause of antepartum bleeding, present with sudden, painless, profuse bleeding after 28 weeks of gestation. *Topic: Placenta previa*

☐ **Correct**   ☐ **Incorrect**

# CHAPTER 9
# INFECTIOUS DISEASE

## EXAMINATION BLUEPRINT TOPICS

**FUNGAL DISEASE**

Candidiasis

Cryptococcosis

Histoplasmosis

Pneumocystis

Systemic fungal infections

**BACTERIAL DISEASE**

Acute rheumatic fever

Botulism

Campylobacter infections

Chlamydia

Cholera

Diphtheria

Gonococcal infections

Methicillin-resistant *Staphylococcus aureus*

Salmonellosis

Shigellosis

Tetanus

**MYCOBACTERIAL DISEASE**

Tuberculosis

Atypical mycobacterial disease

Leprosy (hansen's disease)

**PARASITIC DISEASE**

Amebiasis

Ascariasis

Giardiasis

Hookworms

Malaria

Pinworms

Tapeworms

Toxoplasmosis

**SPIROCHETAL DISEASE**

Lyme disease

Rocky Mountain spotted fever

Syphilis

**VIRAL DISEASE**

Cytomegalovirus (CMV) infections

Epstein-Barr virus (EBV) infections

Erythema infectiosum

Herpes simplex

Human immunodeficiency virus infection

Human papillomavirus (HPV) infections

Influenza

Mumps

Rabies

Roseola

Rubella

Rubeola (Measles)

Varicella-zoster virus infections

Other

**SEPSIS**

General

Clinical manifestations

Diagnosis

Treatment

# FUNGAL DISEASE

## I. CANDIDIASIS
### a. General
   i. Candidiasis is the most common opportunistic fungal infection.
   ii. Most common organism is *Candida albicans*, but also includes *Candida glabrata*, *Candida parapsilosis*, and *Candida tropicalis*.
   iii. Infections range from mucous-membrane infection to life-threatening disseminated disease.
### b. Epidemiology
   i. *Candida* species are normal flora in the gastrointestinal and genitourinary tracts and on the skin.
### c. Clinical Manifestations
   i. Oropharyngeal (thrush) and esophageal infections.

1. White plaques on the buccal mucosa, palate, oropharynx, or tongue.
2. Scraping lesion reveals an erythematous, nonulcerated mucosa.
3. Suspect immune dysfunction (human immunodeficiency virus [HIV]) in an otherwise healthy person.

ii. Vulvovaginitis.
1. Common infection in women of childbearing age.
2. Risk factors include increased estrogen levels, diabetes mellitus, therapy with corticosteroids or antibiotics, and HIV infection.
3. Symptoms include vaginal discomfort, curd-like discharge, and pruritus.
4. Vaginal walls are erythematous and show white plaques.
5. Labia are erythematous and swollen.

iii. Cutaneous infection.
1. Occurs mainly in the intertriginous areas or under large breasts or pannus.
2. Lesions are erythematous with a distinct border, and there are multiple satellite lesions.

iv. Disseminated infection.
1. Most common is candidemia.
    (a) Risk factors include broad-spectrum antibiotics, central intravenous catheters, renal failure, and corticosteroid therapy.
2. Can also cause endocarditis and hepatosplenic infection.

d. **Diagnosis**
i. KOH prep or Gram stain reveals budding yeast and pseudohyphae.
ii. Disseminated disease diagnosed by culture of blood or other sterile body fluid.
1. Imaging studies, such as computed tomography (CT) scan, are also required to determine extent of disease.

e. **Treatment**
i. Thrush treated with clotrimazole troches, nystatin, miconazole, or fluconazole.
ii. Esophagitis treated with fluconazole, itraconazole, clotrimazole, or nystatin.
iii. Vaginitis treated with fluconazole, miconazole, or clotrimazole.
iv. Disseminated disease treated with amphotericin B, fluconazole, voriconazole, or echinocandin (caspofungin). Amphotericin B is nephrotoxic and may cause anemia and cardiac arrhythmias.
v. Cutaneous infection treated with topical barriers and nystatin, clotrimazole, or miconazole.

## II. CRYPTOCOCCOSIS
a. **General**
i. Organism causing infection is yeast called *Cryptococcus neoformans* or *Cryptococcus gattii*.
ii. Infection occurs most often in patients who are immunosuppressed.
iii. Meningitis is the most common clinical presentation but can have pulmonary infection.

b. **Epidemiology**
i. Infections linked to pigeon excreta.
ii. Increased risk of infection with CD4 count <50.

c. **Pathogenesis**
i. Organism is inhaled, causing pulmonary infection first.
ii. If host defenses not adequate, infection can disseminate.

d. **Clinical Manifestations**
i. Central nervous system (CNS) infection.
1. Headache, nuchal rigidity, lethargy, confusion, photophobia, papilledema, nausea, and vomiting.
2. Fever is noted in half of the cases.
ii. Pulmonary infection.
1. Patient typically has underlying chronic obstructive pulmonary disease.
2. Fever, cough, and dyspnea.

e. **Diagnosis**
i. Culture.
ii. Mucicarmine stain or India ink prep: positive.
iii. Antigen testing with latex agglutination or enzyme immunoassay testing for cryptococcal antigen is positive.
iv. Cerebral spinal fluid (CSF) reveals elevated white blood cells (WBCs) (rarely >500/mL) with a predominance of lymphocytes, elevated total protein, and decreased glucose.

f. **Treatment**
i. Amphotericin B plus flucytosine, followed by fluconazole for 6 weeks for CNS infection.
ii. Fluconazole for pulmonary infection.

## III. HISTOPLASMOSIS
a. **General**
i. Caused by *Histoplasma capsulatum*.
1. A dimorphic fungus, a mold at temperatures of less than 35° C and a yeast at 35° C to 37° C.

b. **Epidemiology**
i. Endemic in the Mississippi and Ohio River valleys.
ii. Increased number of organisms in bird or bat guano in caves, soil, and abandoned buildings.

c. **Pathogenesis**
i. Inhale organisms and develop a localized pulmonary infection.

ii. Phagocytized organisms survive and travel within the macrophages to hilar and mediastinal lymph nodes.

iii. Severity of infection based on organism load and immune response.

d. **Clinical Manifestations**

i. Acute pulmonary.

1. Symptoms include fever, chills, fatigue, nonproductive cough, and myalgias.

2. Patchy lobar or multilobed infiltrate noted on chest x-ray film with enlarged hilar or mediastinal lymph nodes.

ii. Chronic pulmonary.

1. Progressive and fatal.

2. Seen in older patients with history of chronic obstructive pulmonary disease.

3. Symptoms include fever, fatigue, anorexia, weight loss, productive cough with purulent sputum, and hemoptysis.

4. Chest x-ray film reveals upper lobe infiltrates with multiple cavities.

iii. Disseminated.

1. Occurs mainly in immunocompromised patients, such as HIV (CD4 counts <200/mL), or post-transplantation or current corticosteroid therapy.

2. Symptoms include fever, chills, anorexia, weight loss, hypotension, dyspnea, and hepatosplenomegaly.

3. Blood test reveals pancytopenia, and diffuse pulmonary infiltrates revealed on chest x-ray film.

e. **Diagnosis**

i. Culture.

1. Can take 6 weeks to grow.

ii. Biopsy stained with methenamine silver.

iii. Wright's stain of peripheral blood.

iv. Enzyme immunoassay antigen test on urine or serum for disseminated disease.

f. **Treatment**

i. Itraconazole for mild to moderate disease.

ii. Amphotericin B for severe disease.

iii. Treatment typically not used for acute pulmonary histoplasmosis unless patient is immunocompromised.

iv. All disseminated disease is treated with amphotericin B or itraconazole.

## IV. PNEUMOCYSTIS

a. **General**

i. Frequent case-defining infection in acquired immunodeficiency syndrome (AIDS).

ii. Disease caused by *Pneumocystis jirovecii*.

1. Eukaryotic microbe with fungal characteristics.

b. **Epidemiology**

i. Exposed early in life, and organism remains latent.

ii. Activated during severe immune system depression.

c. **Clinical Manifestations**

i. Symptoms include hacking, nonproductive cough, fever, and dyspnea.

ii. Lung examination is typically normal but may have rales and wheezing.

d. **Diagnosis**

i. Hypoxemia is most useful marker and predictor of outcome.

ii. Bronchoalveolar lavage with special stains, such as Giemsa stain.

iii. Chest x-ray film typically reveals interstitial infiltrates beginning in the perihilar region and spreading lower in a butterfly pattern.

1. Chest x-ray may be normal early in the disease.

iv. Increased uptake on Gallium scan.

v. Elevated lactate dehydrogenase (LDH) levels.

vi. CD4 counts typically <200 cells/mm$^3$.

vii. Low diffusion capacity noted.

e. **Treatment**

i. Acute disease.

1. Trimethoprim-sulfamethoxazole.

2. Parenteral pentamidine.

3. Clindamycin plus primaquine.

4. Atovaquone.

5. Corticosteroids indicated if PaO2 is less than 70 mm Hg.

ii. Prophylactic treatment.

1. Needed for all patients at high risk.

(a) Prior *Pneumocystis* infection.

(b) CD4 count <200 cells/mm$^3$.

2. Trimethoprim-sulfamethoxazole is primary, other options include the following:

(a) Dapsone.

(b) Aerosolized pentamidine.

## V. SYSTEMIC FUNGAL INFECTIONS

a. **See Table 9.1 for summary of systemic fungal organisms.**

# BACTERIAL DISEASE

## I. ACUTE RHEUMATIC FEVER

a. **General**

i. Inflammatory disease that occurs as a response to an infection due to group A streptococci.

1. Have exudative and proliferative inflammatory lesions on connective tissue, mainly of the heart, joints, and subcutaneous tissue.

**TABLE 9.1**

## Summary of Systemic Fungal Organisms

|  | Histoplasmosis | Blastomycosis | Coccidioidomycosis | Candidiasis | Cryptococcosis | Aspergillosis |
|---|---|---|---|---|---|---|
| Type | Dimorphic | Dimorphic | Dimorphic | Yeast | Yeast | Fungus |
| Epidemiology | Mississippi and Ohio River valleys Soil, caves, and old buildings | North central and south central U.S. Soil or decaying wood | Southwestern U.S. Soil | Normal flora on GI tract, GU tract, and skin | Western U.S. Pigeon excreta | Ubiquitous: water and soil |
| Route of infection | Inhalation | Inhalation | Inhalation | Direct or blood | Inhalation | Inhalation |
| Disease | Pulmonary Disseminated | Pulmonary Disseminated | Pulmonary Disseminated | Vulvovaginitis Esophagitis Cutaneous Oropharyngeal | CNS Pulmonary | Pulmonary |
| Diagnosis | Culture Special stains CF and ID Enzyme assay | Culture Stains | Culture Stains CF | Gram stain KOH prep Culture | Culture Latex agglutination | Culture |
| Treatment | Itraconazole Amphotericin B | Itraconazole Amphotericin B | Ketoconazole Fluconazole Itraconazole Amphotericin B | Clotrimazole Miconazole Fluconazole | Amphotericin B Flucytosine | Amphotericin B Itraconazole |

*GI,* Gastrointestinal; *GU,* genitourinary; *CNS,* central nervous system; *CF,* complement fixation; *ID,* immunodiffusion.

ii. Range of time from infection to onset of symptoms is 1 to 5 weeks.
iii. Mechanism is unknown.
iv. Peak incidence in the 5 to 15 year age group.
  1. Rare in children younger than 3 years or older than 21 years.
b. **Clinical Manifestations**
  i. Major manifestations (Jones criteria).
    1. Carditis.
      (a) Can involve the endocardium, myocardium, or pericardium.
      (b) Present with cardiac murmur, cardiomegaly, pericarditis, and congestive heart failure.
      (c) Cardiac murmur is an apical systolic murmur, blowing and high pitched in nature.
    2. Polyarthritis.
      (a) A migratory arthritis, typically involves larger joints, knees, and ankles.
      (b) Synovial fluid reveals increase in neutrophils, but no bacteria.
    3. Chorea.
      (a) Rapid, purposeless, involuntary movements, involving the face and extremities.
      (b) Speech is slurred; and the tongue, when protruded, retracts involuntarily.
    4. Erythema marginatum.
      (a) Erythematous macule or papule that extends over the skin with central clearing.
    5. Subcutaneous nodules.
      (a) Firm, painless subcutaneous nodules that vary in size from a few millimeters to 2 cm.
      (b) Occur over bony surfaces and tendons of the elbows, knees, and wrists.
    ii. Minor criteria include fever, arthralgia, elevated erythrocyte sedimentation rate or C reactive protein, leukocytosis, prolonged PR interval, first degree heart block, or previous episode of rheumatic fever or inactive heart disease.
c. **Diagnosis**
  i. No laboratory tests are diagnostic for rheumatic fever.
    1. Complete blood count (CBC) reveals a leukocytosis and anemia of chronic disease.
    2. Sedimentation rate and C-reactive protein are elevated.
  ii. Documentation of a recent streptococcal infection is noted.
    1. Includes positive antistreptolysin O (ASO), anti-DNase, or antihyaluronidase titers.
  iii. Diagnosis is based on the Jones criteria.
    1. Two major or one major and two minor manifestations indicate a high probability of acute rheumatic fever.
d. **Treatment**
  i. Bed rest.
  ii. Antibiotics do not modify the course of the disease.
  iii. Antiinflammatory drugs suppress the signs and symptoms but are not curative.

1. Major drugs include aspirin, and corticosteroids if no response to aspirin.
    iv. Decrease risk for disease by prevention with appropriate and timely treatment of streptococcal throat infections.
    v. Secondary prevention of rheumatic fever, prevention of recurrent attacks, includes penicillin G or V, or sulfadiazine.
        1. Erythromycin is used in the penicillin-allergic person.

## II. BOTULISM
a. **General**
    i. Absorbed from gut, lung, or wound.
        1. Does not penetrate intact skin.
    ii. Severe neuroparalytic disease.
    iii. Caused by botulism toxin produced by *Clostridium botulinum*.
        1. A gram-positive, spore-forming obligate anaerobe.
        2. Found in soil, marine environments, and agricultural products.
    iv. Toxin works by binding to receptors and blocks acetylcholine.
b. **Clinical Forms**
    i. Foodborne botulism.
        1. Most common form.
        2. Due to ingestion of preformed toxin in inadequately prepared food (home-canned foods are common).
        3. Occurs in outbreaks.
    ii. Wound botulism.
        1. Unusual form of botulism.
        2. Traumatic wounds with soil contamination.
    iii. Infant botulism.
        1. Due to production of neurotoxin in the gastrointestinal tract, after colonization of *C. botulinum* from the soil or honey.
        2. Typical age is 1 to 9 months.
        3. Symptoms of "floppy baby syndrome" include the following:
            (a) Lethargy.
            (b) Diminished suck.
            (c) Constipation.
            (d) Weakness.
            (e) Diminished spontaneous activity with loss of head control.
    iv. Inhalation botulism.
c. **Clinical Manifestations**
    i. Bulbar musculature affected first, causing diplopia, dysphonia, dysarthria, and dysphagia.
    ii. Decreased salivation, ileus, and urinary retention due to involvement of the cholinergic autonomic nervous system.
    iii. Neurologic.
        1. Bilateral cranial nerve VI palsy.

2. Ptosis.
3. Dilated pupils.
4. Decreased gag reflex.
5. Descending involvement of motor neurons to peripheral muscles, which can lead to respiratory failure.
    iv. Nausea and vomiting.
    v. Afebrile.
d. **Diagnosis**
    i. Analysis of food, serum, stool, and gastric contents for toxin.
    ii. Stool or food culture.
e. **Treatment**
    i. Supportive care monitoring airway.
    ii. Botulinum antitoxin with equine serum heptavalent botulism antitoxin or human-derived botulism immune globulin.
    iii. Antibiotic treatment needed only in wound botulism.
    iv. Prevention.
        1. Destroy spores with heat or irradiation.
        2. Inhibit germination by reducing pH, by refrigerating, by freezing, or by drying.
        3. No honey to infants under age of 1 year.

## III. CAMPYLOBACTER INFECTIONS
a. **General**
    i. Motile, curved, gram-negative bacilli.
    ii. Several human pathogens including *C. jejuni*, *C. coli*, and *C. fetus*.
    iii. Transmitted via contaminated food or water, infected animals, and fecal-oral.
    iv. Presents as a diarrheal illness.
        1. Can lead to Guillain-Barré syndrome.
b. **Clinical Manifestations**
    i. Present with fever, abdominal pain, headache, and myalgias.
    ii. Diarrhea is watery, with occasional blood.
c. **Diagnosis**
    i. Stool culture and blood cultures.
d. **Treatment**
    i. Most cases spontaneously resolve, if not use azithromycin.

## IV. CHLAMYDIA
a. **General**
    i. Obligate intracellular bacteria.
    ii. Organisms.
        1. *Chlamydia trachomatis*.
        2. *Chlamydophila pneumoniae*.
        3. *Chlamydophila psittaci*.
b. **Diseases**
    i. Trachoma.
        1. Most common cause of preventable blindness.
        2. A chronic follicular conjunctivitis.

3. Treated with topical ocular application of tetracycline or oral azithromycin for 6 weeks.

ii. Urethritis/Cervicitis.

1. Causes 30% to 40% of cases of nongonococcal urethritis.

2. Patients present with mild clear or cloudy urethral discharge, urethral discomfort, and mild dysuria.

3. Treat with tetracycline or azithromycin.

iii. Epididymitis/Salpingitis.

1. Spread from urethra to epididymis or fallopian tubes.

2. Male patients present with unilateral testicular pain, scrotal erythema and tenderness, or swelling over the epididymis. Female patients present with low abdominal pain and dyspareunia.

3. Treat with tetracycline or azithromycin.

iv. Atypical pneumonia.

1. Present with nonproductive cough, sore throat, and hoarseness.

2. Crackles are heard on lung examination.

3. Chest x-ray film reveals a pneumonitis.

4. Treat with doxycycline or azithromycin.

v. Psittacosis.

1. Systemic infection transmitted by sick birds.

2. Abrupt febrile illness with shaking chills and fever, headache, myalgias, arthralgias, and nonproductive cough.

3. Chest x-ray film reveals single or multiple localized bronchopneumonic patches.

4. Treat with tetracycline or doxycycline. Second-line drugs include the macrolides.

c. **Table 9.2 summarizes diseases caused by** *Chlamydia.*

## V. CHOLERA

a. **General**

i. Acute, watery "rice water" diarrhea caused by an exotoxin produced by *Vibrio cholerae.*

ii. Patients present with diarrhea after travel to a cholera-endemic area.

iii. Spread via contaminated water and food.

b. **Signs and symptoms are due to the severe water loss**

c. **Diagnosis made by stool culture or rapid detection of cholera antigens**

d. **Treatment**

i. Rehydration via oral route with oral rehydration solution (ORS), Pedialyte, or rice solution.

ii. Antibiotics may be indicated with doxycyline, azithromycin, or ciprofloxacin.

iii. Oral cholera vaccines are available.

## VI. DIPHTHERIA

a. **General**

i. Tonsillopharyngitis and/or laryngitis due to *Corynebacterium diphtheriae.*

ii. Humans are the only natural reservoir, and infection spreads in close-contact settings through respiratory droplets.

b. **Clinical Manifestations**

i. After an incubation period of 2 to 5 days, the illness begins with a sore throat, malaise, cervical lymphadenopathy, and low-grade fever.

ii. Whitish exudate appears on the tonsils and later becomes a grayish membrane.

1. Membrane is very adherent and bleeds easily on attempted removal.

iii. May develop myocarditis, conduction disturbances, and neurologic impairment.

iv. Fatality rate is 3%.

c. **Diagnosis**

i. By gram stain and culture or test for toxin production.

d. **Treatment**

i. Equine diphtheria antitoxin.

ii. Penicillin or erythromycin to limit local infection and prevent transmission.

iii. Prophylactic antibiotics (penicillin or erythromycin) for close contacts.

e. **Prevention**

i. Immunization with diphtheria toxoid.

ii. Doses are given at 2, 4, and 6 months of age; 15 to 18 months of age; 4 to 6 years of age; and 11 to 12 years of age.

## VII. GONOCOCCAL INFECTIONS

a. **General**

i. Sexually transmitted disease due to infection with *Neisseria gonorrhoeae,* a gram-negative diplococcus.

b. **Diseases**

i. Urethritis.

ii. Endocervicitis.

iii. Neonatal conjunctivitis (ophthalmia neonatorum).

**TABLE 9.2**

| Diseases Caused by *Chlamydia* | | | |
|---|---|---|---|
| **Organism** | **Disease** | **Host** | **Transmission** |
| *Chlamydia trachomatis* | Trachoma | Children | Fomites/flies |
| | Urethritis/ Cervicitis | Sexually active people | Direct sexual contact |
| | Epididymitis/ Salpingitis | Sexually active people | Direct sexual contact |
| *Chlamydia psittaci* | Atypical pneumonia | Birds | Aerosol |
| *Chlamydia pneumoniae* | Atypical pneumonia | Humans | Respiratory droplets |

c. **Clinical Manifestations**
   i. Urethritis.
     1. Dysuria and purulent urethral discharge.
   ii. Endocervical.
     1. Vaginal discharge, abnormal vaginal bleeding, and vaginal pruritus.
     2. On examination, cervicitis is noted with mucopurulent discharge present.
     3. Easily induced bleeding with gentle swabbing of the cervix.
   iii. Conjunctivitis.
     1. Mucopurulent discharge on conjunctivae.
     2. Treat with topical antibiotic erythromycin.
d. **Diagnosis**
   i. Gram stain showing intracellular gram-negative diplococci.
     1. Gram stain insensitive in females, culture required.
   ii. Culture.
e. **Treatment**
   i. Table 9.3 lists treatments of gonococcal infections.
   ii. Treat sexual partners.
   iii. Consider HIV and syphilis testing.
f. **Disseminated Gonococcal Disease**
   i. Present with polyarticular tenosynovitis, dermatitis, and/or septic arthritis.
g. **Pelvic Inflammatory Disease**
   i. Due to infection with *Chlamydia* or gonorrhea.
   ii. Patients present with low abdominal pain, fever, malaise, and anorexia.
   iii. On examination, note lower abdominal tenderness, cervical motion tenderness, bilateral adnexal tenderness, and signs of cervicitis or vaginal infection.
   iv. Fallopian scarring may occur and result in infertility or ectopic pregnancy.
   v. Treatment.
     1. IV therapy of cefoxitin or cefotetan plus doxycycline; or clindamycin plus gentamicin.
     2. Oral therapy includes ceftriaxone, cefoxitin, or cefotaxine plus doxycycline with or without metronidazole.
     3. Treatment should be for 14 days total.

**TABLE 9.3**

| Treatment of Uncomplicated Endocervical and Urethral Gonococcal Infections | |
| --- | --- |
| **Treatment of Choice (Initial Single-Dose Treatment)** | **Alternative Treatments** |
| Ceftriaxone 500 mg IM | Gentamicin 240 mg IM plus |
| Cefixime 800 mg PO | Azithromycin 2 gm oral |

VIII. **METHICILLIN-RESISTANT *STAPHYLOCOCCUS AUREUS***
a. **General**
   i. Staphylococci are gram-positive cocci.
   ii. Can cause cellulitis, endocarditis, pneumonia, and osteomyelitis.
b. **Clinical Manifestations**
   i. Symptoms depend on location of infection.
c. **Diagnosis**
   i. Gram stain and culture of the source of infection.
d. **Treatment**
   i. Antibiotic options include vancomycin, linezolid, daptomycin, TMP-SMX, and ceftaroline.

IX. **SALMONELLOSIS**
a. **Typhoid Fever**
   i. General
     1. Caused by *Salmonella enterica* subtype *typhi*.
     2. Transmitted via fecal-oral route through contaminated water or food.
   ii. Clinical Manifestations
     1. At onset, fever, chills, malaise, dry cough, anorexia, and headache that build in intensity, as well as abdominal tenderness.
     2. These are followed by erythematous macules or papules (rose spots) that appear on the shoulders, thorax, and abdomen during the second week of infection.
     3. Intestinal bleeding or perforation may occur.
     4. Relative bradycardia may be noted.
   iii. Diagnosis
     1. Normal or low WBC count with increased bands.
     2. Blood cultures may be positive.
     3. Widal test for agglutinating antibodies against the O and H antigens of *S. typhi* is noted.
   iv. Treatment
     1. Ceftriaxone.
     2. Fluoroquinolones.
     3. Chloramphenicol.
b. **Other *Salmonella* Infections**
   i. General
     1. Most common causes include *S. enteritidis* and *Salmonella typhimurium*.
     2. Infection in humans occurs from consuming food products contaminated with the organisms.
       (a) Sources include poultry, reptiles, and amphibians.
   ii. Clinical manifestations

1. Asymptomatic carrier.
2. Enterocolitis.
   (a) Patients present with crampy abdominal pain and diarrhea.
   (b) Fever.
   (c) WBCs present in the stool with mucus.
3. Enteric fever.
   (a) Similar to typhoid fever.
   (b) Prolonged sustained fever, relative bradycardia, splenomegaly, rose spots, and leukopenia.
4. Bacteremia.
   (a) Fever and chills lasting for days.
   (b) Increased incidence in patients with diseases associated with hemolysis, such as sickle cell disease.
iii. Diagnosis
   1. Stool culture.
   2. Serologic studies are not helpful.
iv. Treatment
   1. Enterocolitis.
      (a) Antibiotic therapy is typically not needed.
   2. Bacteremia and enteric fever.
      (a) Fluoroquinolones or third generation cephalosporins.

## X. SHIGELLOSIS

a. **General**
   i. Infection due to *Shigella* that results in colitis affecting mainly the rectosigmoid colon.
   ii. Transmitted by fecal-oral route and via person-to-person through contaminated hands.
   iii. A small inoculum is needed to cause disease, and the organism is secreted in the stool for up to 6 weeks.
b. **Clinical Manifestations**
   i. Initial presentation is a nonspecific prodrome followed by intestinal symptoms (cramps, loose stools, and watery diarrhea).
   ii. Followed by passage of blood and mucus in the stool, tenesmus, and rectal pain.
   iii. Abdominal pain is located in the left lower quadrant.
   iv. Positive blood cultures are very rare.
c. **Treatment**
   i. Always requires antibiotics.
   ii. Ciprofloxacin in adults and trimethoprim-sulfamethoxazole, ampicillin, or azithromycin in children.
   iii. Do not give agents that decrease intestinal motility, which may worsen symptoms.
d. **Postdysenteric Syndromes**
   i. Proctitis.
   ii. Reiter's syndrome of arthritis, urethritis, and conjunctivitis.

iii. Rectal prolapse.
iv. Toxic megacolon.
v. Hemolytic uremic syndrome.

## XI. TETANUS

a. **General**
   i. A neurologic syndrome due to a neurotoxin produced by *Clostridium tetani*.
   ii. Found in the soil.
b. **Clinical Manifestations: Generalized Tetanus**
   i. Incubation period 7 to 21 days.
   ii. Most common complaint is trismus (lockjaw).
   iii. Other features include irritability, diaphoresis, dysphagia with hydrophobia, and back muscle spasms.
c. **Diagnosis**
   i. Based on clinical findings.
   ii. History of immunization makes tetanus unlikely.
d. **Treatment**
   i. Supportive care and appropriate wound care if indicated.
   ii. Benzodiazepines to control muscle spasms.
   iii. Passive immunization with human tetanus immunoglobulin (TIG).
      1. Not needed with clean, minor wounds or patients up to date with tetanus immunization.
      2. If immunization status unknown or less than three doses, all other wounds should be treated with TIG.
   iv. Active immunization with three doses of tetanus and diphtheria toxoid.
   v. Antibiotic therapy: metronidazole or penicillin.
e. **Prevention**
   i. Active immunization with DPaT (diphtheria and tetanus toxoids and pertussis absorbed).
      1. Given at 2 months, 4 months, 6 months, 15 months, and 4 to 6 years of age.
      2. Tdap (tetanus, diphtheria, and pertussis) booster at age 11 to 12 years.
   ii. Td (tetanus and diphtheria toxoids) or Tdap every 10 years in adults.
   iii. Appropriate wound management.

# MYCOBACTERIAL DISEASE

## I. TUBERCULOSIS

a. **General**
   i. Disease caused by *Mycobacterium tuberculosis*, acid-fast bacillus.
   ii. Humans are only natural reservoir.
   iii. Spread by aerosolized respiratory secretions.

b. **Clinical Manifestations**
  i. Pulmonary disease.
    1. Cough with hemoptysis, fever, and sweating are common.
    2. Other complaints include malaise, fatigue, weight loss, chest pain, and dyspnea.
  ii. Extrapulmonary disease can occur at the following sites:
    1. Lymphatic.
    2. Pleural.
    3. Genitourinary.
    4. Bone or joint.
    5. Disseminated.
    6. Meninges and CNS.
    7. Gastrointestinal.
    8. Pericardial.

c. **Diagnosis**
  i. Chest x-ray film reveals multinodular infiltrate in the upper lung fields (Fig. 9.1).
  ii. Sputum smears and cultures.
    1. Acid-fast or modified acid-fast smears.
    2. Culture is the gold standard.
  iii. Tuberculin skin test and interferon-gamma release blood assay become positive during latent stage.
    1. 5-mm cutoff for positive in patients at high risk of developing active tuberculosis (TB) if infected, such as those who have chest x-ray evidence of past TB, who are immunosuppressed because of HIV infection or drugs, or who are close contacts of patients with infectious TB.

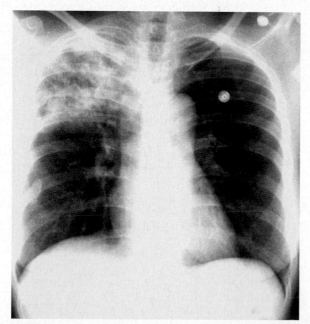

**Fig. 9.1** Chest x-ray: Tuberculosis. *(From Mettler FA: Essentials of Radiology, 2nd ed. Philadelphia: Elsevier Saunders, 2005:84. Fig. 3-49A.)*

    2. 10-mm cutoff for patients with some risk factors, such as injection drug users, recent immigrants from high-prevalence areas, residents of high-risk settings, and patients with certain disorders.
    3. 15-mm cutoff for patients with no risk factors.

d. **Treatment**
  i. All patients with communicable tuberculosis must be treated or quarantined.
  ii. Active tuberculosis patients should receive multiple agents.
  iii. Multiple treatment regimens are available. Drugs include the following:
    1. Isoniazid.
    2. Rifampin.
    3. Rifabutin.
    4. Pyrazinamide.
    5. Ethambutol.
    6. Streptomycin.
  iv. Typical starting four-drug combination includes isoniazid, rifampin, pyrazinamide, and ethambutol.

e. **Prevention**
  i. Treatment of latent infection.
    1. Isoniazid for 9 months as a single agent.
    2. Rifampin for 4 months as a single agent.
    3. Isoniazid plus rifampin for 3 months.

## II. ATYPICAL MYCOBACTERIAL DISEASE

a. *Mycobacterium avium-intracellulare*
  i. Pulmonary infection typically occurs in patients with underlying lung disease.
  ii. Disseminated disease noted in patients with advanced HIV.
  iii. Symptoms include fever, weight loss, anorexia, abdominal pain, and diarrhea.
  iv. Diagnosis made by culture of the organism from the blood, bone marrow, or tissue.
    1. Treatment.
      (a) Azithromycin or clarithromycin, rifabutin or rifampin, and ethambutol.
      (b) Prophylaxis treatment with azithromycin or clarithromycin when CD4 count is less than 100 cells/mL.

## III. LEPROSY (HANSEN'S DISEASE)

a. **Due to the organism** *Mycobacterium leprae*
b. **Mode of transmission is respiratory**
  i. Close contact to those infected and armadillo exposure are risk factors for disease.
c. **Can lead to peripheral nerve damage**
d. **Clinical Manifestations**
  i. Note infiltrative skin lesions, hypoesthesia, and peripheral neuropathy.

e. **Diagnosis**

    i. Microscopic examination of skin biopsy

f. **Treatment**

    i. Treat with dapsone, rifampin, or clofazimine.

# PARASITIC DISEASE

## I. AMEBIASIS

a. **General**

    i. Prevalence is high in many developing countries.

       1. In areas with poor sanitation.

    ii. Caused by *Entamoeba histolytica*.

    iii. May lead to liver abscess formation.

b. **Clinical Manifestations**

    i. Many patients are asymptomatic.

    ii. Patients may present with bloody mucus-containing diarrhea, pain, urgency, and tenesmus.

    iii. Left lower quadrant tenderness is common in acute colitis.

    iv. If liver abscess, note fever and right upper quadrant pain with radiation to right shoulder or back.

       1. Diarrhea is not common in patients with liver abscess.

c. **Diagnosis**

    i. Fecal leukocytes are often absent.

    ii. Diagnosis made with identification of trophozoites or cysts in stool or involved tissue (Fig. 9.2).

    iii. Hepatic ultrasound for evaluation of liver abscess.

    iv. Serology and antigen testing may be helpful.

d. **Treatment**

    i. Antibiotic of choice is metronidazole or tinidazole, which targets trophozoites.

       1. Paromomycin or iodoquinol needed after metronidazole to treat the cyst form.

    ii. Possible drainage for liver abscess.

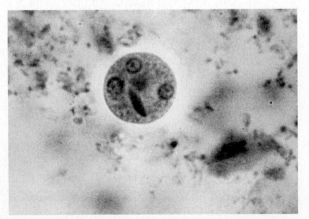

**Fig. 9.2** *Entamoeba histolytica;* mature cyst. *(From Mandell GL: Principle and Practice of Infectious Diseases, 5th ed. 2000:2799, Fig. 262-3.)*

## II. ASCARIASIS

a. **General**

    i. Very common helminthic infection throughout the world.

       1. Noted mainly in southeastern United States.

    ii. Caused by *Ascaris lumbricoides*, a roundworm.

    iii. Found in contaminated soil.

    iv. Once ingested, larvae emerge in the small intestine, migrate to the lung, and then migrate back to the intestine.

b. **Clinical Manifestations**

    i. Typically asymptomatic.

    ii. With heavy exposure, may have cough, dyspnea, or asthma with eosinophilia.

    iii. With intestinal infection, symptoms include abdominal pain, distention, nausea, anorexia, and intermittent diarrhea.

    iv. With heavy worm load, may develop intestinal obstruction or obstruction of the biliary system.

c. **Diagnosis**

    i. Abdominal x-ray film reveals a "whirlpool" pattern of intraluminal worms.

    ii. Diagnose by noting large, brown, tri-layered eggs in the stool.

    iii. Eosinophilia may be noted.

d. **Treatment**

    i. Treat with mebendazole or albendazole.

    ii. Remove patient from contaminated site.

## III. GIARDIASIS

a. **General**

    i. Caused by *Giardia duodenalis*, a flagellated protozoan.

    ii. Acquired from lake or stream water, contaminated food, and personal contact (day care centers).

    iii. Most commonly identified cause of waterborne outbreaks of diarrhea.

b. **Clinical Manifestations**

    i. Incubation period is 1 to 2 weeks.

    ii. Symptoms include bloating, cramping, and flatulence followed by foul-smelling diarrhea.

       1. May develop a malabsorption syndrome.

    iii. Fever is uncommon after the first few days of the disease.

c. **Diagnosis**

    i. Examine stool for presence of trophozoites or cysts (Fig. 9.3).

    ii. Enzyme immunoassay antigen tests.

d. **Treatment**

    i. Drugs of choice are metronidazole, tinidazole, or nitazoxanide..

       1. Paromomycin is used in pregnant women.

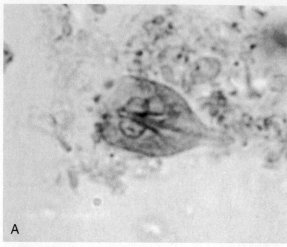

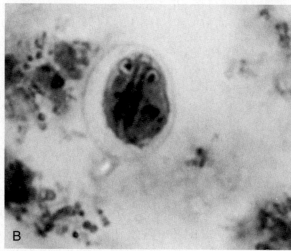

**Fig. 9.3 (A)** and **(B)**, *Giardia duodenalis,* trophozoite, and cyst. *(From Mandell GL: Principle and Practice of Infectious Diseases, 5th ed. Churchill Livingstone. 2005:3199, Fig. 277-1.)*

  **e. Prevention**
   i. Boiling water or iodine-based water treatments will kill organism.
   ii. Cysts resist chlorination but are killed by boiling or by filtration.

## IV. HOOKWORMS
  **a. General**
   i. Worldwide disease; occurs occasionally in southeastern United States.
   ii. Caused by one of two nematodes—*Ancylostoma duodenale* or *Necator americanus.*
   iii. Infection acquired by skin exposure to larvae in soil contaminated by human feces.
    1. Once in the skin, the larvae move to the lung and break into alveoli.
    2. Larvae are coughed up and then swallowed and take up residence in the jejunum.
    3. This cycle takes approximately 4 weeks.

  **b. Clinical Manifestations**
   i. Patients present with a pruritic rash (ground itch) at the site of entry.
   ii. The pulmonary phase is typically asymptomatic, but may have cough, patchy infiltrates, and eosinophilia.
   iii. Intestinal phase symptoms are related to worm burden and may include abdominal pain, nausea, and bloating.
   iv. Anemia may develop later due to blood loss.
   v. Eosinophilia may be noted.
  **c. Diagnosis**
   i. Made by noting eggs in stool sample.
  **d. Treatment**
   i. Drugs of choice include albendazole, mebendazole, or pyrantel pamoate.
   ii. Iron replacement may also be indicated.
   iii. Improve sanitation.

## V. MALARIA
  **a. General**
   i. Any fever in a traveler is malaria until proven otherwise.
   ii. Four *Plasmodium* species cause human malaria.
    1. *P. falciparum.*
    2. *P. vivax.*
    3. *P. ovale.*
    4. *P. malariae.*
   iii. Life cycle.
    1. Female anopheline mosquito bites and infects human with sporozoites.
    2. Evolve from sporozoites to schizonts to merozoites in the liver.
    3. Merozoites are released from the liver and invade the red blood cells, where they multiply.
  **b. Clinical Manifestations**
   i. Fever is manifested by the following three phases:
    1. Cold stage: chills lasting up to several hours.
    2. Hot stage: high fever lasting several hours.
     (a) May be cyclic.
      (i) *P. vivax* and *P. ovale* every 48 hours.
      (ii) *P. malariae* every 72 hours.
      (iii) *P. falciparum* has continuous fevers.
     (b) Fever corresponds to lysis of red blood cells.
    3. Drenching sweats.
   ii. Patients may also present with headache, backache, abdominal pain, nausea and vomiting, hypotension, and altered mental status during hot stage.
   iii. *P. falciparum* may be complicated by coma (cerebral malaria) or renal failure with hemoglobinuria (blackwater fever).

c. **Diagnosis**
   i. Must have high degree of suspicion.
   ii. Examination of thick and thin blood smears for parasite.
d. **Treatment**
   i. Control of the vector very important.
   ii. Chemoprophylaxis with atovaquone-proguanil, doxycycline, mefloquine, chloroquine in chloroquine-sensitive areas.
   iii. Treatment of malaria.
      1. *P. falciparum*, confirmed.
         (a) Chloroquine-resistance: atovaquone-proguanil, artemether-lumefantrine, quinine-sulfate plus doxycycline or clindamycin, or mefloquine.
         (b) Chloroquine-sensitive: chloroquine phosphate or hydroxychloroquine.
      2. *P. vivax* or *P. ovale*, confirmed.
         (a) Chloroquine plus primaquine (screen for glucose-6-phosphate dehydrogenase [G-6-PD] deficiency) or hydroxychloroquine.
      3. *P. malariae*, confirmed.
         (a) Chloroquine or hydroxychloroquine.
   iv. See https://www.cdc.gov/malaria/diagnosis_treatment/indcx.html for the latest treatment guidelines.

## VI. PINWORMS
a. **General**
   i. Most prevalent helminthic infection in the United States.
   ii. Typically affects children in day care centers, institutionalized individuals, and people living in crowded places.
      iii. Caused by *Enterobius vermicularis*.
         1. Adult worms take up residence in the cecum.
         2. Females migrate to the perianal region at night where they lay eggs.
         3. Eggs are infectious for up to 20 days.
b. **Clinical Manifestations**
   i. Most common complaint is perianal or perineal itching and insomnia.
   ii. Infection transmitted by patient's hands.
   iii. May affect multiple family members.
c. **Diagnosis**
   i. Cellophane tape test.
   ii. Diagnosis made by noting ovoid eggs under the microscope.
d. **Treatment**
   i. Treat with mebendazole, pyrantel pamoate, or albendazole as a single dose, repeated in 2 weeks.
   ii. Encourage personal and family hygiene.

## VII. TAPEWORMS
a. **Table 9.4 summarizes tapeworm infections**

## VIII. TOXOPLASMOSIS
a. **General**
   i. Caused by *Toxoplasma gondii*, a protozoan.
   ii. A zoonosis, with the definitive host being cats.
   iii. Two routes of infection.
      1. Oral ingestion of undercooked or raw meat.
      2. Transplacental transmission to fetus.
   iv. An opportunistic pathogen in people with HIV.
b. **Clinical Manifestations**
   i. Primary infection is unrecognized in most cases or presents as a self-limited and nonspecific illness.

**TABLE 9.4**

**Summary of Tapeworms**

| | Taenia Solium | Taenia Saginata | Diphyllobothrium Latum |
|---|---|---|---|
| Disease | Pork tapeworm | Beef tapeworm | Fish tapeworm |
| Location | Mexico, South and Central America, Africa, Southeast Asia, and India | Worldwide, but common in central Asia and eastern Africa | Europe, Canada, Alaska, and Japan |
| Intermediate host | Pigs | Cattle | Fish |
| Signs/Symptoms | Asymptomatic | Asymptomatic | Bloating, abdominal pain, and diarrhea |
| Labs | Eosinophilia | Eosinophilia | Eosinophilia and vitamin $B_{12}$ deficiency |
| Diagnosis | Stool O & P test | Stool O & P test | Stool O & P test |
| Treatment | Praziquantel or niclosamide | Praziquantel or niclosamide | Praziquantel or niclosamide |
| Prevention | Adequate cooking (to >65° C core temperature) of pork and pork products | Adequate cooking (to >65° C core temperature) of beef and beef products. Meat inspection | Adequate cooking or freezing (24–48 hours at −18° C) of fish |

*O & P*, Ova and parasite.

1. May have lymphadenopathy and fatigue without fever.

ii. Immunocompromised patients present with encephalitis, chorioretinitis, pneumonitis, or systemic disease.

**c. Diagnosis**

i. Serology (IgG) to establish exposure.

ii. Identify parasite in tissue.

iii. CT or magnetic resonance imaging (MRI) of the brain for toxoplasmosis of the CNS.
1. Multiple ring-enhancing lesions.

**d. Treatment**

i. Immunocompetent patient.
1. No treatment for lymphadenitis.
2. Systemic disease treated with pyrimethamine, sulfadiazine, and leucovorin (folinic acid).

ii. Immunocompromised patient.
1. Pyrimethamine, sulfadiazine, and folinic acid.
2. Trimethoprim-sulfamethoxazole or dapsone plus pyrimethamine for prophylaxis.
(a) Must be given for the lifetime of the patient.

iii. Prevention.
1. Wash hands, fruits, and vegetables.
2. Avoid contact with materials contaminated with cat feces.

# SPIROCHETAL DISEASE

## I. LYME DISEASE

**a. General**

i. Most common vectorborne disease in the United States.
1. Most cases occur from Maine to Virginia and in Wisconsin and Minnesota.

ii. Caused by a spirochete, *Borrelia burgdorferi*.

iii. Transmitted by ticks of the *Ixodes* genus.

iv. Life cycle involves rodents (white-footed mouse) and larger mammals (deer).

**b. Clinical Manifestations**

i. Three stages.
1. First stage: early localized.
(a) Acute onset of fever, rash, fatigue, headache, myalgias, lymphadenopathy, and fever.
(b) Classic skin lesion is erythema chronicum migrans, which appears about 1 week after the tick bite, most commonly on the trunk, groin, thigh, or axilla.
(c) The lesion is large. The outer border is red with an indurated center.

2. Second stage: early disseminated.
(a) Begins days to weeks after initial infection.
(b) Due to hematogenous spread of the spirochete.
(c) May have multiple erythema migrans lesions.
(i) Lesions are usually annular, smaller, and without indurated centers.
(ii) Can occur anywhere on the body except soles of feet and palms of hands.
(d) Patients may also present with facial nerve palsy, lymphocytic meningitis, arthritis, radiculopathy, or heart block.

3. Third stage: late disease.
(a) Occurs more than a year after initial infection.
(b) Presents with chronic oligoarticular arthritis.

**c. Diagnosis**

i. Based on history of tick bite in an endemic area, classic skin lesion, and other features of the disease.

ii. Serologic testing (enzyme-linked immunosorbent assay [ELISA] followed by Western blot) is commonly used to confirm diagnosis in patients who do not present with clear history of the classic skin lesion.

iii. Polymerase chain reaction (PCR) can be used to aid in the diagnosis of Lyme arthritis.

**d. Treatment**

i. Without treatment, patients may develop cardiac involvement, chronic arthritis, or neurologic disease.

ii. Treatment is typically for 21 to 28 days total.

iii. Table 9.5 covers treatment of Lyme disease.

## II. ROCKY MOUNTAIN SPOTTED FEVER

**a. General**

i. Generalized infection of the vascular endothelium, leading to widespread tissue injury.

**TABLE 9.5**

| Treatment of Lyme Disease | | |
|---|---|---|
| **Early Localized Disease or Early Disseminated Disease** | **Symptoms[a]** | **Arthritis—Early or Late** |
| Doxycycline | Ceftriaxone | Doxycycline |
| Amoxicillin | Penicillin G | Amoxicillin |
| Cefuroxime axetil | | Cefuroxime |
| | | Ceftriaxone |

[a]Symptoms include meningitis, facial nerve palsy with abnormal cerebrospinal fluid, severe neurologic or cardiac disease, and persistent or recurrent arthritis.

ii. Caused by an intracellular bacterium, *Rickettsia rickettsii*.

iii. Transmitted by ticks in the *Dermacentor* genus.

iv. Disease most commonly noted in the South Atlantic regions during the late spring and summer months.

b. **Clinical Manifestations**

i. After a 3- to 12-day incubation period, patients may present with a nonspecific flulike illness with fever (may exceed 39° C), severe headache, and myalgias.

ii. May also note nausea, vomiting, abdominal pain, and diarrhea.

iii. The rash appears between day 1 and day 6 of the illness and is typically maculopapular and/or petechial. Appears first on the wrists or ankles. Appearance of the rash on the palms or soles occurs later, if at all.

c. **Diagnosis**

i. WBC count is normal, but a left shift is present.

ii. Thrombocytopenia is common in rickettsial disease.

iii. Diagnosis is suggested by the typical rash and confirmed with retrospective serologic tests.

1. Other diagnostic tests include biopsy of the rash and PCR testing.

d. **Treatment**

i. Treatment should be started in any patient where the diagnosis is suggested, because of the rash, and before confirmation of the diagnosis.

ii. Doxycycline is the drug of choice.

1. Second line is chloramphenicol.

iii. Mortality rate is 20% if untreated and 4% if treated.

iv. Death occurs due to organ failure.

## III. SYPHILIS

a. **General**

i. Caused by *Treponema pallidum*, a spirochete.

ii. After inoculation through abraded skin or mucous membranes, it attaches to the host cells and spreads in hours to regional lymph nodes.

b. **Clinical Manifestations**

i. Primary.

1. Incubation period 2 to 6 weeks after exposure.

2. Papule develops at site of infection and ulcerates into chancre.

3. Chancre is a painless, indurated ulcer with well-defined borders and a clean base.

(a) Chancre heals in 3 to 6 weeks without treatment.

4. Patients are infectious during this stage.

ii. Secondary.

1. Will develop in 25% of patients with untreated primary syphilis.

2. Occurs 4 to 10 weeks after chancre disappears.

3. Systemic disease with generalized lymphadenopathy, fever, headache, sore throat, and arthralgias.

4. Most common characteristic is the rash. Rash consists of macules and papules on the head, neck, trunk, and extremities, including the palms and soles.

5. Patients are infectious during this stage.

iii. Latent.

1. Defined as a patient having reactive serology in the absence of clinical signs or symptoms.

2. Can be noted between all stages of the disease.

iv. Tertiary.

1. Presentation may include cardiovascular disorders (aortic aneurysm, aortic insufficiency, and coronary stenosis), gummatous lesions (bones and skin), or CNS disorders (general paresis and tabes dorsalis).

v. Neurosyphilis.

1. Can be noted at any time during the disease.

2. People with meningitis may present with headache, nausea, vomiting, stiff neck, cranial nerve palsies, hearing loss, and tinnitus.

3. Meningovascular meningitis can lead to hemiparesis, hemiplegia, aphasia, and seizures.

(a) Tabes dorsalis is the slow, progressive degeneration of the posterior columns and nerve roots.

(b) Develops 20 to 30 years after initial infection and presents with stabbing pain in back and legs with loss of vibratory sensation.

(c) Note Argyll Robertson pupils—pupils that accommodate for near vision but do not respond to light.

c. **Diagnosis**

i. Primary syphilis diagnosed by noting treponemes on dark-field microscopic examination.

ii. Serologic testing.

1. Treponemal: very specific for syphilis.

(a) Fluorescent treponemal antibody absorption test (FTA-ABS).

(b) Microhemagglutination assay—*Treponema pallidum* (MHA-TP).

(c) *Treponema pallidum* particle agglutination assay (TP-PA).

(d) *Treponema pallidum* enzyme immunoassay (TP-EIA).

2. Nontreponemal: detect anticardiolipin antibodies and serve as screening tests.
   (a) Rapid plasma reagin (RPR).
   (b) Venereal Disease Research Laboratory (VDRL) test.
iii. Diagnosis by stage.
   1. Primary: diagnosed with positive treponemal and nontreponemal tests and with the presence of symptoms.
   2. Secondary: diagnosed by a positive RPR and confirmatory test in a patient without signs or symptoms.
   3. Tertiary: diagnosed when syphilitic gumma, cardiovascular disease, or neurologic disease is noted and tests are positive.
   4. Latent: diagnosed with positive tests but with an asymptomatic patient.
   5. Neurosyphilis.
      (a) Diagnosis made based on history and physical, serologic testing, and CSF examination.
      (b) A positive CSF VDRL is highly specific for neurosyphilis.

**d. Treatment**
   i. All positive cases must be reported to the health department, and the partner must be treated.
   ii. All patients with syphilis should be tested for HIV.
   iii. Treatment depends on the stage, but penicillin G is mainstay of therapy for all stages.
      1. Doxycycline, azithromycin, or ceftriaxone are indicated in penicillin-allergic patients.

# VIRAL DISEASE

## I. CYTOMEGALOVIRUS (CMV) INFECTIONS
**a. General**
   i. Member of the *Herpesviridae* family.
   ii. Can be acquired congenitally, perinatally, and via close contact or sexual transmission.
   iii. Leading cause of blindness in patients with AIDS.

**b. Clinical Manifestations**
   i. Immunocompetent patients seldom have any clinical manifestations of infection.
   ii. If symptoms do develop, they are mononucleosis-like.
   iii. Congenital CMV infection.
      1. Typically, asymptomatic at birth but may develop sensory nerve hearing loss and/or psychomotor mental retardation.
      2. While rare, symptomatic signs at birth may include hepatosplenomegaly, jaundice,

anemia, thrombocytopenia, low birth weight, and microencephaly.
   iv. CMV infection in immune-incompetent patient.
      1. Infection may lead to chorioretinitis, gastroenteritis, and neurologic disorders.
      2. Reactivation of disease is common.

**c. Diagnosis**
   i. Detection of CMV cytopathology: "owl eye" cells.
   ii. Cell culture.
   iii. Antibody detection.

**d. Treatment**
   i. Ganciclovir or valganciclovir is used to treat CMV infection in children.
   ii. Ganciclovir or foscarnet is used in adults.
   iii. HIV-positive patients will need prophylactic treatment for CMV infections.

## II. EPSTEIN-BARR VIRUS (EBV) INFECTIONS
**a. General**
   i. Member of the *Herpesviridae* family.
   ii. Cause of infectious mononucleosis and certain lymphoproliferative diseases.
   iii. Transmission requires repeated close contact with infected secretions such as saliva.

**b. Clinical Manifestations**
   i. Fever, malaise, pharyngitis, posterior cervical lymphadenopathy, and splenomegaly.
   ii. A generalized maculopapular rash may also be noted.
   iii. Symptoms may persist for 1 to 2 weeks.

**c. Diagnosis**
   i. CBC reveals a lymphocytosis with many atypical lymphocytes (10%–30%).
   ii. Elevated liver function tests.
   iii. Presence of heterophile antibodies (positive Monospot test).
   iv. Positive EBV-specific serology findings.
   1. See Table 9.6 for the interpretation of EBV serology.

**d. Treatment**
   i. Mainly supportive.
   ii. Corticosteroids can be used in severe disease or if CNS complications.
   iii. Complications.
      1. Contact sports should be avoided to decrease the risk of splenic rupture.
      2. Laryngeal obstruction.
      3. Aseptic meningitis.
      4. Encephalitis.
      5. A rash may develop in patients given ampicillin/amoxicillin.

## III. ERYTHEMA INFECTIOSUM
**a. General**
   i. Also known as "fifth disease."

**TABLE 9.6**

| Serology Results in Epstein-Barr Virus Infection | | | | |
|---|---|---|---|---|
| **Antibody** | **Time of Appearance** | **Persistence** | **Percent of IM Patients with Antibody** | **Note** |
| VCA-IgM | At clinical presentation | 4–6 weeks | 100 | Best indicator of primary infection |
| VCA-IgG | At clinical presentation | Lifelong | 100 | |
| EBNA | 2–4 months after onset | Lifelong | 100 | Presence of EBNA plus VCA-IgG indicates past infection |

*IM*, Infectious mononucleosis; *EBNA*, Epstein-Barr nuclear antigen; *VCA*, viral capsid antigen.

    ii. Caused by the parvovirus B19.

    iii. Spread by respiratory transmission and moderately infectious.

  **b. Clinical Manifestations**

    i. Most cases are asymptomatic or subclinical.

    ii. Develops most often in children younger than age 10.

    iii. Starts with a nonspecific prodrome, then a nonspecific febrile illness with headache, coryza, and diarrhea. This is followed, 2 to 5 days later, by a bright red "slapped-cheek" facial rash.

    iv. Later a maculopapular rash appears on the trunk and extremities.

    v. Adults infected with the virus are more likely to present with arthritis.

  **c. Diagnosis**

    i. Based on clinical findings or by presence of IgM antibodies.

  **d. Treatment**

    i. Usually a self-limited disease.

    ii. Complications.

      1. Infection during pregnancy increases risk of miscarriage.

      2. Aplastic crisis can also develop in patients infected with the virus.

        (a) Treatment of the aplastic crisis includes IV immunoglobulin.

## IV. HERPES SIMPLEX

  **a. General**

    i. Member of the *Herpesviridae* family.

    ii. Humans are the only natural reservoir.

    iii. Direct contact with infected secretions is the major transmission mode.

    iv. Causes both acute and latent infection.

      1. Acute infection consists of development of multinucleated giant cells.

      2. Latent infection can be triggered by fever, trauma, and exposure to ultraviolet light.

  **b. Clinical Manifestations**

    i. Herpes simplex virus-1 (HSV-1).

      1. Grouped or single vesicular lesions that become pustular and form single or multiple ulcers.

      2. Can involve any mucosal surface.

      3. Lesions are very painful and last for 5 to 10 days.

      4. May become latent within sensory nerve root ganglion.

      5. Recurrences are typically unilateral and last about 7 days.

      6. Herpetic whitlow is an HSV infection involving the finger or nail area.

    ii. Herpes simplex virus-2 (HSV-2).

      1. Cause of genital herpes.

      2. Incubation period is 5 days from sexual contact to onset of lesions.

      3. Lesions are small erythematous papules that form into vesicles and then pustules.

      4. With primary disease, the lesions are painful, multiple, and extensive.

        (a) May have systemic symptoms such as fever and myalgias.

      5. Recurrent disease is typically shorter in duration and typically localized to the genital region, without systemic symptoms.

        (a) Prodromal paresthesias may be noted 12 to 24 hours prior to the appearance of the lesions.

  **c. Diagnosis**

    i. Can be made by cell culture, Tzanck smear, antigen detection, and PCR.

      1. Tzanck smear shows multinucleated giant cells.

      2. PCR is the test of choice for diagnosis of HSV encephalitis.

  **d. Treatment**

    i. Use of acyclovir, valacyclovir, or famciclovir is indicated.

      1. IV acyclovir is needed in HSV encephalitis.

    ii. Prophylactic measures include avoidance of contact with HSV-positive secretions and daily acyclovir to suppress recurrences.

    iii. Because of high mortality and morbidity with neonatal HSV infection, cesarean section should be used to prevent transmission to infant from actively infected mother.

## V. HUMAN IMMUNODEFICIENCY VIRUS INFECTION

### a. General

i. Due to infection with HIV-1 virus, most HIV infections worldwide, and HIV-2 virus (infections in West Africa).
  1. A member of the retroviruses.
ii. Uses reverse transcriptase to produce DNA copy from viral RNA, which is incorporated into the host nucleus to produce more viral RNA.
  1. Infects cells with a CD4 receptor (macrophages, T cells, and astrocytes).
iii. Disease is noted worldwide and is spread by parenteral or sexual routes.

### b. Clinical Manifestations

i. After infection, patient develops an acute retroviral syndrome with symptoms like mononucleosis, influenza-like illness, or aseptic meningitis.
ii. Patient is then asymptomatic until development of opportunistic infections, tumors, or wasting syndrome.
iii. During this asymptomatic time frame, patient's CD4 count declines and viral load increases, making them more susceptible to opportunistic infection.
iv. Opportunistic infections.
  1. Table 9.7 lists opportunistic infections seen in HIV.

### c. Diagnosis

i. Antibodies to HIV can be detected within weeks to months after infection.
  1. Anti-HIV is typically detected by the ELISA method within 3 to 6 months of infection.
ii. Positive screening test is confirmed with the Western blot test.
  1. Detects antibodies in the core and envelope of HIV.
iii. Staging of the illness is done with monitoring CD4 cell count and nucleic acid tests for HIV DNA or RNA with the PCR.

### d. Treatment

i. Initial treatment, which should include multiple drugs, should begin before patient develops substantial immunocompromise.
ii. When therapy changes, at least two drugs should be added or substituted to prevent resistance.
iii. During treatment, viral load should be monitored to keep the level below the level of detection and monitor for improvement in CD4 count.
iv. Drugs.
  1. Table 9.8 shows drugs used in treatment of HIV and their side effects.
v. Prophylaxis treatment of opportunistic infections.
  1. Table 9.9 lists treatment options of opportunistic infections seen in HIV.
vi. Prevention.
  1. Avoid high-risk partners and intercourse without condom use.
  2. Transmission to baby from mother can be reduced with the administration of a three-drug regimen, which includes a protease inhibitor or a non–nucleoside reverse transcriptase inhibitor.
  3. Immunizations are important in the care of the HIV-positive patient.
    (a) Indicated immunizations include hepatitis A, hepatitis B, pneumococcus, influenza, and tetanus-diphtheria.
    (b) Contraindicated (live virus) immunizations include varicella; measles, mumps, rubella (MMR); bacille Calmette-Guérin (BCG); and smallpox.

## VI. HUMAN PAPILLOMAVIRUS (HPV) INFECTIONS

### a. General

i. Member of the Papovaviridae family.
ii. Cause warts and genital lesions.
iii. Skin warts are common in children and young adults.
iv. Genital warts are sexually transmitted and are associated with cervical dysplasia and/or neoplasia.

### b. Clinical Manifestations

i. Skin warts.
  1. Two types: flat and plantar.

**TABLE 9.7**

| Opportunistic Infections Noted in Human Immunodeficiency Virus | | | | |
| --- | --- | --- | --- | --- |
| **Bacterial** | **Protozoan** | **Fungal** | **Virus** | **Malignancy** |
| Mycobacterium tuberculosis | Toxoplasma gondii | Candida species | Varicella-zoster | Kaposi's sarcoma |
| Mycobacterium avium-intracellulare | Cryptosporidium parvum | Cryptococcus neoformans | Human papillomavirus | Non-Hodgkin's lymphoma |
| | Isospora belli | Pneumocystis jirovecii | | |
| | Microspora | | | |

**TABLE 9.8**

| Drugs Used in the Treatment of Human Immunodeficiency Virus | | | | |
|---|---|---|---|---|
| **Mechanism of Action** | **Generic Name** | **Trade Name** | **Abbreviation** | **Side Effects** |
| Nucleoside reverse transcriptase inhibitors (NRTIs) | Zidovudine | Retrovir | AZT (ZDV) | Anemia, nausea and vomiting, neutropenia, and myopathy |
| | Abacavir | Ziagen | ABC | Fever, rash, nausea, vomiting, diarrhea, dyspnea, anorexia |
| | Emtricitabine | Emtriva | FTC | Skin hyperpigmentation, , nausea, vomiting, diarrhea, |
| | Stavudine | Zerit | d4T | Peripheral neuropathy |
| | Didanosine | Videx | ddI | Pancreatitis and peripheral neuropathy |
| | Lamivudine | Epivir | 3TC | Nausea, vomiting, headache, and fatigue |
| | Tenofovir | Viread | TDF | Nausea, vomiting, diarrhea, elevated liver function tests |
| Nonnucleoside reverse transcriptase inhibitors (NNRTIs) | Nevirapine | Viramune | NVP | Hepatotoxicity, rash, and nausea |
| | Rilpivirine | Edurant | RPV | Insomnia, headache, rash, nausea, pancytopenia |
| | Etravirine | Intelence | ETR | Anemia, low platelets, life threatening rash |
| | Doravirine | Pifeltro | DOR | Nausea, headache, diarrhea, and fatigue |
| | Efavirenz | Sustiva | EFV | Nightmares, depression |
| Protease inhibitors (PIs) | Saquinavir | Invirase | SQV | Lipodystrophy |
| | Atazanavir | Reyataz | ATV | Nausea, vomiting, diarrhea, rash, jaundice |
| | Darunavir | Prezista | DRV | Nausea, vomiting, diarrhea, rash, jaundice, raised liver function test, elevated amylase, hyperlipidemia |
| | Fosamprenavir | Lexiva | FPV | Diarrhea, headache, dizziness, rash |
| | Ritonavir | Norvir | RTV | Inhibits P450 enzymes, and elevates many drug levels |
| | Indinavir | Crixivan | IDV | Nephrolithiasis |
| | Nelfinavir | Viracept | NFV | Diarrhea |
| Integrase strand transfer inhibitors (INSTIs) | Raltegravir | Isentress | RAL | Elevated liver function tests |
| | Bictegravir | Bictarvy | BIC | Hypersensitivity Rx Headache, insomnia |
| | Elvitegravir | Vitekta | EVG | Nausea, diarrhea |
| | Dolutegravir | Tivicay | DTG | Elevated glucose levels |
| Entry inhibitor | Maraviroc | Selzentry | MVC | Rash, cough |
| | Ibalizumab | Trogarzo | TMB-355 | Infusion reactions Diarrhea Rash |
| Fusion inhibitors | Enfuvirtide | Fuzeon | ENF/T-20 | Hypersensitivity Rx Peripheral neuropathy Loss of appetite |
| PK enhancer | Cobicistat | Tybost | COBI/c | Elevated glucose, insomnia, headache, nausea, diarrhea |
| | Ritonavir | Norvir | RTV/r | Elevated lipid levels, diarrhea |

2. Associated with HPV types 1–4.
3. Infect the keratinized surfaces, typically on the hands and feet.
4. If given time, will regress spontaneously.
ii. Genital warts (*Condyloma acuminata*).
  1. Occur on the squamous epithelium of the external genitalia and perianal area.
  2. Associated with HPV types 6 and 11.

iii. Cervical dysplasia.
  1. HPV types 16 and 18 are associated with intraepithelial cervical dysplasia, neoplasia, and cancer.
c. **Diagnosis**
  i. Confirm by biopsy with the appearance of hyperplasia of prickle cells and production of excess keratin.

**TABLE 9.9**

**Prophylaxis Treatment of Opportunistic Infections in Human Immunodeficiency Virus**

| Pathogen | Primary Prophylaxis | Alternative Prophylaxis |
|---|---|---|
| *Pneumocystis jirovecii* | TMP/SMX | Dapsone Pentamidine |
| *Toxoplasma gondii* | TMP/SMX | Dapsone plus pyrimethamine |
| *Mycobacterium tuberculosis* (INH-sensitive) | INH | Rifabutin plus pyrazinamide |
| *Mycobacterium tuberculosis* (INH-resistant) | Rifampin plus pyrazinamide | Rifampin plus pyrazinamide |
| *Mycobacterium avium* complex | Azithromycin or clarithromycin | Rifabutin |
| Cytomegalovirus retinitis | Ganciclovir | |
| *Cryptococcus neoformans* | Fluconazole | Itraconazole |
| *Histoplasma capsulatum* | Itraconazole | |

*TMP/SMX*, Trimethoprim-sulfamethoxazole; *INH*, isoniazid.

   ii. DNA probes for HPV.
     1. Suggested by the presence of koilocytotic squamous epithelial cells on smear.
  **d. Treatment**
   i. Spontaneous disappearance occurs but may take years.
   ii. Methods of removal include electrocautery, cryotherapy, and chemical (podophyllin or salicylic acid).
   iii. Injection with interferon may also be helpful.
   iv. Best prevention is avoidance of infected tissue.
   v. Two-dose vaccine 6 to 12 months apart is recommended for males and females 11 to 12 years of age. If started at ages 15 to 26 then three-doses are needed.

## VII. INFLUENZA
  **a. General**
   i. Two types of viruses.
     1. Influenza A: the cause of epidemic or pandemic influenza.
      (a) Characterized by envelope glycoproteins known as hemagglutinin (HA) and neuraminidase (N).
      (b) Highly infectious and increased rates of disease are noted in institutional settings.
     2. Influenza B: milder illness.
      (a) Increased incidence in schools and military camps.
  **b. Clinical Manifestations**
   i. Symptoms begin abruptly.
   ii. After a 2- to 4-day incubation period, patient presents with high fever, headache, photophobia, myalgia, pharyngitis, nonproductive cough, and malaise.
   iii. Physical examination findings are nonspecific.
   iv. Symptoms resolve over 2 to 5 days.
  **c. Diagnosis**
   i. Viral culture and antigen detection are available.
  **d. Treatment**
   i. Symptomatic therapy with fluids, rest, and acetaminophen.
   ii. Treat with antivirals.
     1. Neuraminidase inhibitors (zanamivir, oseltamivir, and peramivir).
      (a) Shorten duration of disease if given within the first 48 hours of symptoms.
      (b) Are the drugs of choice.
   iii. Immunization.
     1. Best strategy for prevention.
     2. Recommended for those at increased risk for complications or for those with increased potential to transmit the disease.
   iv. Complications.
     1. Pneumonia.
     2. Reye's syndrome: secondary to use of aspirin in treatment.
     3. Acute myositis and rhabdomyolysis.
     4. *Staphylococcus aureus* superinfection.
     5. Myocarditis and pericarditis.
     6. Encephalitis, transverse myelitis, or Guillain-Barré syndrome.

## VIII. MUMPS
  **a. General**
   i. Mumps virus is a paramyxovirus.
   ii. Spread via respiratory droplets with humans as the only reservoir.
   iii. Incubation period is 14 to 28 days.
   iv. Patient is infectious from 2 days before to 9 days after the development of parotid swelling.
  **b. Clinical Manifestations**
   i. May have a prodromal period, with development of fever, myalgias, and headache.
   ii. Parotid pain and swelling are the hallmarks of the disease.
  **c. Diagnosis**
   i. Based on physical findings and culture or serology results.
   ii. Serum amylase may be elevated.
  **d. Treatment**
   i. Control of symptoms with analgesics and fluids.
   ii. Vaccine given at 12 to 15 months of age with a second dose at 4 to 5 years of age.
  **e. Complications**
   i. Orchitis/Oophoritis.
   ii. Meningoencephalitis.

iii. Deafness.
iv. Arthritis.
v. Pancreatitis

## IX. RABIES
a. **General**
  i. Virus is a bullet-shaped virus of the rhabdovirus group.
  ii. Acute fatal viral illness of the CNS.
  iii. Transmitted by infected secretions between mammals.
  iv. Human exposure to the disease is through infected dogs, cats, skunks, foxes, wolves, raccoons, and bats.
  v. Pathogenesis.
    1. Virus enters epidermis through a bite.
    2. Virus replicates in the striated muscle at the site of inoculation.
    3. Virus enters peripheral nerve and spreads up the nerve to the CNS.
    4. Virus replicates in the gray matter and then passes centrifugally along autonomic nerves to other tissues.
b. **Clinical Manifestations**
  i. Begins as a nonspecific illness with fever, headache, malaise, nausea, and vomiting.
  ii. Onset of encephalitis noted with excess motor activity and agitation.
  iii. Hallucinations, combativeness, muscle spasms, meningeal irritation, seizures, and focal paralysis are noted.
  iv. Increased salivation noted due to autonomic nervous system involvement.
  v. Double vision, facial palsies, and difficulty swallowing noted due to brain stem and cranial nerve dysfunction.
  vi. Hydrophobia also noted.
  vii. With onset of symptoms the survival time is 4 days.
c. **Diagnosis**
  i. Skin biopsy with fluorescent antibody testing.
  ii. Demonstration of the virus in brain tissue at autopsy.
    1. Classic finding is Negri bodies.
d. **Treatment**
  i. Prevention of disease is the key. Done through immunization of animals.
  ii. Preexposure: prophylaxis immunization.
  iii. Postexposure treatment.
    1. Wound care.
    2. Observation of animal for development of signs of rabies.
    3. Treat with vaccine and human rabies immunoglobulin (HRIG) if animal suspected to be rabid.
      (a) HRIG should be injected into the wound site if possible. If not, then give IM.

## X. ROSEOLA
a. **General**
  i. Caused by human herpesviruses 6 and 7.
  ii. Occurs in infancy after an incubation period of 10 days.
b. **Clinical Manifestations**
  i. Patients present with high fever for 3 to 5 days.
  ii. During febrile period, patient is listless and may have cough, diarrhea, lymphadenopathy, or red tympanic membrane.
  iii. Fever resolves, followed by a maculopapular rash on the face or trunk and rapidly spreads over rest of the body.
  iv. Rash lasts only hours or up to 2 days.
c. **Diagnosis**
  i. Based on clinical findings.
d. **Treatment**
  i. Symptomatic treatment only.
  ii. Complications include seizures and rare cases of encephalitis.

## XI. RUBELLA
a. **General**
  i. Due to a *Rubivirus* in the Togaviridae family.
  ii. Transmitted via respiratory droplets.
b. **Clinical Manifestations**
  i. Begins with a sore throat, conjunctivitis, and a low-grade fever.
  ii. On day 2 or 3, a fine macular rash appears on the face and moves downward.
    1. Becomes generalized in 24 hours.
  iii. Fever disappears within 24 hours of the onset of the rash.
  iv. Petechial lesions (Forschheimer's spots) are occasionally noted on the soft palate.
  v. Posterior cervical and occipital lymphadenopathy can be noted.
c. **Diagnosis**
  i. Clinical features seldom permit diagnosis.
  ii. IgM antibodies can be detected to confirm diagnosis.
d. **Treatment**
  i. There is no specific treatment.
  ii. The first dose of immunization is given at 12 to 15 months of age, and the second dose is given at 4 to 6 years of age.
  iii. Immunization status must be checked in all pregnant women.
  iv. Complications.
    1. Congenital rubella.

(a) Can cause a variety of transient, permanent, and developmental problems.

(b) The severity of the illness is related to the time during gestation at which the fetus was infected.

(c) Manifestations include hearing loss, low birth weight, hepatosplenomegaly, meningoencephalitis, mental retardation, and congenital anomalies.

2. Thrombocytopenic purpura.

3. Encephalitis.

## XII. RUBEOLA (MEASLES)

### a. General

i. A paramyxovirus that is highly contagious.

ii. Transmitted by droplets, by person-to-person contact, or by airborne spread.

iii. Incubation period is 10 days.

### b. Clinical Manifestations

i. Prodrome begins with a fever, irritability, malaise, conjunctivitis, and evidence of a respiratory infection.

ii. Koplik's spots appear within several days as small, raised, white or blue-gray lesions on an erythematous base on the buccal mucosa opposite the upper molar.

1. Pathognomonic for measles.

iii. On day 3 or 4, a nonpruritic maculopapular rash begins, starting at the hairline and descending to the trunk and extremities. (See Color Plate 3.)

iv. Fever resolves as the rash appears.

### c. Diagnosis

i. Based on clinical grounds.

ii. IgM antibodies can be detected to confirm diagnosis.

### d. Treatment

i. No specific treatment.

ii. Vitamin A has been reported to reduce the severity of the disease in children.

iii. Immunization.

1. First dose is given at between 12 and 15 months of age, and the second dose is given at 4 to 6 years of age.

iv. Complications.

1. Usually a self-limited disease. Resolves in 7 to 10 days.

2. Complications include pneumonia, bacterial superinfections, otitis media, abnormal liver function tests, postmeasles encephalitis, and subacute sclerosing encephalitis.

## XIII. VARICELLA-ZOSTER VIRUS INFECTIONS

### a. General

i. Causes chickenpox.

### b. Clinical Manifestations

i. Lesions start as erythematous macules that become vesicles and then pustules that crust over.

ii. The hallmark to diagnose chickenpox is the presence of lesions in various stages. (See Color Plate 4.)

1. In smallpox all lesions must be at the same stage of development at a given time.

iii. Lesions can be noted on mucous membranes.

iv. The rash is very pruritic.

### c. Diagnosis

i. Based on clinical presentation.

ii. Laboratory testing includes:

1. PCR for viral DNA.

2. Immunofluorescent antigen detection.

3. Serology testing.

4. Viral culture.

5. Tzanck smear.

### d. Treatment

i. Treatment is symptomatic.

ii. Vaccine is given at 12 to 18 months of age.

iii. Can use acyclovir in immunocompromised patients.

iv. Neonates with perinatal varicella-zoster should be treated with varicella-zoster immune globulin to decrease mortality.

v. Complications

1. Herpes zoster (shingles).

(a) Due to reactivation of latent varicella-zoster virus.

2. Varicella encephalitis.

3. Cerebellar ataxia.

4. Pneumonia.

5. Bacterial superinfection with group A beta-hemolytic *Streptococcus* or *S. aureus*.

## XIV. OTHER

### a. Herpangina

i. Caused by coxsackievirus A.

1. Highly contagious.

2. Affects children aged 3 to 10 years.

ii. Note 1- to 4-mm vesicles on uvula and soft palate.

iii. Patients present with fever and sore throat.

iv. Patients recover in 3 to 5 days.

### b. Hand-Foot-and-Mouth Disease

i. Caused by coxsackievirus A16.

ii. Note small vesicles in anterior part of the mouth and on palms and soles.

iii. Patients present with fever and sore throat.

iv. Patients recover in 1 week.

### c. Zika Virus

i. Mosquito-borne flavivirus, transmitted via blood.

ii. Transmission noted in South and Central America, Mexico, Caribbean Islands, Africa, and Florida.

**TABLE 9.10**

| Viral Disease Infections | | | | | |
|---|---|---|---|---|---|
| **Condition** | **Agent** | **Incubation Period (Days)** | **Prodrome** | **Rash** | **Complications** |
| Chickenpox | Varicella zoster | 10–21 | Rare in children; may present with headache, myalgia, and malaise | Pruritic; vesicles that crust over starting on the face or trunk and spread to the rest of the body | Pneumonia, secondary bacterial infections, and encephalitis |
| Erythema infectiosum | Parvovirus | 12–18 | None | Slapped cheeks | Arthritis and hemolytic anemia |
| Measles | Paramyxovirus | 9–14 | Cough, coryza, conjunctivitis and fever | Confluent, erythematous rash starting at the head and moving caudally | Meningoencephalitis, pneumonia, otitis media, and laryngotracheitis |
| Mumps | Paramyxovirus | 12–25 | Rare; can have fever, myalgia, and a headache | None | Orchitis, deafness |
| Roseola | Human herpesvirus 6 | 10–14 | Fever | Maculopapular rash on the face or trunk and spread over rest of body | Febrile seizures |
| Rubella | Togavirus | 14–21 | Rare, but may have cough, coryza, and lymphadenopathy | Erythematous, maculopapular rash starting on the face and then moving peripherally | Encephalitis and thrombocytopenia |

iii. Presentation is usually asymptomatic but may cause fever, rash, joint pain, or conjunctivitis.

iv. In pregnancy infection can cause microcephaly or other fetal brain or ocular defects.

v. Diagnosis via serologic testing or RT-PCR for viral RNA.

vi. Treatment is supportive care.

## XV. TABLE 9.10 SUMMARIZES VIRAL DISEASE INFECTIONS.

# SEPSIS

## I. GENERAL
a. Dysregulated response to an infection that leads to organ dysfunction
b. Septic shock is a subset of sepsis and presents with persistent hypotension and elevated lactate level despite adequate fluid resuscitation
c. Most common causes are gram-negative bacilli or gram-positive cocci

## II. CLINICAL MANIFESTATIONS
a. Present with fever, tachycardia, diaphoresis, and tachypnea

b. Blood pressure may be normal early in course of disease
c. Signs of organ failure develop in hours
d. qSOFA criteria used to detect organ dysfunction
   i. Respiratory rate ≥22/minute.
   ii. Altered mentation.
   iii. Systolic blood pressure ≤ 100 mm Hg.
   iv. If two or more of these present need further investigation.

## III. DIAGNOSIS
a. White blood cell count can be decreased or increased; left shift noted
b. Respiratory alkalosis develops early followed by metabolic acidosis
c. X-ray and culture to identify source

## IIII. TREATMENT
a. IV fluids improve tissue perfusion and may need pressors (norepinephrine, vasopressin, or epinephrine)
b. Support measures including oxygen
a. Broad spectrum antibiotics

## Antibiotic Table

| Antibiotic | Mechanism of Action | Antimicrobial Activity | Side Effects |
|---|---|---|---|
| **Penicillins** | | | |
| Penicillin G<br>Penicillin V | Cell-wall synthesis inhibitors via penicillin-binding proteins | Anaerobes<br>*Neisseria*<br>*Staphylococcus*<br>*Streptococcus*<br>*Treponema* | Diarrhea<br>Rash<br>Type I hypersensitivity reactions |
| Antistaphylococcal<br>  Nafcillin<br>  Oxacillin<br>  Dicloxacillin<br>  Methicillin | | *Staphylococcus* | |
| Aminopenicillin<br>  Ampicillin<br>  Amoxicillin | | *Escherichia coli*<br>*Haemophilus*<br>*Listeria*<br>*Staphylococcus*<br>*Streptococcus* | |
| Extended spectrum<br>  Penicillin<br>  Piperacillin<br>  Carbenicillin | | Gram-negative bacilli including<br>  *Pseudomonas* | Diarrhea<br>Gastrointestinal upset<br>Platelet dysfunction<br>Type I hypersensitivity reactions<br>Rash |
| **Cephalosporins** | | | |
| First generation<br>  Cefazolin<br>  Cefadroxil<br>  Cephalexin | Cell-wall synthesis inhibitors via penicillin-binding proteins | Anaerobes<br>Gram-negative rods *(Escherichia coli)*<br>*Haemophilus*<br>*Staphylococcus*<br>*Streptococcus* | Diarrhea<br>Hypersensitivity reaction |
| Second generation<br>  Cefotetan<br>  Cefoxitin<br>  Cefuroxime<br>  Cefprozil<br>  Cefaclor | | *Haemophilus*<br>*Streptococcus* | |
| Third generation<br>  Cefotaxime<br>  Ceftazidime<br>  Ceftriaxone<br>  Cefdinir<br>  Cefpodoxime<br>  Cefixime | | Gram-negative bacilli<br>*Haemophilus*<br>*Neisseria*<br>Ceftazidime also covers<br>  *Pseudomonas* | |
| Fourth generation<br>  Cefepime | | Gram-negative bacilli<br>MRSA (methicillin resistant<br>  *Staphylococcus aureus)*<br>*Streptococcus* | |
| Carbapenems<br>  Imipenem/Cilastatin<br>  Meropenem | Cell-wall synthesis inhibitors via penicillin-binding proteins | Gram negatives<br>Gram positives | Seizures |
| Monobactams<br>  Aztreonam | Cell-wall synthesis inhibitors via penicillin-binding proteins | Gram negative, including<br>  *Pseudomonas* | No cross-reaction in patients with penicillin allergy |
| Vancomycin | Cell-wall synthesis inhibitor | *Clostridium*<br>*Corynebacterium*<br>*Staphylococcus*<br>*Streptococcus* | Nephrotoxicity<br>Ototoxicity |
| Rifampin | Inhibits protein synthesis by inhibiting bacterial RNA polymerase | *Haemophilus*<br>*Neisseria meningitidis*<br>*Mycobacterium tuberculosis*<br>*Staphylococcus* | Hepatitis |

### Antibiotic Table—cont'd

| Antibiotic | Mechanism of Action | Antimicrobial Activity | Side Effects |
|---|---|---|---|
| Aminoglycosides<br>Gentamicin<br>Tobramycin<br>Amikacin | Bind to 30S subunit of bacterial ribosome and inhibit synthesis or proteins from mRNA | Aerobic gram negatives | Nephrotoxicity<br>Ototoxicity |
| Macrolides<br>Erythromycin<br>Azithromycin<br>Clarithromycin | Bind to 50S subunit and inhibit protein synthesis | *Streptococcus*<br>*Mycoplasma*<br>*Chlamydia*<br>*Haemophilus*<br>*Legionella* | Cholestatic hepatitis<br>Gastrointestinal upset |
| Ketolide<br>Telithromycin | Binds to 50S subunit and inhibits protein synthesis | *Chlamydia*<br>Gram negatives<br>Gram positives<br>*Legionella*<br>*Mycoplasma* | Dizziness<br>GI upset<br>Headache |
| Tetracyclines<br>Tetracycline<br>Doxycycline<br>Minocycline | Bind to 30S subunit, prevent binding by tRNA molecules, and inhibit protein synthesis | *Chlamydia*<br>Gram negatives<br>Gram positives<br>*Mycoplasma*<br>*Rickettsia*<br>*Spirochetes* | Diarrhea<br>Hepatotoxicity<br>Nausea/Vomiting<br>Teeth discoloration |
| Chloramphenicol | Binds to 50S subunit, prevents binding by tRNA molecules, and inhibits protein synthesis | Anaerobes<br>Gram negatives<br>Gram positives<br>*Rickettsia* | Bone marrow suppression (aplastic anemia)<br>Gray baby syndrome |
| Clindamycin | Binds to 50S subunit of ribosome and inhibits protein synthesis | Anaerobes<br>Gram positives | Pseudomembranous colitis |
| Linezolid | Binds to 50S subunit, prevents formation of first peptide bond, and leads to inhibition of protein synthesis | Gram positives | GI upset<br>Pancytopenia<br>Serotonin syndrome |
| Trimethoprim-sulfamethoxazole | Inhibits bacterial growth by preventing synthesis of tetrahydrofolate, therefore inhibiting DNA synthesis | Gram negatives<br>*Haemophilus*<br>*Listeria*<br>*Streptococcus* | GI upset<br>Hepatitis<br>Leukopenia<br>Rash (Stevens-Johnson)<br>Thrombocytopenia |
| Quinolones<br>Ofloxacin<br>Ciprofloxacin<br>Levofloxacin<br>Moxifloxacin | Inhibit topoisomerases and inhibit DNA supercoiling | Gram negatives<br>Gram positives | Damage to growing cartilage<br>Headache<br>Nausea |
| Metronidazole | Forms free radicals that break DNA molecules and bacterial death | Anaerobes<br>Parasites | Disulfiram reaction |
| Antimycobacterial | Inhibits enzyme needed to synthesize mycolic acid needed for the cell envelope | *Mycobacterium tuberculosis* | |
| Isoniazid | | | Hepatotoxicity<br>Peripheral neuropathy |
| Pyrazinamide | | | Elevated uric acid levels<br>Hepatotoxicity |
| Ethambutol | | | Optic neuritis |

# QUESTIONS

### QUESTION 1
Which of the following physical examination findings is typically noted in patients with diphtheria?
A  Splenomegaly
B  Forschheimer's spots
C  Supraclavicular nodes
D  Papular rash on the trunk
E  Pharyngeal pseudomembrane

### QUESTION 2
Which of the following laboratory results would be expected in a patient with a cytomegalovirus infection?
A  Increased number of atypical lymphocytes
B  Positive heterophil antibody test
C  Elevated cryoglobulins
D  Elevated ASO titer
E  Decreased AST

### QUESTION 3
A patient presents with greasy, malodorous stools and abdominal distention. Which of the following is the most likely diagnosis?
A  Giardiasis
B  Crohn's disease
C  Ogilvie's syndrome
D  Irritable bowel syndrome
E  Pseudomembranous colitis

### QUESTION 4
A 4-year-old patient presents with a 4-day history of fever, irritability, and cough. On examination, there are small, irregular, grayish-white lesions on the upper buccal mucosa, and a maculopapular rash is noted in the hairline. What is the next best step in the management of this patient?
A  Large dose vitamin C
B  Prophylactic antibiotics
C  Antipyretics and analgesics
D  Active immunization
E  High dose IVIG

### QUESTION 5
A 20-year-old female presents with vaginal itching and thick discharge. On physical examination, the vaginal mucosa is inflamed, and patches of white material are noted on the vaginal walls. Which of the following is the best treatment option for this patient?
A  Nystatin
B  Metronidazole
C  Clindamycin
D  Acyclovir
E  Penicillin

### QUESTION 6
The first dose of measles, mumps, and rubella (MMR) vaccine is typically given at what age?
A  Birth
B  2 months
C  12 months
D  18 months
E  24 months

### QUESTION 7
A 40-year-old patient who returned from Japan 4 months ago presents with abdominal pain and diarrhea. Stool cultures are negative. Ova and parasite study reveal bile-stained eggs and proglottids. Which of the following is the most likely infectious agent?
A  *Giardia duodenalis*
B  *Ascaris lumbricoides*
C  *Necator americanus*
D  *Diphyllobothrium latum*
E  *Entamoeba histolytica*

### QUESTION 8
An HIV-positive patient presents with several small, slightly raised, whitish lesions on the lateral aspect of the tongue. The lesions cannot be removed by scraping with a tongue depressor. Which of the following is the most likely diagnosis?
A  Oral candidiasis
B  Kaposi's sarcoma
C  Hairy cell leukoplakia
D  Aphthous ulcers
E  Roth spots

### QUESTION 9
An 8-year-old patient presents with nocturnal perianal itching. Which of the following is the best treatment option for this patient?
A  Acyclovir
B  Penicillin
C  Metronidazole
D  Mebendazole
E  Hydroxychloroquine

### QUESTION 10
A 5-year-old patient presents with postauricular and postoccipital adenopathy and a discrete maculopapular rash that started on the face and has now moved to the trunk. His mother states that it all started after a few days of cold like symptoms. Which of the following is the most likely diagnosis?
A  Rubella
B  Roseola
C  Impetigo
D  Infectious mononucleosis
E  Varicella-zoster infection

# ANSWERS

**1. E**

EXPLANATION: Patients with diphtheria present with fever, malaise, and sore throat. On physical examination, a grayish pseudomembrane that bleeds easily on attempted removal is noted. *Topic: Bacterial disease: diphtheria*

☐ Correct    ☐ Incorrect

**2. A**

EXPLANATION: Patients with cytomegalovirus infection present with atypical lymphocytes. Heterophil antibody is positive in infectious mononucleosis. Elevated cryoglobulins are present in cryoglobulinemia, a plasma cell disorder. Antistreptolysin O (ASO) titer is elevated in streptococcal infections. *Topic: Viral disease: cytomegalovirus infections*

☐ Correct    ☐ Incorrect

**3. A**

EXPLANATION: The clinical features of giardiasis include nausea and bloating, with later symptoms including loose, foul-smelling stools; cramps; and flatulence. Ogilvie's syndrome is severe abdominal distention without diarrhea in postoperative patients or those with severe medical illnesses. In Crohn's disease, the diarrhea is watery and intermittent with right lower quadrant pain. People with irritable bowel syndrome present with a history of diarrhea alternating with constipation. Pseudomembranous colitis presents post antibiotic usage with watery diarrhea and crampy abdominal pain. *Topic: Parasitic disease: giardiasis*

☐ Correct    ☐ Incorrect

**4. C**

EXPLANATION: Patients with rubeola (measles) present with fever, irritability, malaise, and cough. Within days, small, raised white or blue-gray lesions appear on a red base in the buccal mucosa, opposite the upper molars, called Koplik's spots. Antipyretics and analgesics are used to treat symptoms. *Topic: Viral disease: rubeola*

☐ Correct    ☐ Incorrect

**5. A**

EXPLANATION: *Candida* infection of the vagina presents with an inflamed vaginal mucosa and white vaginal discharge. Treatment consists of antifungal agents, such as nystatin. *Topic: Fungal disease: candidiasis*

☐ Correct    ☐ Incorrect

**6. C**

EXPLANATION: Measles, mumps, and rubella (MMR) vaccine is first given at 12 to 15 months of age and repeated at 4 to 6 years of age. *Topic: Viral disease: measles/mumps/rubella*

☐ Correct    ☐ Incorrect

**7. D**

EXPLANATION: The tapeworm, *Diphyllobothrium latum* (fish tapeworm), is more commonly noted in Asia and Japan and is due to consumption of raw seafood/fish. Diagnosis is made by noting bile-stained eggs and proglottids on examination of the stool. *Topic: Parasitic disease: tapeworms*

☐ Correct    ☐ Incorrect

**8. C**

EXPLANATION: Hairy cell leukoplakia, common in immunocompromised patients, presents as whitish plaques on the lateral aspect of the tongue. These lesions may be difficult to remove with a tongue depressor, as opposed to oral candidiasis lesions, which are easy to remove. *Topic: Viral disease: human immunodeficiency virus*

☐ Correct    ☐ Incorrect

**9. D**

EXPLANATION: Perianal itching is noted in pinworm infections. Pinworms are best treated with mebendazole, albendazole, or pyrantel pamoate. *Topic: Parasitic disease: pinworms*

☐ Correct    ☐ Incorrect

**10. A**

EXPLANATION: Children with rubella present with a mild fever, lymphadenopathy, and a fine maculopapular rash that starts on the face and moves to the trunk and extremities. Patients with roseola, due to human herpesvirus type 6 and 7, present with a high fever followed by a fine, small, raised lesion on the trunk and then on the neck and face. Impetigo presents with honey-crusted lesions, and infectious mononucleosis typically presents with fever, pharyngitis, and lymphadenopathy; rash is rare. Varicella-zoster infection presents with very pruritic rash that starts as erythematous macules that become vesicles and pustules. *Topic: Viral disease: rubella*

☐ Correct    ☐ Incorrect

# CHAPTER 10
# PSYCHIATRY/BEHAVIORAL SCIENCE

## EXAMINATION BLUEPRINT TOPICS

**ABUSE AND NEGLECT**

Child abuse and neglect

Domestic violence

Elder abuse

Child sexual abuse

**ANXIETY DISORDERS**

Generalized anxiety disorder

Panic disorder

Phobias

**MOOD DISORDERS**

Bipolar disorder

Cyclothymic disorder

**DEPRESSIVE DISORDERS**

Major depressive disorder

Persistent depressive disorder (dysthymia)

Premenstrual dysphoric disorder

Suicidal behaviors

Homicidal behaviors

**DISRUPTIVE, IMPULSE-CONTROL, AND CONDUCT DISORDERS**

Conduct disorder

Disruptive mood dysregulation disorder (DMDD)

**DISSOCIATIVE DISORDERS**

Dissociative identity disorders

Dissociative amnesia

Depersonalization-derealization disorder

**FEEDING AND EATING DISORDERS**

Anorexia nervosa

Bulimia nervosa

Obesity

**OBSESSIVE-COMPULSIVE AND RELATED DISORDERS**

Obsessive-compulsive disorder (OCD)

Trichotillomania

Hoarding disorder

Dermtillomania

Body dysmorphic disorder

**NEURODEVELOPMNTAL DISORDERS**

Attention-deficit/hyperactivity disorder

Autism spectrum disorder

**PERSONALITY DISORDERS**

General

Types

**SCHIZOPHRENIA SPECTRUM AND OTHER PSYCHOTIC DISORDERS**

Delusional disorder

Schizophrenia

Schizoaffective disorder

Brief psychotic disorder

**SLEEP-WAKE DISORDERS**

Narcolepsy

Parasomnias

**SOMATIC SYMPTOMS AND RELATED DISORDERS**

Somatic symptom disorder

Functional neurological symptom disorder

Illness anxiety disorder

Factitious disorder

Malingering

**SUBSTANCE USE DISORDERS**

General

Alcohol use

Drug use

Tobacco use

**TRAUMA AND STRESSOR-RELATED DISORDERS**

Adjustment

Acute stress disorder

Posttraumatic stress disorder

## ABUSE AND NEGLECT

### I. CHILD ABUSE AND NEGLECT

a. **General**

  i. Defined as an act or omission by a parent or caregiver that results in harm or threat of harm to a child.

   1. Mistreatment includes abuse or neglect.

     (a) Includes physical abuse, emotional abuse, sexual abuse, and human trafficking.

     (b) Neglect (acts of omission) may include failure to provide basic needs such as food, shelter, medicine, education, hygiene, or other necessities.

b. **Clinical Manifestations**

  i. Signs of abuse may include withdrawal, behavioral changes, sleep problems, frequent absences from school. Physical signs may include bruising, old and new fractures, and signs of malnutrition.

  ii. Signs of physical abuse may include unexplained injuries or bruising, injuries that do not match the explanation or are not consistent with the child's developmental stage.

  iii. Signs of neglect may include poor growth, poor hygiene, and lack of appropriate medical care.

c. **Treatment**
  i. Patient safety is paramount.
  ii. Interventions include legal, housing, medical, psychiatric, and social services.
  iii. In general, a report must be made when an individual knows or has reasonable suspicion that a child has been subjected to abuse or neglect.

## II. DOMESTIC VIOLENCE

a. **General**
  i. Behaviors may occur sporadically or continually and include physical violence, psychological abuse, stalking, and sexual abuse.
  ii. Occurs across all socioeconomic, racial, and cultural lines.
    1. Increased risk in families with problems of substance use.

b. **Clinical Manifestations**
  i. The patient may present with vague complaints of anxiety, depression, fatigue, or chronic headaches.
  ii. Injuries or bruising on the body, "accidental injuries," or multiple injuries in various stages of healing may serve as clues to abuse.
  iii. Trauma typically occurs at home and rarely in front of individuals outside the household.
  iv. Victims may blame themselves for the abuse.
  v. An abuser may accompany the patient and not want to leave the patient alone.

c. **Treatment**
  i. Patient safety is paramount.
  ii. Healthcare providers should have a plan for screening, assessing, and referring patients for domestic violence.

## III. ELDER ABUSE

a. **General**
  i. Defined as an act or omission that results in harm or threat to the health or welfare of the elderly.
    1. Mistreatment includes abuse or neglect.
      (a) Abuse may include physical, psychological, financial or material, sexual, or abandonment.
      (b) Acts of omission (neglect) include withholding food, medicine, clothing, or other necessities.
  ii. Family conflicts often underlie elder abuse.

b. **Clinical Manifestations**
  i. Unexplained injuries or bruising on the body, multiple injuries in various stages of healing, dehydration, malnutrition, decubitus ulcers, or poor hygiene may serve as clues to abuse.

c. **Treatment**
  i. Patient safety is paramount.
  ii. Interventions include legal, housing, medical, psychiatric, and social services.

## IV. CHILD SEXUAL ABUSE

a. **General**
  i. Sexual activities imposed on children as an abuse of the caregiver's power over the child.
    1. Perpetrators are commonly male, and the majority have access to the child (relatives or known by the child).

b. **Clinical Manifestations**
  i. Children that demonstrate knowledge of sexual acts, bruises or pain in the genital or anal area, or evidence of a sexually transmitted infection, should increase the index of suspicion for child abuse.
  ii. Forensic evidence collection may be necessary if the abuse was recent and involved exchange of bodily fluids.
  iii. Victims of sexual abuse are at risk for short- and long-term psychological disturbances, such as anxiety, posttraumatic stress disorder (PTSD), and depression.

c. **Treatment**
  i. Patient safety is paramount.
  ii. Interventions include legal, housing, medical, psychiatric, and social services.
  iii. In general, a report must be made when an individual knows or has reasonable suspicion that a child has been sexually abused.

# ANXIETY DISORDERS

## I. GENERALIZED ANXIETY DISORDER

a. **General**
  i. Characterized by tension, worried thoughts, and associated with physical manifestations of anxiety.
  ii. Typical onset in early 20s, and more common in females than in males.
  iii. Comorbidity with major depression or other anxiety disorders in many cases.
  iv. Both genetic and environmental etiologies.

b. **Clinical Manifestations**
  i. Pervasive anxiety and worry excessively about many aspects of their life (job, finances, school, health, relationships, and social situations) occurring most days for at least 6 months.
  ii. Must also have difficulty controlling the worry and must be associated with at least three of the following:
    1. Difficulty concentrating.

2. Easily fatigued.
3. Irritability.
4. Muscle tension.
5. Restlessness.
6. Sleep disturbances.

   iii. Anxiety or physical symptoms cause significant distress and impairment in functioning.

   iv. Symptoms are not attributable to another medical condition, substance use, or other mental health condition.

**c. Treatment**

   i. First-line therapy is selective serotonin reuptake inhibitors (SSRIs) and serotonin norepinephrine reuptake inhibitors (SNRIs).

   ii. Benzodiazepines can be used as short-term therapy while waiting for long-term treatment to take effect (caution for dependence or abuse).

   iii. Buspirone may be adjunct therapy. Beta-blockers may help control autonomic symptoms related to performance anxiety.

   iv. Tricyclic antidepressants (TCAs) and monoamine oxidase (MAO) inhibitors are second-line therapy options.

   v. Psychotherapy: cognitive-behavioral therapy has been proven effective.

## II. PANIC DISORDER

**a. General**

   i. Characterized by recurrent panic attacks (discrete episodes of intense fear, often with autonomic symptoms).

   ii. Typical onset in early 20s, and more common in females than in males.

   iii. Comorbidity with major depression in many cases.

   iv. Agoraphobia (a condition in which patients fear places from which escape may be difficult) is now categorized as a separate entity from panic disorder.

**b. Clinical Manifestations**

   i. Recurrent (at least two), sudden panic attacks (see Table 10.1).

   ii. Onset of panic attack may or may not be triggered, reaches peak within minutes.

   iii. To make the diagnosis, one of the following must occur for at least 1 month.

     1. Persistent concern about future attacks and their consequences.

     2. Significant change in behavior related to the attacks.

   iv. Symptoms are not attributable to another medical condition, substance use, or other mental health condition.

---

**TABLE 10.1**

### DSM5 Panic Attack Specifier

**Note:** Symptoms are presented for the purpose of identifying a panic attack; however, panic attack is not a mental disorder and cannot be coded. Panic attacks can occur in the context of any anxiety disorder as well as other mental disorders (e.g., depressive disorders, posttraumatic stress disorder, substance use disorders) and some medical conditions (e.g., cardiac, respiratory, vestibular, gastrointestinal). When the presence of a panic attack is identified, it should be noted as a specifier (e.g., "posttraumatic stress disorder with panic attacks"). For panic disorder, the presence of panic attack is contained within the criteria for the disorder and panic attack is not used as a specifier

An abrupt surge of intense fear or intense discomfort that reaches a peak within minutes, and during which time four (or more) of the following symptoms occur:

**Note:** The abrupt surge can occur from a calm state or an anxious state.

1. Palpitations, pounding heart, or accelerated heart rate.
2. Sweating.
3. Trembling or shaking.
4. Sensations of shortness of breath or smothering.
5. Feelings of choking.
6. Chest pain or discomfort.
7. Nausea or abdominal distress.
8. Feeling dizzy, unsteady, light-headed, or faint.
9. Chills or heat sensations.
10. Paresthesia (numbness or tingling sensations).
11. Derealization (feelings of unreality) or depersonalization (being detached from oneself).
12. Fear of losing control or "going crazy."
13. Fear of dying.

**Note:** Culture-specific symptoms (e.g., tinnitus, neck soreness, headache, uncontrollable screaming or crying) may be seen. Such symptoms should not count as one of the four required symptoms.

From: *DSM-5*, Diagnostic and Statistical Manual of Mental Disorders, 5th ed. American Psychiatric Association, 2013. Reprinted with permission from the Diagnostic and Statistical Manual of Mental Disorders: DSM5, 5th ed., "Panic Attack Specifier," p. 214 (Copyright © 2013). American Psychiatric Association. All Rights Reserved.

**c. Treatment**

   i. Treatment includes cognitive-behavioral therapy and pharmacotherapy. Use of both psychotherapy and medications is most effective.

     1. Cognitive-behavioral therapy consists of examining behavior, relaxation techniques, and desensitization.

     2. Pharmacotherapy consists of the following medications:

       (a) First-line therapy is SSRIs (e.g., sertraline, fluoxetine, escitalopram).

       (b) Benzodiazepines (e.g., alprazolam, clonazepam) can be used as short-term therapy while waiting for long-term treatment to take effect or for acute attacks (caution for dependence or abuse).

   ii. SNRIs may also be used. TCAs are an option if SSRIs and SNRIs are ineffective.

## III. PHOBIAS

### a. General

i. An anxiety disorder characterized by intense fear of a particular situation (e.g., heights) or object, such as needles.

ii. Onset typically in childhood.

iii. Social anxiety disorder (a disorder in which patients have intense fear of being scrutinized in a social or public setting) is not considered a specific phobia.

### b. Clinical Manifestations

i. An irrational fear of a specific object, place, or situation that is out of proportion to any actual danger.

ii. Consider the following to make the diagnosis:

1. The fear is excessive or out of proportion to any real threat or danger.

2. Exposure must immediately and invariably provoke an anxiety reaction.

3. Everyday activities must be impaired by the avoidance or distress over the feared object or situation.

4. Object or situation is actively avoided or endured with intense anxiety.

5. Specific fear is persistent and lasts longer than 6 months.

6. Symptoms are not attributable to another medical condition, substance use, or other mental health condition.

iii. Specifiers: Animal (e.g., dogs, spiders), blood-injection injury (e.g., needles, blood), natural environment (e.g., heights, water), situational (e.g., tight spaces, airplanes).

### c. Treatment

i. Certain childhood phobias disappear spontaneously with age.

ii. Exposure and desensitization therapy is the treatment of choice.

iii. Medications such as SSRIs (e.g., escitalopram, paroxetine) and benzodiazepines (e.g., alprazolam, diazepam) can be helpful.

# MOOD DISORDERS

## I. BIPOLAR DISORDER

### a. General

i. Subtypes include bipolar I and bipolar II.

1. Bipolar I involves manic episodes with or without major depression or psychosis.

2. Bipolar II involves hypomanic episodes with major depression; no history of manic or mixed episodes.

ii. Bipolar I has equal male-to-female ratios. Family history is the strongest risk factor.

### b. Clinical Manifestations

i. Bipolar I: A manic episode is necessary to meet the criteria.

1. A manic episode is a period of persistent, elevated, or irritable mood accompanied by increased, abnormal, and persistent energy and goal-directed activity.

   (a) Must have a clear period of persistently elevated mood lasting 1 week or severe enough to require hospitalization.

   (b) Symptoms cannot be due to a medical condition.

   (c) Symptoms must cause distress or impairment.

   (d) See Table 10.2 for symptoms of mania.

2. First episode typically occurs in the early 20s–30s.

3. The manic episode may be proceeded or followed by a hypomanic or major depressive episode.

4. The occurrence of mania is not better explained by schizoaffective disorder, schizophreniform disorder, delusional disorder, or other specified or unspecified schizophrenia or psychotic disorder.

ii. Bipolar II: At least one hypomanic episode and one major depressive episode is necessary to meet the criteria.

1. Hypomania is a period of persistent, abnormally elevated, or irritable mood and abnormally and persistently increased energy or activity, lasting at least 4 consecutive days.

2. Hypomania has similar symptoms to mania but causes less impairment and typically does not require hospitalization.

3. No history of a manic episode.

4. Mood and behavioral changes are uncharacteristic of the patient when not symptomatic and noticeable to others.

**TABLE 10.2**

| Criteria for Manic Episode | |
| --- | --- |
| **Criteria** | **Description** |
| Activity | Increased goal-oriented activities or psychomotor agitation |
| Attention | Easily distracted |
| Hedonism | Excessive involvement in pleasurable activities with elevated risk for negative consequences |
| Self-esteem | Highly inflated |
| Sleep | Decreased need for sleep |
| Speech | Pressured or more talkative |
| Thoughts | Racing, flight of ideas |

c. **Treatment**
  i. Mood stabilizers (e.g., lithium, lamotrigine) and second-generation antipsychotics (e.g., aripiprazole or risperidone) are the mainstay of management.
    1. Lithium is considered first-line therapy for acute mania and long-term management. Lithium decreases suicide risk.
    2. Second-generation (atypical) antipsychotics may be used as monotherapy or adjunctive therapy with mood stabilizers.
    3. A combination of mood stabilizers and second-generation antipsychotics is often faster and more effective than monotherapy.
  ii. Mood stabilizers (e.g., lithium, valproic acid) and antipsychotics (e.g., olanzapine or risperidone) for treatment of acute mania.
    1. Antipsychotics or benzodiazepines may be used for acute psychosis or agitation.
  iii. In bipolar, caution should be taken in treatment with monotherapy antidepressants because they may promote severe or frequent hypomania episodes.

## II. CYCLOTHYMIC DISORDER
a. **General**
  i. Symptoms of hypomania and depression but fall short of meeting criteria for full episode of hypomania or depression, respectively.
b. **Clinical Manifestations**
  i. Minimum of at least 2 consecutive years of mild elevations and depressions in mood that do not meet the criteria for full hypomanic episodes or major depressive episodes.
  ii. Over the course of 2 years, patients are symptomatic more days than not and are not symptom-free for more than 2 months.
c. **Treatment**
  i. Mood stabilizers (e.g., lamotrigine, lithium) or second-generation antipsychotics (e.g., aripiprazole or risperidone).
  ii. Psychotherapy.

# DEPRESSIVE DISORDERS

## I. MAJOR DEPRESSIVE DISORDER
a. **General**
  i. A unipolar disorder.
  ii. Female-to-male ratio is 2:1.
  iii. Incidence is greatest between the ages of 20 and 40 years.
  iv. Family history is a risk factor.
b. **Clinical Manifestations**
  i. Diagnosed after a single episode of major depression. Characterized by emotional changes,

**TABLE 10.3**

| Criteria for Major Depression | |
| --- | --- |
| **Criteria** | **Description** |
| Appetite | Increased or decreased with weight loss or gain |
| Concentration | Decreased concentration or increased indecisiveness |
| Energy | Fatigue almost all day |
| Guilt | Feelings of worthlessness or inappropriate guilt |
| Interest | Decrease in interest and pleasure in most activities |
| Mood | Depressed mood almost all day, every day |
| Psychomotor | Agitation or retardation |
| Sleep | Insomnia or hypersomnia |
| Suicide risk | Recurrent thoughts of suicide, death, or suicide attempt |

depressed mood, and vegetative changes, alterations in sleep, appetite, and energy.
    1. Must have five or more depressive symptoms for at least 2 weeks (Table 10.3).
      (a) Must have depressed mood, loss of interest, or loss of pleasure to make diagnosis.
      (b) Symptoms must cause significant distress or impairment of functioning (social, occupational, other).
      (c) No history of manic or hypomanic episode.
      (d) Multiple screening tools are available including the Patient Health Questionnaire (PHQ-2 or PHQ-9) or the Beck Depression Inventory for Primary Care.
    2. Must not be due to a medical condition, bereavement, or substance-induced.
  ii. Is frequently recurrent.
c. **Treatment**
  i. Psychotherapy (e.g., interpersonal therapy, cognitive behavioral therapy).
  ii. SSRIs (e.g., sertraline, escitalopram, fluoxetine) are the first-line medical management.
    1. Second line medications include SNRIs (e.g., venlafaxine, duloxetine) and bupropion.
    2. Tricyclic antidepressants and MAO inhibitors are other alternatives.
  iii. Electroconvulsive therapy can be used in psychotic, severe, or refractory symptoms.

## II. PERSISTENT DEPRESSIVE DISORDER (DYSTHYMIA)
a. **General**
  i. Unipolar mood disorder.
  ii. Loss of interest or pleasure in most activities but do not have symptoms severe enough to meet the diagnosis of major depressive episode.
  iii. More common in females.

b. **Clinical Manifestations**
   i. Essential feature is the chronic nature (greater than 2 years in adults) of the depressed mood present most days.
      1. During the 2-year period, the patient is not free of symptoms for greater than 2 months in a row.
      2. In addition to depressed mood, at least two of the following present:
         (a) Increased or decreased appetite.
         (b) Insomnia or hypersomnia.
         (c) Low energy or fatigue.
         (d) Low self-esteem.
         (e) Impaired concentration or decision making.
         (f) Hopelessness.
   iii. No history of manic or hypomanic episode.
   iv. At times, the patient may have a superimposed major depressive episode.

c. **Treatment**
   i. A combination of pharmacotherapy and psychotherapy is most effective.
      1. SSRIs are the first choice. SNRIs, bupropion, mirtazapine, TCAs and MAO inhibitors.
      2. Interpersonal therapy or cognitive behavioral therapy.

## III. PREMENSTRUAL DYSPHORIC DISORDER
a. **General**
   i. Severe PMS (premenstrual syndrome characterized by physical, behavioral, and mood changes within the luteal phase of the menstrual cycle) with functional impairment including prominent anger, irritability, and internal tension.

b. **Clinical Manifestations**
   i. Symptoms occur 1–2 weeks before menses (luteal phase) and are relieved within 2–3 days of the onset of menses. At least 7 symptom-free days occur during the follicular phase.
   ii. Patients may complain of irritability, anger, anxiety, mood swings, sudden depressed mood, increased sensitivity.
   iii. Physical symptoms may include bloating and fatigue, breast pain or tenderness, weight gain, headache.
   iv. Other symptoms may include changes in appetite, decreased energy, sleep changes, poor concentration, or decreased interest in usual activities.

c. **Treatment**
   i. Lifestyle modifications include stress reduction and exercise.
   ii. SSRIs are first-line pharmacological therapy. May be used continuously or during the luteal phase only.

   iii. Oral contraceptives may be helpful for patients who want contraception or do not want to take SSRIs.

## IV. SUICIDAL BEHAVIORS
a. **General**
   i. Assessing patients for suicidal ideation and plans is important for all depressed patients.
      1. Suicidal ideation consists of thoughts about killing oneself and may or may not include a plan.
   ii. Mortality from suicide is higher in males than females.

b. **Risk Factors**
   i. Previous suicide attempt is the strongest single predictive factor.
   ii. Access to firearms.
   iii. Increasing age.
   iv. Chronic pain or illness.
   v. Organized plan (versus no plan).
   vi. Positive family history of suicide.
   vii. Underlying psychiatric disorders.
   viii. Substance use.
   ix. Marriage and children are protective factors.

c. **Management**
   i. Assess for immediate risk. If concerned for safety of patient, admission and psychiatric evaluation are essential.
   ii. Diagnose and treat underlying mental health disorders.

## V. HOMICIDAL BEHAVIORS
a. **General**
   i. Assessing patients for homicidal ideation is important for all depressed patients.
      1. Assess ideation (thoughts), plan, and intent.
      2. Assess access to means for homicide.
      3. Assess psychotic symptoms, severe anxiety, substance use disorders, history of previous attempts or familial or recent exposure.

b. **Management**
   i. Assess for homicidal ideation and intention. If concerned for the safety of the patient or others, psychiatric hospitalization is indicated.

# DISRUPTIVE, IMPULSE-CONTROL, AND CONDUCT DISORDERS

## I. CONDUCT DISORDER
a. **General**
   i. Pattern of persistent behaviors that deviate from age-appropriate norms and violate the rights of humans and animals.
   ii. Noted in males more than females.

iii. Prevalence 1% to 10%, but increases to 25% to 85% in incarcerated youth.

iv. Age less than 18 years old for diagnosis. May progress to antisocial personality disorder in adulthood.

b. **Diagnosis**

i. Patient aggressive to animals and people.

ii. Destruction of property.

iii. Deceitfulness or theft.

iv. Serious violations of the law.

v. Lack of empathy to victims or remorse for actions.

c. **Treatment**

i. Multisystemic treatment that emphasizes how an individual's problems fit within the broader context.

## II. DISRUPTIVE MOOD DYSREGULATION DISORDER (DMDD)

a. **General**

i. Characterized by severe and recurrent temper outbursts, out of proportion in intensity or duration to the situation.

ii. Diagnosed in children over age 6, less than age 18.

b. **Diagnosis**

i. Severe chronic temper outbursts, verbal aggression, or emotional storms out of proportion to the situation.

ii. Outbursts occur an average of three or more times per week.

iii. Outbursts occur over a period of 12 months or more. No period of 3 or more consecutive months without symptoms.

iv. Persistent irritability does not remit when stressors go away or between episodes, and it is observable by others.

v. Irritability is observed in at least two out of three settings (home, school, with peers) and is severe in at least one setting.

vi. Symptoms present before age 10.

vii. Symptoms are not the result of another disorder.

c. **Treatment**

i. Focus on psychotherapy.

ii. Limit the use of medications.

# DISSOCIATIVE DISORDERS

## I. DISSOCIATIVE IDENTITY DISORDERS

a. **General**

i. Characterized by multiple distinct personality states or identities.

1. Previously referred to as multiple personality disorder.

ii. More common in females.

iii. Psychiatric comorbidities may include PTSD, depression, somatoform disorder, sexual abuse, substance use, and borderline personality disorder.

1. Theorized to be associated with severe childhood trauma and abuse.

b. **Clinical Manifestations**

i. Presence of two or more distinct personality states or identities and gaps in memory or recall of events or personal information.

1. Distinct personality states have different characteristics (e.g., gender, age, sexual orientation), behavior, sense of consciousness, memory, and perception of the world.

ii. Other dissociative symptoms may include:

1. Inability to recall personal or autobiographical information.

2. Dissociative fugue.

3. Depersonalization.

4. Derealization.

iii. Symptoms cause impaired functioning in day-to-day life.

iv. Symptoms may be observed by others and/or self-reported.

c. **Treatment**

i. Psychotherapy is the mainstay of treatment.

## II. DISSOCIATIVE AMNESIA

a. **General**

i. Temporary loss of recall memory caused by disassociation.

1. May last for seconds or years.

ii. Often a result of psychological trauma.

b. **Clinical Manifestations**

i. Inability to recall autobiographical memory usually associated with a stressful or traumatic event.

1. The inability to recall events causes distress.

ii. Types of memory disturbances that can occur in dissociative amnesia:

1. Localized amnesia: failure to recall during a specific period.

2. Selective amnesia: ability to recall some, but not all, parts of a specific period or traumatic event.

3. Systematized amnesia: loss of memory for a particular category of information.

4. Continuous amnesia: loss of memory for each new event as it occurs.

5. Generalized amnesia: complete loss of memory.

iii. Dysfunction in memory is not caused by substance use, dissociative identity disorder, or other physiological causes.

c. **Treatment**
  i. Psychotherapy is the mainstay of treatment.

## III. DEPERSONALIZATION-DEREALIZATION DISORDER

a. **General**
  i. Characterized by the persistence or recurrence of depersonalization and/or derealization.
    1. Depersonalization: a feeling of detachment or estrangement from self.
    2. Derealization: a sense of detachment or unreality with respect to the world around them.
  ii. May be precipitated by acute or chronic traumatic experiences.
  iii. Common comorbidities include depression, anxiety disorders, avoidant and borderline personality disorders.

b. **Clinical Manifestations**
  i. Presence of persistent or recurrent experiences of derealization and/or depersonalization.
    1. Reality testing remains intact.
  ii. Symptoms cause significant distress or impairment of functioning.
  iii. Dysfunction in memory is not caused by substance use, physiological cause, or other psychiatric disorder.

c. **Treatment**
  i. Psychotherapy is the mainstay of treatment.

# FEEDING AND EATING DISORDERS

## I. ANOREXIA NERVOSA

a. **General**
  i. Severe eating disorder characterized by low body weight.
  ii. Diagnosed when body weight falls below 85% of ideal weight or with a body mass index (BMI) less than or equal to 17.5 kg/m². 
    1. Weight loss must be due to behavior directed at maintaining a low weight or body image.
  iii. Average age of onset is 18 and is more common in females.
  iv. Highest mortality rate of psychiatric conditions due to related medical complications.

b. **Clinical Manifestations**
  i. Patients are preoccupied by their weight and body image.
  ii. Symptoms may include amenorrhea, fatigue, weakness, dizziness, irritability, cold intolerance, palpitations, abdominal pain, and constipation.
  iii. Physical exam findings may include hypotension, skin or hair changes, muscle wasting, signs of self-induced vomiting (salivary gland hypertrophy or dental enamel erosion).
  iv. Diagnosis includes the following:
    1. Restriction of calorie intake leading to significantly low body weight (body weight less than 85% of ideal or BMI ≤17.5 kg/m²).
    2. Preoccupation with body image.
    3. Distorted body image.
  v. Methods of weight loss include the following:
    1. Intensive exercise.
    2. Restricting food intake.
    3. Purging.
    4. Misuse of diuretics.

c. **Treatment**
  i. Primary goal is weight gain and treating psychological comorbidities.
    1. Treatment of medical complications is vital.
    2. Medications, such as antidepressants and SSRIs, are used to treat comorbid psychiatric illness.
    3. Psychotherapy, supervised meals, weight monitoring, and disease education are most helpful.

## II. BULIMIA NERVOSA

a. **General**
  i. Eating disorder characterized by recurrent binge eating combined with compensatory behaviors to counteract weight gain.
    1. Usually maintain a normal weight or are overweight.
  ii. More common in females. Age of onset typically in late teens or early adulthood.

b. **Clinical Manifestations**
  i. Patients engage in binge eating and behaviors designed to avoid weight gain.
    1. Recurrent episodes of eating a large amount of food within a discrete timeframe (e.g., 2 hours). Lack of control during binging episodes.
    2. Episodes of binge-eating and compensatory behaviors occur at least once a week for 3 months.
  ii. Compensatory behaviors to counteract overeating and prevent weight gain may include:
    1. Purging: self-induced vomiting, laxatives, diuretics, or enemas.
    2. Restrictive: reduced calorie intake, dieting, fasting, or excessive exercise.
  iv. Patients are overly concerned with body image and preoccupied with becoming fat.

c. **Treatment**
  i. Combination of psychotherapy and pharmacotherapy is most effective.

**TABLE 10.4**

| Medical Complications of Eating Disorders | |
|---|---|
| **Behavior** | **Complication** |
| Binge eating | Gastric distention |
| Diuretic use | Dehydration |
| | Electrolyte abnormalities |
| Laxative use | Constipation |
| | Dehydration |
| | Metabolic acidosis |
| Starvation | Anemia |
| | Bradycardia |
| | Edema |
| | Hypotension |
| | Hypothermia |
| Vomiting | Esophageal rupture |
| | Hypokalemia |
| | Metabolic alkalosis |

**TABLE 10.5**

| Body Mass Index and Weight-Associated Health Risks | | |
|---|---|---|
| **Body Mass Index (kg/m²)** | **Weight** | **Weight-Associated Health Risks** |
| <18.5 | Underweight | Low |
| 18.5–24.9 | Normal | Normal |
| 25–29.9 | Overweight | Low to moderate |
| 30–40 | Obesity | High/Very high |
| >40 | Extreme obesity | Extremely high |

1. Cognitive behavioral therapy can be helpful. Goal is to stop binging and purging behaviors and control the concern about body weight.
2. SSRIs are effective in the treatment of bulimia nervosa. Fluoxetine can reduce the binge-purge cycle.
   ii. Complications: See Table 10.4.

### III. OBESITY
**a. General**
  i. Obesity is the second leading cause of preventable death in the United States.
    1. Obesity increases risk for type 2 diabetes, gallstones, coronary artery disease, breast cancer, and colon cancer.
  ii. About half of obese individuals engage in binge eating.
    1. Obese binge eaters are more likely than non-bingers to suffer from anxiety disorders, social phobias, and alcohol or drug problems.

**b. Clinical Manifestations**
  i. Based on BMI. Recommended screening age 6 years and older.
    1. See Table 10.5.
  ii. Must rule out medical conditions, such as hypothyroidism, as cause of obesity.
  iii. Consider medications as a possible etiology.

**c. Treatment**
  i. Evaluate and treat any medical complications of obesity.
  ii. Behavioral modifications include exercise and dietary changes.
  iii. Diagnose and treat any comorbid psychiatric conditions. Psychotherapy may be beneficial.

  iv. Consider antiobesity medications.
    1. Lorcaserin, a serotonin agonist, or orlistat, which alters fat digestion.
  v. Consider surgical options.
    1. Bariatric surgery, gastric bypass, gastric sleeve, and gastric banding.

## OBSESSIVE-COMPULSIVE AND RELATED DISORDERS

### I. OBSESSIVE-COMPULSIVE DISORDER (OCD)
**a. General**
  i. Anxiety disorder characterized by a combination of thoughts (obsessions) and behaviors (compulsions).
    1. Obsessions: recurrent and persistent thoughts, impulses, or images that are intrusive and inappropriate and that cause anxiety or distress over things that are not real-life problems.
    2. Patient recognizes the obsessions are a product of their own mind.
    3. Compulsions: repetitive behaviors (e.g., hand washing, ordering, checking) or mental acts (e.g., praying, counting, repeating words silently) that the person feels driven to perform in response to an obsession.
  ii. Symptoms can be alienating and time consuming, and often cause severe emotional and economic loss.
  iii. No gender specificity. Average age of onset is around 20 years, many present in childhood or adolescence.

**b. Clinical Manifestations**
  i. Presence of obsessions, compulsions, or both that cause marked distress, that are time consuming, or that significantly interfere with the person's normal routine, occupational (or academic) functioning, or usual social activities or relationships.
  ii. Patterns may involve contamination (e.g., hand-washing, cleaning), doubt or fear of

harm (e.g., checking and rechecking locks, oven off), symmetry (ordering or counting).

iii. Cannot be due to substance use or another medical condition.

c. **Treatment**

i. First-line therapy consists of cognitive behavioral therapy, and medication.

ii. Behavioral and cognitive therapies consist of exposure and response prevention.

iii. Medications include SSRIs (e.g., paroxetine, sertraline, fluoxetine); tricyclic antidepressants, such as clomipramine; and SNRIs, such as venlafaxine.

## II. TRICHOTILLOMANIA

a. **General**

i. Hair-pulling disorder

ii. Most common in females; increased incidence with OCD, skin-picking disorder, and major depressive disorder.

b. **Clinical Manifestations**

i. Decreased hair density, broken hair, short vellus hairs seen in areas of pulling (commonly scalp, eyebrows, or eyelashes but may also include facial or pubic hair).

ii. Repeated attempts to stop hair pulling.

iii. Causes significant stress or interferes with daily functioning.

iv. Cannot be due to substance use or another medical condition.

c. **Treatment**

i. First-line therapy consists of cognitive behavioral therapy.

ii. Medication management includes SSRIs, second generation antipsychotics, N-acetylcysteine, or lithium.

## III. HOARDING DISORDER

a. **General**

i. Persistent difficulty with getting rid of possessions and the perceived need to save items.

ii. Most common in females.

b. **Clinical Manifestations**

i. Diagnostic criteria include:

1. Persistent difficulty with discarding or parting with possessions (regardless of value) resulting in accumulation of possessions.

2. Distress associated with discarding possessions.

3. Possessions accumulate and clutter living areas.

4. Hoarding causes distress or impairment in social, occupational, or other areas of functioning.

5. Not attributed to another medical condition or psychiatric diagnosis.

c. **Treatment**

i. First-line therapy consists of cognitive behavioral therapy specific for hoarding.

ii. For cases initially resistant to CBT, cognitive remediation is recommended over medication management with SSRIs.

## IV. DERMTILLOMANIA

a. **General**

i. Dermtillomania, skin-picking disorder, is characterized by picking at one's own skin (e.g., healthy skin, pimples, scabs, calluses).

ii. Picking at obvious or perceived skin defects, leading to physical damage of the skin.

iii. Most common in females; increased incidence with OCD, skin-picking disorder, and major depressive disorder.

b. **Clinical Manifestations**

i. Some symptoms of skin picking may be common; must reach the criteria for diagnosis:

1. Recurrent skin picking, resulting in physical damage to skin.

2. Repeated attempts to stop or minimize the picking.

3. Causes distress or impairment to daily functioning.

4. Not due to another medication, medical condition, or psychiatric diagnosis.

c. **Treatment**

i. First-line therapy consists of cognitive behavioral therapy.

ii. Medication management includes SSRIs, second generation antipsychotics, N-acetylcysteine.

## V. BODY DYSMORPHIC DISORDER

a. **General**

i. Characterized by extreme preoccupation with one or more perceived flaws or defects in physical appearance.

ii. Causes shame or embarrassment, leading to significant distress or functional impairment.

iii. Age of onset around 15 years; may be associated with anxiety or depression.

b. **Clinical Manifestations**

i. Preoccupation with one or more nonexistent or slight defects in physical appearance.

ii. Concerns about perceived flaw leads to repetitive behaviors (e.g., checking in the mirror, grooming) or mental acts (e.g., comparing self with others).

iii. Preoccupation causes significant distress or impairment.

iv. Preoccupation with appearance not better explained by an eating disorder.
c. **Treatment**
    i. Cognitive behavioral therapy specifically for body dysmorphic disorder.
    ii. Antidepressants (SSRIs); TCAs (Clomipramine) as alternative.

# NEURODEVELOPMENTAL DISORDERS

## I. ATTENTION-DEFICIT/HYPERACTIVITY DISORDER
a. **Characterized by persistent inattention, impulsivity, and/or hyperactivity**
b. **See Pediatrics chapter 14 for additional information**

## II. AUTISM SPECTRUM DISORDER
a. **A spectrum of developmental disorders characterized by impaired communication or social interactions, restricted and repetitive behaviors or interests, and impaired social functioning**
b. **See Pediatrics chapter 14 for additional information**

# PERSONALITY DISORDERS

## I. GENERAL
a. **Three personality disorder clusters (Table 10.6)**
b. **Pattern of symptoms of personality disorders typically established by adolescence or early adulthood**
c. **Patients usually remain in touch with reality**

## II. TYPES
a. **Antisocial**
    i. Characterized by a disregard for rules and laws and rarely experience remorse for their actions.
    ii. High potential for substance use or alcohol use disorder.

**TABLE 10.6**

| Classification of Personality Disorders | | |
| --- | --- | --- |
| **Odd and Eccentric (Cluster A)** | **Dramatic and Emotional (Cluster B)** | **Anxious and Fearful (Cluster C)** |
| Paranoid | Antisocial | Avoidant |
| Schizoid | Borderline | Dependent |
| Schizotypal | Histrionic | Obsessive-compulsive |
| | Narcissistic | |

iii. Diagnostic criteria according to Diagnostic and Statistical Manual of Mental Disorders, Fifth Edition (*DSM-5*):
    1. At least 18 years of age and have a history (by 15 years of age) of violating the rights of others (consistent with conduct disorder).
    2. Includes three or more of the following:
        (a) Doesn't conform with social norms, violates the rights of others, may commit illegal acts.
        (b) Irritable and aggressive towards others.
        (c) Exploits others for personal gain.
        (d) Disregard for the safety of others or self.
        (e) Lack of remorse.
        (f) Impulsivity.
        (g) Difficulty maintaining occupational or financial obligations.
    iv. May benefit from psychotherapy. Management is difficult to achieve.
b. **Avoidant**
    i. *DSM-5* diagnostic criteria:
        1. A pattern of social inhibition because of feeling inadequate and hypersensitive to negative evaluation, beginning in early adulthood.
        2. Presents in a variety of contexts including four or more of the following:
            (a) Avoids occupational activities with social contact because of fears of rejection or criticism.
            (b) Unwilling to socialize unless certain they will be accepted.
            (c) Exhibits caution in intimate relationships due to fear of shame or ridicule.
            (d) Preoccupied with criticism or rejection in social settings.
            (e) Inhibited in new interpersonal situations.
            (f) Low view of self in comparison to others.
            (g) Hesitant to take personal risks or try new activities.
    ii. Primary management with psychotherapy (CBT or group therapy). Interpersonal therapy may be beneficial as well.
c. **Borderline**
    i. Characterized by instability of interpersonal relationships, self-image, moods, reactive affect and poor impulse control.
    ii. *DSM-5* diagnostic criteria:
        1. A pattern of instability of interpersonal relationships, self-image, and moods with poor impulse control, beginning in early adulthood.
        2. Occurs in a variety of contexts including five or more of the following:

(a) Fear of real or imagined abandonment; includes efforts to avoid.

(b) Unstable interpersonal relationships; shifting between idealization and devaluation.

(c) Unstable self-image.

(d) Damaging impulsivity (e.g., substance use, spending money, sex).

(e) Reactivity of mood and affect.

(f) Feelings of emptiness.

(g) Difficulty controlling anger.

(h) Transient dissociation or paranoid ideation.

iii. Primary management with psychotherapy. Antidepressants, mood stabilizers, and antipsychotics have shown limited effectiveness for symptoms of anxiety, depression, and psychotic symptoms.

**d. Dependent**

i. Characterized by needy or submissive behavior, fear of being alone, and difficulty making decisions.

ii. *DSM-5* diagnostic criteria:

1. A pattern of excessive need to be taken care of that leads to submissive, needy behavior and fear of separation or abandonment.

2. Occurs in a variety of contexts including five or more of the following:

(a) Difficulty making everyday decisions without help.

(b) Relies on others to assume responsibility for most aspects of life.

(c) Agreeable for fear of loss of support.

(d) Difficulty initiating projects or doing things on their own.

(f) Exhaustive efforts to obtain approval and support from others.

(g) Helpless when alone; fears of being unable to care for themselves.

(h) When a close relationship ends, quickly seeks another.

(i) Preoccupied with fears about having to care for themselves.

iii. Primary management with psychotherapy (CBT). Antidepressants are used to treat comorbid anxiety or depression.

**e. Histrionic**

i. Characterized by excessive and superficial emotions, overly dramatic, seductive, and a need to be the center of attention.

ii. *DSM-5* diagnostic criteria:

1. A pattern of attention-seeking and excessive emotionality beginning in early adulthood.

2. Present in a variety of contexts including five or more of the following:

(a) Uncomfortable if not the center of attention.

(b) Inappropriate provocative or seductive behavior.

(c) Rapidly changing expressions of emotion.

(d) Uses physical appearance for attention.

(e) Excessively impressionistic speech.

(f) Dramatic, exaggerated expression of emotion.

(g) Easily influenced by others.

(h) Views relationships as more intimate than reality.

iii. Primary management with psychotherapy. Medications for symptoms of anxiety or depression.

**f. Narcissistic**

i. Characterized by self-centeredness, entitlement, need for attention, and a lack of empathy.

ii. *DSM-5* diagnostic criteria:

1. A pattern of grandiosity, need for admiration, exploitative relationships, and lack of empathy.

2. Including five or more of the following:

(a) Exaggerated sense of self-importance.

(b) Preoccupied with thoughts of unlimited money, success, etc.

(c) Believe they are "special" or "unique."

(d) Need for admiration.

(e) Sense of entitlement.

(f) Takes advantage of others.

(g) Lack of empathy.

(h) Envious of others and/or believes others to be envious of them.

(i) Arrogant.

iii. Primary management with psychotherapy.

**g. Obsessive-Compulsive**

i. Characterized by pervasive need for perfectionism and require a great deal of control and order in every aspect of their lives (without obsessions or compulsions).

ii. *DSM-5* diagnostic criteria:

1. A pattern of perfectionism, interpersonal control, and preoccupation with orderliness beginning in early adulthood. Lacking flexibility, openness, and efficiency.

2. Occurs in a variety of contexts including four or more of the following:

(a) Preoccupation with details, rules, schedules, so much so that the primary goal is lost.

(b) Perfectionism interferes with time management.

(c) Work, morals, and productivity take precedence over leisure and social activities.

(d) Inflexible morals, ethics, and values (not accounted for by cultural or religious affiliation).

(e) Inability to get rid of old or useless objects with no sentimental value.

(f) Reluctant to delegate tasks for fear it will be done incorrectly.

(g) Money is difficult to spend; hoards for future needs.

(h) Restricted affect.

iii. Primary management with psychotherapy.

**h. Paranoid**

i. *DSM-5* diagnostic criteria:

1. Pattern of distrust and suspiciousness; anticipate harm, betrayal, and deception.

2. Includes four or more of the following:

(a) Suspects, without evidence, that others are deceiving, harming, or betraying them.

(b) Doubts the loyalty of friends and acquaintances.

(c) Hesitant to confide in others; fears information will be used against them.

(d) Holds grudges.

(e) Read hidden, demeaning, or threatening meanings into benign remarks.

(f) Suspicious regarding fidelity of partner.

ii. Does not occur exclusively as part of another psychiatric disorder and cannot be explained by another medical condition.

iii. May benefit from cognitive behavioral therapy. Group therapy should be avoided.

iv. Short-term antipsychotics if experiencing psychosis.

**i. Schizoid**

i. *DSM-5* diagnostic criteria:

1. Pattern of detachment from social relationships and profound difficulty or restricted range of expressing emotions.

2. Presents in variety of situations and includes four or more of the following:

(a) No desire for close relationships.

(b) Little interest in sexual contact with another person.

(c) Prefers solitary activities.

(d) Takes pleasure in few activities.

(e) Lacks close friends; may have a bond with a first-degree relative.

(f) Indifferent to approval or disapproval of others.

(g) Flattened affect, detachment.

ii. Does not occur exclusively as part of another psychiatric disorder and can not be explained by another medical condition.

iii. May benefit from psychotherapy if willing. Management is difficult.

**j. Schizotypal**

i. Characterized by eccentric and odd behavior and thought patterns similar to schizophrenia but without delusions or hallucinations.

ii. *DSM-5* diagnostic criteria:

1. Includes at least five of the following signs and symptoms:

(a) Cognitive-perceptual: odd beliefs or magical thinking (e.g., telepathy, "sixth sense"), ideas of reference, unusual perceptual experiences, or paranoia.

(b) Oddness: odd thinking and speech, constricted affect, odd behavior or appearance.

(c) Interpersonal: lack of close friends (exception first-degree relatives), social anxiety associated with paranoia.

iii. Psychotherapy is first-line treatment (e.g., CBT, individual, or group). Antipsychotics may help with paranoia.

# SCHIZOPHRENIA SPECTRUM AND OTHER PSYCHOTIC DISORDERS

## I. DELUSIONAL DISORDER

**a. General**

i. Characterized by nonbizarre delusions without other psychotic symptoms.

ii. Disorder is rare and occurs typically in middle to late life.

**b. Clinical Manifestations**

i. At least one nonbizarre delusion (false belief but plausible) present for at least 1 month.

ii. Other than the delusions, the patient's behavior is not odd and there is no significant impairment of function.

iii. Patients must not meet criteria for schizophrenia.

iv. Any manic or depressive episodes have been brief relative to the duration of delusions.

v. Not explained by another psychiatric diagnosis, medical condition, medication or substance use.

vi. Seven subtypes of delusional disorders (Table 10.7).

**c. Treatment**

i. Atypical antipsychotics are first-line treatment.

ii. Adjunctive psychotherapy (e.g., individual, CBT).

## II. SCHIZOPHRENIA

**a. General**

i. Patients have psychotic symptoms and social and/or occupational dysfunction.

ii. Typical onset in the early 20s for men, late 20s for women. Genetic predisposition.

**TABLE 10.7**

| **Subtypes of Delusional Disorders** | |
|---|---|
| **Subtype** | **Description** |
| Erotomanic | Convinced that another person is in love with them. |
| Grandiose | Believe they have special abilities or are more important than reality indicates. |
| Jealous | Suspect that their partner is unfaithful. |
| Persecutory | Convinced that others are observing or looking to harm them, or they are being conspired against. |
| Somatic | Convinced that they have a body function disorder. |
| Mixed | No single delusion is predominant. |
| Unspecific | Cannot be determined or do not match a subtype. |

iii. Etiology is unknown. May be due to hyperactivity in brain dopaminergic pathways.

iv. Better prognosis if later age of onset, acute, positive symptoms.

v. Schizophreniform disorder is schizophrenia that fails to last 6 months and does not involve social withdrawal.

b. **Clinical Manifestations**

i. Two or more of the following symptoms for at least 6 months:
1. Positive symptoms: hallucinations, delusions, disorganized speech, or catatonic behavior.
2. Negative symptoms: flat affect, lack of motivation, poverty of speech, lack of interest.

ii. One symptom must be hallucination, delusion, or disorganized speech and must manifest for at least 1 month.

iii. Impaired functioning in one or more areas of life (e.g., social, occupational, relationships).

iv. Symptoms not attributable to substance use, medication, or another medical diagnosis.

a. **Treatment**

i. Second-generation (atypical) antipsychotic agents are the primary treatments.

ii. Psychosocial treatments are critical to long-term management of patients.

III. **SCHIZOAFFECTIVE DISORDER**

a. **General**

i. Patients have psychotic episodes that resemble schizophrenia but with prominent mood disturbances.

ii. Age of onset is late teens to early 20s.

b. **Clinical Manifestations**

i. Meets the primary criteria for schizophrenia.

ii. Has experienced a major mood episode (mania or major depression) that lasts for an uninterrupted period of time.

iii. Must have had a period of time in which they have psychotic symptoms (2 or more weeks) without a major mood disturbance.

iv. Mood disturbances need to be present for the majority of the illness.

v. Symptoms are not caused by substance use, medications, or other medical diagnoses.

c. **Treatment**

i. Treated with a combination of mood stabilizers and antipsychotic medications.

IV. **BRIEF PSYCHOTIC DISORDER**

a. **General**

i. Presence of one or more psychotic symptoms with onset and remission within 1 month.

ii. Is a rare disorder.

b. **Diagnosis**

i. Presence of one or more of the following:
1. Delusions.
2. Hallucinations.
3. Disorganized speech.
4. Grossly disorganized or catatonic behavior.

ii. Duration more than a day but less than 1 month.

iii. Absence of symptoms comprising a mood disorder.

c. **Treatment**

i. Atypical antipsychotic medications (e.g., risperidone, aripiprazole, quetiapine) may be used.

ii. Psychotherapy; education and reassurance are needed.

# SLEEP-WAKE DISORDERS

I. **NARCOLEPSY**

a. **General**

i. Characterized by long-term inability to regulate sleep-wake cycles.

ii. Typically presents in teens and early 20s.

b. **Clinical Manifestations**

i. Chronic daytime sleepiness; may fall asleep at inappropriate times.

ii. Sudden loss of muscle tone while awake often triggered by sudden, strong emotions (e.g., laughter, fear, anger, stress, or excitement).

iii. Vivid tactile, visual, or auditory hallucinations when falling asleep.

iv. Sleep paralysis immediately before or after falling asleep.

c. **Treatment**

i. Regular sleep schedule, daytime naps.

ii. Modafinil promotes wakefulness during daytime.

iii. REM-suppressing medications (e.g., fluoxetine, venlafaxine) can assist with cataplexy.

iv. Severe sleepiness may be treated with Oxybates. Methylphenidate or amphetamines are alternative options.

## II. PARASOMNIAS
### a. General
i. Characterized by undesirable physical, behavioral, or experiential phenomena that occur with specific sleep stages, or sleep-wake transitions.

### b. Categories
i. Non-rapid eye movement (NREM) sleep arousal disorders.
   1. Sleepwalking: episodes of arising from bed during sleep, difficult to wake, with little or no recall.
      (a) May increase with stress.
      (b) Variants include sleep-related eating and sleep-related sexual behaviors.
      (c) Safety is important.
   2. Sleep terrors: spells of terror, characterized by behaviors of intense fear (e.g., screaming) and autonomic symptoms (e.g., tachycardia, tachypnea, and diaphoresis).
ii. Rapid eye movement (REM) sleep behavior disorder.
   1. Nightmare disorder: repetitive, dysphoric dreams that may involve threats to survival, security, integrity, usually occurring during the second half of sleep.
      (a) Recall is common.
      (b) Psychotherapy may help patients rewrite nightmares. Some benefit from cyproheptadine or prazosin.
   2. REM sleep behavior disorder: repeated episodes of arousal during sleep associated with talking or motor behaviors during REM sleep.
      (a) Melatonin can help with REM sleep behavior disorders.
   3. Isolated sleep paralysis: atonia during REM sleep, often occurring during sleep-wake transitions and can be discomforting or frightening.
      (a) Typically no treatment is needed. Some medications can suppress REM sleep such as fluoxetine and imipramine.

# SOMATIC SYMPTOMS AND RELATED DISORDERS

## I. SOMATIC SYMPTOM DISORDER
### a. General
i. Characterized by presence of physical signs or symptoms without medical cause.
ii. More common in females.

iii. Patients have a complex medical history and often have gone through multiple medical and surgical procedures.

### b. Clinical Manifestations
i. Diagnosed when a patient has multiple medical complaints that are not the result of medical illness.
ii. Symptoms must have begun before age 30 years and have persisted for several years.
   1. Symptom may vary but the state of being symptomatic is persistent.
iii. Diagnostic criteria require the following:
   1. Persistent thoughts, out of proportion to the seriousness of symptoms.
   2. High levels of anxiety about health or symptoms.
   3. Excessive time and energy devoted to symptoms or health concerns.

### c. Treatment
i. Patient support is required.
ii. Avoid opioids.
iii. Psychotherapy is the mainstay of management.

## II. FUNCTIONAL NEUROLOGIC SYMPTOM DISORDER
### a. General
i. Characterized by neurological symptoms (e.g., weakness, nonepileptic seizures) that are inconsistent with neurological disease.
ii. Previously known as conversion disorder.
iii. More common in females.
iv. Commonly comorbid with depression, anxiety or neurological disorder; often preceded by a traumatic event.

### b. Clinical Manifestations
i. At least one neurological symptom that cannot be explained by a neurological condition or other medical or psychiatric diagnosis.
ii. Clinical symptoms and recognized neurologic condition do not align.
iii. Symptom or deficit causes distress, psychosocial impairment or other impaired functioning.
iv. Symptom not better explained by another diagnosis.

### c. Treatment
i. Patient education and supportive care.
ii. Cognitive behavioral therapy.

## III. ILLNESS ANXIETY DISORDER
### a. General
i. Characterized by preoccupation about having or developing a serious medical condition. Previously known as hypochondriasis.
ii. Typically presents in early adulthood; commonly comorbid with anxiety and depressive disorders.

b. **Clinical Manifestations**
  i. Excessive concern about having an illness; persists despite information that shows otherwise (e.g., examinations, laboratory testing) for at least 6 months.
  ii. Physical symptoms of the illness are not present or minimal (may be normal bodily functions).
  iii. High level of anxiety about health, and easily alarmed.
  iv. Excessive health-related behaviors (e.g., checking self) or maladaptive avoidance of situations.

c. **Treatment**
  i. Supportive care. Regularly schedule appointments and reassurance.
  ii. Psychotherapy (CBT) is first-line management. Treat comorbid anxiety or depression.

## IV. FACTICIOUS DISORDER
a. **General**
  i. Purposeful creation or exaggeration of signs or symptoms of medical or psychiatric illness for primary gain (to be seen as ill or injured).
    1. Not for secondary gain (money, to obtain drugs) as seen in malingering.
  ii. More common in females. Associated with personality disorders.

b. **Clinical Manifestations**
  i. Creation or exaggeration of symptoms (e.g., injure themselves purposefully, interfere with diagnostic tests, use substances to make themselves sick).
  ii. May be willing to have surgery or painful tests to obtain sympathy.
  iii. May move to different providers. Often have extensive knowledge about medical conditions.

c. **Treatment**
  i. Collect information from family members or directly from other healthcare providers.
  ii. Contact child or adult protective services if symptoms imposed on another person.

## V. MALINGERING
a. **General**
  i. Intentional falsification of signs and symptoms of medical or psychiatric illness for secondary gain (e.g., insurance money, lawsuits, avoidance of school or work, to obtain drugs).
  ii. NOT a mental illness.

# SUBSTANCE USE DISORDERS

## I. GENERAL
a. *DSM-5* diagnostic criteria for substance use disorder: 11 criteria, or symptoms, that characterize the severity of an individual's addiction
b. **(2–3 symptoms = mild, 4–5 symptoms = moderate, 6 or more symptoms = severe)**
  i. Failure to fulfill major obligations at home, work, or school.
  ii. Recurrent use in situations in which it is hazardous.
  iii. Craving or strong desire to use the substance.
  iv. Recurrent use despite recurrent social and personal problems caused by use.
  v. Tolerance.
  vi. Withdrawal.
  vii. Larger amounts used than intended.
  viii. Persistent failed efforts to decrease use.
  ix. Excessive time spent trying to obtain, use, or recover.
  x. Reduction in important activities.
  xi. Continued use despite awareness that substance is the cause of many problems.

## II. ALCOHOL USE
a. **Alcohol Intoxication**
  i. General
    1. Defined by presence of the following during or shortly after alcohol ingestion.
      (a) Slurred speech.
      (b) Unsteadiness/Incoordination.
      (c) Nystagmus.
      (d) Impaired attention or memory.
      (e) Stupor or coma.
      (f) Maladaptive behavior or psychological changes, such as impaired judgment or inappropriate behavior.
  ii. Diagnosis
    1. Must also consider other possible medical causes, such hypoglycemia or toxicity of other substances.
    2. Diagnosis confirmed with blood alcohol level.
  iii. Treatment
    1. Supportive care.
b. **Alcohol Dependence**
  i. General
    1. Male-to-female ratio for alcohol dependence is 4:1.
    2. Alcohol use becomes dependence when tolerance and withdrawal symptoms develop.
    3. **CAGE Alcohol Screening (two or more equals a positive screen)**
      (a) **C**ut down: "Do you think you should cut down your drinking?"
      (b) **A**nnoyed: "Have people been annoyed by or criticized your drinking?"

(c) **G**uilty: "Have you felt bad about your drinking?"

(d) **E**ye opener: "Have you had a drink to steady your nerves in the morning?"

ii. Clinical manifestations

1. Early diagnosis difficult due to patient denying or minimizing drinking.

2. May present with accidents, falls, blackouts, or difficulties with law enforcement.

3. Information from family may be required to make the diagnosis.

4. Physical examination.

(a) Early findings include acne rosacea, palmar erythema, and hepatomegaly (painless).

(b) Late findings include cirrhosis, jaundice, ascites, testicular atrophy, and gynecomastia.

5. Neuropsychiatric complications of alcoholism include Wernicke-Korsakoff syndrome.

(a) Due to thiamine deficiency.

(b) Wernicke stage consists of nystagmus, ataxia, and mental confusion.

(i) Resolve with thiamine treatment.

(c) Korsakoff stage is anterograde amnesia and confabulation.

(i) May be irreversible in many patients.

6. Other manifestations include alcoholic hallucinations, dementia, peripheral neuropathy, depression, and suicide.

7. In the later stages, social and occupational impairment occur, leading to job loss and family estrangement.

iii. Diagnosis

1. Blood alcohol levels will confirm the presence of alcohol in the blood.

2. Other laboratory changes include elevated mean corpuscular volume (MCV), serum γ-glutamyltransferase (GGT), and high-density lipoprotein (HDL).

iv. Treatment

1. Alcohol intoxication.

(a) Supportive measures: all known alcohol-dependent patients should receive folate and thiamine.

2. Minor alcohol withdrawal.

(a) Begins within 12 to 18 hours after stopping alcohol intake and peaks at 24 to 48 hours.

(i) Untreated, uncomplicated withdrawal lasts 5 to 7 days.

(b) Present with tremors, nausea, vomiting, tachycardia, and hypertension.

(c) Treatment goal is patient comfort and prevention of serious complications.

(i) Treat with chlordiazepoxide or oxazepam.

3. Major alcohol withdrawal.

(a) Alcohol-induced seizures.

(i) Begin within 8 to 36 hours and peak 24 to 48 hours after stopping alcohol intake.

(ii) Treated with IV benzodiazepines and phenytoin.

(b) Alcohol hallucinations.

(i) Begin 48 hours after stopping alcohol intake and may last more than 1 week.

(ii) Characterized by vivid, unpleasant auditory hallucinations in the presence of a clear sensorium.

(iii) Treat with a neuroleptic.

(c) Alcohol withdrawal delirium (delirium tremens).

(i) Life-threatening condition manifested by delirium, autonomic hyperarousal, and mild fever.

(ii) Begins 2 to 3 days after the abrupt stopping of alcohol.

(iii) Treated with IV benzodiazepines and supportive care.

4. Alcohol rehabilitation.

(a) Goals are sobriety and treatment of psychopathology.

(b) Options include the following:

(i) Alcoholics Anonymous.

(ii) Inpatient and residential rehabilitation programs.

(iii) Medications.

(1) Treatment of depression and anxiety.

(2) Disulfiram (Antabuse).

(3) Naltrexone.

## III. DRUG USE

a. **Sedative/Hypnotic/Anxiolytic Use Disorders**

i. General

1. Are cross-tolerant with alcohol.

ii. Clinical manifestations

1. Similar to alcohol manifestations.

2. Withdrawal delirium will start 3 to 4 days after stopping drug.

3. Overdose can cause respiratory compromise.

4. Diagnosed with drug blood levels.

5. Signs and symptoms listed in Table 10.8.

iii. Treatment

1. Detoxification begins with the slow tapering of medication doses.

**TABLE 10.8**

| Signs and Symptoms of Withdrawal From Sedative/Hypnotic/ Anxiolytic Drugs | |
| --- | --- |
| **Minor Withdrawal** | **Major Withdrawal** |
| Anxiety | Coarse tremors |
| Apprehension | Hyperreflexia |
| Restlessness | Nausea and vomiting |
| | Orthostatic hypotension |
| | Seizures |
| | Sweating |
| | Weakness |

2. After detoxification, rehabilitation is required.

b. **Opioid Use Disorder**
   i. General
      1. Opioid drug class includes opiates, opioid peptides, and all synthetic and semisynthetic drugs that mimic the action of opioids.
      2. Withdrawal symptoms typically begin 10 hours after last dose.
   ii. Clinical manifestations
      1. Signs of intoxication occur immediately after use.
         (a) Include pupillary constriction, respiratory depression, slurred speech, hypotension, bradycardia, and hypothermia.
      2. Symptoms of opiate withdrawal (Table 10.9).
      3. Diagnosis confirmed by urine or serum toxicology testing.
   iii. Treatment
      1. Addicted patients should be gradually withdrawn using methadone.
         (a) Withdrawal with short-acting drugs is 7 to 10 days; with long-acting, it is 2 to 3 weeks.

**TABLE 10.9**

| Symptoms of Opiate Withdrawal | |
| --- | --- |
| **Mild Withdrawal** | **Severe Withdrawal** |
| Diarrhea | Abdominal pain/Cramps |
| Dysphoric mood | Anxiety |
| Fever | Hot and cold flashes |
| Hypertension | Muscle aches |
| Insomnia | Nausea and vomiting |
| Pupillary dilation | Seizures (with meperidine |
| Restlessness | withdrawal) |
| Rhinorrhea | |
| Sweating | |
| Tachycardia | |
| Yawning | |

2. Clonidine, a centrally acting alpha-2-agonist, is used to treat the autonomic symptoms of withdrawal.
3. Rehabilitation is needed.
4. Long-term management with methadone maintenance program, Suboxone (Buprenorphine and Naloxone), or Naltrexone.

c. **Central Nervous System (CNS) Stimulant Use Disorder**
   i. General
      1. Includes cocaine and amphetamines.
      2. Cocaine has a rapid onset of action and short half-life and thus requires frequent dosing, whereas amphetamines have a longer onset of action and half-life.
      3. Withdrawal symptoms peak in 2 to 4 days.
   ii. Clinical manifestations
      1. Intoxication characterized by the following:
         (a) Euphoria or hypervigilance.
         (b) Tachycardia or bradycardia.
         (c) Pupillary dilation.
         (d) Hypertension or hypotension.
         (e) Perspiration or chills.
         (f) Nausea and vomiting.
         (g) Weight loss.
         (h) Psychomotor agitation or retardation.
         (i) Confusion, seizures, or coma.
         (j) Respiratory depression and chest pain.
      2. Cocaine intoxication can cause tactile hallucinations, agitation, impaired judgment, and transient psychosis.
      3. Amphetamine can cause agitation, impaired judgment, and transient psychosis.
      4. Withdrawal leads to fatigue, depression, nightmares, headache, sweating, muscle cramps, and hunger.
   iii. Treatment
      1. Treatment consists of supportive care with rehabilitation being the goal.

IV. **TOBACCO USE**
   a. **General**
      i. Tobacco use is the most important modifiable risk factor for death from cancer, cardiovascular disease, and pulmonary disease.
      ii. Tobacco smoke may produce illness through systemic absorption of toxins and/or local pulmonary injury by oxidant gases.
   b. **Clinical Manifestations**
      i. Withdrawal symptoms include anxiety, irritability, difficulty concentrating, restlessness, hunger, craving tobacco, disrupted sleep, and depression.
   c. **Treatment**
      i. Counseling and support systems.

ii. Medications.
  1. Nicotine.
    (a) Replacement products include gum, nasal sprays, inhalers, and transdermal patch.
  2. Bupropion.
    (a) An antidepressant drug; excessive doses can cause seizures, and the drug should not be used in patients with seizures or eating disorders.
    (b) Combination therapy—nicotine replacement plus bupropion—increases likelihood of cessation.
  3. Varenicline.
    (a) Works by blocking the action of nicotine on the appropriate nicotine receptor.

# TRAUMA AND STRESSOR-RELATED DISORDERS

## I. ADJUSTMENT
  a. General
    i. Changes in emotional state or behaviors that occur as a response to an identified stressful event (non-life threatening).
    ii. Examples: breakup or divorce, loss of job, financial issues, health issues.
  b. Clinical Manifestations
    i. Presence of emotional or behavioral symptoms in response to an identifiable stressor(s).
    ii. Response is disproportionate to what would normally be expected within 3 months of the stressor and typically resolves within 6 months of the stressor.
    iii. Symptoms produce significant impairment to daily functioning.
  c. Treatment
    i. Psychotherapy is preferred initial treatment; individual and family therapy are helpful, as are self-help groups.
    ii. Patients often self-medicate themselves with alcohol, caffeine, and over-the-counter medications.
    iii. Treatment of depression or anxiety symptoms with medications is common.

## II. ACUTE STRESS DISORDER
  a. General
    i. Characterized by acute stress reaction in the first month after a traumatic event.
    ii. Lasting 3 to 30 days.
  b. Clinical Manifestations
    i. Similar symptoms to PTSD but event occurred less than 1 month ago.
      (a) May include recurrent intrusions, avoidance of triggers, alterations in mood, or alterations in arousal and reactivity.
    ii. Symptoms cause significant distress or impaired functioning.
    iii. Symptoms not caused by substance use or other medical condition.
  c. Treatment
    i. Cognitive behavioral therapy, especially trauma focused, is first-line treatment.
    ii. Benzodiazepines may be helpful for acute symptoms initially after the traumatic event but use should be limited to 2–4 weeks.
    iii. If symptoms persist greater than 1 month, treat as PTSD.

## III. POSTTRAUMATIC STRESS DISORDER
  a. General
    i. Symptoms that may occur after exposure to a real, threatened, or perceived traumatic event.
      (a) Stressor may have been experienced personally, witnessed, happened to someone close, or through repeated exposure to traumatic events (e.g., first-responders).
    ii. Symptoms last greater than 1 month and/or the event occurred greater than 1 month ago (event can have occurred anytime in the past).
  b. Clinical Manifestations
    i. At least one intrusion symptom: repetitive recollections (e.g., memories, nightmares) or dissociative reactions (e.g., flashbacks) leading to physiologic distress or reactions.
    ii. Avoidance of triggering stimuli.
    iii. At least two negative alterations in cognition and mood (e.g., negative feelings of self, anhedonia, self-blame, shame, anger, dissociation).
    iv. At least two alterations in arousal and reactivity (e.g., irritability, outbursts, reckless behaviors, sleep disturbances, startle response).
    v. Symptoms cause significant distress and functional impairment.
  c. Treatment
    i. Treatment is with cognitive-behavioral therapy; trauma-focused therapy is considered first-line.
    ii. Medications include SSRIs and SNRIs.
    iii. Trazodone may help with insomnia. Prazosin can reduce nightmares.

## Psychiatric Drugs

| Drug Name | Mechanism of Action | Therapeutic Use | Side Effects |
| --- | --- | --- | --- |
| **Antidepressants** | | | |
| Bupropion (Wellbutrin) | Inhibits uptake of dopamine and norepinephrine | Mood disorders<br>Smoking cessation | Risk of seizures |
| Citalopram (Celexa) | Inhibits reuptake of serotonin | Bulimia<br>Mood disorders<br>Panic disorder | Headache<br>Insomnia/Sedation<br>Nausea<br>Sexual dysfunction |
| Desipramine (Norpramin) | Blocks presynaptic uptake of norepinephrine and serotonin | Mood disorders<br>Panic disorder | Cardiac toxicity<br>Orthostatic hypotension<br>Anticholinergic<br>Sexual dysfunction |
| Fluoxetine (Prozac) | Inhibits reuptake of serotonin | Bulimia<br>Mood disorders<br>OCD<br>Panic disorder | Headache<br>Insomnia/Sedation<br>Nausea<br>Sexual dysfunction |
| Fluvoxamine (Luvox) | Inhibits reuptake of serotonin | Bulimia<br>Mood disorders<br>Panic disorder | Headache<br>Insomnia/Sedation<br>Nausea<br>Sexual dysfunction |
| Imipramine (Tofranil) | Blocks presynaptic uptake of norepinephrine and serotonin | Mood disorders<br>Panic disorder | Cardiac toxicity<br>Orthostatic hypotension<br>Anticholinergic<br>Sexual dysfunction |
| Mirtazapine (Remeron) | Modulates norepinephrine | Mood disorders | Sedation |
| Nefazodone (Serzone) | Modulates serotonin | Depression | Postural hypotension<br>Priapism<br>Seizures |
| Nortriptyline (Pamelor) | Blocks presynaptic uptake of norepinephrine and serotonin | Mood disorders<br>Panic disorder | Anticholinergic<br>Cardiac toxicity<br>Orthostatic hypotension<br>Sexual dysfunction |
| Paroxetine (Paxil) | Inhibits reuptake of serotonin | Bulimia<br>Mood disorders<br>Panic disorder | Headache<br>Insomnia/Sedation<br>Nausea<br>Sexual dysfunction |
| Phenelzine (Nardil) | Inhibits presynaptic monoamine oxidase | Mood disorders<br>Panic disorder | Daytime somnolence<br>Hypertensive crisis<br>Orthostatic hypotension |
| Sertraline (Zoloft) | Inhibits reuptake of serotonin | Bulimia<br>Mood disorders<br>Panic disorder | Headache<br>Insomnia/Sedation<br>Nausea<br>Sexual dysfunction |
| Tranylcypromine (Parnate) | Inhibits presynaptic monoamine oxidase | Mood disorders<br>Panic disorder | Hypertensive crisis<br>Insomnia/Agitation<br>Orthostatic hypotension |
| Trazodone (Desyrel) | Modulates serotonin | Depression<br>Insomnia | Priapism<br>Sedation |
| Venlafaxine (Effexor) | Inhibits serotonin and norepinephrine reuptake | Depression<br>Anxiety | Insomnia<br>Seizures |
| **Antipsychotics** | | | |
| Chlorpromazine (Thorazine) | Blocks dopamine receptors | Antipsychotic | Hypotension<br>Sedation |
| Clozapine (Clozaril) | Blocks dopamine and serotonin receptors | Antipsychotic<br>Anticholinergic agranulocytosis | Hypotension<br>Sedation |
| Fluphenazine (Prolixin) | Blocks dopamine receptors | Antipsychotic | Extrapyramidal |

*Continued*

## Psychiatric Drugs—cont'd

| Drug Name | Mechanism of Action | Therapeutic Use | Side Effects |
|---|---|---|---|
| Haloperidol (Haldol) | Blocks dopamine receptors | Antipsychotic | Extrapyramidal |
| Olanzapine (Zyprexa) | Blocks dopamine and serotonin receptors | Antipsychotic | Sedation |
| Perphenazine (Trilafon) | Blocks dopamine receptors | Antipsychotic | Extrapyramidal |
| Quetiapine (Seroquel) | Blocks dopamine and serotonin receptors | Antipsychotic | Cataracts<br>Sedation |
| Risperidone (Risperdal) | Blocks dopamine and serotonin receptors | Antipsychotic | Hypotensive QT prolongation |
| Thioridazine (Mellaril) | Blocks dopamine receptors | Antipsychotic | Anticholinergic<br>Hypotension<br>Pigmentary retinopathy<br>Sedation |
| Trifluoperazine (Stelazine) | Blocks dopamine receptors | Antipsychotic | Extrapyramidal |
| **Anxiolytics** | | | |
| Alprazolam (Xanax) | Agonist at the CNS GABA receptor; augments GABA function | Agitation<br>Akathisia<br>Anxiety disorders<br>Panic disorders | Depress respiratory system<br>Sleepiness |
| Buspirone (BuSpar) | Agonist at the 5-HT receptor | Anxiety | Dizziness<br>Nausea<br>Nervousness |
| Chlordiazepoxide (Librium) | Agonist at the CNS GABA receptor; augments GABA function | Agitation<br>Akathisia<br>Alcohol withdrawal<br>Anxiety disorders | Depress respiratory system<br>Sleepiness |
| Clonazepam (Klonopin) | Agonist at the CNS GABA receptor; augments GABA function | Agitation<br>Akathisia<br>Anxiety disorders<br>Panic disorders | Depress respiratory system<br>Sleepiness |
| Diazepam (Valium) | Agonist at the CNS GABA receptor; augments GABA function | Agitation<br>Akathisia<br>Anxiety disorders<br>Insomnia | Depress respiratory system<br>Sleepiness |
| Lorazepam (Ativan) | Agonist at the CNS GABA receptor; augments GABA function | Agitation<br>Akathisia<br>Anxiety disorders<br>Catatonia | Depress respiratory system<br>Sleepiness |
| Oxazepam (Serax) | Agonist at the CNS GABA receptor; augments GABA function | Agitation<br>Akathisia<br>Alcohol withdrawal<br>Anxiety disorders | Depress respiratory system<br>Sleepiness |
| Temazepam (Restoril) | Agonist at the CNS GABA receptor; augments GABA function | Agitation<br>Akathisia<br>Anxiety disorders<br>Insomnia | Depress respiratory system<br>Sleepiness |
| Triazolam (Halcion) | Agonist at the CNS GABA receptor; augments GABA function | Agitation<br>Akathisia<br>Anxiety disorders<br>Insomnia | Depress respiratory system<br>Sleepiness |
| **Mood Stabilizers** | | | |
| Carbamazepine (Tegretol) | Alters sodium channels | Acute mania<br>Bipolar disorder<br>Seizures | Agranulocytosis<br>Ataxia<br>Dizziness<br>Nausea and vomiting<br>Sedation<br>Somnolence |

## Psychiatric Drugs—cont'd

| Drug Name | Mechanism of Action | Therapeutic Use | Side Effects |
|---|---|---|---|
| Lamotrigine (Lamictal) | Inhibits sodium channels | Bipolar disorder<br>Seizures | Ataxia<br>Blurred vision<br>Dizziness<br>Nausea and vomiting<br>Stevens-Johnson syndrome |
| Lithium (Eskalith) | Alters intracellular messengers | Acute mania<br>Bipolar disorder<br>Depression | Acne exacerbation<br>Ataxia<br>Coarse tremor<br>Confusion<br>Sinus arrest<br>Weight gain |
| Valproate (Depakene) | Augments GABA synthesis | Acute mania<br>Bipolar disorder<br>Seizures | GI distress<br>Mild tremor and ataxia<br>Sedation |
| **Psychostimulants** | | | |
| Dextroamphetamine (Dexedrine) | Facilitates neurotransmitter release in the CNS | Attention deficit disorder<br>Narcolepsy | Anxiety<br>Hypertension<br>Insomnia<br>Tachycardia<br>Weight loss |
| Methylphenidate (Ritalin) | Facilitates neurotransmitter release in the CNS | Attention deficit disorder<br>Narcolepsy | Anxiety<br>Hypertension<br>Insomnia<br>Tachycardia<br>Weight loss |

*CNS*, Central nervous system; *GABA*, γ-aminobutyric acid; *GI*, gastrointestinal; *5-HT*, 5-hydroxytryptamine; *OCD*, obsessive-compulsive disorder.

# QUESTIONS

## QUESTION 1
Which of the following symptoms are likely to be present in a patient with panic disorder?

A  Chest pain and palpitations

B  Shortness of breath and cough

C  Gastric reflux and heartburn

D  Headache and blurry vision

E  Vomiting and diarrhea

## QUESTION 2
Which of the following laboratory findings would most likely be due to alcohol consumption?

A  High glucose

B  High MCV

C  Low GGT

D  Low amylase

E  Low bilirubin

## QUESTION 3
A patient who demonstrates a pattern of excessive attention seeking and emotionality would be diagnosed with which of the following personality disorders?

A  Histrionic

B  Dependent

C  Self-defeating

D  Passive-aggressive

E  Obsessive-compulsive

## QUESTION 4
A 20-year-old patient presents with a 9-month history of poor social skills and social withdrawing. Also noted are hallucinations and delusions. After antipsychotics, which of the following is critical to the long-term management of this patient?

A  Self-help group therapy

B  Psychosocial therapy

C  Electroshock therapy

D  Biofeedback therapy

E  Aversion therapy

*Continued*

## QUESTIONS—cont'd

### QUESTION 5
Which of the following medications is used in the treatment of schizophrenia?
A Lamotrigine (Lamictal)
B Bupropion (Wellbutrin)
C Fluoxetine (Prozac)
D Risperidone (Risperdal)
E Clonazepam (Klonopin)

### QUESTION 6
Which of the following medications should not be taken with consumption of aged cheeses and meats?
A Serotonin-norepinephrine reuptake inhibitors
B Selective serotonin reuptake inhibitor
C Monoamine oxidase inhibitor
D Tricyclic antidepressant
E Neuroleptic

### QUESTION 7
Which of the following metabolic abnormalities is most commonly noted in patients with anorexia nervosa?
A Hypokalemia
B Hyponatremia
C Respiratory alkalosis
D Hypermagnesemia
E Hypercalcemia

### QUESTION 8
A 54-year-old female presents 3 weeks after witnessing a car hit a pedestrian in the street. She has had trouble sleeping and continues to have nightmares about the accident. She has avoided driving her own car since the event. She endorses feeling detached and uninvolved in daily activities. Which of the following is the most likely diagnosis?
A Posttraumatic stress disorder
B Major depressive disorder
C Acute stress disorder
D Normal grief
E Dysthymia

### QUESTION 9
Which of the following medications used in smoking cessation works by blocking the action of nicotine on the appropriate receptor?
A Bupropion (Zyban)
B Varenicline (Chantix)
C Clonidine (Catapres)
D Naltrexone (Vivitrol)
E Fomepizole (Antizol)

### QUESTION 10
Which of the following personality disorders is characterized by a yearning to be cared for and a clinging behavior?
A Dependent
B Narcissistic
C Borderline
D Avoidant
E Schizoid

## ANSWERS

1. A
EXPLANATION: *DSM-5* criteria for panic attacks include palpitations, sweating, shaking, shortness of breath, chest pain, dizziness, and a feeling of unreality or fear of losing control. ***Topic: Anxiety disorders***
☐ Correct  ☐ Incorrect

2. B
EXPLANATION: Common laboratory changes in patients with alcohol dependence include elevated MCV, elevated serum GGT, and elevated HDL. ***Topic: Alcohol use***
☐ Correct  ☐ Incorrect

3. A
EXPLANATION: Histrionic personality disorder is characterized by excessive and superficial emotionality and the need to be the center of attention. ***Topic: Personality disorders***
☐ Correct  ☐ Incorrect

## ANSWERS—cont'd

**4.  B**

EXPLANATION: Schizophrenia is most common in patients in their 20s, and people with schizophrenia present with at least a 6-month history of abnormal premorbid functioning, hallucinations, and delusions. Treatment consists of antipsychotic medications and psychosocial therapy, such as psychotherapy and skills training. *Topic: Schizophrenia*

☐ Correct   ☐ Incorrect

**5.  D**

EXPLANATION: Treatment of schizophrenia consists of antipsychotic drugs, such as perphenazine, risperidone, and olanzapine. *Topic: Schizophrenia*

☐ Correct   ☐ Incorrect

**6.  C**

EXPLANATION: MAOIs inhibit the catabolism of dietary amines. When foods containing tyramine (aged cheeses and meats) are consumed, the patient may suffer from hypertensive crisis. *Topic: Mood disorders*

☐ Correct   ☐ Incorrect

**7.  A**

EXPLANATION. Eating disorders can lead to a number of medical complications, including hypokalemia, metabolic acidosis or alkalosis, and anemia. *Topic: Anorexia nervosa*

☐ Correct   ☐ Incorrect

**8.  C**

EXPLANATION: Acute stress disorder is characterized by symptoms similar to PTSD that occur after a traumatic event lasting for 3 to 30 days. *Topic: Trauma and stressor-related disorders*

☐ Correct   ☐ Incorrect

**9.  B**

EXPLANATION: Varenicline is used in smoking cessation and works by blocking the action of nicotine on the appropriate nicotine receptor. *Topic: Tobacco use*

☐ Correct   ☐ Incorrect

**10.  A**

EXPLANATION: Dependent personality disorder is characterized by extreme dependence on others, yearning to be cared for, clinging behavior, and living in fear of separation. *Topic: Personality disorders*

☐ Correct   ☐ Incorrect

# CHAPTER 11
# DERMATOLOGIC SYSTEM

## EXAMINATION BLUEPRINT TOPICS

**ACNEIFORM LESIONS**

Acne vulgaris

Folliculitis

Rosacea

**DESQUAMATION**

Erythema multiforme

Stevens-Johnson syndrome

Toxic epidermal necrolysis

**DISEASES/DISORDERS OF THE HAIR AND NAILS**

Alopecia areata

Androgenetic alopecia

Onychomycosis

Paronychia

**SPIDER BITES**

Black widow and brown recluse spiders

**EXANTHEMS**

Hand-foot-and-mouth disease

**INFECTIOUS DISEASE**

**BACTERIAL**

Cellulitis

Erysipelas (St. Anthony's Fire)

Impetigo

**FUNGAL**

Candidiasis

Tinea versicolor

Tinea corporis

Tinea pedis

**PARASITIC**

Lice

Scabies

**VIRAL**

Condyloma acuminatum (venereal warts)

Herpes simplex

Molluscum contagiosum

Varicella-zoster virus infections (shingles)

Verrucae (warts)

**KERATOTIC DISORDERS**

Actinic keratosis (AK)

Seborrheic keratosis

**NEOPLASMS**

Basal cell carcinoma

Kaposi's sarcoma

Melanoma

Squamous cell carcinoma

**ECZEMATIC AND PAPULOSQUAMOUS DISORDERS**

**ECZEMATOUS DISORDERS**

Eczema

Contact dermatitis

Nummular eczematous dermatitis

Perioral dermatitis

Seborrheic dermatitis

Dyshidrotic eczema (pompholyx)

Lichen simplex chronicus

**PAPULOSQUAMOUS DISORDERS**

Drug eruptions

Lichen planus

Pityriasis rosea

Psoriasis

**PIGMENT DISORDERS**

Melasma

Vitiligo

**SKIN INTEGRITY**

Burns

Decubitus ulcers

Stasis dermatitis

**VASCULAR ABNORMALITIES**

Cherry angioma

Telangiectasia

**VESICULOBULLOUS DISEASE**

Pemphigoid

Pemphigus

**OTHER DERMATOLOGIC DISORDERS**

Acanthosis nigricans

Hidradenitis suppurative (acne inversa)

Lipomas

Epidermal inclusion cysts (epidermoid cysts)

Photosensitivity reactions

Pilonidal disease

Urticaria (hives)

---

## ACNEIFORM LESIONS

### I. ACNE VULGARIS
    a. **General**
        i. One of the most common skin disorders.
        ii. Common between ages 10 and 15 years and lasts 5 to 10 years.
        iii. Disease due to epidermal sloughing, increased sebum production, growth of sebaceous glands, and increased concentrations of *Propionibacterium acnes*.
        iv. Other etiologies include polycystic ovarian syndrome (PCOS) and medications, such as glucocorticoids, phenytoin, lithium, and isoniazid.

b. **Clinical Manifestations**
  i. Two types of lesions.
   1. Inflammatory.
    (a) Consist of papules (<5 mm in diameter), pustules (central core of purulent material), and nodules/cysts (>5 mm in diameter).
   2. Noninflammatory.
    (a) Consist of open (blackheads) and closed (whiteheads) comedones.
   3. See Color Plate 5.
  ii. Disease severity based on number of lesions.
   1. Table 11.1 shows grading criteria.
c. **Diagnosis**
  i. Based on history and clinical findings.
d. **Treatment**
  i. Treatment is continual, not curative.
   1. Therapy should take into account medical and psychosocial issues.
   2. Response to therapy requires 6 to 8 weeks. Follow-up visits should be planned accordingly for compliance with treatment.
   3. Treatment is usually considered "set-up" in nature.
  ii. Treatment varies with type of lesions and severity of disease.
   1. Comedones.
    (a) Use agents that cause mild drying and peeling, including the following:
     (i) Benzoyl peroxide.
      (1) Side effects include allergic contact dermatitis.
     (ii) Retinoids.
      (1) Include azelaic acid, tretinoin (Retin-A), and tazarotene.
      (2) Side effects include facial dryness and erythema.
      (3) Response to treatment typically occurs within 4 to 6 weeks.
   2. Papules and pustules.
    (a) The above agents that are used for comedones are used along with the following:
     (i) Topical antibiotics.
      (1) Clindamycin.
      (2) Erythromycin.
     (ii) Oral antibiotics.
      (1) Tetracycline.
      (2) Erythromycin.
      (3) Doxycycline.
      (4) Minocycline.
     (iii) Antibiotics must be taken for 6 to 8 weeks before evaluation of treatment success, and then must be tapered to the lowest possible dose to keep the skin clear.
     (iv) Must use topical therapy in conjunction with oral antibiotics to prevent antibiotic resistance.
   3. Nodules and cysts.
    (a) Isotretinoin (Accutane) is very effective.
     (i) Related to vitamin A.
     (ii) A potent teratogen and induces an elevation in triglycerides.
     (iii) Therapy is typically 16 to 20 weeks in length.
    (b) Triamcinolone, a steroid, can be injected into the cysts.
    (c) Prednisone is used if Accutane causes an initial flare but is not indicated for any usual acne treatment.
     (i) Patients should be on an oral retinoid if oral steroids are used.
  iii. Hormonal treatment includes the following:
   1. Oral contraceptives (estrogen plus progestin).
   2. Spironolactone.

## II. FOLLICULITIS
a. **General**
  i. Infection and inflammation of the follicular unit.
  ii. A number of different types.
   1. Mechanical: results from persistent trauma.
   2. Bacterial.
    (a) Can be spread by trauma, scratching, and shaving.
    (b) Most common cause is *S. aureus* infection.
    (c) *Pseudomonas* is indicated in "hot-tub folliculitis."
   3. Fungal.
  iii. A furuncle (boil) is an infection of a hair follicle with purulent material from the dermis into subcutaneous tissue.
  iv. A carbuncle is a group of inflamed follicles into a single mass with purulent drainage.
b. **Clinical Manifestations**
  i. Present with dome-shaped pustules with erythematous halos in the follicle.

**TABLE 11.1**

| Acne Severity Grading | | |
| --- | --- | --- |
| **Severity** | **Papules/Pustules** | **Nodules** |
| Mild | Few to several | None |
| Moderate | Several to many | Few to several |
| Severe | Many and/or extensive | Many |

ii. Lesions may be tender and may itch.

iii. Typically no systemic symptoms.

c. **Diagnosis**

i. Based on history and clinical findings.

d. **Treatment**

i. Predisposing factors must be eliminated and can be discovered through a comprehensive history. Discontinue use of topical steroids to the area and all over-the-counter (OTC) medications previously applied to the affected area.

ii. Mupirocin (Bactroban) can be used for superficial disease.

1. Does not have activity against *Pseudomonas*.

iii. Oral antistaphylococcal antibiotics are indicated for extensive or spreading disease.

1. Antibiotics include oxacillin, dicloxacillin, and cefuroxime.

## III. ROSACEA

a. **General**

i. A chronic inflammatory acneiform disorder.

ii. Typically affects females more than males, and age of onset is typically after age 30.

iii. Symptoms wax and wane with variation and intensity in each patient.

iv. Cause is unknown.

1. No comedones are noted.

b. **Clinical Manifestations**

i. Intermittent flushing erythema and recurrent appearance of papules, pustules, and telangiectasia.

ii. Noted mainly on cheeks, nose, brow, and chin.

iii. Patients may note burning and itching.

iv. Can progress to rhinophyma, a bulbous appearance of the nose due to sebaceous hyperplasia.

c. **Diagnosis**

i. Based on history and clinical findings.

d. **Treatment**

i. Avoidance of triggers is the mainstay of treatment; hot beverages, hot/cold weather changes, spicy foods, or psychological stress can induce flares.

ii. Maintenance therapy is with the following topical antibiotics: metronidazole, sulfacetamide, clindamycin.

iii. Oral antibiotics are used in severe cases, tetracycline, Bactrim, and minocycline.

# DESQUAMATION

## I. ERYTHEMA MULTIFORME

a. **General**

i. A common, acute inflammatory disease.

ii. Often associated with herpes simplex virus (HSV), *M. pneumoniae*, and medications (NSAIDs, sulfonamides, antiepileptics, and antibiotics).

b. **Clinical Manifestations**

i. Characterized by many different lesions, including target-shaped skin lesions, erythematous macules and papules, urticaria-like lesions, vesicles, and bullae. (See Color Plate 6.)

ii. Targetoid lesions are dusky red, round papules and macules that may itch.

1. Lesions are 1 to 3 cm in size with a central dark red area surrounded by a pale edematous area.

iii. Appear on the acral areas, which are the palms, soles, and dorsal aspects of the hands and feet. Lesions also occur on the extensor surfaces of the forearms and legs.

c. **Diagnosis**

i. Based on history and clinical findings.

d. **Treatment**

i. Typically resolves within 1 month.

ii. Avoidance of offending agent(s).

iii. Pruritus is managed with topical steroids if needed.

## II. STEVENS-JOHNSON SYNDROME

a. **General**

i. A severe blistering mucocutaneous syndrome, involving at least two mucous membranes.

ii. More common in young adults and children.

iii. Associated with *Mycoplasma pneumoniae* and cytomegalovirus (CMV) infections and drugs, such as allopurinol, phenytoin, phenobarbital, sulfonamides, and aminopenicillins.

b. **Clinical Manifestations**

i. Acutely have erythematous papules, dusky-appearing vesicles, and target lesions.

1. Involves less than 10% to 15% of the body surface area (BSA).

ii. Lesions typically noted on the trunk and face, including the oral mucosa.

iii. Oral, genital, and perianal mucosa often develop bullae and erosions.

iv. Lesions may become eroded, and secondary infections may occur.

v. Patients often note skin to be tender and burning.

c. **Diagnosis**

i. Based on history and clinical findings.

ii. Skin biopsy shows full-thickness epidermal necrosis sparing the dermis. Disruption is in the dermal-epidermal junction.

d. **Treatment**

   i. Uncomplicated cases typically resolve within 1 month.

   ii. Treatment focuses on removing the offending agent, and maintaining nutritional and fluid requirements.

   iii. Children have a slightly better prognosis than adults.

   iv. Mortality is about 5% to 10%.

## III. TOXIC EPIDERMAL NECROLYSIS

a. **General**

   i. Rare, life-threatening disease with widespread blistering and sloughing of skin.

     1. Involves greater than 30% of BSA.

   ii. Typically related to drug ingestion, recent immunization, viral infection, *Mycoplasma* infection, streptococcal infection, or syphilis.

     1. Common precipitating drugs include the following:

       (a) Sulfonamides.

       (b) Antimalarials.

       (c) Anticonvulsants.

       (d) Nonsteroidal antiinflammatory drugs (NSAIDs).

       (e) Allopurinol.

b. **Clinical Manifestations**

   i. Present with a diffuse, erythematous, sun-burned appearance, with scattered target lesions and bullae in no specific distribution.

   ii. Bullae join together and result in widespread skin sloughing.

   iii. Gentle pressure easily produces epidermal detachment, leaving a tender, glistening, raw surface.

c. **Diagnosis**

   i. Based on history and clinical findings.

   ii. Skin biopsy reveals a full-thickness necrotic epidermis.

d. **Treatment**

   i. Overall mortality rate is 40% to 50%.

   ii. Treatment focuses on pain control, removal of possible offending agent(s), maintaining fluid balance, and local wound care.

   iii. Patients should wear a medical alert bracelet indicating their reaction if a triggering agent is identified.

# DISEASES/DISORDERS OF THE HAIR AND NAILS

## I. ALOPECIA AREATA

a. **General**

   i. Nonscarring hair loss of rapid onset and in a sharply defined area.

   ii. A chronic, autoimmune condition due to T-cell–mediated inflammation that disrupts the normal hair cycle.

   iii. Most common in children and young adults with onset frequently before age 30 years.

   iv. Associated with thyroid disease and vitiligo.

b. **Clinical Manifestations**

   i. The pattern of hair loss is patchy.

     1. Areas of hair loss are typically 1 to 4 cm in size and smooth, circular, discrete areas of complete hair loss.

   ii. Skin is very smooth or may have short stubs of hair.

     1. Remaining hair is described as having an "exclamation point" appearance as the shaft is fractured distally and tapers toward the scalp.

   iii. Superficial nail pitting or nail fragility (trachyonychia) may be present.

c. **Diagnosis**

   i. Based on history and clinical findings.

d. **Treatment**

   i. Most hair regrows, and treatment is not needed.

   ii. If treatment is needed, intradermal triamcinolone or topical immunotherapy can be used with varying response rates.

   iii. It can progress to alopecia totalis, which should prompt evaluation for additional autoimmune processes.

## II. ANDROGENETIC ALOPECIA

a. **General**

   i. A common, genetically predetermined form of hair loss found in both men and women.

     1. In men, it is often called "male-patterned baldness."

   ii. Typically begins after puberty and is fully expressed by the time the patient is in their mid-40s.

b. **Clinical Manifestations**

   i. Hair loss occurs in a well-defined pattern, characteristically beginning above the temples bilaterally.

   ii. This progresses to a receding hairline, resulting in an 'M' shape of remaining hair.

   iii. Later, total hair loss is noted in the central scalp.

   iv. The exposed scalp is typically smooth and shiny in appearance.

c. **Diagnosis**

   i. Based on history and clinical findings.

d. **Treatment**

   i. Topical minoxidil (Rogaine).

     1. Promotes hair growth by increasing anagen (growth phase of hair), shortening telogen

(resting phase when hair lost), and enlarging follicles.

2. Regrowth takes 8 to 12 months.
3. Rare side effects include contact and irritant dermatitis.
4. It can subsequently be used for management of hypertension.

ii. Oral finasteride (Propecia).
1. Works by blocking 5-alpha-reductase, thereby inhibiting conversion of testosterone to dihydrotestosterone (DHT).
2. Side effects include decreased libido and erectile dysfunction.
3. It should not be used by females due to the risk of teratogenicity secondary to the conversion of testosterone to DHT, resulting in defects in male genital development in utero.

iii. Hair transplantation.

## III. ONYCHOMYCOSIS
a. **General**
   i. A fungal infection (tinea) of the nail plate.
   ii. Risk factors include older age, swimming, tinea pedis, psoriasis, and diabetes mellitus.

b. **Clinical Manifestations**
   i. Four clinical patterns are observed.
   1. Distal subungual.
      (a) Distal plate appears yellow or white, and the nail rises and separates from the underlying bed.
   2. White superficial.
      (a) The nail is soft, dry, and powdery.
      (b) The nail plate is not thickened and remains adherent to the bed.
   3. Proximal subungual.
      (a) The surface of the nail plate remains intact, but hyperkeratotic debris causes the nail to separate.
      (b) Relatively uncommon compared to other clinical patterns.
   4. *Candida*.
      (a) Nail plate is thick and turns yellow to brown.

c. **Diagnosis**
   i. Potassium hydroxide (KOH) examination.
   1. Hyphae and/or arthrospores are present.
   ii. Fungal culture.
   iii. Histopathological examination of nail clippings.

d. **Treatment**
   i. Systemic antifungal agents are more effective than topical agents.
   ii. Antifungal agents include the following:
   1. Terbinafine.

2. Itraconazole.
3. Fluconazole.
4. Griseofulvin.

iii. Topical and systemic agents are used for 6 weeks for fingernails and 12 weeks for toenails.

## IV. PARONYCHIA
a. **General**
   i. A bacterial or fungal infection of the proximal and/or lateral nail fold.
   ii. It can be an acute or chronic disease.
   1. Acute infection is due to trauma and manipulation.
      (a) Infection due to *S. aureus* and *Streptococcus pyogenes*.
   2. Chronic infection is due to contact irritant exposure.
      (a) Infection due to *Candida* species.

b. **Clinical Manifestations**
   i. In acute infection, the patient presents with nail pain and swelling, typically of a single nail.
   1. Pus accumulates behind the cuticle or deeper in the lateral nail folds.
   ii. In chronic infection, many or all fingers are involved.
   1. Tenderness, erythema, and mild swelling may be noted.
   2. The nail plate is distorted but uninfected.

c. **Diagnosis**
   i. Diagnosis is based on clinical findings and history of trauma to the digits or nail folds.

d. **Treatment**
   i. Acute infection is treated with local care (warm compresses or soaks) and antistaphylococcal antibiotics.
   1. Incision and drainage may be necessary.
   2. Prevention of recurrent trauma and maintenance of normal cuticles is helpful to prevent recurrence.
   ii. Chronic disease is treated with local care and topical corticosteroids.

# SPIDER BITES

## I. BLACK WIDOW AND BROWN RECLUSE SPIDERS
a. **General**
   i. Spider bites are common; however, of the 50 species of spiders in the United States, only the black widow and brown recluse spider produce severe reactions.
   ii. Black widow spider is 3 to 4 cm in length and has a red hourglass-shaped marking on the ventral surface of the abdomen.

1. Disease is due to the envenomation of a neurotoxin.
2. Black widow spiders are typically encountered near woodpiles, logs, or barns or in shoes.
iii. Brown recluse spider is 1.5 cm in length; is yellow, tan, or brown; and has a dark-brown, violin-shaped marking on its thorax.
   1. Typically noted in the south central United States and found in woodpiles, attics, garages, and basements.
b. **Clinical Manifestations**
   i. Black widow spider bites typically reveal mild erythema or swelling at the bite site.
      1. A local hive-like reaction followed by cyanosis and expanding necrosis may occur.
   ii. Brown recluse spider bites present with local pain and burning due to vasospasm.
c. **Diagnosis**
   i. Based on clinical findings and having a high degree of suspicion.
d. **Treatment**
   i. Black widow spider bites are treated with ice to restrict the spread of venom.
      1. Antivenom can be given for acute symptoms if available.
   ii. Brown recluse spider bites are treated with supportive care.
      1. Red-brown fang marks may be noted at the site of the lesion.
      2. Severe reactions can present with cramping abdominal pain, hypertension, muscle complaints, irritability, and agitation.
      3. Systemic symptoms can include fever, chills, vomiting, weakness, and muscle and joint pain.
      4. With severe necrosis, local wound care and antibiotics are needed.

# EXANTHEMS

## I. HAND-FOOT-AND-MOUTH DISEASE
a. **General**
   i. A common, highly contagious illness caused by coxsackievirus A16.
   ii. Fecal oral transmission.
   iii. Common in young children in daycare centers and schools.
b. **Clinical Manifestations**
   i. Patients have an initial prodrome of fever, malaise, and throat pain.
   ii. Rash presents as small vesicles on a small erythematous base.
   iii. Vesicles rupture, creating ulcers surrounded by erythema.

iv. The rash is typically found on the oral mucosa as well as the hands and feet (including the palms and soles), but can also spread to the genitals and surrounding skin.
c. **Diagnosis**
   i. Typically a clinical diagnosis.
   ii. Light microscopy of vesicle biopsy can be used to differentiate HFM from other vesicular rashes.
d. **Treatment**
   i. Management is primarily supportive in nature.
   ii. NSAIDs can be used to manage fever and any associated pain.
   iii. Hydration status should be monitored as patients often refuse oral intake secondary to pain.

# INFECTIOUS DISEASE

## BACTERIAL

### I. CELLULITIS
a. **General**
   i. Infection of the deep dermis and subcutaneous tissue.
   ii. Increased risk in patients with diabetes mellitus, cirrhosis, renal failure, malnutrition, cancer, or history of IV drug use.
b. **Clinical Manifestations**
   i. Present with fever, chills, malaise, erythema, edema, and pain.
   ii. On examination, an expanding red, swollen, tender, or painful plaque or patch with an ill-defined, nonpalpable border.
   iii. Regional lymphadenopathy may occur.
c. **Diagnosis**
   i. Laboratory tests reveal leukocytosis.
   ii. Most often caused by group A *Streptococcus* and *S. aureus*.
      1. Other agents include the following:
         (a) *Erysipelothrix rhusiopathiae*: most common among fish handlers, butchers, and farmers.
         (b) *Aeromonas hydrophila*: most common after swimming in fresh water.
         (c) *Vibrio* species: most common after swimming in salt water.
         (d) *Pasteurella multocida*: most common after animal bite or scratch.
d. **Treatment**
   i. Empiric antibiotic therapy should be directed against staphylococcal and streptococcal organisms.
      1. Antibiotic choices include the following:
         (a) Penicillinase-resistant penicillin (dicloxacillin).

(b) Clindamycin.

(c) First-generation cephalosporin (cephalexin).

(d) Azithromycin or clarithromycin.

(e) Amoxicillin.

## II. ERYSIPELAS (ST. ANTHONY'S FIRE)

a. **General**

i. Infection of the dermis with lymphatic involvement.

ii. *S. pyogenes* is the most common etiologic agent, followed by *S. aureus*, *Pneumococcus*, *Klebsiella pneumoniae*, and *Yersinia enterocolitica*.

iii. Affects the very young, the very old, and the debilitated, and those with a history of lymphedema or chronic cutaneous ulcers.

iv. Incidence of erysipelas is higher in the summer months and has increased dramatically since the 1980s.

b. **Clinical Manifestations**

i. Onset is sudden with prodromal symptoms of malaise, fever, chills, nausea, and myalgias.

ii. Adenopathy and lymphangitis may also occur.

iii. One or more red, tender, and firm spots that rapidly increase in size.

1. Form a tense, deeply erythematous, hot, sharply demarcated, elevated, shiny patch.

iv. Most commonly located on the lower leg.

v. Red, painful streaks of lymphangitis may or may not be noted extending toward regional lymph nodes.

c. **Diagnosis**

i. Based on clinical findings.

ii. White blood cell count is elevated with a left shift.

d. **Treatment**

i. Antibiotic options include penicillin V, amoxicillin, azithromycin, or clarithromycin.

ii. If systemic signs such as fever and chills, need IV antibiotics such as ceftriaxone or cefazolin.

## III. IMPETIGO

a. **General**

i. Primarily affects children and is a common, contagious, superficial skin infection.

ii. Produced by *S. aureus* or group A beta-hemolytic *Streptococcus*.

iii. Transmission is by skin-skin contact.

iv. Predisposing factors are warm temperatures, high humidity, and poor hygiene.

b. **Clinical Manifestations**

i. Lesions most commonly noted on the face.

ii. Two forms: bullous and nonbullous.

1. Bullous.

(a) Commonly occurs in young children.

(b) Associated with weakness, fever, and diarrhea.

(c) Vesicles may occur on the face, trunk, buttocks, perineum, or extremities.

(d) Vesicles enlarge into flaccid, translucent bullae that can be as large as 5 cm, and can easily rupture leaving a shiny, dry erosion.

(e) Bullous impetigo heals quicker than nonbullous impetigo.

2. Nonbullous.

(a) Accounts for 70% of all cases of impetigo.

(b) Appearance of a 2- to 4-mm erythematous macule that evolves into a vesicle or pustule.

(c) Results in a superficial erosion with the "honey-colored crust" as the end result.

(d) Occurs on the face, around the nose and mouth, and on the extremities.

(e) 5% of nonbullous impetigo is caused by *S. pyogenes*.

3. See Color Plate 7.

c. **Diagnosis**

i. Based on clinical findings.

d. **Treatment**

i. Mupirocin ointment or cream (Bactroban) is used for limited, localized infection.

ii. Severe infections are treated concurrently with topical mupirocin and oral antibiotics.

1. Dicloxacillin, cephalexin, or clindamycin.

iii. Local cleansing, removal of crusts, and application of wet dressings are important.

iv. Recurrent infections require evaluation of nasal and/or perineal carriage of *S. aureus*.

# FUNGAL

## I. CANDIDIASIS

a. **General**

i. Inflammatory condition of two closely opposed skin surfaces.

ii. Superficial infection due to *Candida*.

iii. Risk factors include obesity, occlusive clothing, incontinence, diabetes, use of glucocorticoids, HIV, and chemotherapy.

b. **Clinical Manifestations**

i. Presents as erythematous, macerated plaques and erosions with peripheral scaling and erythematous satellite lesions.

ii. Common locations include inguinal folds, axillae, scrotum, intergluteal folds, web spaces of digits, and abdominal folds.

**c. Diagnosis**

　i. Potassium hydroxide (KOH) prep reveals budding yeast.

**d. Treatment**

　i. Ameliorate predisposing factors.

　ii. Topical antifungals include nystatin, miconazole, clotrimazole, and ketoconazole.

## II. TINEA VERSICOLOR

**a. General**

　i. Infection caused by the yeast, *Malassezia (Pityrosporum)*.

　　1. Part of normal skin flora.

　　2. Increased risk for infection with excess heat and humidity and with oily skin.

**b. Clinical Manifestations**

　i. Present with many small, circular, tan–to-pink, scaling papules on the upper trunk.

　ii. Hypopigmentation is common and symptoms may become more apparent in the summer months.

**c. Diagnosis**

　i. Based on history and clinical findings.

　ii. Potassium hydroxide (KOH) examination of the scales reveals hyphae and round spores, a "spaghetti and meatballs" pattern.

　iii. Wood's lamp reveals a yellow to yellow-green fluorescence.

**d. Treatment**

　i. Topical treatments include the following:

　　1. Selenium sulfide lotion.

　　2. Ketoconazole shampoo.

　　3. Miconazole, clotrimazole, or econazole.

　ii. Oral antifungals may also be helpful.

## III. TINEA CORPORIS

**a. General**

　i. Dermatophyte infection of the body.

　　1. Dermatophytes infect and survive only in dead keratin (stratum corneum, hair, and nails).

　ii. Epidemics occur among wrestlers through direct contact as well as contact with the mat.

　iii. There are three dermatophytes.

　　1. *Microsporum*.

　　2. *Trichophyton*.

　　3. *Epidermophyton*.

**b. Clinical Manifestations**

　i. Two patterns.

　　1. Round annular lesions (ringworm).

　　　(a) Begin as flat, scaly papules that slowly develop a raised border.

　　　(b) Central area becomes brown or hypopigmented.

　　　(c) Extend in all directions.

　　2. Deep inflammatory lesions.

　　　(a) Round, inflamed, elevated lesion with a red, boggy, pustular surface.

　　　(b) Due to infection that extends into the hair follicle.

**c. Diagnosis**

　i. Potassium hydroxide examination reveals hyphae.

　ii. Culture may be needed to identify specific organisms, but this is often not necessary to initiate treatment.

**d. Treatment**

　i. Antifungal cream (terbinafine, clotrimazole, miconazole) for at least 1 week after resolution of the infection.

　ii. Oral antifungals may be needed for severe or resistant cases.

　　1. Griseofulvin.

　　2. Itraconazole.

　　3. Fluconazole.

## IV. TINEA PEDIS

**a. General**

　i. The most common area infected by dermatophytes.

　ii. Also known as athlete's foot.

　iii. Common in young and middle-aged adults.

　iv. More common in males than in females.

　v. Predisposing factors include shoe wearing creating a warm, moist environment; locker room floors; and communal baths.

**b. Clinical Manifestations**

　i. Three classic presentations.

　　1. Interdigital.

　　　(a) Web space is dry, scaly, and fissured.

　　　(b) Itching is profuse.

　　2. Chronic scaling of the plantar surface.

　　　(a) Entire sole is covered with fine, silvery-white scales.

　　　(b) Itching is profuse.

　　3. Acute vesicular.

　　　(a) Present with pruritic sterile vesicles that are due to an allergic response to the fungus.

**c. Diagnosis**

　i. Potassium hydroxide examination reveals fungal elements.

**d. Treatment**

　i. Topical medications include terbinafine or naftifine.

　ii. Acute vesicular responds to Burow's wet dressings several times a day with topical antifungal creams.

　iii. Oral or topical antifungal agents may be needed.

**d. Table 11.2 summarizes tinea infections**

**TABLE 11.2**

| Tinea Infections | |
|---|---|
| **Body Location** | **Name** |
| Beard | Tinea barbae |
| Body | Tinea corporis |
| Face | Tinea faciei |
| Foot | Tinea pedis |
| Groin | Tinea cruris |
| Hand | Tinea manuum |
| Nails | Onychomycosis |
| Scalp | Tinea capitis |

# PARASITIC

### I. LICE
  **a. General**
    i. Lice are flat, wingless insects that infest the hair of the scalp, body, and pubic region.
      1. *Pediculus humanus capitis* infects the head.
      2. *Pediculus humanus corporis* causes body lice.
      3. *Phthirus pubis* infects the pubic hair.
    ii. Attached to the skin, feed off human blood, and lay nits on the hair shaft.
      1. Nits are the white, hard, oval lice eggs.
    iii. Transmission via close personal contact or contact with hats, hair brushes, or combs.
    iv. They require a human host for survival.
  **b. Clinical Manifestations**
    i. Lice are 3 to 4 mm in length and can be seen on the scalp and hair shafts.
    ii. Nits are small white eggs attached to the hair shaft.
      1. These can be differentiated from dandruff as they are not easily brushed away from the hair shaft.
    iii. Lice feces can be seen on the skin as small, rust-colored flecks.
    iv. Pruritus is common and bacterial infection secondary to excoriations may occur.
    v. Posterior cervical adenopathy may be noted.
  **c. Diagnosis**
    i. Based on identification of the lice or nits.
  **d. Treatment**
    i. Topical treatments.
      1. Permethrin (Elimite).
      2. Lindane (Kwell).
        (a) It can cause neurotoxicity and possible seizures and is not recommended for use in treating lice.
      3. Malathion (Ovide).

      (a) Contraindicated for neonates and infants due to increased scalp permeability and subsequent drug absorption.
      4. Treatment should be repeated in 1 week.
      5. All household contacts must be treated along with the patient.
    ii. Oral treatments for refractory cases.
      1. Ivermectin.
        (a) Repeat in 10 days.
    iii. Manual nit removal.
      1. This step is essential and requires a specific nit comb.
    iv. Infested clothing and bedding should be washed in hot water.

### II. SCABIES
  **a. General**
    i. Caused by *Sarcoptes scabiei* var. *hominis*.
      1. The mite is 3 mm long and has a flattened, oval body with eight legs.
    ii. It is very contagious.
  **b. Clinical Manifestations**
    i. Patient presents with severe itching that is typically worse at night.
    ii. Classic lesion is a burrow that is linear, curved, or S-shaped and is a slightly elevated vesicle or papule.
      1. Commonly found in the finger webs, wrists, sides of hands and feet, penis, buttocks, and scrotum.
    iii. Rash appears about 3 to 6 weeks after exposure.
  **c. Diagnosis**
    i. Clinical suspicion based on history.
    ii. Microscopic identification of mite, mite eggs, or feces from skin lesions.
  **d. Treatment**
    i. Permethrin (Elimite) can be applied to the skin from the neck down and repeated in 1 week.
      1. Permethrin is preferred in children.
      2. Lindane (Kwell) can cause neurotoxicity and possible seizures and is not recommended for use in treating scabies.
    ii. Oral ivermectin can be used in most patients and should be repeated in 2 weeks.
    iii. All clothes and bedding should be washed in hot water to kill mites and eggs.

# VIRAL

### I. CONDYLOMA ACUMINATUM (VENEREAL WARTS)
  **a. General**
    i. Infection of the genital or anal skin by human papillomavirus (HPV).

1. Genital warts are most commonly caused by HPV 6 and 11.
   ii. Warts spread rapidly over moist areas.
   iii. Risk factors include multiple sexual partners, history of sexually transmitted infection (STI), and immunosuppression.

b. **Clinical Manifestations**
   i. The lesions are asymptomatic and patients may not know they are present.
      1. Some patients may note pruritus, bleeding, and burning.
   ii. Lesion appearance will vary from person to person.
   iii. Lesions may be pale pink to white, rough, barely raised papules or have projections on a broad base.
   iv. Lesion surface may be smooth, velvety, and moist and lack the hyperkeratosis.
   v. Lesions may coalesce and form a large, cauliflower-like mass.

c. **Diagnosis**
   i. Based on clinical findings.
      1. Acetic acid applied to the wart will cause most lesions to turn white or blanch and can be a helpful screening tool.

d. **Treatment**
   i. First-line treatment for genital warts is topical imiquimod.
   ii. Liquid nitrogen cryotherapy can be performed.
      1. Treatment may be painful and may cause scarring.
   iii. Electrocautery and curettage can be used for a few isolated lesions.
   iv. Podofilox can be used for external genital warts.
      1. Adverse effects include pain, burning, and inflammation.
   v. Condoms may reduce, but not eliminate, transmission to partners.
   vi. HPV infection increases the risk for cervical, anal, and oropharyngeal cancer.

## II. HERPES SIMPLEX

a. **General**
   i. Transmission is almost always due to direct contact with infected secretions.
      1. Humans are the only natural reservoirs.
      2. Transmission can occur with viral shedding when vesicles are not visible.
   ii. Infection is both acute and latent.
      1. Acute infection is manifested by onset of a prodrome of tingling or burning followed by painful burning vesicles that

rupture to cause ulcerations, followed by scabbing.
      (a) Giant cells can be seen in fluid from the vesicles.
      (b) Once infected, the virus remains in a latent state, but latent infection can result in recurrent outbreaks in the same location.
      2. Recurrent infection can be triggered by fever, trauma, and exposure to ultraviolet light.
      (a) Recurrent outbreaks tend to be less severe and resolve faster over time.

b. **Clinical Manifestations**
   i. HSV type 1.
      1. Grouped or single vesicular lesions that become pustular and form single or multiple ulcers.
      2. Symptoms typically occur 3 to 7 days after exposure.
      3. Can involve any mucosal surface, but are most common in the oral mucosa.
      4. Lesions are very painful and last for 5 to 10 days.
      5. May become latent within sensory nerve root ganglion.
      6. Recurrences, average four per year, are typically unilateral and last about 7 days.
      7. Herpetic whitlow is HSV infection involving the finger or nail folds.
      8. Herpes gladiatorum is cutaneous herpes in athletes involved in contact sports.
   ii. HSV type 2.
      1. Often called genital herpes.
      2. Incubation period is typically less than 20 days from sexual contact to onset of lesions.
      (a) In some cases, exposure may be years prior to the initial outbreak.
      3. Lesions are small erythematous papules that form into vesicles and then pustules that rupture and ulcerate.
      4. With primary disease, the lesions are painful, multiple, and extensive.
      (a) May have systemic symptoms such as fever, headache, and myalgias.
      (b) Symptoms may last 2–4 weeks in the initial outbreak.
      5. Recurrent disease is typically shorter in duration and is localized to the genital region, without systemic symptoms.
      (a) Prodromal paresthesias may be noted 12 to 24 hours before the appearance of the lesions.

**c. Diagnosis**
  i. Can be made by cell culture, Tzanck smear, antibody detection, and polymerase chain reaction (PCR).
    1. Tzanck smear shows multinucleated giant cells.
    2. PCR is the test of choice for diagnosis of HSV encephalitis.
    3. Antibody detection can reveal history of infection but it does not differentiate between acute and chronic disease.

**d. Treatment**
  i. Use of acyclovir, valacyclovir, or famciclovir is indicated.
    1. Intravenous (IV) acyclovir is needed in HSV encephalitis.
  ii. Prophylactic measures include avoidance of contact with HSV-positive secretions and daily antivirals to suppress recurrences.
    1. Antivirals used include acyclovir, famciclovir, and valacyclovir.
  iii. Because of high mortality and morbidity with neonatal HSV infection, cesarean birth should be used to prevent transmission to an infant born from an actively infected mother.
    1. Prophylactic valacyclovir starting at 36 weeks' gestation is often indicated for pregnant mothers where HSV2 antibodies are detected, regardless of presence of symptoms.

## III. MOLLUSCUM CONTAGIOSUM
  **a. General**
    i. Molluscum contagiosum virus is a poxvirus.
      1. Humans are the only known hosts.
    ii. Spread by skin-skin contact. Spreading by fomite-skin is less common, but does occur
    iii. Common in children with atopy.
    iv. In adults, considered a sexually transmitted infection (STI).

  **b. Clinical Manifestations**
    i. Lesions are usually asymptomatic, but may be in an area of pruritus and therefore appear excoriated and inflamed. (See Color Plate 8.)
      1. Can occur anywhere on the body, except for palms of the hands and the soles of the feet.
    ii. Lesions are firm, umbilicated pearly papules with a waxy surface. Number of lesions varies from 1 to greater than 20, they may be condensed to one area or spread across the body, and they are from 2 to 5 mm in diameter.
    iii. Immunocompromised patients will have >100 lesions and are very susceptible to this virus.

**c. Diagnosis**
  i. Based on history and clinical findings.
**d. Treatment**
  i. Lesions may resolve spontaneously in 6 to 9 months, but may take over 12–18 months in some individuals.
  ii. Prior to resolution, lesions may become inflamed and pus-filled before rupturing, bleeding, and scabbing.
    1. This is sometimes referred to as the "BOTE" (beginning of the end) sign.
  iii. Skin-skin contact or sharing of towels or bedding should be avoided.
  iv. Curettage or cryosurgery can be used to remove the central infectious core but may result in scarring; however, ruptured lesions may also result in scarring.
  v. Options for topical agents include cantharidin solution (blistering agent), imiquimod cream (immunomodulator), and tretinoin (retinoid) cream applied directly to the lesion with care to avoid the surrounding skin.

## IV. VARICELLA-ZOSTER VIRUS INFECTIONS (SHINGLES)
  **a. General**
    i. Viral infection of the skin involving a single or multiple dermatomes.
    ii. Results from reactivation of latent varicella zoster virus in the sensory ganglia.
    iii. Increased likelihood of unknown malignancy in patients with zoster as symptoms may arise due to immunosuppression.
    iv. Zoster vaccine (Zostavax) is indicated for patients 60 years and older whether or not they have had a previous outbreak.
      1. It is a live vaccine.
      2. May be given earlier for patients with immunosuppression.
      3. Vaccination is contraindicated during pregnancy.

  **b. Clinical Manifestations**
    i. Systemic symptoms include headache, photophobia, and malaise.
    ii. Prodrome of intense pain, pruritus, and tingling; hyperesthesia occurs in >90% of patients.
    iii. Pain and burning in the affected dermatome may precede rash by 3 to 5 days.
      1. Most common dermatomes involve the thoracic and lumbar regions.
    iv. Grouped vesicles on an erythematous base are presentations of herpes zoster. (See Color Plate 9.)
    v. Vesicles umbilicate or rupture before forming crusts.
      1. Crusts fall off in 2 to 3 weeks.

vi. Ophthalmic zoster.
    1. Involves any branch of the ophthalmic nerve.
    2. Vesicles on the side or tip of the nose (Hutchinson's sign) are associated with corneal involvement.
        (a) Due to involvement of the nasociliary (first) branch of the trigeminal nerve.
    3. Should be treated emergently by an ophthalmologist to prevent permanent vision loss.
vii. Ramsay Hunt syndrome.
    1. Linked to reactivation of latent disease in the geniculate ganglion.
    2. Present with ipsilateral facial paralysis (CN VII), ear pain, and vesicles in the auditory canal and auricle.

**c. Diagnosis**
    i. Based on history and clinical findings.
    ii. Tzanck smear may be positive.

**d. Treatment**
    i. Topical therapy (wet dressings) or oral steroids decrease the acute pain and improve rash resolution.
        1. Oral steroids have no effect on postherpetic neuralgia.
    ii. Oral antiviral agents decrease acute pain, inflammation, and viral shedding.
        1. Most effective if started within the first 48 hours.
        2. Agents include acyclovir, valacyclovir, or famciclovir.
        3. Topical antivirals are not indicated in treatment of herpes zoster.
    iii. Complications.
        1. Postherpetic neuralgia.
            (a) Pain in the associated dermatome persists more than 30 days after the rash.
                (i) Most commonly noted in patients over 60 years of age.
            (b) Pain is severe and intractable.
            (c) Treatment.
                (i) Amitriptyline can be used for prevention.
                (ii) Treatment of acute symptoms consists of oral analgesics, topical lidocaine patch, tricyclic antidepressants, gabapentin, steroids, or topical capsaicin cream.
                (iii) Consultation with a pain management specialist may be needed.

## V. VERRUCAE (WARTS)
**a. General**
    i. There are greater than 150 genotypes of HPV, all which can cause verrucae.

    ii. Transmission is by the following:
        1. Direct skin–skin contact of clinically infected or subclinically infected humans.
        2. Indirectly by contaminated surfaces.
        3. Autoinoculation.

**b. Clinical Manifestations**
    i. Flesh-colored papules evolve into dome-shaped, gray-to-brown, hyperkeratotic, rough papules.
    ii. Common sites include the hands, periungual skin, elbows, knees, and plantar surfaces.

**c. Diagnosis**
    i. Based on clinical findings.
    ii. Biopsy may be needed to rule out squamous cell carcinoma.

**d. Treatment**
    i. Approximately two-thirds spontaneously resolve within 2 years.
    ii. Over-the-counter preparations (salicylic acid) are safe and effective.
    iii. 5-Fluorouracil and imiquimod (approved for genital warts) can be used as well.
    iv. Cryotherapy, liquid nitrogen can be effective.
        1. Pain and blistering may be noted after treatment.

# KERATOTIC DISORDERS

## I. ACTINIC KERATOSIS (AK)
**a. General**
    i. Common, persistent, keratotic lesion with malignant potential.
    ii. Formation is secondary to years of sun exposure.
    iii. Lesions are more common after 40 years of age.
    iv. About 10% to 20% of lesions progress to squamous cell carcinoma.

**b. Clinical Manifestations**
    i. Lesions typically found on sun-exposed areas of elderly patients.
    ii. Lesions found mainly on the face, neck, head, and hands.
        1. Typically 3 to 6 mm in size; may be as large as 2 cm.
    iii. Present as a poorly defined area of erythema and have a rough surface; tender papules, crusts, or plaques can occur. Morphology varies. (See Color Plate 10.)

**c. Diagnosis**
    i. Based on clinical findings and biopsy results.

**d. Treatment**
    i. Regular follow-up with complete skin examinations.

1. Patients with AKs have a higher risk for developing other cutaneous malignancies.
ii. Single lesions can be treated with cryotherapy (liquid nitrogen).
iii. Topical 5-fluorouracil or imiquimod can be used to decrease the number of superficial lesions.
iv. Sun protection and exposure prevention measures should be discussed with patients.

## II. SEBORRHEIC KERATOSIS
### a. General
i. Common, benign, persistent epidermal lesion.
ii. Often confused with cutaneous malignancies.
  1. Associated with basal cell carcinoma and melanoma.
iii. Typically noted after 50 years of age.
### b. Clinical Manifestations
i. Most lesions are 0.2 to 3 cm in diameter. Lesions may be flat or raised and may be smooth, velvety, or verrucous. Some have an umbilicated surface.
  1. A well-circumscribed border with a "stuck-on" appearance.
  2. Surface crumbles when excoriated.
ii. Color varies; white, pink, brown, and black may be noted.
iii. Presence of horn cysts on the surface assists in the diagnosis.
iv. Lesions can arise on any part of the body, except lips, palms, and soles.
  1. Common on areola of both males and females.
### c. Diagnosis
i. Based on history and clinical findings.
ii. Sudden onset of numerous lesions may be associated with internal malignancy.
### d. Treatment
i. Cryosurgery is used for flat or slightly raised lesions.
ii. Cautery and curettage are needed for thicker lesions.

# NEOPLASMS

## I. BASAL CELL CARCINOMA
### a. General
i. The most common cutaneous malignancy.
  1. Incidence rises after age 40 years.
ii. Locally invasive, slow growing and rarely metastasizes.
iii. Risk factors include long-term sun exposure and prior ionizing radiation.
### b. Clinical Manifestations
i. Lesions are most common on sun exposed areas including the face, scalp, ears, and neck.

ii. Individual lesions are pearly-white, dome-shaped papules with overlying telangiectasias. (See Color Plate 11.)
iii. Lesions can ulcerate, bleed, and develop a crusted center.
iv. Lesions vary in color, from flesh colored to the dark brown-black color of a pigmented basal cell carcinoma, including red, pink, gray, white, and brown.
### c. Diagnosis
i. Initial suspicion is based on clinical findings.
ii. Diagnosis requires confirmation with a shave or punch biopsy.
### d. Treatment
i. The goal of treatment is elimination of the tumor with clear margins.
ii. Options for treatment include the following:
  1. Electrosurgery (electrodesiccation and curettage).
    (a) A 5-year cure rate is 92% for primary tumors.
  2. Office excision.
    (a) A 5-year cure rate is 90% for primary tumors.
  3. Mohs' surgery.
    (a) A 5-year cure rate is 99% for primary tumors.
    (b) Useful for tumors that have a high recurrence rate or located in cosmetically sensitive areas.
  4. Radiation therapy.
    (a) A 5-year cure rate is 90% for primary tumors.

## II. KAPOSI'S SARCOMA
### a. General
i. Angioproliferative disorder due to infection with human herpesvirus-8 (HHV-8).
ii. Most common tumor in HIV-infected patients.
iii. CD4 count is typically less than $100/mm^3$.
  1. Since the widespread use of antiretroviral therapy, the incidence has decreased markedly.
### b. Clinical Manifestations
i. Lesions most often appear on the lower extremities, face, oral mucosa, and genitalia.
ii. Lesions are elliptical and in a linear form.
iii. Lesions are of various colors including pink, red, purple, or brown.
iv. Lesions are papular and range in size from 5 mm to 5 cm.
### c. Diagnosis
i. Based on appearance of lesions but confirmed by biopsy.

d. **Treatment**
   i. There is no cure available and management is directed at reducing symptoms and slowing disease progression.
   ii. Combination antiretroviral therapy will decrease incidence and severity of disease.
   iii. Surgical removal including local excision, electrodesiccation, or curettage.
   iv. Intralesional chemotherapy with vinblastine.
   v. Radiation therapy for extensive disease.

## III. MELANOMA
a. **General**
   i. Malignancy of the melanocytes.
   ii. Most common over the age of 50 years, however, incidence in young females is steadily rising.
   iii. Risk factors.
      1. Fair skin.
      2. Presence of atypical nevi.
      3. Personal history of melanoma.
      4. Positive family history of atypical nevi or melanoma.
      5. History of severe blistering sunburn before age 14.
      6. Congenital nevi.
      7. Repeated exposure to intense UV radiation (such as tanning bulbs).

b. **Clinical Manifestations**
   i. Most common early symptom is itching at the site of the lesion; later tenderness, bleeding, and ulceration may develop.
   ii. Early signs also include increase in size, change in color, or change in shape of the lesion.
      1. Consideration should be given to any new, changing, or growing nevi as well as nevi that do not appear similar to other nevi present on the individual.
   iii. Appearance of melanoma varies considerably and a low index of suspicion is necessary.
      1. See Color Plate 12.
      2. See Table 11.3.

c. **Diagnosis**
   i. Diagnosis made by punch biopsy.
      1. Shave biopsy is not indicated.
   ii. Prognosis varies with certain conditions.
      1. Prognosis is better with the following:

         (a) Thin melanoma.
         (b) Melanoma on the extremity.
         (c) Localized disease.
         (d) Female and younger patients.

d. **Treatment**
   i. Survival rates and treatment options vary with the stage of the disease.
   ii. Frequent follow-up is required.
   iii. Treatment by stages.
      1. Stage I is treated with surgical intervention.
      2. Stages II and III are treated with surgical intervention and adjuvant immunotherapy treatment.

         (a) Immunotherapy consists of interleukin-2 and monoclonal antibody (ipilimumab).
   iv. The following are 5-year survival rates by SEER stage.
      1. Localized: 99%.
      2. Regional: 68%.
      3. Distant: 30%.
      4. All SEER stages combined: 93%.

## IV. SQUAMOUS CELL CARCINOMA
a. **General**
   i. Arise from keratinocytes of the skin or mucosal surfaces.
      1. Second most common type of skin cancer.
   ii. Most commonly noted on sun-exposed areas including the lips, hands, neck, and head (when hair is absent or sparse).
   iii. Risk factors include the following:
      1. Ultraviolet light exposure.
      2. Chemicals (hydrocarbons and arsenic).
      3. Tobacco.
      4. Chronic infections.
      5. Human papillomavirus (HPV).

b. **Clinical Manifestations**
   i. Lesions are typically found on sun-damaged skin.
   ii. Early lesions have the appearance of actinic keratosis (rough, sandpaper-like lesions that are typically flesh colored or slightly yellow-brown).
   iii. Mature lesions have a red, poorly defined base with an adherent yellow-white scale. (See Color Plate 13.)
   iv. Over time, the lesions become larger and more raised and develop a firm, red nodule with a necrotic center.
   v. Regional lymph nodes must be examined as SCC can metastasize.

c. **Diagnosis**
   i. Skin biopsy (excisional) is required.
   ii. Risk factors for metastasis include the following:
      1. Tumor greater than 2 cm in diameter.

**TABLE 11.3**

| ABCDEs of Malignant Melanoma | |
| --- | --- |
| Asymmetry | Diameter >6 cm |
| Border irregularity | Evolution/Enlargement |
| Color variation | |

2. Decreased degree of differentiation.
3. Recurrent lesions.
4. Tumor arising from a scar or chronic wound.
5. Location.
   (a) Increased risk with lesions on the ear or lip.

   d. **Treatment**
      i. Long-term prognosis for nonmetastatic, adequately treated cancer is excellent.
      ii. Treatment of primary lesions is wide local excision.
         1. Mohs' surgery is an option if tissue sparing is important, primarily used in cosmetically sensitive areas.
      iii. Radiation is a treatment option.

# ECZEMATOUS AND PAPULOSQUAMOUS DISORDERS

## ECZEMATOUS DISORDERS

### I. ECZEMA
   a. **General**
      i. Pruritic inflammation of the dermis and epidermis.
      ii. Often associated with a personal or family history of asthma and/or allergic rhinitis.
         1. 80% of children with atopic dermatitis will develop asthma or allergic rhinitis later in life.
      iii. Onset is typically between 3 and 6 months of life with approximately 60% of patients developing symptoms before 12 months.
      iv. Mechanism of disease is due to impaired epidermal barrier function, alterations in cell mediated immune responses, IgE mediated hypersensitivity, and environment.
   b. **Clinical Manifestations**
      i. In adults, an erythematous scaling patchy rash is noted in the flexural regions.
      ii. In infants and young children, the rash is papulovesicular or erythematous, lichenification secondary to the scratching may be noted, and it most commonly affects the face and extensor surfaces.
      iii. The primary complaint in both adults and children is pruritus and dry skin.
         1. It is triggered by contact with irritants such as dust mites, pollens, detergents, soaps, sweating, stress, and scratching.
      iv. White or red dermatographism may be present.
   c. **Diagnosis**
      i. Based on history and clinical findings.
      ii. In infants, atopic dermatitis must be differentiated from seborrheic dermatitis.

**TABLE 11.4**

| Comparison of Atopic Dermatitis and Seborrheic Dermatitis | | |
| --- | --- | --- |
| | **Atopic Dermatitis** | **Seborrheic Dermatitis** |
| Duration | Chronic | About 6 weeks |
| Family history | Positive for atopy | Negative family history |
| Location | Children: face, extensor surfaces | Children: axilla, diaper area |
| | Adult: generalized | Adults: central face, posterior auricular |
| Pruritus | Yes | Children: no |
| | | Adults: yes |

1. Table 11.4 summarizes atopic dermatitis and seborrheic dermatitis.
   d. **Treatment**
      i. Educate patients to avoid scratching and triggers, including frequent bathing and scented soaps, lotions, and detergents.
      ii. Decrease pruritus with hydroxyzine or diphenhydramine.
      iii. Hydration of skin with hydrated petrolatum, Eucerin cream, or Lac-Hydrin.
      iv. Topical steroids are used to decrease inflammation.
         1. Side effects of chronic use include skin atrophy and suppression of the hypothalamic–pituitary–adrenal (HPA) axis in children and adults, as well as osteoporosis in adults.
      v. Skin infections, typically secondary to *Staphylococcus aureus*, are common and may require treatment with oral antibiotics, such as erythromycin, dicloxacillin, or first-generation cephalosporins.

### II. CONTACT DERMATITIS
   a. **General**
      i. Inflammatory skin reaction of the dermis and epidermis secondary to an external agent.
         1. If the agent directly damages the skin, the reaction is irritant contact dermatitis.
         2. If the reaction is immunologic in nature, the reaction is allergic contact dermatitis due to a delayed (type IV) cell-mediated hypersensitivity reaction.
         3. Table 11.5 lists common irritants and allergens.
   b. **Clinical Manifestations**
      i. History of exposure to an irritant is a primary finding.
         1. Exposures may be related to the patient's occupation. Nickel found in jewelry and belt buckles is also a common irritant.

**TABLE 11.5**

| Common Irritants and Allergens | |
|---|---|
| **Irritants** | **Allergens** |
| Cement | Bacitracin |
| Ethylene oxide | Formaldehyde |
| Fiberglass | Fragrance |
| Industrial solvents | Neomycin |
| Plants | Nickel |
| Soaps/Detergents | Plants (poison ivy/oak) |
| Wool | Thimerosal |

    ii. Patients with irritant contact dermatitis will typically complain of burning and itching within minutes after exposure.
       1. Skin may turn red and become edematous; vesicular eruption occurs that can coalesce into patches with serous fluid drainage.
    iii. Acute allergic contact dermatitis has sharply demarcated areas, edema, and vesicular lesions.
       1. These lesions are frequently linear if due to plant exposure (poison ivy). (See Color Plate 14.)
    iv. Chronic contact dermatitis can lead to dry, thick skin with lichenification.

**c. Diagnosis**
    i. Based on history and clinical findings

**d. Treatment**
    i. Most important step in management is removal of the irritant.
    ii. Topical or systemic steroids may be needed for irritation and pruritus if present.
    iii. Supportive measures include cool compresses or oatmeal baths.

## III. NUMMULAR ECZEMATOUS DERMATITIS

**a. General**
    i. Chronic, pruritic, inflammatory dermatitis.
    ii. Primarily occurs in young adulthood or older age.
    iii. Common on lower legs and trunk.
    iv. Associated with atopy.

**b. Clinical Manifestations**
    i. Presents with coin-shaped plaques (4 to 5 cm in diameter) composed of papulomacular patches on an erythematous base.
    ii. Very pruritic.
    iii. May have central clearing so differentiation from tinea and psoriasis is necessary.

**c. Diagnosis**
    i. Based on history and clinical findings.

**d. Treatment**
    i. Skin hydration with hydrated petrolatum or moisturizing cream.
    ii. Potent topical steroids.

## IV. PERIORAL DERMATITIS

**a. General**
    i. Occurs mainly in young women, 16 to 45 years of age.

**b. Clinical Manifestations**
    i. Presents with irregularly grouped, discrete erythematous papulopustules on an erythematous base.
    ii. Initially perioral and lasts weeks to months.
       1. Sparing of the vermilion border is noted.
    iii. Flares may be associated with mint or fluoride containing products such as gum or toothpaste.

**c. Diagnosis**
    i. Based on history and clinical findings.
    ii. Must be differentiated from rosacea.

**d. Treatment**
    i. Topical steroids and skin care products should be avoided.
    ii. Antibiotics are required.
       1. Topical antibiotics include metronidazole, clindamycin, or erythromycin gels.
       2. Systemic antibiotics in addition to topical gels for refractory cases include minocycline, doxycycline, or tetracycline.
         (a) Pregnant patients can take oral erythromycin.
    iii. Topical calcineurin inhibitors (Pimecrolimus) will decrease disease severity.

## V. SEBORRHEIC DERMATITIS

**a. General**
    i. A common, chronic, inflammatory papulosquamous disease.
    ii. All ages are affected, including infants.
       1. In infants, it is often referred to as "cradle cap."

**b. Clinical Manifestations**
    i. Papules are moist, transparent to pink-orange-red patches that are macerated, +/− scale, with sharp delineated margins.
    ii. More common in areas with numerous sebaceous glands, such as the scalp margins, central face, and the sternal area.
       1. Classic locations include the eyebrows, base of eyelashes, nasolabial folds, and external ear canal.
    iii. It may itch, mainly when it involves the scalp.
    iv. Cradle cap is yellow, greasy adherent scales on the vertex of the scalp in infants.

**c. Diagnosis**
    i. Based on history and clinical findings.

**d. Treatment**
    i. Daily shampooing with dandruff shampoos.
       1. Shampoos should contain selenium sulfide or zinc pyrithione.

2. In infants, the scalp should be washed with baby oil or petroleum jelly prior to washing with baby shampoo. After washing, light combing with a washcloth or comb of the area can remove papules.

ii. Hydrocortisone 1% to decrease itching and redness.

iii. Topical antifungals, such as ketoconazole or ciclopirox, can be helpful in mild to moderate non-scalp cases.

iv. If there is no response to treatment in infants or adults, consider possible zinc deficiency or immunocompromised state.

## VI. DYSHIDROTIC ECZEMA (POMPHOLYX)
   a. **General**
   i. Chronic, relapsing disease of unknown etiology.
   ii. More common in patients with atopic dermatitis and/or allergic rhinitis.
   b. **Clinical Manifestations**
   i. Presents with highly pruritic, symmetric vesicles on the palms, lateral fingers, or plantar surface of the feet.
   ii. Vesicles are 1 to 5 mm in diameter, monomorphic, deep seated, and filled with clear tapioca-like fluid.
   iii. Resolves slowly over 1 to 3 weeks, leaving a red, cracked base with brown spots.
   c. **Diagnosis**
   i. Based on history and clinical findings.
   d. **Treatment**
   i. Wet dressings, with Burow's solution (10% aluminum acetate in a 1:40 dilution), are the initial treatment.
   ii. Medium- or high-potency topical steroids are alternated with the wet dressings.
   iii. Oral steroids may be needed in severe cases.

## VII. LICHEN SIMPLEX CHRONICUS
   a. **General**
   i. A localized form of lichenified, circumscribed plaques that results from repeated rubbing and scratching.
   ii. Frequently involves the wrists, ankles, scrotum, and back of the neck.
   iii. More common in adults and can last for decades.
   b. **Clinical Manifestations**
   i. Skin examination reveals sharply demarcated light red to dark violet patches or plaques that are thickened with accentuated skin lines.
   c. **Diagnosis**
   i. Based on history and clinical findings.
   ii. Must rule out tinea infection.
   d. **Treatment**
   i. Stopping the itch-scratch cycle is imperative. Occlusive dressings may be needed at night.

ii. Water soaks followed by medium- to high-potency topical steroids.

1. Low-potency steroids should be used on the face and genitals without occlusion.

# PAPULOSQUAMOUS DISORDERS

## I. DRUG ERUPTIONS
   a. **General**
   i. A common complication of drug therapy.
   ii. There is a wide range in severity of reactions.
   b. **Clinical Manifestations**
   i. May present with fever and, hours later, a diffuse maculopapular rash, hives, and/or pruritus may occur.
   c. **Drug Reaction Types**
   i. Morbilliform eruptions.
   1. Most frequent and appear very similar to viral exanthems.
   2. Commonly due to ampicillin, isoniazid, phenytoin, quinidine, sulfonamides, or thiazides.
   3. Typically occurs 7 to 10 days after starting the drug.
      (a) Occurrence may not occur on the first use.
      (b) Subsequent uses may produce a more rapid and/or more severe reaction.
   4. Maculopapular eruption, red macules, and papules become confluent and often spare the face.
   5. Pruritus is common.
   6. Treatment includes antihistamines and cooling lotions.
   ii. Urticarial drug reactions.
   1. Due to an anaphylactic immunoglobulin E (IgE)–dependent reaction that occurs within minutes to hours of administration.
   2. Due to commonly used drugs such as aspirin and penicillin, as well as blood products.
   3. Treatment includes antihistamines and cooling lotions.
      (a) Epinephrine may be needed in severe reactions.
   iii. Fixed drug eruptions.
   1. Present with single or multiple, round, demarcated red plaques that appear soon after the drug exposure and reappear in the same site each time the drug is taken.
   2. Preceded by itching and burning.
   3. May occur on any part of the body.
   4. Length of time from reexposure to onset of symptoms is typically 30 minutes to 6 hours.
   5. Commonly due to tetracycline or co-trimoxazole.
   iv. Drug-induced hyperpigmentation.

**TABLE 11.6**

| Common Drug-Induced Hyperpigmentation | |
|---|---|
| **Drug** | **Color Change** |
| Amiodarone | Dusky red on photodistributed areas |
| Antimalarial agents | Brown discoloration on shins |
| Bleomycin | Streaking hyperpigmentation on trunk and extremities |
| Hydantoin | Brown pigmentation on the face |
| Minocycline | Blue-gray on skin and gingiva |
| Oral contraceptives | Brown pigmentation on the cheeks and central face |
| Zidovudine | Brown discoloration on nails and lips |

1. Caused by many different drugs and typically fades with time.
   (a) Table 11.6 lists drug pigmentation changes.
  v. Chemotherapy-induced acral erythema.
   1. Presents with tingling of palms of hands and soles of feet followed within a few days by painful, well-defined symmetric swelling and erythema.
   2. Commonly noted with use of cytosine arabinoside, fluorouracil, and doxorubicin.
   3. Treatment is supportive.

## II. LICHEN PLANUS
### a. General
   i. Uncommon, inflammatory papulosquamous disorder of unknown cause.
   ii. More common in middle-aged adults.
   iii. A lichen planus–like reaction is noted with certain drugs, such as gold salts, beta blockers, antimalarials, thiazide, and furosemide.
   1. Can be related to hepatitis C; if there is a possible exposure, screening should be ordered.
   iv. The following are the 6 Ps of lichen planus:
   1. *Pruritic.*
   2. *Planar.*
   3. *Polygonal.*
   4. *Papules.*
   5. *Purple.*
   6. *Plaques*
### b. Clinical Manifestations
   i. Pruritus is variable.
   ii. Lesions are 2- to 10-mm flat-topped, violaceous papules with irregular angulated borders and Wickham's striae.
   1. Wickham's striae are white lines seen with magnification of the lesions.
   2. Helpful to differentiate these lesions from verrucae when located on the penile surface.
   iii. New lesions are purple or pink, but over time become violaceous.

  iv. Mainly noted on the flexor surface of the wrists, shins, scalp, glans penis, and mouth.
   1. See Color Plate 15.
### c. Diagnosis
   i. Based on history and clinical findings.
### d. Treatment
   i. Antihistamines to control pruritus if present.
   ii. Topical steroids are the initial treatment for localized disease.
   iii. Intralesional triamcinolone acetonide is used for hypertrophic lesions.
   iv. Oral steroids are used in generalized, severe skin involvement.
   v. Severe cases may also require systemic retinoids or cyclosporine.

## III. PITYRIASIS ROSEA
### a. General
   i. Most cases are in patients between the ages of 10 and 40 years.
   ii. May note a history of an upper respiratory infection (URI) within a month of onset.
### b. Clinical Manifestations
   i. Lesions are salmon-colored oval plaques, 1 to 2 cm in diameter, with fine scale at periphery, typically located first on the trunk.
   1. The first lesion is called the *herald patch*.
   2. Children may show lesions on the scalp, face, groin, elbows, and knees.
   3. See Color Plate 16.
   ii. Multiple smaller lesions appear following the *herald patch* on the trunk and give a Christmas tree–pattern appearance.
   iii. Lesions typically clear spontaneously in 4 to 12 weeks.
### c. Diagnosis
   i. Based on history and clinical findings.
   ii. The herald patch must be differentiated from a tinea infection.
   iii. May be confused with secondary syphilis.
   iv. Rapid plasma reagin and/or Venereal Disease Research Laboratory (RPR/VDRL) testing will be negative in the absence of syphilis.
### d. Treatment
   i. Self-limiting and asymptomatic.
   ii. Ultraviolet B (UVB) light may quicken resolution of the lesions.

## IV. PSORIASIS
### a. General
   i. A common, chronic, inflammatory papulosquamous disease.
   ii. Secondary to abnormal T-lymphocyte function.
   iii. The skin, nails, and joints can be affected.
   iv. Age of onset peaks during 20s and again in late 50s.

**b. Clinical Manifestations**
  i. Presents with red, sharply defined, scaling papules/plaques that form stable, round-to-oval plaques.
  ii. The scales are silvery white and reveal bleeding when scratched or removed (Auspitz's sign). (See Color Plate 17.)
  iii. Lesions are typically noted on the extensor surfaces of the extremities (elbows and knees), scalp, and sacrum.
    1. The palms of the hands, soles of the feet, and the face are typically spared.
    2. Nail pitting is common, but not always present.
**c. Diagnosis**
  i. Based on history and clinical findings.
  ii. Punch biopsy shows thickening of the epidermis (acanthosis).
**d. Treatment**
  i. Psychosocial impact can be severe.
  ii. There are three main categories of treatment.
    1. Topical.
      (a) Includes topical tar preparations, steroids, anthralin, calcipotriene, and tazarotene.
    2. Phototherapy.
      (a) Ultraviolet B is a very effective treatment and often used in conjunction with topical treatment.
      (b) Patients may note symptoms improve in the summer months or after periods of high sun exposure.
    3. Systemic.
      (a) Used in patients who are very uncomfortable, who have lesions over more than 20% of their body, or whose symptoms are refractory to topical management.
      (b) Utilizes a rotational therapy, best managed by a dermatologist.
      (c) Agents include the following:
        (i) Methotrexate.
          (1) Side effects include nausea, fatigue, leukopenia, hepatic fibrosis, and cirrhosis.
        (ii) Cyclosporine.
          (1) Side effects include hypertension and nephrotoxicity.
        (iii) Acitretin.
          (1) Side effects include teratogenicity, hepatitis, and increased cholesterol.
        (iv) Biologicals.
          (1) Inhibit tumor necrosis factor.
          (2) Include infliximab and etanercept.
          (3) Side effects include increased risk of infection and lymphoma.

# PIGMENT DISORDERS

**I. MELASMA**
  **a. General**
    i. Acquired brown pigmentation of the face and neck.
    ii. More common in women with darker skin tones.
    iii. Most commonly occurs during the second and third trimester of pregnancy, during use of oral contraceptives, or from extensive sun exposure in genetically predisposed females.
  **b. Clinical Manifestations**
    i. More common on forehead, malar eminences, upper lip, and chin.
    ii. Symmetric macular brown hyperpigmentation is noted.
  **c. Diagnosis**
    i. Based on clinical findings.
  **d. Treatment**
    i. Sun protection is helpful in reducing the visibility of pigmentation.
    ii. Usually fades after discontinuing oral contraceptives or at the end of pregnancy.
    iii. Physical ultraviolet (UV) blockers are recommended. Avoid UV light. If not pregnant, consider skin-lightening agents (hydroquinone or azelaic acid).

**II. VITILIGO**
  **a. General**
    i. Affects 1% of the general population worldwide.
    ii. Average age of onset is 20.
    iii. Without evidence, most patients with vitiligo attribute the onset with physical injury, sunburn, emotional injury, illness, or pregnancy.
    iv. Genetic predisposition with multiple loci involved and most likely inheritance is autosomal recessive.
    v. Due to an autoimmune process against melanocytes.
      1. Linked to other autoimmune diseases so presence of comorbid autoimmune disorders is common.
  **b. Clinical Manifestations**
    i. There are two types.
      1. Type A: generalized.

(a) Fairly symmetric pattern of white, depigmented, 0.5- to 5.0-cm macules and patches.

(b) Common locations include dorsal hands, fingers, face, body folds, axillae, and genitalia.

2. Type B: segmental.

(a) Limited to one segment of the body.

**c. Diagnosis**

i. Biopsy of lesions shows absence of melanocytes.

ii. Wood's lamp accentuates hyperpigmentation.

**d. Treatment**

i. Goals are repigmentation and stabilization of the depigmentation process, including the following:

1. Corticosteroids: mid- to low-potency agents.

2. Calcineurin inhibitors (tacrolimus).

3. Narrow-band UVB.

4. Topical vitamin D analogues.

ii. Repigmentation efforts are typically unsuccessful.

# SKIN INTEGRITY

## I. BURNS

**a. General**

i. Classified into six groups based on the mechanism of injury.

1. Scalds.

(a) Child abuse accounts for a large number of immersion scald burns.

2. Contact burns.

3. Fire.

4. Chemical.

5. Electrical.

6. Radiation.

ii. Highest incidence of burns occurs during the first few years of life and between the ages of 20 and 29 years.

**b. Clinical Manifestations**

i. Skin is the largest organ of the body.

1. Three major layers.

(a) Epidermis: outermost layer.

(i) Four distinct layers.

(ii) Function is protection from environment, water homeostasis, and immunologic surveillance.

(b) Dermis.

(i) Type I collagen is the majority of dermis.

(ii) Contains pilosebaceous unit, apocrine gland, exocrine gland, melanocytes, nerve end organs, and Merkel and Langerhans cells.

(iii) Provides communication from the skin to the immunologic and nervous systems.

(c) Subcutaneous tissue.

(i) Contains fat cells and provides a cushion for the dermis.

(ii) Thickness varies depending on total body fat.

ii. Depth of burns classified according to degrees.

1. Superficial (first-degree) burns.

(a) Minor epithelial damage of epidermis.

(b) Redness, tenderness, and pain are present.

(c) No blistering is present and two-point discrimination remains intact.

(d) Healing takes several days and occurs without scarring.

(e) Most common causes are flash burns and sunburns.

2. Partial-thickness (second-degree) burns.

(a) Superficial partial-thickness burns

(i) Involve epidermis and superficial dermis layers.

(ii) Skin appears pink, moist, and soft, and thin-walled blisters are present.

(iii) Skin is very tender to touch.

(iv) Typically heal in 2 to 3 weeks without scarring.

(b) Deep partial-thickness burns.

(i) Involve the epidermis and extend into the lower (reticular) dermis layer.

(ii) Skin appears red with blanched white areas and thick-walled blisters.

(iii) Typically heal in 3 to 6 weeks; scarring is possible with the development of contractions across joints.

(c) Second-degree burns are typically due to splash scalds.

3. Full-thickness (third-degree) burns.

(a) Burn that destroys the full thickness of the epidermis and dermis.

(b) Skin is white or leathery with underlying clotted vessels, and destruction of sensory nerve endings results in anesthesia of the affected area.

(c) Skin grafting is needed unless the burn is small (<1 cm in diameter).

(d) Caused by immersion scalds, flame burns, and chemical and high-voltage electrical injuries.

4. Fourth-degree.

(a) Full-thickness destruction of skin, subcutaneous tissue, fascia, muscle, bone, and other structures.

(b) Treatment requires débridement and reconstruction of tissues.

(c) Result from prolonged exposure to causes of third-degree burns.

c. **Diagnosis**
i. Burn wound assessment.
1. Rule of nines.
(a) Adult's body surface area (BSA) allocation.
(i) 9% to head and neck.
(ii) 9% to each upper extremity.
(iii) 18% to anterior portion of trunk.
(iv) 18% to posterior portion of trunk.
(v) 18% to each lower extremity.
(vi) 1% to perineum and genitalia.
(b) Child's BSA allocation is different to account for larger head size in relation to the body.
(i) 18% to head and neck.
(ii) 9% to each upper extremity.
(iii) 18% to anterior portion of trunk.
(iv) 18% to posterior portion of trunk.
(v) 14% to each lower extremity.
(vi) 1% to perineum and genitalia.
(c) Fig. 11.1 illustrates the rule of nines.
2. Palm method.
(a) Size of entire volar surface of a patient's hand is approximately equivalent to 1% of the patient's BSA.

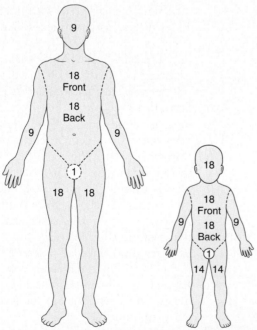

**Fig. 11.1** Rule of nines for estimating percentage of burn area. *(From Roberts JR, Hedges JR, Vroucher D, et al: Clinical Procedures in Emergency Medicine, 4th ed. Philadelphia: WB Saunders 2004:751, Fig. 39-1.)*

ii. Carboxyhemoglobin.
1. Carbon monoxide level should be obtained.
2. Treat with 100% oxygen until the level is less than 10%.
(a) Hyperbaric oxygen may be needed if there is the presence of metabolic acidosis, history of neurologic deficits, pregnancy, or cardiac abnormalities or in the very young or very old.
iii. Cyanide.
1. Inhalation injury may lead to cyanide poisoning.
2. Treat with nitrite-thiosulfate antidote.

d. **Treatment**
i. Early response to burn incidents has a great influence on the magnitude of injury.
ii. Prehospital care.
1. Evaluate for signs of inhalation injury.
(a) Includes dyspnea, burns on mouth and nose, soot in posterior pharynx, singed nasal hairs, sooty sputum, and cough.
(b) Treat with humidified oxygen, nonrebreathing mask at 10 to 12 L/minute.
2. All burned clothing and skin should be washed with cool water.
(a) Inhibits lactate production and acidosis.
(b) Limits vascular permeability.
(c) Decreases dermal ischemia.
iii. Hospital care.
1. Fluid resuscitation.
(a) Tremendous fluid loss occurs with burns.
(b) Adequate fluid resuscitation is evidenced by normal urine output.
(i) 1 mL/kg/hour in those younger than 2 years old.
(ii) 0.5 mL/kg/hour in older children.
(iii) 30 to 40 mL/hour in adults.
(c) Parkland formula for fluid resuscitation.
(i) Uses lactated Ringer's solution.
(ii) Total volume given is 4 mL/kg/% BSA burned during the first 24 hours.
(1) One half of the total is given the first 8 hours, and the rest is given over the next 16 hours.
(d) Galveston formula for fluid resuscitation.
(i) Used in children.
(ii) Uses 5% dextrose in lactated Ringer's solution.
(iii) Total volume given is 5000 mL/m$^2$ of % BSA burned plus 2000 mL/m$^2$ during the first 24 hours.

(1) One half of the total is given the first 8 hours, and the rest is given over the next 16 hours.

(2) Dextrose is added to prevent hypoglycemia.

2. Pain management.

(a) Requirement for pain medications is inversely related to depth of burn injury.

(i) Full-thickness burns are painless, due to sensory nerve damage however, many patients have concurrent less severe burns that require pain control.

(b) Morphine is the medication of choice.

3. Escharotomy.

(a) Full-thickness circumferential burn of an extremity may result in vascular compromise.

(b) May note loss of pulses and increase in tissue compartment pressures.

(c) Escharotomy prevents ischemic injury.

## II. DECUBITUS ULCERS

### a. General

i. Due to prolonged pressure on areas of the skin, resulting in tissue damage.

ii. Typically occur on bony prominences, such as the hip, sacrum, or lateral malleolus.

iii. Require three forces: pressure, shear, and friction.

iv. Predisposing conditions include the following:

1. Paraplegia/quadriplegia.

2. Diabetes mellitus.

3. Peripheral vascular disease.

4. Peripheral neuropathy.

5. Immobility.

### b. Clinical Manifestations

i. Detection requires complete skin examination.

ii. Patients present with painless open sores.

iii. Lesions vary in size and depth.

iv. May note presence of tissue damage, necrotic tissue, and exudate.

v. Varying stages of ulcers are listed in Table 11.7.

### c. Diagnosis

i. Based on clinical findings.

### d. Treatment

i. Management involves prevention, early recognition, and aggressive treatment.

ii. Stages I and II are best treated with local care and pain management.

iii. Stages III and IV often require surgical intervention.

1. Debridement of necrotic tissue and wound care with wet-to-dry dressings are often required.

**TABLE 11.7**

| Stages of Decubitus Ulcers | |
|---|---|
| **Stage** | **Description** |
| I | Erythema of intact skin |
| II | Partial-thickness skin loss of epidermis and dermis |
| III | Full-thickness skin loss<br>Does not extend through fascia |
| IV | Full-thickness skin loss with extensive destruction<br>Damage through the fascia, often involving the muscle and bone<br>Sinus tracts are common |

iv. Antibiotics are required if complications of sepsis or osteomyelitis are suspected.

v. Prevention is critical for many patients as treatment can be difficult.

## III. STASIS DERMATITIS

### a. General

i. Eczematous dermatitis of the legs, associated with edema, varicose veins, and hyperpigmentation.

ii. Chronic disease with frequent relapse is common.

iii. Most commonly occurs on the lower legs.

### b. Clinical Manifestations

i. Often, a history of deep vein thrombosis (DVT), surgery, or ulceration is present.

ii. The skin appears dry, fissured, and erythematous.

iii. Pruritus, edema, and brown discoloration of the skin are common.

### c. Diagnosis

i. Based on history and clinical findings.

### d. Treatment

i. Elevation and compression of the legs will decrease edema and stasis.

ii. Cool water dressings for acute exudative inflammation.

iii. Topical or oral steroids may be required.

iv. Lubrication with bland emollients can help with dryness.

v. Oral antihistamines may be needed for pruritus.

# VASCULAR ABNORMALITIES

## I. CHERRY ANGIOMA

### a. General

i. Small, benign skin growth that typically presents after age 30 and is most commonly found on the trunk.

b. **Clinical Manifestations**
   i. Bright red, pin-sized lesion that is typically under 0.25 inches in diameter.
c. **Diagnosis**
   i. Clinical diagnosis is typically sufficient.
d. **Treatment**
   i. Are typically only removed for cosmetic reasons.
   ii. Electrocautery, cryotherapy, or shave excision can be used if desired.

## II. TELANGIECTASIA

a. **General**
   i. Often referred to as "spider veins."
   ii. They may be harmless, present in chronically sun-exposed areas, or be associated with underlying conditions such as rosacea, scleroderma, systemic lupus erythematosus, or hepatic disease.
b. **Clinical Manifestations**
   i. Small, red lesion with thread-like projections.
   ii. Often located near the nasolabial folds.
c. **Diagnosis**
   i. Clinical diagnosis.
d. **Treatment**
   i. Telangiectasias are not harmful but may be removed for cosmetic purposes.
      1. Removal techniques include laser therapy and electrodessication.
   ii. Sun protection, mild cleansers, and minimization of exposure to extreme temperatures can help prevent development.

# VESICULOBULLOUS DISEASE

## I. PEMPHIGOID

a. **General**
   i. An uncommon, autoimmune blistering disease that primarily affects the elderly population (>60 years of age).
   ii. Due to immunoglobulin G (IgG) autoantibodies directed against the epithelial basement membrane zone.
   iii. Can also be drug-induced secondary to sulfa drugs, furosemide, or penicillamine.
b. **Clinical Manifestations**
   i. Begins with localized areas of erythema or pruritic papules that form plaques.
      1. Generally noted in the skin folds and in the flexural areas.
      2. Rare on the head and face.
   ii. Plaques turn dark red in 1 to 3 weeks as the vesicles and bullae rapidly appear.
   iii. Bullae are tense and rupture in 1 week, leaving an eroded base that heals rapidly.

iv. Itchiness is moderate to severe.
c. **Diagnosis**
   i. Biopsy is required for diagnosis.
   ii. Skin biopsy shows subepidermal bulla with infiltration of eosinophils.
d. **Treatment**
   i. Goal of treatment is to stop blistering, decrease itching, and protect against secondary infection.
   ii. Oral steroids are the best initial treatment; immunosuppressive agents may be required.
   iii. Minocycline has also been shown to be effective.
   iv. In localized disease and for maintenance therapy following oral prednisone, topical steroids can be used.

## II. PEMPHIGUS

a. **General**
   i. A rare autoimmune disorder causes intraepidermal blisters and erosions.
   ii. Most often seen in middle-aged adults and is a chronic, potentially life-threatening condition.
b. **Clinical Manifestations**
   i. Begins with vesicles on the oral mucosa before extending to the skin and/or genital mucous membranes.
   ii. Vesicles are painful and are typically not pruritic
   iii. Secondary skin infections can occur.
c. **Diagnosis**
   i. Biopsy with direct immunofluorescence.
d. **Treatment**
   i. Mild cases can be treated with a combination of topical and oral corticosteroids.
   ii. Immunosuppressants (azathioprine or mycophenolate mofetil).
   iii. Wound care is necessary to prevent secondary infection.

# OTHER DERMATOLOGIC DISORDERS

## I. ACANTHOSIS NIGRICANS

a. **General**
   i. Thickened, velvety hyperpigmented plaques.
      1. Primarily in the posterior neck folds, axilla, and antecubital fossa.
   ii. Associated with obesity, insulin resistance, and diabetes.
   iii. Associated with adenocarcinoma of the gastrointestinal (GI) tract.
   iv. Can be caused by medications, such as estrogen, nicotinic acid, glucocorticoids, and protease inhibitors.

**b. Clinical Manifestations**

    i. Patient complaint of an asymptomatic, "dirty" appearance to the skin folds.

    ii. Skin examination shows symmetric, velvety, black-brown changes.

**c. Diagnosis**

    i. Based on clinical findings.

**d. Treatment**

    i. Treat underlying etiology.

    ii. Aimed at cosmetic improvement of skin texture; topical retinoids or vitamin D analogue products provide desquamation and improve the texture and lighten the color.

    iii. Evaluate all patients for insulin resistance by checking hemoglobin A1c or fasting blood glucose.

    iv. If insulin resistance is not present, consider the association with GI malignancy and work up accordingly.

## II. HIDRADENITIS SUPPURATIVA (ACNE INVERSA)

**a. General**

    i. Inflammatory disorder of the apocrine gland–bearing skin in the axillae, anogenital, and inframammary regions.

    ii. Onset is after puberty; more women are affected than men by 3:1.

      1. More common in obese patients.

      2. Cigarette smoking is a major triggering factor.

    iii. A disease of the follicular infundibula followed by rupture of follicular contents.

      1. Androgens contribute to the development of disease.

**b. Clinical Manifestations**

    i. Classic finding is a double comedo with sinus tracts developing and with subsequent scarring.

    ii. Disease will progress with development of deep, dermal inflammation and development of large, painful abscesses.

    iii. Disease onset typically in the second and third decades of life.

**c. Diagnosis**

    i. Based on history and clinical findings.

**d. Treatment**

    i. Large cysts should be incised and drained.

    ii. Small cysts can be injected with triamcinolone acetonide.

    iii. Antibiotics are the mainstay of therapy.

      1. Long-term therapy with oral tetracycline, erythromycin, doxycycline, minocycline, or clindamycin with rifampin.

    iv. Topical clindamycin is effective for control.

    v. With oral retinoids, isotretinoin is not effective; but acitretin has shown efficacy.

    vi. Combination therapy of cyproterone acetate plus ethinyl estradiol is more effective than isotretinoin.

## III. LIPOMAS

**a. General**

    i. Subcutaneous tumors of adipose tissue.

**b. Clinical Manifestations**

    i. Typically located on the trunk, neck, and proximal limbs.

    ii. Soft, symmetric, and easily movable over deeper structures.

      1. May be described as a golf ball under the skin.

    iii. May be single or multiple and vary in size.

**c. Diagnosis**

    i. Based on clinical findings.

**d. Treatment**

    i. If a cosmetic defect is evident, lipomas may be surgically removed.

    ii. There is no medical reason for removal.

## IV. EPIDERMAL INCLUSION CYSTS (EPIDERMOID CYSTS)

**a. General**

    i. Most common cause of cutaneous cysts.

    ii. Consist of normal epidermis that produces keratin.

    iii. May remain stable or may enlarge.

**b. Clinical Manifestations**

    i. Are discrete, freely movable cysts or nodules.

    ii. Often have a central punctum.

    iii. May become infected and enlarge.

**c. Diagnosis**

    i. Ultrasound may be helpful in determining contents of the cyst.

    ii. Punch biopsy is necessary for diagnosis.

**d. Treatment**

    i. Steroid injection into the cyst can reduce inflammation.

    ii. Cyst excision may be needed as a small percentage can have malignant transformation.

    iii. Antibiotics are typically not needed.

      1. If needed, use amoxicillin-clavulanate.

## V. PHOTOSENSITIVITY REACTIONS

**a. General**

    i. Heightened skin sensitivity secondary to UV radiation.

    ii. This typically occurs secondary to systemic medication use, underlying conditions such as lupus, or skin care products that contain retinols, glycolic acid, or benzoyl peroxide.

**b. Clinical Manifestations**

    i. A red, painful rash appears on the skin similar to a sunburn.

ii. It may occur within minutes to hours after sun exposure and does not typically spread beyond the sun-exposed region.

c. **Diagnosis**

i. Clinical diagnosis with thorough medication review.

d. **Treatment**

i. Discontinue associated medication or product use.

ii. Symptomatic management of pain if present with NSAIDs.

## VI. PILONIDAL DISEASE

a. **General**

i. A chronic skin condition forming pilonidal cavities that can cause sinus tracts along the gluteal cleft.

ii. Occurs in males more than females with a 3:1 ratio.

iii. Risk factors include sedentary lifestyle, local trauma, family history, and obesity.

b. **Clinical Manifestations**

i. Clinical presentation is often varied.

ii. An acute abscess typically presents first, with a localized reaction.

iii. Chronic abscesses can cause sinus tracts to form, resulting in drainage.

c. **Diagnosis**

i. Digital rectal examination with rigid proctoscopy.

d. **Treatment**

i. Individualized management is necessary.

ii. Surgical intervention is common with approaches varying by severity. Incision and drainage may suffice in mild disease, while unroofing to allow secondary healing may be required in more advanced disease.

1. Medications
   (a) Oral corticosteroids (Table 11.8).
   (b) Topical steroids (Table 11.9).

**TABLE 11.8**

| Oral Corticosteroids Comparison | |
| --- | --- |
| **Generic Name** | **Equivalent Dose (mg)** |
| Cortisone | 25 |
| Hydrocortisone | 20 |
| Prednisolone | 5 |
| Prednisone | 5 |
| Triamcinolone | 4 |
| Methylprednisolone | 4 |
| Dexamethasone | 0.75 |
| Betamethasone | 0.60 |

**TABLE 11.9**

| Topical Steroids | | |
| --- | --- | --- |
| **Group** | **Generic** | **Percentage** |
| I (Super) | Clobetasol propionate | 0.05 |
| | Halobetasol propionate | 0.05 |
| II (High) | Betamethasone dipropionate | 0.05 |
| | Halcinonide | 0.1 |
| | Fluocinonide | 0.05 |
| III (Medium) | Betamethasone dipropionate | 0.05 |
| | Triamcinolone acetonide | 0.5 |
| | Amcinonide | 0.1 |
| IV (Medium) | Triamcinolone acetonide | 0.1 |
| | Mometasone furoate | 0.1 |
| | Hydrocortisone | 0.2 |
| V (Medium) | Triamcinolone acetonide | 0.1 |
| | Desonide | 0.05 |
| | Hydrocortisone butyrate | 0.1 |
| | Fluocinolone acetonide | 0.025 |
| | Hydrocortisone valerate | 0.2 |
| VI (Low) | Prednicarbate | 0.05 |
| | Triamcinolone acetonide | 0.025 |
| | Fluocinolone acetonide | 0.01 |
| VII (Low) | Hydrocortisone acetate | 1.0 |
| | Hydrocortisone | 1.0 |

## VII. URTICARIA (HIVES)

a. **General**

i. Urticaria is divided into acute, chronic, and physical.

ii. Acute

1. Individual lesions last less than 24 hours and recurrence of lesions last less than 6 weeks.
2. More common in individuals with a history of atopia.
3. Due to histamine release from mast cells, mediated by IgE.

iii. Chronic

1. Individual lesions last less than 24 hours and recurrence of lesions last greater than 6 weeks.
2. Patients should be evaluated for the five Is:
   (a) *I*ngestants: foods, additives, antibiotics.
   (b) *I*nhalants: dust, pollen.
   (c) *I*njectants: drugs, stings, bites.
   (d) *I*nfections: bacterial, viral, fungal, parasitic.
   (e) *I*nternal disease: chronic infections, systemic lupus erythematosus (SLE), thyroid disease.

iv. Physical

1. Brief attack of urticaria induced by physical stimuli.

2. Most attacks last 1 to 6 hours.
3. Types.
    (a) Dermatographism: produced by rubbing or stroking of skin leaving visible lines.
    (b) Pressure: due to pressure from walking, standing, or wearing tight garments.
    (c) Cholinergic: due to overheating from exercise.
    (d) Cold: due to sudden drop in air temperature or sudden exposure to cold water.
    (e) Solar: due to exposure to UV light.
  b. **Clinical Manifestations**
    i. Pruritus is very common.
    ii. Plaques are pink, red, or flesh colored, often with central pallor, nonpitting, and edematous.
    iii. Vary in size from a few millimeters to several centimeters.
    iv. Linear lesions suggest physical urticaria.
    v. As old lesions resolve, new lesions appear.
  c. **Diagnosis**
    i. Based on clinical findings.
  d. **Treatment**
    i. All suspected triggers should be avoided.
    ii. Antihistamines are used initially.
      1. Histamine-1 blockers such as hydroxyzine work best.
      2. Nonsedating histamine-1 blockers (second-generation agents), such as loratadine and cetirizine, are first-line agents.
    iii. Prednisone is used in cases not controlled by antihistamines.
      1. Prednisone may not be helpful in chronic urticaria.
    iv. Epinephrine is used in extensive, severe cases.
    v. Identifying a cause for chronic cases may be difficult.

# QUESTIONS

### QUESTION 1

Which of the following best describes the rash of pityriasis rosea?

A  Salmon-colored oval plaques

B  Purple-colored flat papules

C  Clear fluid-filled vesicles

D  Red, raised scales

E  Indurated macule

### QUESTION 2

A 16-year-old wrestler presents with three round, scaly papules that have raised borders. Which of the following laboratory tests would assist in making the correct diagnosis?

A  Tzanck smear

B  Gram stain

C  KOH prep

D  Wright's stain

E  Eosinophil count

### QUESTION 3

On physical examination of a 21-year-old male, the physician assistant notes a cluster of verrucous lesions on the corona of the penis. Which of the following is the most likely diagnosis?

A  Condyloma acuminatum

B  Candidiasis balanitis

C  Syphilitic chancre

D  Herpes genitalis

E  Chancroid

### QUESTION 4

Which of the following is the best treatment option for a patient with stage I melanoma?

A  Radiation therapy

B  Surgical excision

C  Subcutaneous (SQ) vincristine

D  IV alpha interferon

E  Oral ipilimumab

### QUESTION 5

A 20-year-old patient presents with severe itching between their fingers. On physical examination linear elevated vesicles are noted in the finger webs. Which of the following is the treatment of choice for this patient?

A  Minocycline (Minocin)

B  Fluconazole (Diflucan)

C  Mebendazole (Vermox)

D  Permethrin (Elimite)

E  Cefazolin (Ancef)

### QUESTION 6

A 4-year-old presents with lesions on his cheeks and around his nose. On physical examination, several large, thin-roofed bullae are noted on the cheeks and around the nose. Which of the following is the treatment of choice?

A  Oral amoxicillin

B  Oral doxycycline

C  Bacitracin ointment

D  Mupirocin ointment

E  IV ceftaroline

*Continued*

## QUESTIONS—cont'd

### QUESTION 7
Stevens-Johnson syndrome is most commonly linked to exposure of which of the following medications?
A  Levofloxacin (Levaquin)
B  Glucophage (Metformin)
C  Phenytoin (Dilantin)
D  Amiodarone (Cordarone)
E  Acetaminophen (Tylenol)

### QUESTION 8
A 65-year-old female presents with yellow, greasy-appearing eruptions on her face. Which of the following is the most likely diagnosis?
A  Rosacea
B  Psoriasis
C  Lichen planus
D  Pityriasis rosea
E  Seborrheic dermatitis

### QUESTION 9
Which of the following best describes the lesion of seborrheic keratosis?
A  Waxy texture with a stuck-on appearance
B  Benign fleshy papules in the skinfolds
C  Discrete umbilicated papule
D  Red, target-shaped lesions
E  Fluid-filled vesicles

### QUESTION 10
A 6-year-old male presents with numerous small white eggs attached to the shafts of the scalp hair. Which of the following is the treatment of choice?
A  Tea tree oil
B  Dapsone (DDS)
C  Permethrin (Elimite)
D  Minocycline (Minocin)
E  Griseofulvin (Grifulvin)

## ANSWERS

**1.  A**
EXPLANATION: Pityriasis rosea lesions are described as salmon-colored oval plaques, 2 cm in diameter, with fine scales at the periphery. Multiple smaller lesions on the trunk give a Christmas tree pattern. *Topic: Pityriasis rosea*
☐ Correct  ☐ Incorrect

**2.  C**
EXPLANATION: Tinea corporis, a dermatophyte infection of the body, is common among wrestlers and presents as flat, scaly papules that develop a raised border with the center becoming brown or hypopigmented. Diagnosis is made by noting the presence of hyphae on KOH prep. *Topic: Tinea corporis*
☐ Correct  ☐ Incorrect

**3.  A**
EXPLANATION: Condyloma acuminatum, or venereal warts, varies from pale to white, rough, barely raised papules to large raised lesions on a broad base. *Topic: Condyloma acuminatum*
☐ Correct  ☐ Incorrect

**4.  B**
EXPLANATION: Treatment of melanoma, malignancy of the melanocytes, varies with the stage. Stage I is treated with surgical excision and stages II through IV are treated with both surgical intervention and high-dose interferon. *Topic: Melanoma*
☐ Correct  ☐ Incorrect

**5.  D**
EXPLANATION: Scabies, caused by *Sarcoptes scabiei,* presents with severe itching that is worse at night. The classic lesion is a burrow that is linear, curved, or S-shaped and a slightly elevated vesicle or papule. Typically found in the finger webs, wrists, penis, buttocks, and scrotum. Treatment of choice is permethrin or lindane. *Topic: Scabies*
☐ Correct  ☐ Incorrect

**6.  D**
EXPLANATION: Bullous impetigo presents as thin-roofed bullae primarily on the face. For localized infections the treatment of choice is mupirocin (Bactroban) ointment. *Topic: Infectious disease: Bacterial*
☐ Correct  ☐ Incorrect

**7.  C**
EXPLANATION: Stevens-Johnson syndrome, a desquamation syndrome, is associated with *Mycoplasma pneumoniae* infection and medications such as phenytoin, phenobarbital, sulfonamides, allopurinol, and aminopenicillins. *Topic: Stevens-Johnson syndrome*
☐ Correct  ☐ Incorrect

**8.  E**
EXPLANATION: Patients with seborrheic dermatitis, an acute or chronic papulosquamous dermatitis, present with dry scales or greasy yellow eruptions on the face, scalp, chest, eyelid margins, and body folds. *Topic: Seborrheic dermatitis*
☐ Correct  ☐ Incorrect

## ANSWERS—cont'd

**9.   A**

EXPLANATION: Seborrheic keratosis is a benign growth and is best described as having a waxy texture and a stuck-on appearance. ***Topic: Seborrheic keratosis***

☐ **Correct**   ☐ **Incorrect**

**10.   C**

EXPLANATION: Patients with head lice present with many small, white eggs firmly attached to the hair (nits) or with the presence of lice (3–4 mm in length) on the hair shaft or scalp. Treatment consists of permethrin, pyrethrin, or lindane. ***Topic: Lice***

☐ **Correct**   ☐ **Incorrect**

# CHAPTER 12
# HEMATOLOGIC SYSTEM

## EXAMINATION BLUEPRINT TOPICS

**ANEMIA**

General

Iron-deficiency anemia

Thalassemia

Sideroblastic anemia

Vitamin $B_{12}$ deficiency

Folate deficiency

Anemia of chronic disease

Hemolytic anemia

Aplastic anemia

**MALIGNANCIES**

Acute lymphocytic leukemia (ALL)

Chronic lymphocytic leukemia (CLL)

Acute myelogenous leukemia (AML)

Chronic myelogenous leukemia (CML)

Hairy cell leukemia

Lymphoma

Multiple myeloma

Myelodysplastic syndrome

Polycythemia vera

Oncologic emergencies

**COAGULATION DISORDERS**

Hemostasis

Factor VIII disorder

Factor IX disorder

Factor XI disorder

Hypercoagulable states

Thrombocytopenia

Thrombocytosis

Transfusion reactions

Hemochromatosis

# ANEMIA

## I. GENERAL
### a. Definition
  i. Any condition resulting from a significant decrease in the total erythrocyte mass.
  ii. A hemoglobin of less than 12 g/dL in females and less than 14 g/dL in males or a hematocrit of less than 36% in females and less than 42% in males.
### b. Erythropoiesis
  i. Definition.
    1. A series of events during which the hematopoietic cells mature into functional red blood cells.
  ii. Controlled by many different factors, including erythropoietin, granulocyte-macrophage colony-stimulating factor (GM-CSF), and cytokines such as interleukin-3.
  iii. Normal red blood cell.
    1. Biconcave disk with a life span of approximately 120 days.
  iv. Reticulocyte.
    1. A cell that remains after the nucleus is lost from an orthochromic erythroblast.
    2. Contains RNA and other cellular remnants that stain blue with methylene blue stain.

3. Reticulocyte index or corrected reticulocyte count.
    (a) Used to correct for degree of anemia.
    (b) Formula (Fig. 12.1).
4. Normal range: 1% to 2% or an absolute reticulocyte count of 50,000 to 60,000/mL.
5. Interpretation.
    (a) Elevated reticulocyte count and index noted in anemia secondary to increased destruction of red blood cells.
    (b) Decreased reticulocyte count and index noted in anemia secondary to decreased production of red blood cells.
### c. Clinical Manifestations
  i. Due to decreased oxygen transport.
    1. Fatigue.
    2. Dyspnea.
    3. Angina.
  ii. Due to decreased blood volume.
    1. Pallor.
    2. Postural hypotension.
    3. Syncope.
    4. Headache.
    5. Tinnitus.
  iii. Due to increased cardiac output.
    1. Tachycardia.
    2. Systolic ejection heart murmur.
    3. Lightheadedness.

$$\text{Observed reticulocyte count (\%)} \times \frac{\text{Patient's Hematocrit}}{\text{Normal Hematocrit}} = \text{Reticulocyte Index}$$

**Fig. 12.1** Formula for reticulocyte index.

iv. Due to hemolysis of red blood cells.
    1. Jaundice.
    2. Splenomegaly.
**d. Classifications**
  i. Cytochromic classifications.
    1. Microcytic (mean corpuscular volume [MCV] <80 fL).
      (a) Iron-deficiency anemia.
      (b) Thalassemia.
      (c) Anemia of chronic disease.
      (d) Lead poisoning.
      (e) Sideroblastic anemia.
    2. Normocytic (MCV = 80 − 100 fL).
      (a) Anemia of chronic disease.
      (b) Hemolytic anemia.
      (c) Anemia of acute hemorrhage.
      (d) Aplastic anemia.
    3. Macrocytic (MCV > 100 fL).
      (a) Vitamin $B_{12}$ deficiency.
      (b) Folate deficiency.
      (c) Preleukemia.
      (d) Liver disease.
      (e) Drugs such as zidovudine and hydroxy-urea.
**e. Normal Ranges (Table 12.1)**
**f. Anemia Flowchart (Fig. 12.2)**

## II. IRON-DEFICIENCY ANEMIA
**a. Normal Iron Metabolism**
  i. Daily intake and loss are small, unless increased blood loss with bleeding or hemolysis of red blood cells.
  ii. Absorption occurs in the duodenum and upper jejunum.
  iii. Transported by transferrin and stored as ferritin.
**b. Etiologies**
  i. Blood loss.
    1. Gastrointestinal (GI), menstruation, pulmonary, or urinary sources.
    2. Evaluate for GI blood loss in older males with iron deficiency.
  ii. Increased iron demand.
    1. Due to pregnancy, lactation, and rapid growth and development.
  iii. Malabsorption.
    1. Due to gastrectomy, pancreatic insufficiency, sprue, or short bowel syndrome.
  iv. Poor dietary intake.
  v. Hemolysis.
**c. Clinical Manifestations**
  i. See clinical manifestations earlier in section I.
  ii. Pica syndrome: appetite for substances not fit as food (clay, starch, ice).
  iii. Angular stomatitis and atrophy of tongue mucosa secondary to impaired epithelial function.
  iv. Spooning or curling of nails (koilonychia).
**d. Laboratory Features**
  i. Cell morphology.
    1. Typically microcytic, hypochromic.
      (a) Will vary with degree of iron deficiency.
      (b) See Color Plate 18.
  ii. Iron studies (Table 12.2).
**e. Treatment**
  i. Identify and correct underlying cause.
  ii. Transfusion.
    1. Reserved for those with cardiovascular instability, with continued blood loss, or in need of immediate intervention.
  iii. Iron therapy.
    1. Oral.
      (a) Treat with 300 mg of elemental iron per day.
        (i) Ferrous sulfate 325 mg, orally (PO) three times a day (TID).
      (b) Complications include GI distress, such as abdominal pain, nausea, vomiting, or constipation.
      (c) Monitor response to therapy by noting increased reticulocyte count in 7 to 10 days and increase in hemoglobin/hematocrit in 2 to 3 weeks.

**TABLE 12.1**

| Normal Ranges | | |
| --- | --- | --- |
| | **Male** | **Female** |
| White blood cell count | 5,000–10,500/μL | 5,000–10,500/μL |
| Red blood cell count | 4.5–5.5 × 10⁶/μL | 4.1–5.1 × 10⁶/μL |
| Hemoglobin | 14–16 g/dL | 12–14 g/dL |
| Hematocrit | 42–48% | 36–42% |
| Mean corpuscular volume (MCV) | 80–100 fL | 80–100 fL |
| Mean corpuscular hemoglobin (MCH) | 26–34 pg/cell | 26–34 pg/cell |
| Mean corpuscular hemoglobin concentration (MCHC) | 31–36 g/dL | 31–36 g/dL |
| Platelet count | 150,000–450,000/μL | 150,000–450,000/μL |

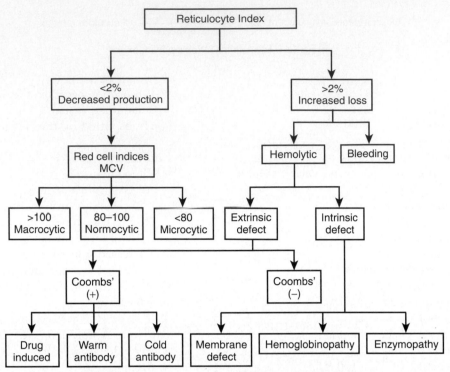

**Fig. 12.2** Anemia flowchart. *MCV*, Mean corpuscular volume.

**TABLE 12.2**

| Comparison of Iron Studies in Various Disorders | | | | | |
|---|---|---|---|---|---|
| | **Total Serum Iron (μg/dL)** | **Total Iron Binding Capacity (μg/dL)** | **Percentage Saturation** | **Ferritin (μ/L)** | **Bone Marrow Iron Stores** |
| Normal | 50–150 | 300–360 | 30–50 | 50–200 | Normal |
| Iron-deficiency anemia | <30 | >360 | <10 | <15 | Decreased |
| Inflammation | <50 | <300 | 10–20 | Normal | Normal |
| Thalassemia | Normal | Normal | 30–80 | 50–300 | Normal |
| Sideroblastic anemia | Normal to high | Normal | 30–80 | 50–300 | Increased |

    (d) If patient fails to respond to treatment, evaluate for possible patient noncompliance, incorrect diagnosis (thalassemia), poor absorption, erythropoietin deficiency, or other concurrent anemia.

  2. Parenteral.

    (a) Used in those unable to tolerate oral therapy.

    (b) Major complication is allergic reaction and anaphylaxis.

## III. THALASSEMIA

  **a. Etiology**

    i. A group of hereditary disorders in which there is a defect in the synthesis of one or more of the globin polypeptide chains in hemoglobin.

      1. Mature adult hemoglobin is a tetramer of two alpha chains and two beta chains.

      2. If ratio is not correct, hemoglobin may precipitate out in the red blood cell.

    ii. Leads to absent or decreased synthesis of the affected globin chain and development of nonfunctioning hemoglobin.

    iii. Primarily affects people of Mediterranean, African, or Asian ancestry.

      1. Especially common where malaria is endemic.

  **b. Types**

    i. Alpha-thalassemia.

      1. Defect in the alpha-chain synthesis, results in excess of beta chains.

      2. Four types.

(a) Silent carrier.
   (i) Deletion of one alpha gene.
(b) Alpha-thalassemia trait.
   (i) Deletion of two alpha genes.
   (ii) Mild anemia.
(c) Hemoglobin H.
   (i) Deletion of three alpha genes.
   (ii) Severe anemia with signs of hemolysis.
(d) Hydrops fetalis.
   (i) Deletion of all four alpha genes.
   (ii) Leads to death in utero.
  ii. Beta-thalassemia.
    1. Defect in the beta-chain synthesis, results in excess alpha chains.
    2. Two types.
     (a) Beta-thalassemia minor.
      (i) Microcytic anemia.
     (b) Beta-thalassemia major (Cooley's anemia).
      (i) Severe anemia with bone changes.
      (ii) Copper-colored skin.
      (iii) Jaundice and hepatosplenomegaly.

**c. Laboratory Features**
  i. Microcytic, hypochromic red blood cells.
    1. Target and teardrop cells are common on microscopic evaluation of the blood.
  ii. MCV is low, typically less than 70 fL.
  iii. Normal iron studies.
  iv. Hemoglobin electrophoresis is diagnostic.
    1. Beta-thalassemia note increased hemoglobin $A_2$ and F.
    2. Alpha-thalassemia note increased hemoglobin H and Barts.

**d. Treatment**
  i. Transfuse as needed.
    1. Watch for iron overload with multiple transfusions.
  ii. Commonly misdiagnosed as iron-deficiency anemia and treated with iron supplements.
    1. Can lead to iron overload.
  iii. Splenectomy may be needed in beta-thalassemia major and hemoglobin H disease.
  iv. All patients diagnosed with thalassemia should undergo genetic counseling.

## IV. SIDEROBLASTIC ANEMIA
**a. Etiology**
  i. Due to a mitochondrial defect that prevents the incorporation of iron into hemoglobin.
  ii. Iron then accumulates in the mitochondria around the red blood cell nucleus forming a ringed sideroblast.

**b. Classification**
  i. Acquired.

    1. Secondary to prolonged exposure to toxins or drugs.
     (a) Seen with ethanol, lead, and isoniazid.
    2. Typically noted in patients older than 65 years.
  ii. Hereditary.
    1. X-linked recessive.
    2. Seen in both men and women, typically diagnosed during first three decades of life.
  iii. Idiopathic.
    1. A type of myelodysplastic syndrome.

**c. Laboratory Features**
  i. Blood smear.
    1. Dimorphic cell population, microcytic, hypochromia with normocytic or macrocytic cells.
  ii. Mild anemia with increased serum iron and ferritin. Total iron-binding capacity (TIBC) is normal or decreased, and transferrin is decreased.
  iii. Low reticulocyte count.
  iv. Bone marrow.
    1. Ringed sideroblasts noted on bone marrow examination when stained with Prussian blue stain.

**d. Treatment**
  i. Treat the underlying cause.
  ii. Red blood cell transfusions for severe anemia.
    1. May require an iron-chelating agent (desferrioxamine) after numerous transfusions to avoid iron overload.

## V. VITAMIN B₁₂ DEFICIENCY
**a. Normal Vitamin $B_{12}$ Metabolism**
  i. Vitamin $B_{12}$ is required for normal nuclear maturation and DNA synthesis.
  ii. Obtained only through dietary sources, such as meats, cheese, milk, and eggs.
  iii. Absorbed in terminal ileum and stored in the liver.
    1. Liver stores will last for 7–10 years.

**b. Etiologies**
  i. Decreased intake of vitamin $B_{12}$.
    1. Seen in strict vegetarians and vegans.
  ii. Impaired absorption of vitamin $B_{12}$.
    1. Lack of intrinsic factor or autoimmune destruction of parietal cells (pernicious anemia).
     (a) Pernicious anemia also associated with other autoimmune disorders such as Graves' disease, thyroiditis, and adrenal insufficiency.
    2. Malabsorption in patients with sprue or inflammatory bowel disease.
    3. Competitive absorption problem due to bacterial overgrowth or fish tapeworm (*Diphyllobothrium latum*).

iii. Increased requirement for vitamin $B_{12}$.
    1. Uncommon because of large stores of vitamin $B_{12}$ but can be seen in pregnancy and patients with neoplastic disorders.
iv. Impaired utilization of vitamin $B_{12}$.

**c. Clinical Manifestations**
  i. See anemia clinical manifestations earlier in section I.
  ii. Red, beefy tongue.
  iii. May have the following neurologic signs and symptoms:
    1. Loss of memory.
    2. Paresthesia and numbness in the extremities.
      (a) This is the earliest neurologic sign.
    3. Diminished position or vibratory sense.
    4. Weakness and ataxia.

**d. Laboratory Features**
  i. Red blood cells are macrocytic (MCV > 110 fL) and oval in shape.
    1. See Color Plate 19.
  ii. White blood cells are hypersegmented with more than five lobes.
  iii. Platelets are large and decreased in number.
  iv. Low reticulocyte count.
  v. Decreased serum vitamin $B_{12}$ levels (<200 pg/mL).
    1. Values less than 100 indicate significant deficiency.
  vi. Homocysteine and methylmalonic acid (MMA) levels are elevated.
    1. Vitamin $B_{12}$ functions as a cofactor for two enzymes.
      (a) Methionine synthase and L-methylmalonyl-CoA mutase.
    2. Methionine synthase catalyzes the conversion of homocysteine to the amino acid methionine.
    3. False elevations in renal insufficiency, hypothyroidism, and hypovolemia.
  vii. Schilling test.
    1. Interpretation (Table 12.3).
  viii. Anti–intrinsic factor antibody or anti–parietal cell antibodies may be present in pernicious anemia.

**e. Treatment**
  i. Treat underlying cause.
  ii. Vitamin $B_{12}$ supplements.
  iii. Monitor response by checking for increase in reticulocyte count in 7 days.
  iv. Neurologic symptoms may not resolve.
  v. Pernicious anemia patients at increased risk for gastric cancer.

## VI. FOLATE DEFICIENCY
**a. Normal Folate Metabolism**
  i. Folate required for synthesis of nuclear proteins.

**TABLE 12.3**

| Interpretation of Schilling Test | | |
|---|---|---|
| Condition | $^{57}$Co-labeled Vitamin $B_{12}$ without Intrinsic Factor | $^{57}$Co-labeled Vitamin $B_{12}$ with Intrinsic Factor |
| Normal | ≥8% | ≥8% |
| Pernicious anemia | Decreased | Corrected |
| Vitamin $B_{12}$ malabsorption | Decreased | Not Corrected |

    1. Vitamin $B_{12}$ is a required cofactor for folate metabolism.
  ii. Obtained through dietary sources, such as green leafy vegetables, liver, and eggs.
  iii. Absorbed in proximal jejunum and stored in the liver.
    1. Liver stores last only 4 months.

**b. Etiologies**
  i. Decreased intake of folate.
    1. Seen in patients with poor diets and alcoholism.
  ii. Impaired absorption of folate.
    1. Due to intestinal bypass surgery, malabsorption syndromes, and phenytoin (Dilantin) use.
  iii. Increased requirement for folate.
    1. Seen in pregnancy, children, hyperthyroidism, and neoplasia.
  iv. Impaired utilization.
    1. Seen with folate antagonists such as trimethoprim-sulfamethoxazole (Bactrim).
    2. Alcohol impairs utilization of folate in the bone marrow.

**c. Clinical Manifestations**
  i. Same signs and symptoms as vitamin $B_{12}$ deficiency EXCEPT no neurologic abnormalities.
  ii. Also note diarrhea, cheilosis, and glossitis.

**d. Laboratory Features**
  i. Macrocytic (MCV > 100 fL) red blood cells.
  ii. Hypersegmented neutrophils.
  iii. Platelets are large and decreased in number.
  iv. Low reticulocyte count.
  v. Serum folate levels are low (≤4 ng/mL).
  vi. Homocysteine levels elevated.

**e. Treatment**
  i. Treat with replacement therapy.
    1. Folate 1 to 5 mg/day PO.
  ii. Monitor response by checking for increase in reticulocyte count in 7 days.
  iii. Folate deficiency increases the risk of neural tube defects in pregnancy.

## VII. ANEMIA OF CHRONIC DISEASE

a. **Etiology**
  i. Most common cause of anemia in the hospitalized or chronically ill patient.
  ii. Seen in patients with chronic:
    1. Infection.
    2. Inflammatory disease.
    3. Malignancy.
    4. Renal disease.

b. **Clinical Manifestations**
  i. Same as anemia listed earlier in section III.
  ii. Will also have the signs and symptoms of the underlying etiology.

c. **Laboratory Features**
  i. Red blood cells are normocytic, normochromic or microcytic, hypochromic.
  ii. Decreased reticulocyte count.
  iii. Increased erythrocyte sedimentation rate (ESR).
  iv. Decreased serum iron but normal or increased serum ferritin.

d. **Treatment**
  i. Treat underlying cause.
  ii. Erythropoietin helpful in treating anemia due to chronic renal disease.

## VIII. HEMOLYTIC ANEMIA

a. **General**
  i. Only a hemolytic process or acute blood loss will cause the hemoglobin to abruptly drop.
  ii. The red blood cell has three components that may be involved in a hemolytic process.
    1. Metabolic machinery (enzymes).
    2. Hemoglobin.
    3. Red cell membrane.
  iii. Reticulocyte count is elevated in hemolytic anemia.

b. **Etiology**
  i. Acquired hemolytic anemia.
  ii. Congenital hemolytic anemia.
    1. Membrane abnormalities.
    2. Hemoglobinopathies.
    3. Enzyme deficiency.

c. **Clinical Manifestations**
  i. Splenomegaly and jaundice are common on physical examination.
  ii. Laboratory features.
    1. In general, may note the following:
      (a) Increased lactate dehydrogenase (LDH).
      (b) Hemoglobinuria.
      (c) Increased indirect bilirubin.
      (d) Decreased haptoglobin in intravascular hemolysis.

      (i) Haptoglobin is a carrier protein that binds free hemoglobin in the bloodstream.
      (e) Blood smear may show spherocytes, schistocytes, or helmet cells.
    2. Coombs' test.
      (a) Direct.
        (i) Detects antibody on red blood cell surface.
          (1) Used in the evaluation of acquired hemolytic anemia.
          (2) Detects antiimmunoglobulin (IgG) or anticomplement (C3).
      (b) Indirect.
        (i) Detects antibody in the plasma.
        (ii) Used in the cross-matching of blood products.

d. **Specific Hemolytic Disorders**
  i. Acquired hemolytic anemia.
    1. Distinguished by results of the Coombs' test.
    2. Coombs' negative.
      (a) Hypersplenism.
        (i) Have increased removal of cellular elements by the spleen.
        (ii) Causes:
          (1) Primary (idiopathic).
          (2) Secondary.
            [a] Acute/Chronic infections.
              [i] Malaria, tuberculosis, hepatitis.
            [b] Chronic inflammatory disease.
              [i] Systemic lupus erythematosus (SLE), sarcoidosis.
            [c] Congestive splenomegaly.
            [d] Myeloproliferative disorders.
            [e] Leukemia/Lymphoma.
        (iii) Diagnosed by demonstrating shortened red blood cell survival and splenic sequestration.
        (iv) Treat underlying cause or splenectomy.
      (b) Microangiopathic.
        (i) Mechanical disruption of the red blood cells.
        (ii) Must see schistocytes on peripheral blood smear.
        (iii) Seen with disseminated intravascular coagulation (DIC), thrombotic thrombocytopenic purpura (TTP), and hemolytic uremic syndrome (HUS).

(c) Chemical.
  (i) Noted with lead poisoning and freshwater drowning.
(d) Physical.
  (i) Noted with second- or third-degree burns over greater than 20% body.
(e) Infectious.
  (i) Common with malaria, viral infections such as parvovirus B19, and *Clostridium welchii* infection.
3. Coombs' positive.
  (a) Drug-induced.
    (i) Three mechanisms.
      (1) Hapten type.
        [a] Coombs' positive for anti-IgG.
      (2) Immune complex.
        [a] Coombs' positive for C3.
      (3) Autoantibody.
        [a] Coombs' positive for anti-IgG.
        [b] May last for months, even after stopping medications.
    (ii) See Table 12.4.
    (iii) Treatment.
      (1) Stop drugs.
      (2) Autoantibody type may need treatment with steroids.
  (b) Warm autoantibody.
    (i) Usually IgG antibody.
    (ii) Primary (idiopathic) or secondary due to tumor infection or autoimmune disorder (SLE).
    (iii) Treat with steroids and splenectomy.
  (c) Cold autoantibody.
    (i) Usually IgM antibody.

**TABLE 12.4**

| **Summary of Drug-Induced Hemolytic Anemias** | | | |
|---|---|---|---|
| **Mechanism** | **Hapten** | **Immune Complex** | **Autoantibody** |
| Example | Penicillin | Quinidine | Methyldopa |
| Coombs' test | Positive | Positive | Positive |
| Anti-IgG | Positive | Rarely positive | Positive |
| Anti-C3d | Rarely positive | Positive | Negative |
| Drugs | Cephalothin | Hydrochlorothiazide | L-Dopa |
| | Ampicillin | Antihistamines | Ibuprofen |
| | Methicillin | Rifampin | Diclofenac |
| | | Isoniazid | Interferon-alpha |
| | | Sulfonamides | |
| | | Insulin | |
| | | Tylenol | |

  (ii) Causes intravascular hemolysis.
  (iii) Cold agglutinins secondary to viral or mycoplasmal infection.
    (1) May have elevated mean corpuscular hemoglobin concentration (MCHC > 36 g/dL).
    (2) MCHC will be normal after warming of blood and retesting.
  (iv) Poor response to steroids.
ii. Congenital hemolytic anemia.
  1. Membrane abnormalities.
    (a) Hereditary spherocytosis.
      (i) Autosomal dominant disorder.
      (ii) Due to a deficiency in the proteins that maintain adherence between the cytoskeleton and bilipid membrane, this results in loss of cell surface area.
      (iii) Most common congenital hemolytic anemia in the White population.
      (iv) Features include splenomegaly and numerous spherocytes on peripheral smear.
      (v) Will have a positive osmotic fragility test, negative Coombs' test, and an elevated MCHC.
      (vi) Treatment includes splenectomy if indicated and folic acid to decrease risk for folate deficiency.
    (b) Hereditary elliptocytosis.
      (i) Rare autosomal dominant disorder.
      (ii) Due to weakness of the cytoskeletal of the cell.
      (iii) Present with 40% to 60% elliptocytes on peripheral smear.
      (iv) Treatment, if needed, is splenectomy.
  2. Enzyme deficiency.
    (a) Glucose-6-phosphate dehydrogenase (G-6-PD) deficiency.
      (i) Sex-linked disorder.
        (1) Commonly of African or Mediterranean descent.
      (ii) Defect in hexose-monophosphate shunt.
      (iii) Hemolysis is intravascular (red blood cell lysis secondary to stress) and extravascular (red blood cells age prematurely).
      (iv) Due to stress-induced hemolysis secondary to sulfonamides, antimalarials, vitamin K, infection, or fava beans.
      (v) Labs include hemoglobinuria and decreased G-6-PD activity level

and may note Heinz bodies on peripheral smear.
  (1) Heinz bodies are due to oxida-
      tion of hemoglobin.
  (vi) Treatment.
      (1) Avoid medications that stress
          red blood cells.
      (2) Folate supplements.
(b) Pyruvate kinase deficiency.
  (i) Very rare disorder, commonly seen
      in children.
  (ii) Defect in Embden-Meyerhof
       pathway.
  (iii) Patients present with anemia, jaun-
        dice, and splenomegaly.
  (iv) Diagnose by checking enzyme
       activity.
  (v) Treatment.
      (1) Transfusion as needed.
      (2) Folate supplement.
3. Hemoglobinopathies.
  (a) Sickle cell anemia.
    (i) Inherited disorder resulting in pro-
        duction of defective hemoglobin.
        (1) Decreased solubility in deoxy-
            genated form; this leads to
            sickling.
    (ii) Due to substitution of valine for
         glutamic acid at position six on the
         beta chain.
    (iii) Very common in Black population
          (0.3%).
          (1) Homozygotes have sickle cell
              disease.
    (iv) Signs and Symptoms.
         (1) Anemia: pallor and fatigue.
         (2) Hemolysis: jaundice and gall-
             stones.
         (3) Dactylitis.
         (4) Leg ulcers.
         (5) Priapism.
         (6) Pulmonary, cerebral, and
             splenic emboli.
         (7) Retinal artery obstruction
             leading to blindness.
         (8) Sickle cell crisis.
             [a] Skeletal pain.
             [b] Fever.
             [c] Anemia.
             [d] Jaundice.
             [e] Note: Look for infection as
                 source of sickle cell crisis.
    (v) Laboratory features.
        (1) Microcytic hypochromic or
            normocytic anemia.

        (2) Elevated reticulocyte count.
        (3) Sickle cells noted on peripheral
            blood smear. (See Color
            Plate 20.)
        (4) Elevated indirect bilirubin.
        (5) Hemoglobin electrophoresis.
            [a] Diagnostic with elevated
                sickle cell hemoglobin (HbS)
                in sickle cell disease.
    (vi) Treatment.
         (1) Avoid triggers.
         (2) Good nutrition.
         (3) Folic acid supplements.
         (4) Vaccines: *Haemophilus influen-
             zae* type b and pneumococcal.
         (5) Hydroxyurea increases hemo-
             globin F levels, reduces sickling
             deformities of the red blood
             cells, and improves blood flow.
         (6) Crisis.
             [a] Pain control.
             [b] Transfusions.
             [c] Antibiotics for infection.
    (vii) Outcomes.
          (1) Survival depends on number of
              crises per year.
  (b) Sickle cell trait.
    (i) Heterozygotes are carriers of sickle
        cell trait.
    (ii) May have mild anemia and typi-
         cally asymptomatic.
    (iii) Laboratory features.
          (1) Hemoglobin electrophoresis.
              [a] 50% HbS in sickle cell car-
                  riers.
  (c) Hemoglobin SC disease.
    (i) Patient has milder symptoms than
        with sickle cell disease.
    (ii) Retinopathy and splenomegaly are
         noted.
    (iii) Hemoglobin electrophoresis re-
          veals equal amounts of hemoglobin
          S and hemoglobin C.
  (d) Hemoglobin C disease.
    (i) Mild to moderate anemia.
    (ii) Note hemoglobin crystals and tar-
         get cells on peripheral smear.
    (iii) Diagnose with hemoglobin elec-
          trophoresis.
    (iv) In most patients no treatment is
         required.

## IX. APLASTIC ANEMIA
### a. General
   i. Pancytopenia with bone marrow hypocellularity.

b. **Etiologies**
i. Acquired.
1. Idiopathic.
2. Radiation.
3. Chemicals such as benzene.
4. Drugs such as chemotherapy agents, chloramphenicol, heavy metals, and insecticide.
5. Viruses such as hepatitis and parvovirus B19.
6. Immune diseases.
7. Paroxysmal nocturnal hemoglobinuria.
(a) Rare acquired disorder.
(b) Clinical features include variable hemoglobinuria and pancytopenia.
(c) Laboratory features include increased reticulocytes and negative direct Coombs' test.
(d) Ham's test or sucrose lysis test is positive.
ii. Inherited.
1. Fanconi's anemia.
2. Preleukemia.

c. **Clinical Manifestations**
i. Bleeding is common early in this disease.
ii. Symptoms of anemia (see section I).
iii. Patients typically look and feel well despite the pancytopenia.

d. **Laboratory Features**
i. Significant pancytopenia.
ii. Bone marrow is hypocellular and fatty.

e. **Treatment**
i. Bone marrow transplantation.
ii. Immunosuppression.

# MALIGNANCIES

## I. ACUTE LYMPHOCYTIC LEUKEMIA (ALL)
a. **General**
i. Most common leukemia in childhood; uncommon in adults.
ii. Immature lymphocytes or lymphoblasts are produced with no further differentiation.

b. **Etiologies**
i. Radiation exposure, benzene, and previous chemotherapy linked to development of ALL.

c. **Clinical Manifestations**
i. Abrupt onset of fatigue, malaise, bone pain, sweats, bleeding, and easy bruising.
ii. Physical examination reveals lymphadenopathy, pallor, petechiae, and ecchymoses.

d. **Laboratory Features**
i. Pancytopenia develops secondary to marrow replacement by tumor cells.
ii. Elevated white cell count in two-thirds of patients.

iii. Elevated uric acid and lactate dehydrogenase (LDH).
iv. Increased blasts noted in bone marrow.
1. 30% to 100% blasts.
v. May have a t(9; 22) translocation (Philadelphia chromosome [Ph[1]]).
1. Presence of this translocation indicates a poorer prognosis.
vi. World Health Organization divides ALL into B-cell lymphoblastic leukemia or T-cell lymphoblastic leukemia.
1. Immunophenotyping used to classify disease.

e. **Treatment**
i. Remission induction.
1. Chemotherapy with vincristine, prednisone, L–asparaginase, and anthracycline. 2. A tyrosine kinase inhibitor, such as imatinib, is added in for patients who are positive for Philadelphia chromosome.
ii. Postremission therapy.
1. Consolidation chemotherapy utilizes a wide variety of chemotherapy agents.
2. Maintenance therapy utilizes oral 6-mercaptopurine or methotrexate.
iii. Central nervous system (CNS) prophylaxis required.
1. Intrathecal methotrexate or brain radiation.
iv. Bone marrow transplantation.

## II. CHRONIC LYMPHOCYTIC LEUKEMIA (CLL)
a. **General**
i. An indolent lymphoproliferative disorder characterized by lymphocytosis, lymphadenopathy, and splenomegaly.
ii. Most common adult leukemia, typically around 70 years of age.

b. **Etiology**
i. Cause of CLL is unknown.
ii. Affects the B-cells.

c. **Clinical Manifestations**
i. Most patients are asymptomatic.
ii. May present with fatigue, lethargy, weight loss, and decreased exercise tolerance.
iii. Physical examination reveals enlarged lymph nodes, mainly cervical, and splenomegaly is rare until late in the disease.

d. **Laboratory Features**
i. An absolute lymphocytosis in the peripheral blood.
1. Absolute lymphocyte count greater than 5,000/mcL.
2. Smudge cells present.
ii. Anemia and thrombocytopenia may be present.

e. Treatment
  i. Chemotherapy.
     1. Fludarabine, chlorambucil, and rituximab in combination are used.
  ii. Radiation therapy.
     1. Used for localized lymphadenopathy and splenomegaly that do not respond to chemotherapy.
  iii. Monoclonal antibodies.
  iv. Bone marrow transplantation.

## III. ACUTE MYELOGENEOUS LEUKEMIA (AML)

a. **General**
  i. Group of heterogeneous disorders characterized by uncontrolled proliferation of primitive hematopoietic cells.
  ii. Increased incidence with age.
     1. Most common adult leukemia.
  iii. Classification.
     1. AML with recurrent genetic abnormalities.
     2. AML with myelodysplastic-related features.
     3. Therapy-related AML with myelodysplastic syndrome.
     4. AML, not otherwise specified.
b. **Etiologies**
  i. Strong link to toxin exposure, such as benzene and carbon tetrachloride, and alkylating agents, such as melphalan and nitrosoureas.
  ii. Increased risk with ionizing radiation.
  iii. Increased risk with trisomy 21 (Down syndrome).
  iv. The most common risk factor is myelodysplastic syndrome.
c. **Clinical Manifestations**
  i. Abrupt onset of fatigue, malaise, bone pain, sweats, bleeding, easy bruising, or signs of infection.
  ii. Physical examination reveals pallor, petechiae, and ecchymoses.
d. **Laboratory Features**
  i. 30% to 100% blasts noted in bone marrow.
     1. Auer rods present in blasts are virtually pathognomonic for AML.
  ii. Anemia and thrombocytopenia are present.
  iii. Elevations in uric acid and LDH are noted.
e. **Treatment**
  i. Remission induction.
     1. Chemotherapy with daunorubicin and cytarabine.
     2. Watch for severe myelosuppression and infection.
  ii. Postremission therapy.
     1. Intensive consolidation chemotherapy.
     2. No CNS prophylaxis is needed.
  iii. Bone marrow transplantation.

## IV. CHRONIC MYELOGENOUS LEUKEMIA (CML)

a. **General**
  i. A chronic myeloproliferative disorder characterized by excessive growth and development of differentiated cells.
  ii. Incidence of CML increases with age.
b. **Etiology**
  i. No etiologic agent has been identified.
c. **Clinical Manifestations**
  i. Symptoms include fatigue, weight loss, night sweats, and malaise.
  ii. Physical examination reveals marked splenomegaly.
  iii. Lymphadenopathy is rare.
d. **Laboratory Features**
  i. Elevated white blood cell count with presence of complete cell line from blasts to mature neutrophils.
     1. Basophilia may be present.
  ii. Philadelphia (Ph[1]) chromosome is present in 95% of CML cases.
  iii. Increased uric acid noted in most patients.
     1. May lead to a gouty arthritis after treatment.
  iv. Low leukocyte alkaline phosphatase (LAP) score.
     1. This will assist in separating CML from leukemoid reaction.
e. **Treatment**
  i. Based on age and phase of disease.
  ii. Tyrosine kinase inhibitors are not curative but effective in the asymptomatic chronic phase and are the initial treatment choice for patients in this phase.
  iii. Palliation therapy in CML includes the use of hydroxyurea, busulfan, and recombinant interferon or pegylated interferon.
     1. Hydroxyurea is a debulking agent to decrease white blood cell count.
  iv. Transplantation therapy.
     1. Allogenic stem cell transplantation.

## V. HAIRY CELL LEUKEMIA

a. **General**
  i. A chronic B-cell disorder.
  ii. More common in elderly people, with males affected more than females.
b. **Clinical Manifestations**
  i. May have hepatosplenomegaly.
  ii. Peripheral lymphadenopathy is rare.
c. **Laboratory Features**
  i. Pancytopenia is present.
  ii. Lymphocytes have hairlike, cytoplasmic projections.
d. **Treatment**

i. Splenectomy.

ii. Purine analogs such as 2-chlorodeoxyadenosine (Cladribine) produce remission in 90% of cases.

## VI. LYMPHOMA

### a. Hodgkin's Lymphoma

i. General.

1. Malignant disorder of the lymphatic system that mainly affects the lymph nodes.

2. Onset of disease has a bimodal distribution.

   (a) First peak is in the second and third decades of life.

   (b) Second peak after age 50 years.

3. More common in males and less common in Black people.

4. Have contiguous spread from lymph node to lymph node, with a central distribution of affected nodes.

ii. Etiology.

1. May be a link to Epstein-Barr virus.

iii. Clinical Manifestations.

1. Localized lymphadenopathy is common.

   (a) Lymph nodes are firm, freely mobile, and nontender.

2. Chronic pruritus may be seen.

3. Disulfiram-like reaction and pain with alcohol ingestion may be noted.

4. May have fever, weight loss, and night sweats (B symptoms).

   (a) Presence of B symptoms is poor prognostic indicator.

iv. Laboratory features.

1. Noting Reed-Sternberg cells in lymph node tissue makes diagnosis.

   (a) Reed-Sternberg cells are large, binucleated cells with prominent nucleoli.

2. Mild to moderate anemia may be present.

3. ESR is elevated.

v. Treatment.

1. Staging of disease is very important for treatment and prognosis.

   (a) Staging should include lymph node biopsy, chest x-ray, computed tomography (CT) scan of chest and abdomen, complete blood count (CBC), ESR, and chemistry profile including liver function tests.

   (b) Ann Arbor staging.

      (i) Stage I: only one lymph node region or structure.

      (ii) Stage II: two or more lymph node regions on same side of the diaphragm.

      (iii) Stage III: lymph node regions or structures on both sides of the diaphragm are involved.

      (iv) Stage IV: involvement of other organs such as liver, bone marrow, and CNS.

2. Treatment includes radiation therapy and chemotherapy (Adriamycin, bleomycin, dacarbazine, and vincristine).

   (a) 85% curable with treatment.

### b. Non-Hodgkin's Lymphoma

i. General

1. Solid tumor of the immune system.

2. Classified as indolent or aggressive.

3. 90% are B cell in origin.

ii. Etiology

1. Unknown, although immune system abnormalities, infectious agents, and environmental and occupational exposure have been implicated.

iii. Clinical Manifestations

1. Symptoms include chest pain, cough, superior vena cava syndrome, abdominal and back pain, and spinal cord compression.

   (a) Due to lymphadenopathy in the mediastinum or retroperitoneum.

2. Patients may also present with fatigue, fever, weight loss, and night sweats.

3. Most common presentation is asymptomatic lymphadenopathy.

   (a) Noted in the cervical, axillary, or inguinal region.

   (b) Nodes are firm and nontender and greater than 1 cm in size.

iv. Laboratory features

1. Biopsy results vary depending on type of non-Hodgkin's lymphoma.

v. Treatment

1. Surgical excision.

2. Radiation therapy.

3. Chemotherapy.

4. Immunotherapy.

5. Targeted drugs

## VII. MULTIPLE MYELOMA

### a. General

i. Neoplastic proliferation of a single clone of plasma cells (B cells).

ii. Seen more commonly in patients older than 65 years.

iii. Twice the incidence in Black people compared with White people.

### b. Etiology

i. Cause is unclear; may be linked to organic solvents, herbicides, and insecticides.

c. **Clinical Manifestations**
   i. Symptoms include bone pain (mainly the back and chest), weakness, and fatigue.
   ii. May also develop symptoms due to development of acute infection, renal insufficiency, and hypercalcemia.

d. **Laboratory Features**
   i. Normocytic, normochromic anemia.
   ii. Serum protein electrophoresis shows a peak or localized band.
      1. IgG M protein is most common.
      2. Light chain (Bence Jones protein) may be noted in the urine.
   iii. Increase in number of plasma cells and red blood cell rouleaux noted.
   iv. X-ray film of bones reveals punched-out lytic lesions.
      1. Compression and pathologic fractures are common.
      2. See Fig. 12.3.
   v. Diagnostic criteria.
      1. Bone marrow greater than 10% plasma cells or a plasmacytoma and one of the following:
         (a) M protein in the serum (usually >3 g/dL).
         (b) M protein in the urine.
         (c) Lytic bone lesions.

e. **Treatment**
   i. Chemotherapy with melphalan, proteasome inhibitor (bortezomib) or immunomodulatory (lenalidomide), and prednisone.
   ii. Autologous stem cell transplantation.
   iii. Patients are very prone to infection.
   iv. Vaccinations and antibiotics may be required.

## VIII. MYELODYSPLASTIC SYNDROME
   a. **General**

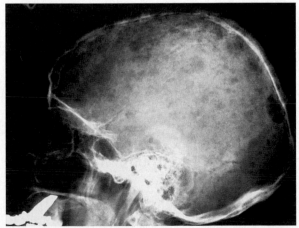

**Fig. 12.3** Skull x-ray in a patient with multiple myeloma. *(From Mettler F: Essentials of Radiology, 2nd ed. Philadelphia: Elsevier Saunders, 2005:17, Fig. 2-3.)*

   i. Group of clonal hematopoietic stem cell disorders.
   ii. Etiology is unknown.
   iii. Include the following:
      1. Refractory anemia.
      2. Refractory anemia with ringed sideroblasts.
      3. Refractory cytopenia with multilineage dysplasia with or without ringed sideroblasts.
      4. Refractory anemia with excess blasts.
      5. Myelodysplastic syndrome unclassified.
      6. Myelodysplastic syndrome with isolated del(5q).
      7. Chronic myelomonocytic leukemia.
      8. Chronic neutrophilic leukemia.

b. **Clinical Manifestations**
   i. Symptoms vary depending on cell line involved.
   ii. Anemia leads to fatigue, weakness, and pallor.
   iii. Neutropenia leads to fever and increased risk of infection.
   iv. Thrombocytopenia leads to bleeding and bruising.

c. **Diagnosis**
   i. Check complete blood count, peripheral smear, and bone marrow aspiration and biopsy.

d. **Treatment**
   i. Supportive care, transfusion and erythrocyte-stimulating agents.
   ii. Chemotherapy with azacitidine, decitabine, or lenalidomide.
   iii. Stem cell transplantation.

## IX. POLYCYTHEMIA VERA
   a. **General**
      i. A chronic myeloproliferative neoplasm characterized by an elevated red blood cell mass.
      ii. Increased risk of developing myelofibrosis and acute myelogenous leukemia.

b. **Clinical Manifestations**
   i. Ruddy complexion, splenomegaly, and left upper quadrant pain noted.
   ii. Signs of arterial and venous thromboses noted.
   iii. Laboratory findings include elevated red cell mass, elevated hemoglobin/hematocrit, and decreased erythropoietin.

c. **Diagnosis**
   i. Criteria for diagnosis.
      1. Major.
         (a) Increased hemoglobin level.
         (b) Bone marrow showing hypercellularity.
         (c) JAK2 V617F or JAK2 exon 12 mutation.
      2. Minor.
         (a) Decreased serum erythropoietin level.

3. To make diagnosis, must have all three major or first two major and the minor criteria.

d. **Treatment**
   i. Periodic phlebotomy to maintain hematocrit less than 45%.
   ii. Aspirin to decrease microvascular events.
   iii. Myelosuppressive therapy with pegylated interferon alfa-2B or interferon alfa-2A, or the nonspecific JAK inhibitor Ruxolitinib.

## IX. ONCOLOGIC EMERGENCIES

a. **Tumor Lysis Syndrome**
   i. General
      1. Incidence unknown but in some disorders is as high as 40%.
         (a) Commonly associated with ALL and non-Hodgkin's lymphoma.
      2. Seen with administration of chemotherapy, corticosteroids, radiation, and hormonal agents.
      3. Etiology
         (a) Results from intracellular release of ions and metabolites from malignant cells before and after cytotoxic therapy.
         (b) Can lead to seizures, arrhythmias, acute renal failure, and sudden death.
   ii. Diagnosis
      1. Criteria for diagnosis includes:
         (a) Acute kidney injury
         (b) Hypocalcemia (calcium < 7 mg/dL)
         (c) Hyperuricemia (uric acid > 8 mg/dL)
         (d) Hyperphosphatemia (phosphorus > 6.5 mg/dL)
         (e) Hyperkalemia (potassium > 6 mEq/L)
   iii. Treatment
      1. Prevention and recognition of patients at risk is most important.
         (a) Increased risk with large tumor mass, preexisting renal insufficiency, and elevated LDH.
      2. Treatment consists of intravenous (IV) fluids and allopurinol or rasburicase before tumor therapy started.
         (a) Alkalinization of urine is not indicated.
      3. Severe complications may be treated with hemodialysis.

b. **Spinal Cord Compression**
   i. General
      1. Seen in 30% of patients with disseminated cancer.
      2. Due to compression from epidurally located tumors or bony fragments from pathologic fractures.
   ii. Clinical manifestations

1. Most common symptom is back pain.
   (a) Almost always precedes neurologic signs.
2. Neurologic signs and symptoms depend on location of compression, but include reflex abnormalities, weakness, numbness, and bowel or bladder dysfunction.
   iii. Diagnosis
      1. Emergent magnetic resonance imaging (MRI) of the spine or CT myelogram for diagnosis.
   iv. Treatment
      1. Corticosteroids, radiation therapy, and decompressive surgery are the mainstays of treatment.
      2. If treatment delayed loss of function may be irreversible.

c. **Superior Vena Cava Syndrome**
   i. General
      1. Due to thin-walled, low-pressure superior vena cava being obstructed by a variety of mediastinal components.
      2. Typically due to a neoplastic process.
         (a) Mainly primary lung carcinoma, non-Hodgkin's lymphoma, and metastatic tumors.
         (b) May also be seen as a complication of central venous access.
   ii. Clinical manifestations
      1. Typical symptoms include head fullness, dyspnea, cough, and chest pain.
      2. Physical examination findings include swelling of the neck and face.
   iii. Diagnosis
      1. Chest x-ray film reveals mediastinal widening, with a mass often seen in the region of the superior vena cava.
      2. CT scan will identify the mass and collateral flow.
   iv. Treatment
      1. If unknown primary, do biopsy for histologic diagnosis before treatment.
      2. Treatment includes radiation therapy with or without chemotherapy.

d. **Chemotherapy Toxicity**
   i. See Table 12.5 for list of chemotherapy toxicities.

# COAGULATION DISORDERS

## I. HEMOSTASIS
a. **Fig. 12.4 shows coagulation cascade.**

## II. FACTOR VIII DISORDER
a. **General**

**TABLE 12.5**

| Chemotherapeutic Agent Toxicity | |
|---|---|
| **Drug** | **Toxicity** |
| Bleomycin | Pulmonary fibrosis |
| Cisplatin | Hearing loss |
| | Nephrotoxicity |
| Cyclophosphamide | Hemorrhagic cystitis |
| Daunorubicin | Cardiomyopathy |
| Fluorouracil | Diarrhea |
| | Oral/GI ulcers |
| Methotrexate | Oral/GI ulcers |
| | Pulmonary fibrosis |
| | Cirrhosis |
| Vincristine | Peripheral neuropathy |
| Gemcitabine | Fever |
| | Flulike symptoms |
| Imatinib mesylate | Nausea/Vomiting |
| | Fluid retention |
| Paclitaxel | Peripheral neuropathy |
| | Nausea/Vomiting |
| | Allergic reactions |

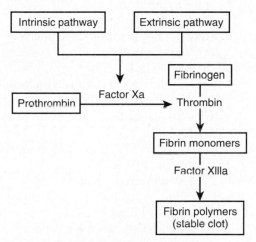

**Fig. 12.4** Coagulation cascade.

i. Hemophilia A is a deficiency in factor VIII (antihemophilic factor).
ii. Sex-linked recessive disorder.
iii. Seen in 1 per 5000 male births.

**b. Clinical Manifestations**
   i. Severity of signs and symptoms vary with circulating levels of the factor.
   ii. Delayed bleeding after trauma or surgery.
      1. Due to inability to stabilize platelet plug.
   iii. Hemarthroses are spontaneous or follow trauma.
   iv. Retroperitoneal hematomas.
   v. CNS bleeds may occur without trauma.

**c. Laboratory Features**
   i. Prolonged partial thromboplastin time (PTT).

ii. Prothrombin time (PT), platelet count, and bleeding time are normal.
iii. Decreased activity level of factor VIII.

**d. Treatment**
   i. Prevent trauma.
   ii. Avoid aspirin and other antiplatelet medications.
   iii. Supplement coagulation factor.
      1. Factor VIII concentrate.
      2. Desmopressin.
      3. Fresh frozen plasma or cryoprecipitate.
   iv. Emicizumab, a recombinant humanized bispecific monoclonal antibody, is an effective treatment for hemophilia A.
   v. Aminocaproic acid, an antifibrinolytic agent, can be used as adjunctive therapy to suppress fibrinolysis and prevent late bleeding after oropharyngeal mucosal trauma.
   vi. Genetic counseling for family.

**III. FACTOR IX DISORDER**
   **a. General**
      i. Hemophilia B is a deficiency in factor IX (antihemophilic factor B or Christmas factor).
      ii. Sex-linked recessive disorder.
      iii. Seen in 1 per 30,000 male births.
   **b. Clinical Manifestations**
      i. Signs and symptoms are no different from those seen in factor VIII deficiency.
      ii. Severity of signs and symptoms vary with circulating levels of the factor.
      iii. Delayed bleeding after trauma or surgery.
         1. Due to inability to stabilize platelet plug.
         2. Patients may present with excessive bleeding at circumcision.
      iv. Hemarthroses are spontaneous or follow trauma.
      v. Retroperitoneal hematomas.
      vi. CNS bleeds may occur without trauma.
   **c. Laboratory Features**
      i. Prolonged PTT.
      ii. PT, platelet count, and bleeding time are normal.
      iii. Decreased activity level of factor IX.
   **d. Treatment**
      i. Prevent trauma.
      ii. Avoid aspirin and other antiplatelet medications.
      iii. Supplement coagulation factor.
         1. Factor IX concentrate.
         2. Fresh frozen plasma or cryoprecipitate.
      iv. Aminocaproic acid, an antifibrinolytic agent, can be used as adjunctive therapy to suppress fibrinolysis and prevent late bleeding after oropharyngeal mucosal trauma.
      v. Genetic counseling to family.

## IV. FACTOR XI DISORDER

a. **General**

  i. Rare disorder but more common in Ashkenazi Jews.

  ii. Autosomal disorder; either recessive or dominant patterns noted.

  iii. Factor XI is a component of the contact phase of the coagulation system.

b. **Etiology**

  i. Bleeding is not as severe as with factor VIII or IX deficiency.

c. **Clinical Manifestations**

  i. Spontaneous bleeding and hemarthroses are uncommon.

  ii. Patients undergoing basic surgery, such as tonsillectomy or dental extraction, are at high risk for bleeding unless replacement therapy is given.

d. **Laboratory Features**

  i. Prolonged PTT, normal PT, and decreased factor XI activity.

e. **Treatment**

  i. Factor XI concentrate.

  ii. Fresh frozen plasma is the mainstay of treatment.

  iii. Antifibrinolytic therapy.

## V. HYPERCOAGULABLE STATES

a. **General**

  i. Group of hereditary and acquired conditions that confer and increase risk to develop thrombi.

  ii. Disorders include the following:

    1. Antiphospholipid syndrome.

    2. Factor V Leiden syndrome.

    3. Prothrombin gene G20210A mutation.

    4. Elevated factor VIII.

    5. Hyperhomocysteinemia.

    6. Deficiencies in antithrombin, protein C, and protein S.

b. **Diagnosis**

  i. Testing is indicated in the following patients:

    1. Idiopathic or recurrent venous thromboembolism (VTE).

    2. VTE at age <40 years.

    3. VTE with strong family history.

    4. VTE in unusual vascular sites.

    5. Warfarin-induced skin necrosis.

    6. Recurrent pregnancy loss.

  ii. Initial screening tests.

    1. PT/PTT/Fibrinogen.

    2. Anticardiolipin antibody assay.

    3. Protein C and S.

    4. Antithrombin level.

    5. C-reactive protein (CRP).

    6. Homocysteine.

c. **Treatment**

  i. Treat like any other thrombotic event.

  ii. Anticoagulants such as warfarin, heparin, and direct oral anticoagulant inhibitors are indicated.

  iii. Heparin is used in pregnancy.

## VI. THROMBOCYTOPENIA

a. **Idiopathic Thrombocytopenic Purpura (ITP)**

  i. General

    1. Autoimmune bleeding disorder in which patients develop antibodies against their own platelets.

  ii. Etiology

    1. Childhood ITP is usually acute and follows a viral infection.

    2. In adults, onset is more gradual, without a preceding illness, and is chronic in course.

  iii. Clinical manifestations

    1. No splenomegaly.

    2. Superficial bleeding of skin, mucous membranes, and genitourinary tract.

  iv. Laboratory features

    1. Decreased platelet count.

    2. Rule out pseudothrombocytopenia.

      (a) Pseudothrombocytopenia due to the following:

        (i) Artifact of automated cell counting.

        (ii) Platelet satellitism.

    3. Check coagulation studies to rule out DIC.

  v. Treatment

    1. Acute disease is self-limited.

      (a) Asymptomatic patients with platelet count >30,000/mcL and no bleeding are monitored.

    2. Chronic disease, platelet count <30,000/mcL, or patients bleeding will need IV immunoglobulin, platelets, high-dose steroids and possible splenectomy.

    3. Second-line medical therapies include thrombopoietin receptor agonists (romiplostim), rituximab, fostamatinib, or other immunosuppressive drugs.

    4. Stop all drugs that may be worsening thrombocytopenia.

      (a) Drugs include trimethoprim-sulfamethoxazole, quinine, penicillins, furosemide, phenytoin, cimetidine, and many others.

b. **Thrombotic Thrombocytopenic Purpura (TTP)**

  i. General

    1. Characterized by severe thrombocytopenia, microangiopathic hemolytic anemia, fever,

renal insufficiency, and neurologic abnormalities.

2. HUS, commonly seen in infants and children, is similar to TTP.
   (a) Patients typically present with GI signs and symptoms, abdominal pain, and diarrhea.
   (b) Microangiopathic hemolytic anemia.
   (c) Thrombocytopenia is mild to moderate.
   (d) No neurologic abnormalities.
   (e) Acute renal failure is common.
   (f) Severe hypertension is seen.

ii. Etiology
   1. Congenital or acquired deficient activity of the plasma enzyme ADAMTS13.

iii. Clinical manifestations
   1. Fever.
   2. Neurologic abnormalities, including headache, aphasia, or stupor.

iv. Laboratory features
   1. Thrombocytopenia.
   2. Schistocytes on peripheral blood smear.
   3. Increased reticulocyte count.
   4. Increased LDH.
   5. Normal PT, PTT, and fibrinogen levels.
   6. ADAMTS13 levels <10% with the presence of antibody against ADAMTS13 is characteristic of most adults with TTP.

v. Treatment
   1. Large-volume plasmapheresis and corticosteroids.

c. **von Willebrand's Disease**
   i. General
      1. von Willebrand's protein normally binds to factor VIII, delivering it to sites of coagulation and preventing its clearance from the circulation.
      2. A platelet function disorder.
      3. Most common inherited bleeding disorder.
   ii. Etiology
      1. Absence of von Willebrand's factor (vWF) results in failure to form a primary platelet plug.
      2. Types.
         (a) Type I: autosomal dominant with a deficiency of vWF.
         (b) Type II: autosomal dominant with defective vWF.
         (c) Type III: autosomal recessive with complete absence of vWF.
   iii. Clinical manifestations
      1. Symptoms include easy bruising and mucosal surface bleeding.
         (a) Symptoms may worsen with aspirin or nonsteroidal antiinflammatory drug (NSAID) ingestion.

2. Menorrhagia.
3. Hemarthrosis and retroperitoneal bleeding are rare, except in type III.

iv. Laboratory features
   1. Prolonged bleeding time.
   2. Prolonged PTT.
      (a) Due to factor VIII deficiency.
   3. Plasma von Willebrand's factor antigen.
   4. Plasma von Willebrand's factor activity decreased.
   5. Factor VIII activity decreased.

v. Treatment
   1. Administer factor VIII concentrates.
   2. DDAVP, a synthetic analogue of antidiuretic hormone (ADH), induces the release of vWF.
   3. Oral tranexamic acid used in women with excessive menstrual bleeding.

d. **Disseminated Intravascular Coagulation (DIC)**
   i. General
      1. Condition in which coagulation factors are activated and degraded simultaneously.
      2. Patient will present with both bleeding and thrombosis.
   ii. Etiology
      1. Triggered by endothelial cell injury or release of tissue factors that activate the coagulation cascade (Fig. 12.5).
      2. Can be caused by the following:
         (a) Obstetric complications.
            (i) Amniotic fluid embolism.
            (ii) Retained dead fetus.
            (iii) Abruptio placentae.
         (b) Transfusion reactions.
         (c) Malignancy.
            (i) Pancreatic carcinoma.
            (ii) Adenocarcinoma.
            (iii) Acute promyelocytic leukemia.

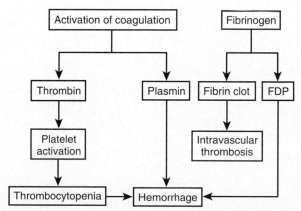

**Fig. 12.5** Pathogenesis of disseminated intravascular coagulation. *FDP,* Fibrin degradation products.

(d) Trauma.
  (i) Brain injury.
  (ii) Crush injury.
  (iii) Burns.
(e) Infection or sepsis.
  (i) Gram-negative sepsis.
(f) Acute pancreatitis
(g) Adult respiratory distress syndrome (ARDS).

iii. Clinical manifestations
1. Bleeding is the most common clinical finding.
  (a) Bleeding from skin and mucous membranes.
2. May develop small purpuric to large ecchymoses.
3. Thrombotic events include gangrenous digits and nose, as well as hemorrhagic necrosis of the skin.

iv. Laboratory features
1. Prolonged PT, PTT, and thrombin time.
  (a) Due to coagulation factor consumption.
2. Thrombocytopenia due to platelet consumption.
3. Elevated fibrin degradation products (FDPs) or D-dimer due to fibrinolysis.
4. Fibrinogen level is decreased.
5. Elevated D-dimer level.

v. Treatment
1. Must treat underlying cause of the DIC.
2. Control major symptoms.
  (a) For bleeding, give fresh frozen plasma and platelets.
  (b) For thrombosis, give IV heparin.

## VII. THROMBOCYTOSIS

### a. Essential Thrombocythemia
i. A myeloproliferative neoplasm.
ii. Have overproduction of platelets.
iii. No correlation between the platelet count and risk of thrombosis.
iv. Extremely elevated platelet counts can develop bleeding due to loss of von Willebrand's factor multimers.

### b. Reactive Thrombocytosis
i. Due to platelet overproduction in response to another disorder.
1. Other disorders include:
  (a) Acute infection.
  (b) Chronic inflammatory disorders.
  (c) Iron deficiency.
  (d) Cancer.
  (e) Splenectomy.
ii. Congenital familial thrombocytosis due to thrombopoietin and thrombopoietin receptor gene mutation.

iii. Platelet function is normal.
iv. Not associated with an increased risk of bleeding or thrombosis.
v. Treat the underlying condition.

## VIII. TRANSFUSION REACTIONS

### a. General
i. RBC transfusion is unnecessary in hospitalized, hemodynamically stable patients unless the hemoglobin concentration is <7 g/dL.
ii. In patients with acute MI or unstable myocardial ischemia, RBC transfusion can be considered at hemoglobin concentration <8 g/dL.
iii. Transfusion complications include:
1. Febrile nonhemolytic reaction.
2. Acute hemolytic reaction.
3. Graft versus host disease.
4. Transfusion-associated circulatory overload.
5. Transfusion-related acute lung injury.
6. Infection.

### b. Diagnosis
i. Early recognition is key.
ii. Symptoms include chills, rigors, fever, dyspnea, urticaria, and itching.

### c. Types
i. Febrile nonhemolytic transfusion reaction.
1. Due to reaction to donor white blood cells in transfusion.
2. Symptoms include fever and chills.
3. Treat with acetaminophen and use leukocyte-poor blood units.
ii. Acute hemolytic transfusion reaction.
1. Due to recipient plasma antibodies reacting with donor red blood cell antigens.
2. Causes intravascular hemolysis leading to hemoglobinuria.
  (a) Can lead to acute kidney injury and disseminated intravascular coagulation.
3. Symptoms include dyspnea, fever, chills, and lumbar back pain.
  (a) Severe reaction can develop signs of shock.
4. Direct antiglobulin test will be positive, elevated LDH, and increased free hemoglobin.
5. Stop transfusion immediately and start supportive care with intravenous fluid and furosemide to maintain renal output.
iii. Graft versus host disease.
1. Due to transfusion containing immunocompetent lymphocytes to an immunocompromised host.
  (a) Donor cells attack host tissues.
2. Symptoms include fever, rash, vomiting, diarrhea, and pancytopenia.

3. Treatment includes stopping transfusion and corticosteroids or other immunosuppressants.
    (a) Preventive of disease by using irradiated blood products.
  iv. Transfusion-associated circulatory overload.
    1. Most common cause of transfusion related death.
    2. High osmotic load of blood products causes fluid to move to intravascular space.
    3. Presents with signs of fluid overload.
    4. Treatment includes transfusing slowly and diuretic therapy.
  v. Transfusion-related acute lung injury.
    1. Rare, caused by anti-HLA or antigranulocyte donor plasma antibodies that affect the recipient white blood cells.
      (a) Second most common cause of transfusion-related death.
    2. Symptoms include acute respiratory edema.
    3. Chest x-ray reveals noncardiogenic pulmonary edema.

4. Treatment is supportive.
    (a) Diuretics should be avoided.
  vi. Infection.
    1. Rare complication. More common in platelet concentrates; 1:25500 transfusions.
    2. Infections include syphilis, hepatitis, HIV, CMV, and Zika virus.

## IX. HEMOCHROMATOSIS
  a. **General**
    i. Genetic disorder with excessive iron that accumulates in various tissues.
    ii. Can lead to cirrhosis, cardiomyopathy, diabetes, and arthropathy.
  b. **Symptoms**
    i. Do not develop symptoms until there is significant organ damage.
  c. **Diagnosis**
    i. Will have an elevated ferritin iron, and transferrin saturation level.
  d. **Treatment**
    i. Serial phlebotomies.

# QUESTIONS

## QUESTION 1
A 67-year-old male presents with melena and weight loss. CBC reveals hemoglobin of 8.9 g/dL, hematocrit 27%, and an MCV 74 fL. Which related cardiac sign is most likely to be noted on physical examination?

A  Bradycardia
B  II/VI systolic murmur
C  Midsystolic click
D  Displaced PMI
E  $S_4$ gallop

## QUESTION 2
A 60-year-old patient presents with fatigue. On examination, his tongue is noted to be red and fissured, and decreased vibratory sensation is noted in the lower extremities. CBC reveals the following:

A.  WBC $8.1 \times 10^9$/L
B.  Hgb 10.1 g/dL
C.  Hct 31%
D.  MCV 124 fL
E.  Platelet 160,000/μL

Examination of the blood smear reveals anisocytosis, poikilocytosis, and hypersegmented neutrophils. Which of the following tests would be helpful in the evaluation of this patient?

A  Direct Coombs' test
B  Serum vitamin $B_{12}$ level
C  Serum ferritin level
D  Erythrocyte sedimentation rate
E  Erythrocyte protoporphyrin level

## QUESTION 3
A patient presents with thrombocytopenia, schistocytes, fever, and headache. Which of the following is the most likely diagnosis?

A  von Willebrand's disease
B  Idiopathic thrombocytopenic purpura
C  Disseminated intravascular coagulation
D  Thrombotic thrombocytopenic purpura
E  Henoch-Schönlein purpura

## QUESTION 4
A 52-year-old male presents with a painless 3-cm mass in his neck. He has also noted night sweats. Which of the following is the next best step in the evaluation of this patient?

A  Erythrocyte sedimentation rate
B  Complete blood count
C  Bone marrow biopsy
D  Lymph node biopsy
E  Chest CT scan

*Continued*

## QUESTIONS—cont'd

### QUESTION 5

A patient currently taking Coumadin presents with spontaneous nosebleeds. Laboratory tests reveal a prothrombin time of 45 seconds and INR 6.9. Which of the following is the treatment of choice for this patient?

A   Heparin

B   Salicylate

C   Vitamin K

D   Protamine sulfate

E   Vasopressin (DDAVP)

### QUESTION 6

Which of the following tests is most useful in monitoring effective response to treatment in patients with iron-deficiency anemia?

A   Hemoglobin level

B   Hematocrit level

C   Reticulocyte count

D   Iron level

E   Ferritin

### QUESTION 7

In hemophilia B, which of the following coagulation factors is deficient?

A   VI

B   VII

C   VIII

D   IX

E   X

### QUESTION 8

In which of the following disorders are the pneumococcal and Hemophilus *influenzae* type b vaccines indicated?

A   Sickle cell anemia

B   Sideroblastic anemia

C   Iron-deficiency anemia

D   Essential thrombocytosis

E   Paroxysmal nocturnal hemoglobinuria

### QUESTION 9

Which of the following is the treatment of choice for thrombotic thrombocytopenic purpura?

A   Plasma exchange

B   Corticosteroids

C   Splenectomy

D   Vincristine

E   Heparin

### QUESTION 10

A 55-year-old nonsmoking male presents with hemoglobin of 18.0 g/dL and hematocrit of 56%. Splenomegaly is noted on examination. Which of the following is the most likely diagnosis?

A   Polycythemia vera

B   Idiopathic myelofibrosis

C   Secondary erythrocytosis

D   Myelodysplastic syndrome

E   Chronic myelogenous leukemia

## ANSWERS

**1.   B**

EXPLANATION: Clinical signs of anemia include tachycardia and a systolic ejection heart murmur due to increased cardiac output. Pallor and postural hypotension may be noted due to decreased blood volume. *Topic: Anemia*

☐ Correct    ☐ Incorrect

**2.   B**

EXPLANATION: Vitamin $B_{12}$ deficiency presents with red, beefy tongue and neurologic complaints, such as paresthesia and numbness of the extremities. CBC results reveal an elevated MCV, thrombocytopenia, and hypersegmented neutrophils. Diagnosis is made by measuring serum vitamin $B_{12}$ levels. *Topic: Vitamin $B_{12}$ deficiency*

☐ Correct    ☐ Incorrect

**3.   D**

EXPLANATION: Patients with thrombotic thrombocytopenic purpura present with severe thrombocytopenia, microangiopathic hemolytic anemia (have presence of schistocytes), and neurologic abnormalities. *Topic: Thrombocytopenia*

☐ Correct    ☐ Incorrect

**4.   D**

EXPLANATION: Hodgkin's lymphoma is common after age 50 years and the patient presents with a nontender, firm lymph node. B-symptoms—such as fever, weight loss, and night sweats—may also be noted. Evaluation of this patient consists of lymph node biopsy. *Topic: Lymphoma*

☐ Correct    ☐ Incorrect

**5.   C**

EXPLANATION: Overdose of Coumadin is treated with vitamin K or fresh frozen plasma. Protamine sulfate is used to treat overdose of heparin. *Topic: Coagulation disorders*

☐ Correct    ☐ Incorrect

# ANSWERS—cont'd

**6. C**

EXPLANATION: Iron-deficiency anemia is treated with ferrous sulfate, and response to therapy can be measured by elevation in reticulocyte count 7 to 10 days after starting treatment.
*Topic: Iron-deficiency anemia*
☐ Correct   ☐ Incorrect

**7. D**

EXPLANATION: Hemophilia B (Christmas disease) is due to a deficiency of factor IX. Hemophilia A is due to deficiency of factor VIII. *Topic: Factor IX disorder*
☐ Correct   ☐ Incorrect

**8. A**

EXPLANATION: Patients with sickle cell anemia have a decreased immune response secondary to asplenism. These patients should be vaccinated for bacterial infections such as pneumococcus and *Haemophilus influenzae* type b.
*Topic: Anemia: hemolytic anemia*
☐ Correct   ☐ Incorrect

**9. A**

EXPLANATION: Thrombotic thrombocytopenic purpura is best treated by plasma exchange with fresh frozen plasma. Corticosteroids, splenectomy, and vincristine are secondary treatments. *Topic: Thrombocytopenia*
☐ Correct   ☐ Incorrect

**10. A**

EXPLANATION: Polycythemia vera is a myeloproliferative disorder with a hematocrit typically greater than 54% in males. On physical examination, plethora and splenomegaly are noted. Secondary erythrocytosis is an increase in hematocrit secondary to smoking or to living at high altitudes. *Topic: Polycythemia vera*
☐ Correct   ☐ Incorrect

# CHAPTER 13
# GENITOURINARY AND RENAL SYSTEMS

## EXAMINATION BLUEPRINT TOPICS

**BENIGN CONDITIONS OF THE GENITOURINARY TRACT**

Benign prostatic hypertrophy (BPH)

Erectile dysfunction

Varicocele

Incontinence

Nephrolithiasis

Paraphimosis/Phimosis

Testicular torsion

Urethral stricture

Urethrocele

Congenital abnormalities

**INFECTIOUS/INFLAMMATORY CONDITIONS**

Cystitis

Epididymitis

Orchitis

Prostatitis

Pyelonephritis

Urethritis

**NEOPLASTIC DISEASES**

Bladder carcinoma

Prostate carcinoma

Renal cell carcinoma

Testicular carcinoma

**RENAL DISEASES**

Acute renal failure

Chronic renal failure

Glomerulonephritis

Hydronephrosis

Nephrotic syndrome

Polycystic kidney disease

Renal vascular disease

**ELECTROLYTE AND ACID-BASE DISORDERS**

Hyponatremia

Hypernatremia

Hypokalemia

Hyperkalemia

Hypocalcemia

Hypercalcemia

Hypomagnesemia

Acid-base disorders

Volume depletion

Volume excess

Urinalysis

## BENIGN CONDITIONS OF THE GENITOURINARY TRACT

### I. BENIGN PROSTATIC HYPERTROPHY (BPH)
a. **General**
   i. Process begins in the 30s, and by age 80 more than 80% of men have BPH.
   ii. Risk factors are increasing age and functioning testes.
b. **Clinical Manifestations**
   i. Have lower urinary tract symptoms such as hesitancy, straining, urgency, sense of incomplete voiding, weak stream, and dribbling.
      1. Symptoms appear slowly and progress gradually over years.
   ii. On digital rectal examination, the prostate is enlarged and firm.
   iii. Neurologic examination needed to rule out neuropathic bladder, caused by peripheral neuropathy or saddle-area anesthesia, as a cause of these symptoms.
c. **Diagnosis**
   i. Prostate-specific antigen (PSA) should be obtained to evaluate for possible prostate cancer if life expectancy is greater than 10 years.
      1. Urinalysis to rule out infection.
   ii. Bladder outlet obstruction diagnosed by showing increased bladder pressure relative to urine flow with pressure-flow studies.
d. **Treatment**
   i. Medical therapy.
      1. Alpha-1-adrenergic blockers (terazosin, tamsulosin, doxazosin).
         (a) Relax smooth muscle in the bladder neck, prostate capsule, and prostatic urethra.
         (b) Side effects include hypotension, dizziness, retrograde ejaculation, and asthenia.
      2. 5-α-reductase inhibitors (finasteride, dutasteride).

(a) Inhibit conversion of testosterone to dihydrotestosterone and decrease prostate size.

(b) Side effects include sexual ejaculatory dysfunction.

(i) May also reduce PSA levels.

3. Phosphodiesterase-5 inhibitors.

(a) Approved for use in men with both urinary symptoms and erectile dysfunction.

ii. Surgical therapy.

1. Transurethral prostatectomy (TURP), resection of the prostate, is the gold standard.

## II. ERECTILE DYSFUNCTION

a. **General**

i. Defined as the consistent inability to maintain or achieve an erection sufficient to allow penetration and sexual intercourse.

ii. Most cases have organic causes rather than psychogenic (depression, stress).

iii. Etiologies include arterial, venous, neurogenic, or psychogenic causes.

iv. Antihypertensives such as centrally acting sympatholytics may alter erections, and beta-blockers and spironolactone alter libido.

1. Other drugs include selective serotonin reuptake inhibitors (SSRIs), ketoconazole, cimetidine, alcohol, and cocaine.

b. **Clinical Manifestations**

i. Problems with erectile dysfunction must be separated from problems with ejaculation, libido, and orgasm.

ii. History of systemic diseases.

1. History of hyperlipidemia, vascular disease, diabetes, and hypertension linked to erectile dysfunction.

c. **Diagnosis**

i. Laboratory testing should be obtained to rule out systemic disease.

ii. Hormone levels such as testosterone, prolactin, follicle-stimulating hormone (FSH), and luteinizing hormone (LH) should be obtained.

iii. Nocturnal tumescence testing should be completed to separate organic from psychogenic etiologies.

d. **Treatment**

i. Varies with etiology.

1. Hormonal replacement.

(a) Testosterone injections given in cases of androgen deficiency.

2. Vacuum constriction device.

3. Vasoactive therapy.

(a) Sildenafil inhibits phosphodiesterase 5, a vasoconstrictor; allows cyclic guanosine

monophosphate (cGMP) to function unopposed; and allows sustained blood flow to the penis.

(i) Patients taking nitrates may develop hypotension.

4. Penile prosthesis.

5. Vascular reconstruction.

6. Lifestyle modifications.

## III. VARICOCELE

a. **General**

i. Abnormal dilation of the pampiniform plexus in the scrotum.

1. Due to incompetent valves in the spermatic vein.

ii. Common cause of infertility.

iii. Rare in boys younger than 10 years of age.

b. **Clinical Manifestations**

i. Occurs mainly on the left side. If on the right side and the boy is less than 10 years old, this may indicate an abdominal or renal mass.

ii. Patients may complain of a dull ache in the testis.

iii. On physical examination, a painless testicular mass is noted.

1. Described as a cord mass or "bag of worms."

2. Testis on the affected side may be atrophic.

iv. On standing, a varicocele will become more prominent and disappears in a recumbent position.

c. **Treatment**

i. Ligation of the spermatic vein, varicocelectomy, is indicated to increase chance for fertility.

## IV. INCONTINENCE

a. **General**

i. Common in older females.

ii. Occurs when urine leaks involuntarily.

iii. Classified into one of four groups.

1. Mixed incontinence.

(a) Combination of other types of incontinence.

(b) Results from loss of sphincter efficiency or abnormal connection between the urinary tract and skin (fistulas).

2. Stress incontinence.

(a) Loss of urine with activities that increase intraabdominal pressure (coughing, lifting).

(b) Patients do not leak in the supine position.

(c) Due to laxity in the pelvic floor muscles.

3. Urge incontinence.

(a) Uncontrolled loss of urine that is preceded by a strong, unexpected urge to void.

(b) Unrelated to position or activity.

(c) Due to detrusor hyperreflexia or sphincter dysfunction.

(d) Seen in inflammatory conditions or neurogenic disorders.

4. Overflow incontinence.

(a) Due to chronic urinary retention.

(i) Seen in BPH and urethral strictures.

(b) Results from a chronically distended bladder.

**b. Clinical Manifestations**

i. History is most important with a voiding diary.

ii. On physical examination, note presence of fistula, neurologic abnormalities, or distended bladder.

iii. Rectal examination needed to determine rectal tone.

iv. Laboratory testing should be completed to rule out urinary tract infection (UTI).

**c. Diagnosis**

i. Urodynamic evaluation should be completed.

**d. Treatment**

i. Varies with etiology.

1. Mixed incontinence.

(a) Treat the underlying cause.

2. Stress incontinence.

(a) Topical estrogens.

(b) Drug therapy to increase urethral resistance.

3. Urge incontinence.

(a) Medical therapy with antispasmodic agents, anticholinergic agents, or tricyclic antidepressants.

4. Overflow incontinence.

(a) Urethral catheter is both diagnostic and therapeutic.

(b) Treatment of underlying cause.

## V. NEPHROLITHIASIS

**a. General**

i. A crystalline mass within the urinary tract.

1. Most common are calcium oxalate.

ii. More common in males than in females; very uncommon in Black people and Asians.

iii. Struvite calculi associated with *Proteus* causing UTI and urine pH greater than 7.0.

1. May increase in size and become a staghorn calculus.

**b. Clinical Manifestations**

i. Sudden onset of unbearable, colicky pain.

1. May have nausea and vomiting associated with the pain.

ii. Pain begins in the flank and moves anteriorly toward the groin and is referred to the testes or labia.

iii. Hematuria is common.

**c. Diagnosis**

i. Abdominal x-ray film will allow detection of most stones (Fig. 13.1).

1. Cystine and uric acid stones are not detected on x-ray film.

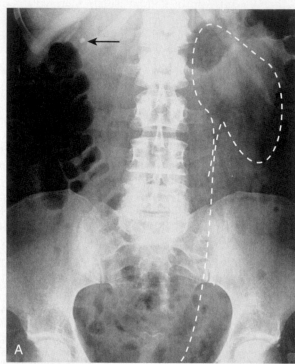
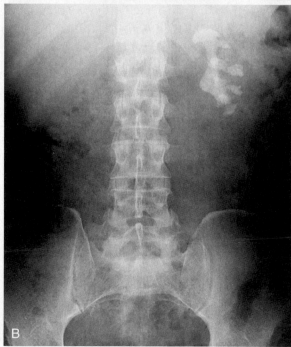

**Fig. 13.1** Kidney stones on abdominal x-ray film. **(A)** Right renal calculi *(arrow)* in the right upper quadrant. Hatched line outlines the right kidney. **(B)** Calcification in the collecting system of the left kidney, called a staghorn calculus. *(From Mettler FA: Essentials of Radiology, 2nd ed. Philadelphia: Elsevier Saunders, 2005:221, Fig. 7-11.)*

ii. Helical computed tomography (CT) scan has replaced intravenous pyelogram (IVP) as test of choice for diagnosis of nephrolithiasis.

d. **Treatment**

   i. Pain relief with NSAIDs has been shown to be as effective as opioids.

   ii. Intravenous (IV) fluid hydration.

   iii. Most stones <5 mm will pass without intervention.

   iv. Extracorporeal shock wave lithotripsy (ESWL) is used to remove stones from 5 mm to 2 cm in size.

      1. Cystoscopy may be needed with stent placement to temporarily relieve obstruction.

   v. Percutaneous nephrolithotomy is used to treat stones larger than 2 cm.

   vi. Prevention of recurrent stones.

      1. Evaluation of stone composition.

         (a) 24-hour urine for calcium, potassium, magnesium, sodium, phosphorus, citrate, oxalate, uric acid, and creatinine.

         (b) Serum studies include electrolytes, calcium, phosphorus, and parathyroid hormone.

      2. Prevention therapy.

         (a) Increased fluid intake.

         (b) Diets with reduced sodium, oxalate, and protein.

         (c) Thiazide diuretics: lower calcium excretion in the urine.

## VI. PARAPHIMOSIS/PHIMOSIS

a. **General**

   i. Paraphimosis is the painful swelling of the foreskin and penis distal to a phimotic ring.

      1. Occurs if the foreskin remains retracted for a prolonged period of time.

   ii. Phimosis is the inability to retract the foreskin.

      1. Can result from repeated episodes of balanitis, which is inflammation of the glans penis as a result of poor hygiene.

         (a) In older patients, balanitis may be a presenting sign for diabetes.

b. **Treatment**

   i. Applying steady, gentle pressure to the foreskin to decrease the swelling can reduce paraphimosis.

      1. Condition can reoccur; dorsal slit or a circumcision should be done.

   ii. Phimosis is treated with topical corticosteroids or circumcision.

## VII. TESTICULAR TORSION

a. **General**

   i. A urologic emergency. Diagnosis and treatment must be prompt to save the testis.

   ii. Most common cause of testicular pain in boys older than 12 years of age.

      1. Torsion of the appendix of the testis is the most common cause of testicular pain in boys between ages 2 and 11 years.

   iii. Due to inadequate fixation of the testis within the scrotum.

      1. Abnormal attachment is called a bell-clapper deformity.

b. **Clinical Manifestations**

   i. With acute testicular torsion, the patient presents with acute testicular pain and swelling of the scrotum.

      1. On examination, the scrotum is swollen and tender. The cremasteric reflex is absent.

   ii. With torsion of the appendix of the testis, the patient presents with gradual onset of testicular pain and scrotal erythema.

      1. On examination, palpation of the testis reveals a 3- to 5-mm tender indurated mass on the upper pole.

         (a) This mass may be visible through the scrotum and is called the blue-dot sign.

   iii. Testis is high riding and epididymis is posterior.

c. **Diagnosis**

   i. Testicular flow scan or color Doppler ultrasound is required to separate testicular torsion from torsion of the appendix of the testis.

d. **Treatment**

   i. Testicular torsion is treated with prompt surgical exploration and detorsion.

      1. If completed within 6 hours, excellent survival chance for testicular tissue.

      2. After detorsion, the testes should each be fixed to the scrotum by scrotal orchiopexy.

   ii. Torsion of the appendix of the testis will typically resolve in 3 to 10 days.

      1. No surgery is needed.

      2. Pain control is very important.

## VIII. URETHRAL STRICTURE

a. **General**

   i. Narrowing of the urethra secondary to scarring.

      1. May be secondary to instrumentation of the urethra, intermittent or long-term use of catheters, trauma, enlarged prostate, cancer, sexually transmitted infections, and radiation therapy.

   ii. Clinical Manifestations

      1. Symptoms include decreased urine stream, incomplete bladder emptying, dysuria, urinary urgency and frequency, urinary tract infections.

   iii. Diagnosis

1. Retrograde urethrogram or cystoscopy can confirm diagnosis.
   iv. Treatment
   1. Short strictures can be treated initially with urethral dilations or internal urethrotomy.
   2. Severe cases are treated with urethral reconstruction.

## IX. URETHROCELE
a. **General**
   i. Circumferential protrusion of the distal urethra through the external urethral meatus.
   ii. Rare condition that is most common in prepubescent females and postmenopausal women.
b. **Clinical Manifestations**
   i. Vaginal bleeding is the most common symptom of urethral prolapse.
   ii. A round, doughnut-shaped protrusion of mucosa can be observed obscuring the urethral opening on physical examination.
c. **Diagnosis**
   i. Diagnosis is made primarily through physical examination. Cystourethroscopy can be used to confirm the diagnosis.
d. **Treatment**
   i. Mild cases can be treated conservatively by addressing the underlying causes, using sitz water baths and maintaining good hygiene.
   ii. Surgical repair is required for severe cases.

## X. CONGENITAL ABNORMALITIES
a. **Vesicoureteral Reflux**
   i. General.
   1. Retrograde passage of urine from the bladder into the upper urinary tract.
   2. Seen in 1% of newborns.
   ii. Categories.
   1. Primary: most common, due to incompetent/inadequate closure of ureterovesical junction (UVJ).
   2. Secondary: result of abnormally high pressure in the bladder resulting in failure to close the UVJ.
      (a) Often due to anatomic or functional bladder obstruction.
   iii. Diagnosis.
   1. Note hydronephrosis on renal ultrasound.
   2. Contrast voiding cystourethrogram (VCUG) is abnormal.
   iv. Treatment.
   1. Medical treatment with antibiotics for possible infection.
   2. Surgery.
b. **Penile Abnormalities**
   i. Epispadias.
   1. Urethral meatus is located on the dorsal side of the penis.
   2. Associated with bladder exstrophy.
   3. Treatment is surgical repair.
   ii. Hypospadias.
   1. Abnormal ventral placement of the urethral opening.
   2. Location can range from glans, shaft of penis, scrotum, and perineum.
   3. Treatment is surgical repair.
   iii. Peyronie disease.
   1. Benign fibrotic disorder of the penis.
   2. Results in pain, abnormal penile curvature or deformity, and sexual dysfunction.
   3. Treatment includes surgery and injectable collagenase *Clostridium histolyticum*.
   iv. Penile fracture.
   1. Due to a tear in the tunica albuginea secondary to trauma to the penis.
   2. Forceful bending of the erect penis during intercourse is the most common cause.
   3. Symptoms include severe pain, immediate loss of erection, and bruising.
   4. Treatment requires surgical repair of the tunica albuginea.
c. **Renal Agenesis**
   i. Absence of kidney—unilateral or bilateral.
   ii. Diagnosis made by ultrasound.
   1. May be diagnosed as early as 10 to 12 weeks of gestation.
   iii. Bilateral renal agenesis is incompatible with extrauterine life.
d. **Horseshoe Kidney**
   i. Congenital abnormality when two kidneys are fused together.
   1. More common in males than females.
   ii. Symptoms include abdominal pain, nausea, renal calculi, and urinary tract infection.
   iii. Diagnosis is made by ultrasound.
   iv. Treatment is supportive.

# INFECTIOUS/INFLAMMATORY CONDITIONS

## I. CYSTITIS
a. **General**
   i. Infection of the bladder.
   ii. Typically due to gram-negative rods (*Escherichia coli*) and, at times, gram-positive cocci (*Enterococcus*).
   iii. Route of infection is up through the urethra.
   1. In women, symptoms may appear after sexual intercourse.
b. **Clinical Manifestations**

i. Present with frequency, urgency, dysuria, and suprapubic pain.
   1. No fever or chills.
   2. Women may present with hematuria.
ii. On physical examination, suprapubic tenderness may be noted.

**c. Diagnosis**
  i. Urinalysis reveals pyuria and bacteriuria.
  ii. Urine culture is positive for bacteria.

**d. Treatment**
  i. A short course of antibiotics, such as trimethoprim-sulfamethoxazole, nitrofurantoin, or fosfomycin.

## II. EPIDIDYMITIS

**a. General**
  i. Most cases are infectious and are divided into two groups based on age distribution.
    1. Younger than 40 years old.
      (a) Typically sexually transmitted and due to *Chlamydia trachomatis* or *Neisseria gonorrhoeae*.
    2. Older than 40 years old.
      (a) Typically nonsexually transmitted and caused by a gram-negative rod from a UTI or prostatitis.

**b. Clinical Manifestations**
  i. Symptoms of urethritis (pain at tip of the penis and urethral discharge) and cystitis (frequency, urgency, and dysuria) are noted.
  ii. Fever and scrotal swelling may be noted.

**c. Diagnosis**
  i. Laboratory tests may reveal leukocytosis with a left shift.
  ii. Gram stain of the discharge shows increased white blood cells and/or gram-negative diplococci in patients with gonorrhea.
  iii. Urinalysis and culture are positive in nonsexually transmitted cases.

**d. Treatment**
  i. Supportive care with bed rest and scrotal elevation.
  ii. Antibiotic therapy varies with route of transmission.
    1. Sexually transmitted cases treated with single-dose ceftriaxone and doxycycline for 10 days.
    2. Nonsexually transmitted cases treated with fluoroquinolones for 10 days.
  iii. Scrotal abscess is possible if not adequately treated.

## III. ORCHITIS

**a. General**
  i. Due to Coxsackie B or the mumps virus.

ii. A more common complication after mumps in adolescents and adults.
iii. Trauma may also cause orchitis.

**b. Clinical Manifestations**
  i. Typically follows parotitis within 8 days.
  ii. Abrupt onset with fever, chills, nausea, and lower abdominal pain.
  iii. Affected testicle becomes tender and swollen.

**c. Treatment**
  i. Supportive care with pain control.
  ii. About one-third of affected testicles will atrophy.
  iii. Infertility is rare.

## IV. PROSTATITIS

**a. General**
  i. Etiology varies with type of prostatitis.
    1. Table 13.1 lists causes of prostatitis and Table 13.2 compares etiologies.

**b. Clinical Manifestations**
  i. Acute bacterial prostatitis presents with high fever, chills, and malaise.
    1. Urinary symptoms include dysuria, frequency, and urgency.
    2. On physical examination, if performed, a very tender prostate is noted on digital rectal examination.
  ii. Chronic bacterial prostatitis is typically noted in elderly men and associated with recurrent UTIs.
    1. Symptoms are similar to acute bacterial infection but are less severe.
    2. On digital rectal examination, the prostate is normal, swollen, firm, or tender.

**TABLE 13.1**

| Causes of Prostatitis | | |
| --- | --- | --- |
| **Type** | **Definition** | **Etiology** |
| Acute bacterial | Acute infection of the prostate | *Escherichia coli* *Pseudomonas aeruginosa* *Serratia* *Klebsiella* *Proteus* *Enterococcus* |
| Chronic bacterial | Recurrent infection of the prostate | *E. coli* *P. aeruginosa* *Serratia* *Klebsiella* *Proteus* *Enterococcus* |
| Chronic noninflammatory | No sign of infection | *Mycoplasma hominis* *Ureaplasma* *Trichomonas* *Chlamydia* |

**TABLE 13.2**

**Comparison of Prostatitis Etiologies**

| | Acute Bacterial | Chronic Bacterial | Chronic Noninflammatory | Asymptomatic Inflammatory |
|---|---|---|---|---|
| Fever | Yes | No | No | No |
| Urinalysis | Positive | Negative | Negative | Negative |
| Expressed prostatic secretions | Contraindicated | Positive | Positive | Negative |
| Culture-bacteria | Positive | Positive | Negative | Negative |
| Treatment | Trimethoprim-sulfamethoxazole or a fluoroquinolone | Trimethoprim-sulfamethoxazole or a fluoroquinolone | Doxycycline or Erythromycin | Alpha-blocking agents |

iii. Chronic abacterial prostatitis presents with pelvic pain and UTI symptoms and pain during or after ejaculation.

c. **Diagnosis**
   i. Acute bacterial prostatitis is diagnosed based on clinical findings and a positive urine culture.
      1. Prostate massage with digital rectal examination is contraindicated due to risk of sepsis.
   ii. Chronic bacterial and chronic noninflammatory prostatitis are diagnosed with the two- or four-glass test.
      1. With the four-glass test, culture initial stream urine, the midstream urine, the expressed prostate excretions after massage, and the postmassage stream urine.
      2. With the two-glass test, culture urine before and after prostate massage.

d. **Treatment**
   i. Acute bacterial prostatitis treated with antibiotics; IV needed for severe disease.
      1. Ampicillin and aminoglycoside for parenteral antibiotics.
      2. Fluoroquinolones for oral antibiotics.
      3. Treat for 4–6 weeks.
   ii. Chronic bacterial infection treated with antibiotics.
      1. Fluoroquinolones and trimethoprim-sulfamethoxazole are indicated.
      2. Treat for 4–6 weeks.
      3. Alpha-blocker may be tried to improve symptoms and to reduce recurrences.
   iii. Chronic inflammatory infection is difficult to treat.
      1. Antibiotics may be tried, but success is low.
      2. Symptomatic relief may be provided by NSAIDs and alpha-blockers.

V. **PYELONEPHRITIS**
   a. **General**
      i. An infectious inflammatory condition involving the kidney/renal pelvis.

   ii. Etiology is most commonly gram-negative rods such as *E. coli*, *Proteus*, or *Klebsiella*.
   iii. Route of the infection is ascending from the lower urinary tract.

b. **Clinical Manifestations**
   i. Symptoms include fever, chills, flank pain, urgency, dysuria, and frequency.
   ii. On physical examination, vital signs reveal fever and tachycardia; costovertebral angle tenderness is noted.

c. **Diagnosis**
   i. Complete blood count reveals a leukocytosis with a left shift.
   ii. Pyuria, bacteriuria, and hematuria are noted on the urinalysis.
      1. On microscopic examination of the urine, white blood cell casts are noted.
   iii. Urine culture is positive for bacteria.

d. **Treatment**
   i. Empiric antibiotic coverage with ceftriaxone, ciprofloxacin, ampicillin-sulbactam, or imipenem and then guided to culture sensitivity.
   ii. Treat for a total of 7 to 14 days.
   iii. Complications include sepsis with shock.

VI. **URETHRITIS**
   a. **General**
      i. Refers to inflammation of the urethra.
      ii. Most cases are acquired through sexual intercourse.
      iii. There are two types of urethritis.
         1. Gonococcal.
            (a) Etiology is *N. gonorrhoeae*.
         2. Nongonococcal.
            (a) Etiology is *C. trachomatis* or *Ureaplasma urealyticum*.
         3. Table 13.3 compares types of urethritis.

   b. **Clinical Manifestations**
      i. Gonococcal.
         1. Produces thick, purulent urethral discharge and burning with urination.

**TABLE 13.3**

| Comparison of Gonococcal and Nongonococcal Urethritis | | |
| --- | --- | --- |
| | Gonococcal | Nongonococcal |
| Organism | *Neisseria gonorrhoeae* | *Chlamydia trachomatis* |
| Incubation period | 3–10 days | 7–30 days |
| Discharge | Profuse, purulent | Scant, watery |
| Diagnosis | Gram stain Culture | Immunoassay |
| Treatment | Ceftriaxone | Doxycycline or azithromycin |

ii. Nongonococcal.

   1. Presents with dysuria and scant urethral discharge.

**c. Diagnosis**

  i. Urethritis may be suggested if urine dipstick test for leukocyte esterase is positive and no bladder infection is present.

  ii. Gonococcal.

   1. Gram stain reveals gram-negative diplococci and many white blood cells.

   2. Culture is used to make the diagnosis.

  iii. Nongonococcal.

   1. Demonstration of urethritis and exclusion of *N. gonorrhoeae* are required for diagnosis.

   2. Gram stain shows many white blood cells but no bacteria.

   3. Direct fluorescent antibody testing and enzyme immunoassay are also used to make the diagnosis.

**d. Treatment**

  i. Urethritis can be prevented through the use of condoms.

   1. Gonococcal.

    (a) Antibiotic of choice is ceftriaxone.

    (b) If concerned about concurrent infection with *C. trachomatis*, then doxycycline, azithromycin, or ofloxacin should also be used.

   2. Nongonococcal.

    (a) Doxycycline is the antibiotic of choice.

     (i) Azithromycin, levofloxacin, or ofloxacin can also be used.

  ii. Complications.

   1. Complications in males are rare, but include urethral strictures.

   2. In females, complications include pelvic inflammatory disease (PID), infertility, and ectopic pregnancy.

# NEOPLASTIC DISEASES

## I. BLADDER CARCINOMA

  **a. General**

   i. Male-to-female ratio is 3:1.

   ii. Incidence increases with age, with the median age of diagnosis at 70 years.

   iii. Risk factors include smoking and occupational exposure to arylamine (dye, rubber, or leather workers).

   v. Transitional cell is the most common histologic type.

  **b. Clinical Manifestations**

   i. Present with hematuria—gross or microscopic.

    1. Blood remains throughout urination.

   ii. May have abdominal or flank pain.

   iii. May have irritative voiding symptoms.

   iv. Physical examination is typically normal.

  **c. Diagnosis**

   i. Flexible cystoscopy is the most important test.

    1. Transurethral resection with cystoscopy and bladder biopsy.

   ii. CT scan obtained to evaluate for metastatic disease.

  **d. Treatment**

   i. Transurethral resection for superficial disease.

    1. Flexible cystoscopy required every 3 months for monitoring disease.

   ii. With muscle-invasive disease, radical cystectomy with radiation or chemotherapy.

## II. PROSTATE CARCINOMA

  **a. General**

   i. Most prostate cancers are adenocarcinoma.

   ii. Risk factors include advancing age, positive family history for prostate cancer, and Black race.

   iii. No increased risk with BPH.

  **b. Clinical Manifestations**

   i. Patients with early-stage disease are typically asymptomatic.

   ii. Develop obstructive voiding symptoms as disease advances.

   iii. Can also develop hematuria with advanced disease.

   iv. Prostate nodules or asymmetric areas of induration may be noted on digital rectal examination.

  **c. Diagnosis**

   i. Many cases are diagnosed with elevated PSA testing.

    1. In patients with values greater than 4 ng/mL, biopsy should be considered.

2. Other causes of elevated PSA include BPH, prostatic inflammation, and perineal trauma.

ii. Diagnosis made on transrectal ultrasound with biopsy.

**d. Treatment**

i. Treatment options include the following:
1. Watchful waiting.
2. Androgen deprivation.
3. Radical prostatectomy.
4. Radiation therapy.

ii. Low- or intermediate-risk disease is treated with watchful waiting, radical prostatectomy or local radiation therapy.

iii. High-risk patients are treated with aggressive local therapy and androgen deprivation.

iv. Patients with metastatic disease are treated with androgen deprivation after radical prostatectomy.

## III. RENAL CELL CARCINOMA

**a. General**

i. Male-to-female ratio is 3:1.

ii. Most common cell type is clear cell.

iii. Risk factors include obesity, hypertension, smoking, and occupational exposure (cadmium, asbestos).

**b. Clinical Manifestations**

i. Classic triad of flank pain, abdominal mass, and hematuria.

ii. May also note weight loss, fatigue, and anorexia.

**c. Diagnosis**

i. Ultrasound or CT scan needed for diagnosis.

ii. Staging required to determine treatment and prognosis.

**d. Treatment**

i. Localized disease treated with surgical removal of tumor.

ii. Immunomodulatory therapy with high-dose interleukin-2 effective in metastatic disease.

iii. Poor response with radiation or chemotherapy.

iv. The 5-year survival rate is 60% to 70%.

## IV. TESTICULAR CARCINOMA

**a. General**

i. Primary age of onset is 15 to 35 years.

ii. Increased risk with a history of cryptorchidism.

**b. Clinical Manifestations**

i. Present with testicular pain or testicular mass.

ii. With metastatic disease, can present with flank pain.

iii. On physical examination, a testicular mass is noted.

**c. Diagnosis**

i. Testicular ultrasound to evaluate the mass.
1. CT scan to evaluate for metastatic disease.

ii. Serum beta-human chorionic gonadotropin (beta-hCG) and/or alpha-fetoprotein levels are elevated.

**d. Treatment**

i. Orchiectomy with radiation therapy is used in stage I and II disease.

ii. With metastatic disease, chemotherapy is added after surgery.

iii. The 5-year survival rate is over 95%.

# RENAL DISEASES

## I. ACUTE RENAL FAILURE

**a. General**

i. Sudden reduction in kidney function.
1. Defined as low glomerular filtration rate (GFR) and fall in urine output.

ii. Causes of acute renal failure (Table 13.4).

iii. Acute kidney injury (AKI) is abrupt (within 48 hours) reduction in kidney function with retention of nitrogen waste products.

**b. Clinical Manifestations**

i. Symptoms develop with the development of uremia and its effects on other organ systems.
1. Weight gain and edema are common.
2. Table 13.5 shows symptoms of uremia.

ii. Laboratory results.
1. Typically elevated blood urea nitrogen (BUN) or creatinine.

**TABLE 13.4**

| Causes of Acute Renal Failure | | |
| --- | --- | --- |
| **Prerenal** | **Renal** | **Postrenal** |
| ↓**Intravascular Volume** | Ischemic | **Obstruction** |
| Hemorrhage | Postoperative shock | Stones |
| Vomiting | | Tumors |
| Diarrhea | **Nephrotoxic** | Benign |
| Burns | Aminoglycosides | prostatic |
| | Contrast agents | hypertrophy |
| ↓**Intravascular Capacity** | **Inflammatory** | |
| Sepsis | Interstitial nephritis | |
| Vasodilators | Acute glomerulonephritis | |
| Anaphylaxis | Vasculitis | |
| Myocardial failure | | |
| Myocardial infarction | **Pregnancy Related** | |
| Pulmonary embolism | Eclampsia | |
| Congestive heart failure | Abruptio placentae | |
| Hepatorenal syndrome | | |
| | **Renovascular Disease** | |
| | Renal artery thrombosis | |

**TABLE 13.5**

| Symptoms of Uremia | |
| --- | --- |
| **Organ System** | **Symptoms** |
| Cardiovascular | Dyspnea on exertion, pericarditis |
| Gastrointestinal | Anorexia, nausea and vomiting |
| General | Fatigue and weakness |
| Genitourinary | Nocturia |
| Neurologic | Change in mental status |
| Pulmonary | Shortness of breath |
| Skin | Pruritus and easy bruising |

2. Criteria for acute renal dysfunction.
   (a) Risk: increase in creatinine 1.5× normal, decrease in GFR by >25%, or urine output <0.5 mL/kg/hour for 6 hours.
   (b) Injury: increase in creatinine 2× normal, decrease in GFR by >50%, or urine output <0.5 mL/kg/hour for 12 hours.
   (c) Failure: increase in creatinine 3× normal, decrease in GFR by >75%, or urine output <0.3 mL/kg/hour for 24 hours or anuria for 12 hours.

c. **Diagnosis**
   i. Typically the first abnormality is elevated serum creatinine.
   ii. Microscopic examination of the urine may reveal cellular debris.
   iii. Urine studies can be used to separate prerenal from renal.
      1. Table 13.6 summarizes urine study results.
   iv. Ultrasound of the kidney needed to rule out obstruction as possible etiology.

d. **Treatment**
   i. Determine the cause.
   ii. Restore blood pressure and correct intravascular volume status.
   iii. Dialysis may be required until renal recovery.
   iv. In oliguric renal failure, a trial of loop diuretics may be tried to convert to nonoliguric failure.
   v. Remove possible etiologic agents, such as drugs and obstruction.

**TABLE 13.6**

| Urine Study Results in Acute Renal Failure | | |
| --- | --- | --- |
| **Test** | **Prerenal** | **Renal** |
| Urine sodium | <20 | >20 |
| Urine to plasma | >20 | <20 creatinine ratio |
| Fractional sodium | <1 | >1 excretion |

## II. CHRONIC RENAL FAILURE

a. **General**
   i. Slow, progressive decline in kidney function.
   ii. CKD-EPI Creatinine Equation 2021 should be used to estimate GFR.
      1. $eGFR_{cr} = 142 \times min(S_{cr}/\kappa, 1)^{\alpha} \times max(S_{cr}/\kappa, 1)^{-1.200} \times 0.9938^{Age} \times 1.012$ [if female]
         (a) $S_{cr}$ = serum creatinine in mg/dL
         (b) $\kappa$ = 0.7 (females) or 0.9 (males)
         (c) $\alpha$ = −0.241 (female) or −0.302 (male)
         (d) $min(S_{cr}/\kappa, 1)$ is the minimum of $S_{cr}/\kappa$ or 1.0
         (e) $max(S_{cr}/\kappa, 1)$ is the maximum of $S_{cr}/\kappa$ or 1.0
         (f) Age (years)
   iii. Stages.
      1. Stage 1 (slight reduction): GFR >90 mL/min, but presence of markers of kidney disease (blood, urine, or imaging studies).
      2. Stage 2 (mild reduction): GFR 60–89 mL/min with presence of markers of kidney damage.
      3. Stage 3a (mild to moderate reduction): GFR 45–59 mL/min.
      4. Stage 3b (moderate to severe reduction): GFR 30–44 mL/min.
      5. Stage 4 (severe reduction): GFR 15–29 mL/min.
      6. Stage 5 (kidney failure): GFR <15 mL/min or permanent replacement therapy.
      7. Watch for acute exacerbations in chronic disease due to use of angiotensin-converting enzyme (ACE) inhibitors, aminoglycosides, and contrast media.
      8. Table 13.7 shows etiologies of chronic renal failure.

**TABLE 13.7**

| Causes of Chronic Renal Failure |
| --- |
| Diabetes glomerulosclerosis |
| Hypertensive glomerulosclerosis |
| Glomerular disease |
|    Glomerulonephritis |
|    Systemic lupus erythematosus |
|    Wegener's granulomatosis |
| Tubulointerstitial disease |
|    Obstructive nephropathy |
|    Analgesic nephropathy |
|    Chronic pyelonephritis |
|    Myeloma kidney |
| Vascular disease |
|    Scleroderma |
|    Vasculitis |
| Cystic disease |
|    Polycystic kidney disease |

b. **Clinical Manifestations**
   i. Symptoms develop with the development of uremia and its effects on other organ systems.
      1. Typically markedly elevated BUN or creatinine.
   ii. Anemia due to decreased production of erythropoietin.
   iii. Renal osteodystrophy due to hyperparathyroidism.
      1. Increased risk for fracture and bone pain.
c. **Diagnosis**
   i. Microscopic examination of the urine may reveal waxy casts.
   ii. Ultrasound of the kidney may reveal small or polycystic kidneys.
d. **Treatment**
   i. Monitor progression of renal failure through measurement of serum creatinine and creatinine ratio on spot urine (UACR).
   ii. Control blood pressure, blood glucose levels, and diet with protein restrictions, and avoid renal toxic drugs.
      1. ACE inhibitors slow progression of renal failure.
         (a) Monitor potassium level when starting an ACE inhibitor.
   iii. Treat anemia with erythropoietin.
      1. Maintain hemoglobin at 11–12 g/dL.
   iv. Calcium, vitamin D, and bicarbonate supplement to avoid bone disease.
      1. Also restrict dietary phosphate.
   v. Dialysis needed in end-stage renal disease.
      1. Kidney transplantation provides the most complete correction of end-stage disease.
   vi. Complications.
      1. Hyperkalemia
      2. Acid-base disorders.

3. Hypertension.
4. Pericarditis.
5. Anemia.
6. Encephalopathy.
7. Renal osteodystrophy.

## III. GLOMERULONEPHRITIS
a. **General**
   i. Acute glomerulonephritis is an uncommon cause of acute renal failure.
   ii. Due to immune complex deposits in the kidney.
   iii. Etiologies include the following:
      1. Immunoglobulin A (IgA) nephropathy (Berger's disease).
      2. Postinfectious glomerulonephritis.
      3. Lupus nephritis.
      4. Pauci-immune glomerulonephritis.
         (a) Wegener's granulomatosis disease.
      5. Goodpasture's syndrome.
      6. Table 13.8 summarizes glomerulonephritis.
b. **Clinical Manifestations**
   i. Edema is noted in periorbital and scrotal regions.
   ii. Hypertension may be present.
c. **Diagnosis**
   i. Serologic markers.
      1. Antineutrophil cytoplasmic autoantibodies (ANCAs).
      2. Antiglomerular basement membrane autoantibodies (anti-GBMs).
   ii. Urinalysis.
      1. Dysmorphic red blood cells and red blood cell casts are common.
      2. Proteinuria is also noted.
   iii. Biopsy for definitive diagnosis.
d. **Treatment**
   i. Correction of hypertension and fluid overload.

**TABLE 13.8**

| Summary of Glomerulonephritis | | | | |
|---|---|---|---|---|
| **Disease** | **Signs and Symptoms** | **Serologic Markers** | **Treatment** | **Notes** |
| Poststreptococcal glomerulonephritis | Oliguric Edema | High ASO titer | Supportive | Occurs after pharyngitis and impetigo |
| IgA nephropathy | Gross hematuria | Elevated IgA levels | Corticosteroids | Associated with URI or flulike illness |
| Wegener's granulomatosis | Fever, malaise, weight loss | ANCA positive | Corticosteroids Cyclophosphamide | Respiratory tract symptoms common |
| Goodpasture's syndrome | Hemoptysis | Anti-GBM antibodies positive | Plasma exchange Steroids | Lung injury is common |
| Lupus nephritis | Rash | ANA positive | Steroids Mycophenolate mofetil Cyclophosphamide | |

*ANA*, Antinuclear antibody; *ANCA*, antineutrophil cytoplasmic antibody; *anti-GBM*, antiglomerular basement membrane; *ASO*, antistreptolysin O; *IgA*, immunoglobulin A; *URI*, upper respiratory infection.

ii. Corticosteroids and cytotoxic agents may be needed.

## IV. HYDRONEPHROSIS
a. **General**
   i. Distention and dilation of the kidney.
   ii. Caused by obstruction of urine flow.
   iii. Etiologies.
      1. Stones.
      2. Blood clots.
      3. Prostatic enlargement.
      4. Congenital.
b. **Clinical**
   i. Flank pain, nausea, and vomiting may be noted.
c. **Diagnosis**
   i. CT scan or ultrasound.
d. **Treatment**
   i. Treat the underlying cause.

## V. NEPHROTIC SYNDROME
a. **General**
   i. Seen in patients with systemic renal disease, diabetes mellitus, amyloidosis, systemic lupus erythematosus (SLE), or idiopathic nephrotic syndrome.
   ii. Urine protein excretion greater than 3.5 g/24 hours.
b. **Clinical Manifestations**
   i. Peripheral edema is the classic finding.
   ii. May note dyspnea due to pulmonary edema or abdominal fullness due to ascites.
   iii. Anasarca is common with nephrotic syndrome.
c. **Diagnosis**
   i. Urinalysis reveals proteinuria with little or no cellular elements noted on microscopic examination.
   ii. Serum albumin is decreased, along with total protein.
   iii. As proteinuria increases, the frequency of hyperlipidemia increases.
   iv. Renal biopsy needed to classify disease.
d. **Treatment**
   i. Protein restriction to limit adverse effects on renal function.
   ii. Salt restriction to manage edema.
   iii. Treatment of hyperlipidemia with medications and dietary management.
   iv. Steroids needed in minimal change disease, focal segmental glomerulosclerosis, and membranous nephropathy.
   v. In diabetic nephropathy, the rate of progression of disease can be controlled by strict glycemic control.
   vi. ACE inhibitor for proteinuria.

## VI. POLYCYSTIC KIDNEY DISEASE
a. **General**
   i. One of the more common hereditary disorders.
      1. Autosomal dominant: most common, with symptoms typically developing between ages 30 and 40.
      2. Autosomal recessive: rare, symptoms begin the first few months of life.
   ii. A history of UTI and nephrolithiasis is common.
   iii. Family history is positive.
b. **Clinical Manifestations**
   i. Presents with abdominal or flank pain and hematuria—microscopic or gross.
   ii. Hypertension is common.
   iii. On physical examination, kidneys may be palpable.
c. **Diagnosis**
   i. Ultrasound of the kidney reveals more than five cysts.
   ii. Cysts also noted on CT scan.
d. **Treatment**
   i. Aggressive treatment of hypertension.
   ii. Statins for hyperlipidemia.
   iii. Bed rest and analgesics for pain and hematuria.
   iv. Dialysis or transplant when end-stage renal disease develops.

## VII. RENAL VASCULAR DISEASE
a. **General**
   i. Caused by a variety of conditions that affect the blood flow into or out of the kidneys.
      1. Atherosclerosis.
      2. Diabetes.
      3. Hypertension.
      4. Morbid obesity.
      5. Fibromuscular dysplasia.
      6. Injury.
      7. Infection.
   ii. Types of renal vascular disease include:
      1. Renal artery stenosis.
      2. Renal artery thrombosis.
      3. Renal vein thrombosis.
      4. Renal artery aneurysm.
      5. Atheroembolic renal disease.
b. **Clinical Manifestations**
   i. Typically asymptomatic until advanced stages of the underlying disease process.
   ii. Hypertension is common.
c. **Diagnosis**
   i. Made by angiography, duplex ultrasound, renography and magnetic resonance angiography.
d. **Treatment**
   i. Aimed at correcting the underlying cause.

# ELECTROLYTE AND ACID-BASE DISORDERS

## I. HYPONATREMIA
  **a. General**
    i. Defined as a serum sodium less than 130 mEq/L.
  **b. Clinical Manifestations**
    i. Most patients are asymptomatic.
    ii. May present with lethargy, weakness, confusion, and seizures.
  **c. Diagnosis**
    i. Begins with serum osmolality and volume status.
    ii. Urine sodium levels needed in patients with low osmolality and hypovolemia.
    iii. See Fig. 13.2.
  **d. Treatment**
    i. Symptomatic patient.
      1. Usually seen in patients with sodium of less than 120 mEq/L.
      2. Increase sodium by only 1 to 2 mEq/L/hour to decrease risk for demyelination of central nervous system (CNS) (osmotic demyelination).
      3. Treat with saline plus furosemide.
    ii. Asymptomatic patient.
      1. Correct sodium at rate of 0.5 mEq/L/hour.
      2. Water restriction to approximately 1 L/day.
      3. Normal saline with furosemide.
      4. Demeclocycline may be used, inhibiting effects of antidiuretic hormone (ADH) on distal tubule.
        (a) May require a week to see onset of action.

## II. HYPERNATREMIA
  **a. General**
    i. An intact thirst mechanism typically prevents hypernatremia.
      1. Excess water loss will only cause hypernatremia when appropriate water intake is not possible.

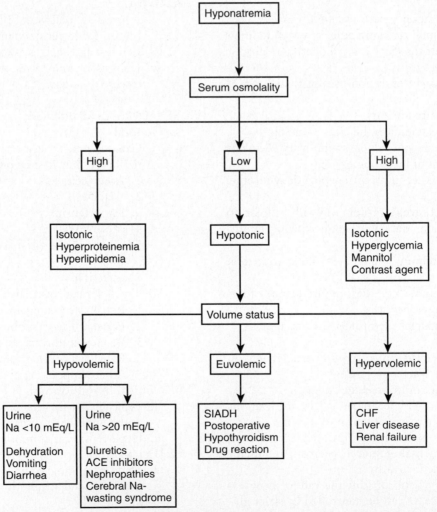

**Fig. 13.2** Diagnosis of hyponatremia. *ACE*, Angiotensin-converting enzyme; *CHF*, congestive heart failure; *SIADH*, syndrome of inappropriate antidiuretic hormone.

2. Etiologies.
   (a) Dehydration.
   (b) Lactulose.
   (c) Mannitol therapy.
   (d) Diabetes insipidus.
   (e) Excessive sodium intake.
   (f) Primary aldosteronism.
b. **Clinical Manifestations**
   i. Orthostatic hypotension and oliguria are typical.
   ii. Mental status changes such as delirium and coma are seen in severe hypernatremia.
c. **Diagnosis**
   i. If urine osmolality is greater than 400 mOsm/kg, then renal water-conserving ability is intact.
      1. Due to nonrenal losses (sweating, diarrhea) or renal losses.
   ii. If urine osmolality is less than 250 mOsm/kg, then consider diabetes insipidus.
d. **Treatment**
   i. Treatment of the underlying cause and replacement of water.
   ii. Correct slowly to reduce risk for cerebral edema and neurologic impairment.
      1. Decrease sodium by 0.5 mEq/L/hour.

## III. HYPOKALEMIA
a. **General**
   i. Normal range is 3.5 to 5.5 mEq/L.
   ii. Etiology.
      1. Trauma.
      2. Increased aldosterone.
      3. Diuretics.
      4. Hypomagnesemia.
      5. Renal tubular acidosis.
      6. Extrarenal loss: diarrhea, vomiting, laxative abuse.
      7. Metabolic alkalosis.
b. **Clinical Manifestations**
   i. In mild to moderate disease, note muscle weakness, fatigue, and muscle cramps.
   ii. In severe disease, note flaccid paralysis, hyporeflexia, tetany, and rhabdomyolysis.
c. **Diagnosis**
   i. Labs reveal potassium of less than 3.5 mEq/L.
   ii. On electrocardiogram (EKG), note decreasing size and broadening of T waves.
      1. Increased risk of digitalis toxicity in hypokalemia.
d. **Treatment**
   i. Oral potassium supplement for mild to moderate deficiency.
   ii. IV potassium for severe deficiency (potassium less than 3.0 mEq/L).

iii. Concurrent deficiency in magnesium may make potassium correction more difficult.

## IV. HYPERKALEMIA
a. **General**
   i. Typically associated with acidosis.
   ii. Etiologies.
      1. Hemolysis of red blood cells.
      2. Thrombocytosis or leukocytosis (pseudo-hyperkalemia).
      3. Renal failure.
      4. Drugs: heparin, spironolactone, ACE inhibitors, nonsteroidal antiinflammatory drugs (NSAIDs).
      5. Burns.
      6. Metabolic acidosis: diabetic ketoacidosis (DKA), lactic acid.
      7. Excessive intake.
      8. Rhabdomyolysis.
      9. Tumor lysis syndrome.
b. **Clinical Manifestations**
   i. May produce muscle weakness and flaccid paralysis, abdominal distention, and diarrhea.
c. **Diagnosis**
   i. Labs reveal potassium greater than 5.5 mEq/L.
   ii. On EKG, note peaked T waves and widening QRS.
d. **Treatment**
   i. Severe hyperkalemia.
      1. Concern about cardiac toxicity and EKG changes.
      2. Treatment consists of distributing potassium back into the cells via albuterol, insulin, or bicarbonate.
   ii. Nonemergent hyperkalemia.
      1. Withhold potassium and give cation exchange resins.
         (a) Sodium polystyrene, ion exchange resin, can be given orally or rectally.
      2. Loop diuretics and dialysis can also be used to decrease potassium.

## V. HYPOCALCEMIA
a. **General**
   i. Etiologies include the following:
      1. Malabsorption.
      2. Vitamin D deficiency.
      3. Alcoholism.
      4. Diuretic therapy.
      5. Hypoparathyroidism.
      6. Renal failure.
      7. Drugs: aminoglycosides.
b. **Clinical Manifestations**
   i. May produce muscle spasm, tetany, seizures, and arrhythmias.

ii. Positive Chvostek's and Trousseau's signs.
c. **Diagnosis**
   i. On EKG, note the prolonged QT interval.
   ii. Calcium level of less than 8.5 mg/dL.
d. **Treatment**
   i. In severe deficiency cases, calcium gluconate is given IV.
   ii. In asymptomatic cases, oral calcium with vitamin D supplements is indicated.

## VI. HYPERCALCEMIA
a. **General**
   i. Etiologies include the following:
      1. Primary hyperparathyroidism.
      2. Neoplastic disease.
      3. Thiazide diuretics.
      4. Sarcoidosis.
b. **Clinical Manifestations**
   i. Major symptoms include constipation and polyuria.
   ii. In severe hypercalcemia, may note stupor, coma, and azotemia.
c. **Diagnosis**
   i. Symptoms occur with levels greater than 12 mg/dL.
   ii. EKG reveals shortened QT interval.
d. **Treatment**
   i. Treat the underlying cause.
   ii. Normal saline is an emergency treatment of choice.
   iii. In malignancy, bisphosphonates (zoledronic acid or pamidronate) are safe and effective.
   iv. Calcitonin.

## VII. HYPOMAGNESEMIA
a. **General**
   i. Most of the body's magnesium is in the skeleton and soft tissue.
   ii. Most magnesium comes from green leafy vegetables.
   iii. Results from decreased intestinal absorption or increased losses in urine or stool.
   iv. Etiology. Table 13.9 shows causes of hypomagnesemia.
b. **Clinical Manifestations**
   i. Symptoms include weakness, anorexia, cardiac arrhythmias, tetany, and seizures.
   ii. Hypokalemia often accompanies hypomagnesemia.
c. **Diagnosis**
   i. Serum magnesium levels are less than 1.6 mEq/L.
d. **Treatment**
   i. Mild or moderate deficiency treated with oral magnesium oxide or chloride supplement.

**TABLE 13.9**

| Causes of Hypomagnesemia |
| --- |
| **Gastrointestinal** |
| Malabsorption |
| Severe diarrhea |
| Small bowel resection |
| **Renal** |
| Bartter's syndrome |
| Postobstructive diuresis |
| Volume expansion |
| Diabetic ketoacidosis |
| Diuretics |
| **Body Fluid Loss** |
| Burns |
| **Other** |
| Alcoholism |
| Thyrotoxicosis |

ii. Severe disease treated with IV magnesium sulfate.

## VIII. ACID-BASE DISORDERS
a. **General**
   i. See Table 13.10 for normal ranges for acid-base disorders.
   ii. Interpretation.
      1. Acidosis versus alkalosis.
         (a) If arterial blood pH is less than 7.40, the patient is acidemic.
         (b) If arterial blood pH is greater than 7.40, the patient is alkalemic.
      2. Determine primary process.
         (a) After evaluating pH, look at $P_{CO_2}$ and bicarbonate.
            (i) If pH is acidemic and $P_{CO_2}$ is greater than 45 mm Hg, the primary process is respiratory; if bicarbonate is less than 22, the primary process is metabolic.
            (ii) If pH is alkalemic and the $P_{CO_2}$ is less than 35 mm Hg, the primary process is respiratory; if bicarbonate

**TABLE 13.10**

| Normal Ranges for Acid-Base Disorders | |
| --- | --- |
| **Test** | **Normal Range** |
| pH | 7.35–7.45 |
| $P_{CO_2}$ | 35–45 mm Hg |
| Bicarbonate | 22–26 mmol/L |
| Sodium | 135–145 mEq/L |
| Potassium | 3.5–5.0 mEq/L |
| Chloride | 98–108 mmol/L |
| $P_{O_2}$ | 80–100 mm Hg |

**TABLE 13.11**

| Primary Acid-Base Disorders | | | |
|---|---|---|---|
| Test | Primary Disorder | Normal Range | Primary Disorder |
| pH | Acidemia | ← 7.35 to 7.45 → | Alkalemia |
| $P_{CO_2}$ | Respiratory alkalosis | ← 35 to 45 → | Respiratory acidosis |
| Bicarbonate | Metabolic acidosis | ← 22 to 26 → | Metabolic alkalosis |

**TABLE 13.12**

| Etiology of Metabolic Acidosis | |
|---|---|
| Normal Anion Gap | Elevated Anion Gap |
| Carbonic anhydrase inhibitors | Ethylene glycol intoxication |
| Early renal failure | Uremia |
| Gastrointestinal bicarbonate loss (diarrhea, ureteral diversions) | Lactic acidosis |
| Hydrochloric acid administration | Salicylate intoxication |
| Post-hypocapnia | Methanol ingestion |
| Renal tubular acidosis | Diabetic ketoacidosis |

is greater than 26, the primary process is metabolic.

(b) See Table 13.11 and Fig. 13.3.

3. Anion gap.

(a) Difference between the major cations and anions.

(b) If elevated, suspect presence of excess organic acids or acidic foreign substances.

(c) Calculation.

(i) Anion gap = $Na^+ - (Cl^- + HCO_3^-)$.

(d) Normal range is 10 to 14 mEq/L.

(e) Used to separate different causes of metabolic acidosis.

**b. Disorders**

i. Metabolic acidosis.

1. Etiology.

(a) Separated based on anion gap.

(b) Table 13.12 shows causes of metabolic acidosis.

2. Clinical manifestations.

(a) Dyspnea on exertion and nausea and vomiting are common.

(b) On physical examination, labored deep respirations with use of accessory muscles may be noted.

ii. Metabolic alkalosis.

1. Etiology

(a) Causes separated based on urine chloride.

(b) Table 13.13 shows causes of metabolic alkalosis.

2. Clinical manifestations.

(a) CNS symptoms such as confusion, obtundation, delirium, and coma can be noted.

(b) Cardiac arrhythmias and hypotension can also be noted.

iii. Respiratory acidosis.

1. Etiology

(a) Can be acute or chronic respiratory acidosis.

(b) Table 13.14 shows causes of respiratory acidosis.

2. Clinical manifestations.

(a) Related to degree and duration of acidosis and presence of hypoxia.

**TABLE 13.13**

| Etiology of Metabolic Alkalosis | |
|---|---|
| Low Urine Chloride | Normal or High Urine Chloride |
| Vomiting or nasogastric suctioning | Cushing's syndrome |
| Diuretic use in past | Conn's syndrome |
| Post-hypercapnia | Exogenous steroids |
| | Bartter's syndrome |
| | Current or recent diuretic use |

**TABLE 13.14**

| Etiology of Respiratory Acidosis | |
|---|---|
| Acute | Chronic |
| Acute airway obstruction | Chronic respiratory center depression |
| Central nervous system depression (drugs, CNS event) | Chronic lung disease |
| Hemothorax, pneumothorax | Chronic neuromuscular disease |
| Neuromuscular disorders | |
| Severe pneumonia or pulmonary edema | |
| Ventilator dysfunction | |

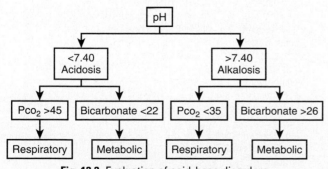

**Fig. 13.3** Evaluation of acid-base disorders.

(b) In acute disease, CNS symptoms such as confusion, anxiety, psychosis, and seizures may be noted.

(c) In chronic disease, note lethargy, fatigue, and confusion.

iv. Respiratory alkalosis.
1. Etiology.
   (a) Anxiety.
   (b) Hypoxia.
   (c) CNS disease.
   (d) Drug use: salicylates.
   (e) Pregnancy.
   (f) Sepsis.
   (g) Hepatic encephalopathy.
   (h) Mechanical ventilation.
2. Clinical manifestations.
   (a) May cause dizziness, perioral paresthesias, confusion, hypotension, seizures, and coma.

## IX. VOLUME DEPLETION

a. **General**
   i. Defined as reduced total body water.
   ii. Occurs when the rate of salt and water intake is less than the combined rates of renal and extrarenal losses.
   iii. Etiologies grouped into decreased fluid intake or increased fluid loss.
      1. Increased loss grouped into renal or extrarenal causes.
      2. Table 13.15 shows causes of volume depletion.

b. **Clinical Manifestations**
   i. Signs and symptoms vary with degree of depletion.

ii. Orthostatic hypotension and tachycardia are common.

iii. On physical examination, note decreased skin turgor and dry mucous membranes.

c. **Diagnosis**
   i. Orthostatic hypotension, with a 20 mm Hg drop in systolic pressure or a 10 mm Hg drop in diastolic pressure.
   ii. Positive response to a fluid challenge.

d. **Treatment**
   i. Fluid replacement with normal saline.
   ii. Most potent fluid replacement substance is blood.
      1. Used typically in cases of hemorrhage.

## X. VOLUME EXCESS

a. **General**
   i. Increase in total body water.
   ii. Occurs when the rate of salt and water intake exceeds renal and extrarenal losses.
      1. Table 13.16 shows causes of volume excess.

b. **Clinical Manifestations**
   i. Symptoms related to cause of volume excess.
   ii. Cases due to reduced effective circulating volume will have edema.

c. **Diagnosis**
   i. Varies with underlying cause.

d. **Treatment**
   i. Diuretics are the treatment of choice.
      1. Table 13.17 lists effects of diuretics.

## XI. URINALYSIS

a. **Table 13.18 summarizes common findings on urinalysis**

**TABLE 13.15**

| Causes of Volume Depletion | |
| --- | --- |
| **Renal Losses** | **Extrarenal Losses** |
| **Hormonal Deficit** | Hemorrhage |
| Primary diabetes insipidus | Sweating and burns |
| Aldosterone insufficiency | Vomiting |
| | Diarrhea |
| **Renal Deficit** | Tube drainage |
| Renal tubular acidosis | |
| Bartter's syndrome | |
| Secondary diabetes insipidus | |
| Diuretic abuse | |
| Osmotic diuresis | |
| Chronic renal failure | |
| Interstitial nephritis | |

**TABLE 13.16**

| Causes of Volume Excess | | |
| --- | --- | --- |
| **Reduced Effective Circulating Volume** | **Primary Hormone Excess** | **Primary Renal Sodium Retention** |
| Systemic increase in venous pressure | Primary aldosteronism | Renal failure |
| Right-sided heart failure | Cushing's syndrome | |
| Constrictive pericarditis | Syndrome of inappropriate antidiuretic hormone | |
| Local increase in venous pressure | | |
| Left-sided heart failure | | |
| Vena cava obstruction | | |
| Reduced oncotic pressure | | |
| Nephrotic syndrome | | |
| Hypoalbuminemia | | |
| Cirrhosis | | |

**TABLE 13.17**

## Effects of Diuretics

| Diuretic | Primary Effect | Side Effect |
|---|---|---|
| **Proximal Diuretic** | | |
| Acetazolamide | ↓ Na$^+$/H$^+$ | Hypokalemic, hyper-chloremic acidosis |
| **Loop Diuretic** | | |
| Furosemide | ↓ Na$^+$/K$^+$:2Cl$^-$ absorption | Hypokalemic alkalosis Bumetanide Hearing deficits |
| **Early Distal Diuretic** | | |
| Thiazide | ↓ NaCl absorption | Hypokalemic alkalosis Hyperglycemia |
| **Late Distal Diuretic** | | |
| Spironolactone Triamterene | ↓ Na$^+$ absorption | Hyperkalemic acidosis |

**TABLE 13.18**

## Common Findings on Urinalysis

| Test | Disease State |
|---|---|
| **Macroscopic** | |
| Specific gravity | Dehydration or fluid overload |
| Protein | Functional: severe muscle exertion, pregnancy |
| | Organic: fever, hypertension, glomerulone-phritis, nephrotic syndrome, infection |
| Glucose | Diabetes mellitus |
| Ketones | Diabetic ketoacidosis, starvation |
| Blood | Stones, infection, tumor, tuberculosis, glomerulonephritis |
| Nitrite | Infection |
| Leukocyte esterase | Infection |
| **Microscopic** | |
| Red blood cells | Stones, infection, tumor, tuberculosis, glomerulonephritis |
| White blood cells | Infection |
| **Casts** | |
| Red blood cell cast | Acute glomerulonephritis |
| White blood cell cast | Pyelonephritis |
| Waxy cast | Renal failure |

# QUESTIONS

## QUESTION 1
Which of the following is the most common symptom of bladder cancer?

A  Incontinence
B  Urinary retention
C  Suprapubic pain
D  Hematuria
E  Dysuria

## QUESTION 2
Which of the following is the first step in the evaluation of the patient with an increasing serum creatinine?

A  Abdominal x-ray of kidney, ureter, and bladder (KUB)
B  Intravenous pyelogram
C  24-hour urine volume
D  Abdominal CT scan
E  Renal ultrasound

## QUESTION 3
A 20-year-old patient presents with gradual onset of scrotal pain and swelling. The patient's temperature is 38.3° C. Urinalysis reveals many white blood cells and bacteria. Which of the following is the most likely diagnosis?

A  Urinary tract infection
B  Testicular torsion
C  Inguinal hernia
D  Epididymitis
E  Prostatitis

## QUESTION 4
A 35-year-old patient presents with nausea, hematuria, and right flank pain with radiation to the right testicle. Urinalysis reveals 50 to 100 red blood cells, 0 to 1 white blood cells, and many calcium oxalate crystals. Which of the following is the most appropriate clinical intervention?

A  IV antibiotics
B  Hemiacidrin (Renacidin)
C  Extracorporeal lithotripsy and thiazide diuretics
D  Support care with fluids and pain medications
E  Tamsulosin and cystoscopy

*Continued*

## QUESTIONS—cont'd

### QUESTION 5

A 25-year-old male presents with fever and dysuria. On physical examination, the prostate is noted to be very tender, enlarged, and indurated. Urinalysis reveals many white blood cells. Which of the following would be the best treatment option for this patient?

A  Finasteride (Proscar)

B  Ibuprofen (Motrin)

C  Ciprofloxacin (Cipro)

D  Phenazopyridine (Pyridium)

E  Lisinopril (Zestril)

### QUESTION 6

How frequently should a patient perform a self-testicular examination to screen for testicular cancer?

A  Daily

B  Weekly

C  Monthly

D  Biannually

E  Yearly

### QUESTION 7

A patient presents with the following labs:

Sodium: 138 mEq/L        Glucose: 230 mg/dL

Potassium: 5.2 mEq/L      Creatinine: 1.4 mg/dL

Chloride: 100 mEq/L       BUN: 45 mg/dL

Bicarb: 13 mmol/L

What is the anion gap for this patient?

A  12

B  20

C  25

D  35

E  40

### QUESTION 8

A 17-year-old male presents with right groin pain for the past 2 hours. Elevation of the scrotum relieves the pain. The patient has been sexually active with multiple partners over the past 2 years. On physical examination, the right scrotum is acutely tender, swollen, and erythematous. Which of the following is the most likely diagnosis?

A  Prostatitis

B  Epididymitis

C  Incarcerated hernia

D  Torsion of the testicle

E  Fournier's gangrene

### QUESTION 9

Which of the following is a common characteristic feature of nephrotic syndrome?

A  Hematuria

B  Proteinuria

C  Hypolipidemia

D  Hyperalbuminemia

E  Vitamin D deficiency

### QUESTION 10

Which of the following is the primary effect of aldosterone on the distal renal tubules?

A  Reabsorption of potassium

B  Reabsorption of sodium

C  Reabsorption of chloride

D  Secretion of sodium

E  Secretion of chloride

## ANSWERS

**1.  D**

EXPLANATION: Bladder cancer is typically noted in males with a median age of 70 years. Typical presentation is painful hematuria and possible abdominal or flank pain. ***Topic: Bladder carcinoma***

☐ Correct   ☐ Incorrect

**2.  E**

EXPLANATION: Elevation of serum creatinine may be the first finding of acute renal failure. Renal ultrasound and avoidance of renal toxic medications are the first steps in the evaluation of these patients. ***Topic: Acute renal failure***

☐ Correct   ☐ Incorrect

**3.  D**

EXPLANATION: Patients with epididymitis typically present with fever, scrotal swelling, and symptoms of urethritis. Urinalysis reveals an increased number of white blood cells and bacteria. ***Topic: Epididymitis***

☐ Correct   ☐ Incorrect

**4.  D**

EXPLANATION: Nephrolithiasis presents with colicky flank pain radiating to the testes or labia. Hematuria is common. Treatment of acute disease consists of support care with IV fluids and pain control. ***Topic: Nephrolithiasis***

☐ Correct   ☐ Incorrect

## ANSWERS—cont'd

**5. C**

EXPLANATION: Acute prostatitis presents with fever, chills, and dysuria. On physical examination, the prostate is noted to be very tender. Urinalysis reveals many white blood cells. Treatment consists of antibiotics, such as fluoroquinolones ciprofloxacin, or trimethoprim-sulfamethoxazole. *Topic: Prostatitis*

☐ Correct   ☐ Incorrect

**6. C**

EXPLANATION: Testicular cancer screening with self-testicular examination should be completed each month. *Topic: Testicular carcinoma*

☐ Correct   ☐ Incorrect

**7. C**

EXPLANATION: Anion gap is calculated by adding the serum chloride and bicarbonate and then subtracting this total from the serum sodium. Anion gap for this patient is 25 mEq/L. *Topic: Acid-base disorders*

☐ Correct   ☐ Incorrect

**8. B**

EXPLANATION: Patients with epididymitis present with fever and irritative voiding symptoms. Symptoms may follow acute physical strain or sexual activity. On physical examination, pain is noted to improve with elevation of the scrotum and the scrotum is tender, swollen, and erythematous. *Topic: Epididymitis*

☐ Correct   ☐ Incorrect

**9. B**

EXPLANATION: Nephrotic syndrome presents with proteinuria, hypoalbuminemia, hyperlipidemia, and peripheral edema. *Topic: Nephrotic syndrome*

☐ Correct   ☐ Incorrect

**10. B**

EXPLANATION: Aldosterone, secreted by the adrenal gland, causes sodium reabsorption in the distal tubules and collecting ducts. *Topic: Volume depletion*

☐ Correct   ☐ Incorrect

# CHAPTER 14
# PEDIATRICS

## EXAMINATION BLUEPRINT TOPICS

**IMMUNIZATIONS**

Schedules

**GROWTH AND DEVELOPMENT**

Tanner stages

Developmental milestones

**THE NEWBORN INFANT**

Evaluation

Nutrition

**GENETIC DISORDERS**

General

Congenital hypothyroidism (Cretinism)

Cystic fibrosis

Down syndrome (Trisomy 21)

Klinefelter's syndrome

Trisomy 13 (Patau syndrome)

Trisomy 18 (Edwards syndrome)

Turner's syndrome

**CARDIAC DISEASES**

General

Congenital heart disease

**EYES, EARS, NOSE, AND THROAT/PULMONARY**

Acute bronchiolitis

Acute epiglottitis

Croup (laryngotracheitis)

Hyaline membrane disease (respiratory distress syndrome)

Foreign body aspiration

Kawasaki's disease

Meconium aspiration

Acute otitis media

Pharyngitis

Pertussis

Sudden infant death syndrome

**GASTROENTEROLOGY**

Colic

Duodenal atresia

Jaundice

Inborn errors of metabolism

Intussusception

Pyloric stenosis

Volvulus (malrotation)

**MUSCULOSKELETAL**

Developmental hip dysplasia

Juvenile rheumatoid arthritis

Osgood-Schlatter disease

Slipped capital femoral epiphysis

**NEUROLOGY**

Cerebral palsy

Coma

Neuroblastoma

Seizures

**PSYCHIATRY**

Attention-deficit disorder

Autism spectrum disorder

Child abuse

**GENITOURINARY**

Cryptorchidism

Hydrocele

Wilms' tumor (nephroblastoma)

**DERMATOLOGY**

Diaper dermatitis

## IMMUNIZATIONS

### I. SCHEDULES
   a. See Figs 14.1 and 14.2 for immunization and catch-up schedules.

## GROWTH AND DEVELOPMENT

### I. TANNER STAGES
   a. See Table 14.1 and Fig. 14.3 for description of stages

### II. DEVELOPMENTAL MILESTONES
   a. Table 14.2 lists developmental milestones
   b. Table 14.3 covers screening for developmental delays

## THE NEWBORN INFANT

### I. EVALUATION
   a. **Apgar Scoring**
      i. Rapid scoring system based on response to the birth process.

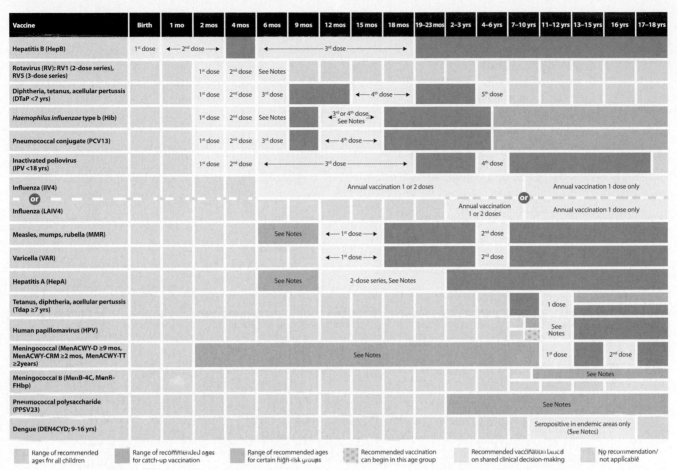

| Vaccine | Birth | 1 mo | 2 mos | 4 mos | 6 mos | 9 mos | 12 mos | 15 mos | 18 mos | 19–23 mos | 2–3 yrs | 4–6 yrs | 7–10 yrs | 11–12 yrs | 13–15 yrs | 16 yrs | 17–18 yrs |
|---|---|---|---|---|---|---|---|---|---|---|---|---|---|---|---|---|---|
| Hepatitis B (HepB) | 1st dose | ←— 2nd dose —→ | | | ←————————— 3rd dose —————————→ | | | | | | | | | | | | |
| Rotavirus (RV): RV1 (2-dose series), RV5 (3-dose series) | | | 1st dose | 2nd dose | See Notes | | | | | | | | | | | | |
| Diphtheria, tetanus, acellular pertussis (DTaP <7 yrs) | | | 1st dose | 2nd dose | 3rd dose | | ←— 4th dose —→ | | | | | 5th dose | | | | | |
| Haemophilus influenzae type b (Hib) | | | 1st dose | 2nd dose | See Notes | | 3rd or 4th dose, See Notes → | | | | | | | | | | |
| Pneumococcal conjugate (PCV13) | | | 1st dose | 2nd dose | 3rd dose | | ←— 4th dose —→ | | | | | | | | | | |
| Inactivated poliovirus (IPV <18 yrs) | | | 1st dose | 2nd dose | ←————————— 3rd dose —————————→ | | | | | | | 4th dose | | | | | |
| Influenza (IIV4) | | | | | | | Annual vaccination 1 or 2 doses | | | | | | | Annual vaccination 1 dose only | | | |
| or Influenza (LAIV4) | | | | | | | | | | | | Annual vaccination 1 or 2 doses | | or Annual vaccination 1 dose only | | | |
| Measles, mumps, rubella (MMR) | | | | | See Notes | | ←— 1st dose —→ | | | | | 2nd dose | | | | | |
| Varicella (VAR) | | | | | | | ←— 1st dose —→ | | | | | 2nd dose | | | | | |
| Hepatitis A (HepA) | | | | | See Notes | | 2-dose series, See Notes | | | | | | | | | | |
| Tetanus, diphtheria, acellular pertussis (Tdap ≥7 yrs) | | | | | | | | | | | | | | 1 dose | | | |
| Human papillomavirus (HPV) | | | | | | | | | | | | | | See Notes | | | |
| Meningococcal (MenACWY-D ≥9 mos, MenACWY-CRM ≥2 mos, MenACWY-TT ≥2years) | | | | | | | | See Notes | | | | | | 1st dose | | 2nd dose | |
| Meningococcal B (MenB-4C, MenB-FHbp) | | | | | | | | | | | | | | | See Notes | | |
| Pneumococcal polysaccharide (PPSV23) | | | | | | | | | | | | | | See Notes | | | |
| Dengue (DEN4CYD; 9-16 yrs) | | | | | | | | | | | | | | Seropositive in endemic areas only (See Notes) | | | |

Range of recommended ages for all children ■ Range of recommended ages for catch-up vaccination ■ Range of recommended ages for certain high-risk groups ■ Recommended vaccination can begin in this age group ■ Recommended vaccination based on shared clinical decision-making ■ No recommendation/ not applicable

**Fig. 14.1** Immunization schedule for ages 0 through 18 years—United States, 2022. For the footnotes found in the figure, please go to the following website: https://www.cdc.gov/vaccines/schedules/downloads/child/0-18yrs-child-combined-schedule.pdf

ii. Measured at 1- and 5-minute intervals after birth.

iii. Table 14.4 summarizes the Apgar scoring table.

    1. A 1-minute score provides information related to labor and delivery.

iv. Scoring.

    1. Normal: 7–10.

    2. Low: 4–6, may require medical care.

    3. Critically low: less than 3, will need immediate medical care.

**b. Newborn Examination**

  i. General.

    1. Vitals.

      (a) Heart rate: normal 120–140 beats per minute (BPM).

      (b) Respiratory rate: normal 30–60 breaths per minute.

      (c) Temperature: normal 36.4–37.0° C (97.5–98.6° F) axillary.

      (d) Blood pressure: normal 50–70 mm Hg systolic and 25–50 mm Hg diastolic.

      (e) Head circumference: normal 13–14.5 inches (33–37 cm).

      (f) Chest circumference: normally 2–3 cm smaller than the head circumference.

  ii. Skin.

    1. Preterm infants redder in color because of less subcutaneous fat.

    2. Acrocyanosis is harmless cyanosis of the hands and feet.

    3. Harlequin color change is a benign condition in which half of the body is red and the other half is pale.

    4. Jaundice is noted in almost 50% of term newborns by third or fourth day of life.

      (a) Abnormal if noted on first day of life.

    5. Lanugo hair is soft, fine, immature hair on the scalp, brow, and face of preterm infants.

(a) Replaced by vellus hair in term infants.

6. Vernix caseosa is a soft, white, creamy covering on the skin of the preterm infant that disappears by term.

7. Congenital skin conditions.

(a) Port wine stain: flat, pink to purple macular lesions caused by dilated capillaries. Vary in size and can cover any part of the body.

(i) If eye is involved, should rule out glaucoma.

(b) Dermal melanocytosis (Mongolian spots): large, slate blue, well-demarcated areas of pigmentation near the buttocks.

(i) Will fade and disappear over time.

(ii) Often mistaken for abuse.

(c) Capillary hemangioma: bright red, protuberant lesion seen on the face, scalp, back, or anogenital area.

(i) Typically develops within first 2 months of life.

(ii) 95% will disappear by 9 years of age.

iii. Head, eyes, ears, nose, and throat.

1. Head.

(a) Shape of head and molding will resolve 2 to 3 days after vaginal delivery.

(b) Fontanels.

| Vaccine | Minimum Age for Dose 1 | Minimum Interval Between Doses | | | | |
|---|---|---|---|---|---|---|
| **Children age 4 months through 6 years** | | | | | | |
| | | Dose 1 to Dose 2 | Dose 2 to Dose 3 | | Dose 3 to Dose 4 | Dose 4 to Dose 5 |
| Hepatitis B | Birth | 4 weeks | **8 weeks and at least 16 weeks after first dose** minimum age for the final dose is 24 weeks | | | |
| Rotavirus | 6 weeks Maximum age for first dose is 14 weeks, 6 days. | 4 weeks | **4 weeks** maximum age for final dose is 8 months, 0 days | | | |
| Diphtheria, tetanus, and acellular pertussis | 6 weeks | 4 weeks | 4 weeks | | 6 months | 6 months |
| Haemophilus influenzae type b | 6 weeks | **No further doses needed** if first dose was administered at age 15 months or older. **4 weeks** if first dose was administered before the 1st birthday. **8 weeks (as final dose)** if first dose was administered at age 12 through 14 months. | **No further doses needed** if previous dose was administered at age 15 months or older **4 weeks** if current age is younger than 12 months and first dose was administered at younger than age 7 months and at least 1 previous dose was PRP-T (ActHib®, Pentacel®, Hiberix®), Vaxelis® or unknown **8 weeks and age 12 through 59 months (as final dose)** if current age is younger than 12 months and first dose was administered at age 7 through 11 months; OR if current age is 12 through 59 months and first dose was administered before the 1st birthday and second dose was administered at younger than age 15 months; OR If both doses were PedvaxHIB® and were administered before the 1st birthday | | **8 weeks (as final dose)** This dose only necessary for children age 12 through 59 months who received 3 doses before the 1st birthday. | |
| Pneumococcal conjugate | 6 weeks | **No further doses needed** for healthy children if first dose was administered at age 24 months or older. **4 weeks** if first dose was administered before the 1st birthday **8 weeks (as final dose for healthy children)** if first dose was administered at the 1st birthday or after | **No further doses needed** for healthy children if previous dose was administered at age 24 months or older **4 weeks** if current age is younger than 12 months and previous dose was administered at <7 months old **8 weeks (as final dose for healthy children)** if previous dose was administered between 7–11 months (wait until at least 12 months old); OR if current age is 12 months or older and at least 1 dose was administered before age 12 months | | **8 weeks (as final dose)** This dose only necessary for children age 12 through 59 months who received 3 doses before age 12 months or for children at high risk who received 3 doses at any age. | |
| Inactivated poliovirus | 6 weeks | **4 weeks** | **4 weeks** if current age is <4 years **6 months (as final dose)** if current age is 4 years or older | | **6 months (minimum age 4 years for final dose)** | |
| Measles, mumps, rubella | 12 months | 4 weeks | | | | |
| Varicella | 12 months | 3 months | | | | |
| Hepatitis A | 12 months | 6 months | | | | |
| Meningococcal ACWY | 2 months MenACWY-CRM 9 months MenACWY-D 2 years MenACWY-TT | 8 weeks | See Notes | | See Notes | |
| **Children and adolescents age 7 through 18 years** | | | | | | |
| Meningococcal ACWY | Not applicable (N/A) | 8 weeks | | | | |
| Tetanus, diphtheria; tetanus, diphtheria, and acellular pertussis | 7 years | 4 weeks | **4 weeks** if first dose of DTaP/DT was administered before the 1st birthday **6 months (as final dose)** if first dose of DTaP/DT or Tdap/Td was administered at or after the 1st birthday | | **6 months** if first dose of DTaP/DT was administered before the 1st birthday | |
| Human papillomavirus | 9 years | **Routine dosing intervals are recommended.** | | | | |
| Hepatitis A | N/A | 6 months | | | | |
| Hepatitis B | N/A | 4 weeks | **8 weeks and at least 16 weeks after first dose** | | | |
| Inactivated poliovirus | N/A | 4 weeks | **6 months** A fourth dose is not necessary if the third dose was administered at age 4 years or older and at least 6 months after the previous dose. | | A fourth dose of IPV is indicated if all previous doses were administered at <4 years or if the third dose was administered <6 months after the second dose. | |
| Measles, mumps, rubella | N/A | 4 weeks | | | | |
| Varicella | N/A | **3 months** if younger than age 13 years. **4 weeks** if age 13 years or older | | | | |
| Dengue | 9 years | 6 months | 6 months | | | |

**Fig. 14.2** Catch-up immunization schedule for ages 4 months through 18 years—United States, 2022. For the footnotes found in the figure, please go to the following website: https://www.cdc.gov/vaccines/schedules/downloads/child/0-18yrs-child-combined-schedule.pdf

**TABLE 14.1**

| Tanner Stages | | |
|---|---|---|

| *Breast Development* | | |
|---|---|---|
| **Stage** | **Average Age (Years)** | **Description** |
| Stage 1 | | Preadolescent; elevation of papilla only |
| Stage 2 | 9–13.4 | Breast bud stage; elevation of breast and papilla; areolar enlargement |
| Stage 3 | 10–14.3 | Further enlargement of breast and areola without separation of contour |
| Stage 4 | 10.8–15.4 | Projection of areola and papilla to form the secondary mound |
| Stage 5 | 11.9–18.8 | Mature stage; projection of papilla only as areola recesses to breast contour |

| *Pubic Hair (Male and Female)* | | |
|---|---|---|
| **Stage** | **Average Age (Years)** | **Description** |
| Stage 1 | Preadolescent | No pubic hair |
| Stage 2 | M 11.3–15.1<br>F 9.3–14.1 | Sparse growth of long, slightly pigmented downy hair, mainly at base of penis or along labia |
| Stage 3 | M 11.8–16<br>F 10.2–14.6 | Darker, coarser, curled hair spread sparsely over junction of pubes |
| Stage 4 | M 12.2–16.5<br>F 10.8–15.1 | Hair resembles adult in type; distribution smaller than in adult; no spread to medial surface of thighs |
| Stage 5 | M 12.2–17.3<br>F 12.2–16.7 | Adult in quantity and type of distribution of the horizontal pattern |

| *Genital Development (Male)* | | |
|---|---|---|
| **Stage** | **Average Age (Years)** | **Description** |
| Stage 1 | Preadolescent | Testes, scrotum, and penis same size and proportion as early childhood |
| Stage 2 | 10.6–12.7 | Enlargement of scrotum and testes; skin of scrotum darkens and changes texture; penis has little or no change |
| Stage 3 | 11.8–13.9 | Enlargement of penis, first in length; testes and scrotum grow further |
| Stage 4 | 12.8–14.8 | Increased size of penis; growth in breadth and development of glans; darkening of scrotal skin; and enlargement of testes and scrotum |
| Stage 5 | 13.8–16.0 | Adult size and shape |

(i) Anterior: diamond shaped and located midline at the junction of the coronal and sagittal sutures.
   (1) Anterior fontanel is typically 10–30 mm in size. Anterior fontanel is larger than the posterior fontanel.
   (2) Increased diameter in the following:
      [a] Achondroplasia.
      [b] Hydrocephaly.
      [c] Apert syndrome.
      [d] Osteogenesis imperfecta.
      [e] Prematurity.
      [f] Vitamin D deficiency.
      [g] Intrauterine growth restriction.
   (3) Typically closes by 18 months of age.

(ii) Posterior: located at the intersection of the occipital and parietal bones.
   (1) May be closed at birth but, if open, should close by 2 months of age.
(iii) If fontanels are bulging, may indicate increased intracranial pressure.
(iv) The presence of a third fontanel suggests trisomy 21 but may be seen in preterm infants.

2. Eyes.
   (a) Epicanthal fold: if flat, may be a sign of Down syndrome.
   (b) Pupillary reflexes: present after 28 to 30 weeks of gestation.
      (i) Cornea larger than 1 cm in diameter in a term infant suggests congenital glaucoma.

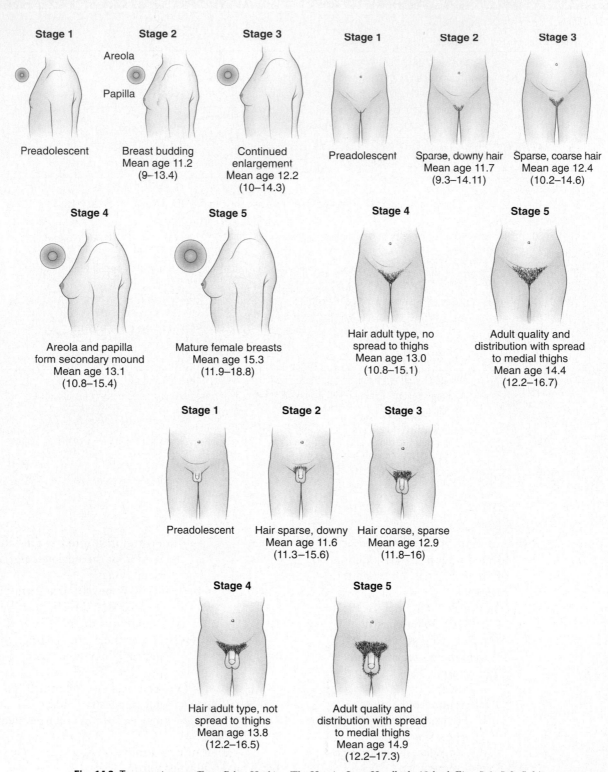

**Stage 1**

Preadolescent

**Stage 2**

Areola

Papilla

Breast budding
Mean age 11.2
(9–13.4)

**Stage 3**

Continued
enlargement
Mean age 12.2
(10–14.3)

**Stage 1**

Preadolescent

**Stage 2**

Sparse, downy hair
Mean age 11.7
(9.3–14.11)

**Stage 3**

Sparse, coarse hair
Mean age 12.4
(10.2–14.6)

**Stage 4**

Areola and papilla
form secondary mound
Mean age 13.1
(10.8–15.4)

**Stage 5**

Mature female breasts
Mean age 15.3
(11.9–18.8)

**Stage 4**

Hair adult type, no
spread to thighs
Mean age 13.0
(10.8–15.1)

**Stage 5**

Adult quality and
distribution with spread
to medial thighs
Mean age 14.4
(12.2–16.7)

**Stage 1**

Preadolescent

**Stage 2**

Hair sparse, downy
Mean age 11.6
(11.3–15.6)

**Stage 3**

Hair coarse, sparse
Mean age 12.9
(11.8–16)

**Stage 4**

Hair adult type, not
spread to thighs
Mean age 13.8
(12.2–16.5)

**Stage 5**

Adult quality and
distribution with spread
to medial thighs
Mean age 14.9
(12.2–17.3)

**Fig. 14.3** Tanner stages. *(From Johns Hopkins: The Harriet Lane Handbook, 18th ed. Figs. 5-1, 5-2, 5-3.)*

**TABLE 14.2**

| Developmental Milestones | | |
|---|---|---|
| **Age** | **Gross Motor** | **Visual Motor** |
| 1 month | Raises head slightly from prone<br>Lifts chin up | Tight grasp<br>Follows to midline |
| 2 months | Lifts chest off table | Follows objects past midline |
| 3 months | Supports self on forearms in prone<br>Holds head up steadily | Follows in a circular pattern |
| 6 months | Sits well unsupported | Reaches with either hand<br>Grasps |
| 9 months | Creeps and crawls<br>Pulls to stand | Uses pincer grasp<br>Holds bottle<br>Finger feeds |
| 12 months | Walks alone | Throws objects<br>Lets go of objects |
| 18 months | Runs<br>Throws toy without falling | Turns 2–3 pages<br>Fills spoon<br>Feeds self |
| 24 months | Walks up and down stairs without assistance | Turns page one at a time<br>Removes clothes |
| 36 months | Pedals tricycle<br>Alternates feet when going up stairs | Partially dresses and undresses<br>Draws a circle |
| 4 years | Hops and skips<br>Alternates feet when going down stairs | Buttons clothes<br>Catches ball |
| 5 years | Skips<br>Jumps over low objects | Ties shoes<br>Spreads with knife |

(ii) Presence of a red reflex suggests the absence of cataracts.

(iii) Leukokoria: white pupillary reflex and suggests cataracts, tumor, chorioretinitis, or retinopathy.

3. Ears.

(a) Low-set ears suggest Down syndrome.

4. Throat/Mouth.

(a) Check for cleft lip and palate.

(b) Natal teeth may be present in the lower incisor position. They are shed before the deciduous teeth erupt.

(c) White material on the throat or tongue may indicate thrush.

iv. Neck.

1. Clavicle fracture may be noted due to birth trauma.

2. Webbing of the neck may indicate Turner's syndrome.

v. Chest/Lungs.

1. Watch for periods of apnea and periodic breathing.

2. Breast hypertrophy may be noted.

(a) Milk should not be expressed.

3. Grunting during expiration may indicate serious cardiopulmonary disease or sepsis.

vi. Heart.

1. Heart rate may vary with crying and sleep, but a heart rate below 90 is of concern.

2. Transient murmurs are common and benign.

3. Point of maximal impulse may be over the xiphoid process for the first 48 hours.

vii. Abdomen.

1. Diastasis recti is incomplete closure of the rectus muscles.

2. Umbilical cord.

(a) Consists of two ventrally placed arteries and one dorsally placed vein.

(b) If oozing blood, consider a bleeding disorder.

(c) Umbilical hernia is common in Black infants.

(i) May regress spontaneously by 5 years of age.

viii. Genitalia.

1. Males.

(a) Testis should be descended at birth.

(i) In most cases, the testes descend by the third month.

**TABLE 14.3**

| Screening for Developmental Delays (Upper Range of Development) | | | | |
|---|---|---|---|---|
| **Age (Months)** | **Gross Motor** | **Fine Motor** | **Social Skills** | **Language** |
| 3 | Supports weight on forearms | Opens hands spontaneously | Smiles appropriately | Coos, laughs |
| 6 | Sits momentarily | Transfers objects | Shows likes and dislikes | Babbles |
| 9 | Pulls to stand | Pincer grasp | Plays pat-a-cake, peek-a-boo | Imitates sounds |
| 12 | Walks with one hand held | Releases an object on command | Comes when called | 1–2 meaningful words |
| 18 | Walks up stairs with assistance | Feeds with a spoon | Mimics actions of others | At least 6 words |
| 24 | Runs | Builds a tower of 6 blocks | Plays with others | 2–3 word sentences |

From Kliegman R: Nelson Textbook of Pediatrics, 2007:2434, Table 591-1.

**TABLE 14.4**

| Apgar Scoring System | | | | |
| --- | --- | --- | --- | --- |
| | Sign | 0 | 1 | 2 |
| A | Activity (muscle tone) | Absent | Arms/legs flexed | Active movement |
| P | Pulse (BPM) | Absent | <100 | >100 |
| G | Grimace (irritability) | No response | Grimace | Coughs, pulls away |
| A | Appearance (skin color) | Pale all over | Pink, except extremities | Pink all over |
| R | Respirations | Absent | Slow | Good, crying |

*BPM,* Beats per minute.

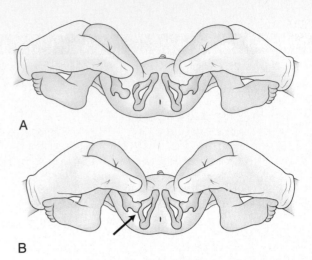

**Fig. 14.4 (A)** and **(B)** Ortolani's maneuver.

    (ii) Cryptorchidism is more common in preterm infants.

  (b) Check for hypospadias—meatus located in abnormal ventral position.

    (i) Is a contraindication to circumcision.

  (c) Congenital phimosis is common. Foreskin should not be forcefully retracted.

  2. Females.

    (a) A white serosanguineous vaginal discharge may be noted during the first few days of life due to estrogen effect.

ix. Extremities.

  1. Single transverse palmar crease is a single palmar crease that is present in some normal infants or common in Down syndrome.

  2. Hip examination.

    (a) Ortolani's test: presence of an audible click with abduction of the hips to almost 90 degrees is a positive Ortolani's sign.

      (i) Indicates dysplasia or a dislocated hip.

      (ii) See Fig. 14.4.

x. Neurologic.

  1. Brachial plexus injury may cause paralysis of upper arm.

    (a) May result from traction on the head and neck during delivery.

  2. Erb's palsy: inability to abduct the arm at the shoulder, to rotate the arm externally, and to supinate the forearm due to injury to the fifth and sixth cervical nerves.

  3. Reflexes.

    (a) Rooting response.

      (i) Method: on touching a corner of the mouth or cheek, the head turns to the same side and the mouth opens.

      (ii) Indicates: a primitive response to ensure nursing.

        (1) Absent in severe central nervous system (CNS) disease.

      (iii) Timing: presents at 32 weeks of gestation and disappears after 3 to 4 months.

    (b) Parachute reaction.

      (i) Method: suspend the child by the trunk and then forward flex as if to fall. Normal response is extension of all extremities.

      (ii) Indicates: important in facial protection when falling.

      (iii) Timing: appears at 5 to 8 months.

    (c) Palmar grasp.

      (i) Method: stimulate the palm by placing index finger in palm. The normal response is to grasp the finger.

      (ii) Indicates: absence of this response in the newborn or persistence after 5 months suggests cerebral disease.

      (iii) Timing: appears at 32 weeks' gestation and disappears after 3 to 5 months.

    (d) Moro's (startle) reflex.

      (i) Method: support infant's body and then allow head to drop a few centimeters. Response is symmetrical abduction of the upper extremities at the shoulders and extension of the fingers.

      (ii) Indicates: normal response indicates an intact CNS.

      (iii) Timing: present at 28 weeks' gestation and disappears at 4 to 6 months of age.

(e) Galant's reflex.
  (i) Method: elicited by stroking one side of the back along a paravertebral line 2–3 cm from the midline from the shoulder to the buttocks. Normal response is lateral curvature of the trunk toward the stimulated side with shoulder and hip moving toward the side stroked.
  (ii) Indicates: absent in infants with transverse spinal cord lesions.
  (iii) Timing: normally disappears at 2 to 3 months.
(f) Placing (stepping) response.
  (i) Method: allow the dorsum of the infant's feet to lightly touch the surface of a table. Normal response is to flex the knee and hip and to place the stimulated foot on top of the table.
  (ii) Indicates: absence indicates paresis of the lower extremities.
  (iii) Timing: normally noted after 4 to 5 days of life and disappears after 4 to 6 months.

## II. NUTRITION
a. **General**
  i. Normal full-term infant passes meconium in the first 24 hours and voids within the first 12 hours.
  ii. It is normal to lose 5% to 10% of weight over the first 5 days.
  iii. Feedings.
    1. Breast-fed infants typically feed 10 to 15 minutes on each side every 2 to 3 hours.
    2. Bottle-fed infants eat ½ to 1 oz every 2 to 4 hours.
  iv. Weight–gestational age relationship.
    1. Appropriate for gestational age (AGA): 2500–4000 g.
    2. Small for gestational age (SGA).
      (a) Moderately low birth weight (MLBW): 1501–2500 g.
      (b) Very low birth weight (VLBW): 1001–1500 g.
      (c) Extremely low birth weight (ELBW): <1000 g.
    3. Large for gestational age (LGA): >4000 g.
  v. Growth rates.
    1. Age 0 to 2 months: 30 g (1 oz)/day.
    2. Age 2 to 6 months: 20 g/day.
      (a) Weight should double by 4–6 months.
    3. Age 12 months: by 1 year, the birth weight should have tripled.

4. Age 30 months: child should weigh 30 pounds.
5. Age 4 years: child should weigh 40 pounds.

# GENETIC DISORDERS

## I. GENERAL
a. **Table 14.5 summarizes inheritance patterns**

## II. CONGENITAL HYPOTHYROIDISM (CRETINISM)
a. **General**
  i. Incidence is 1 in 2000–3000 live births.
    1. Rate lower in Black and higher in Hispanic and Asian infants.
  ii. All states require screening for hypothyroidism.
  iii. Etiologies.
    1. Due to hypoplasia or aplasia of the thyroid gland.
    2. Failure to secrete hormone secondary to enzyme deficiency.
b. **Clinical Manifestations**
  i. Note typical signs and symptoms of hypothyroidism including bradycardia; dry, coarse hair; poor muscle tone; constipation; pale, cool skin; and intellectual disability.
c. **Diagnosis**
  i. Screening test will reveal an elevated thyroid stimulating hormone (TSH).
    1. Serum testing reveals a low free thyroxine (Free $T_4$) and elevated TSH.
d. **Treatment**
  i. The sooner treatment is started, the better the prognosis.
  ii. Treatment consists of levothyroxine at 10 µg/kg/day.
    1. Monitor therapy with $T_4$ or free thyroxine ($FT_4$) and TSH.
      (a) Check every 1–2 months for the first 6 months, then every 3 to 4 months until age 3.
      (b) Then check every 6 to 12 months until growth is complete.

## III. CYSTIC FIBROSIS
a. **General**
  i. Autosomal recessive disease and most common lethal inherited disease in White American population.
    1. Incidence is 1 in 2000–3000 live births.
    2. 10% of patients diagnosed in the preteen years.
    3. Due to defect in cystic fibrosis transmembrane conductance regulator (CFTR) on chromosome 7.

**TABLE 14.5**

## Summary of Inheritance Patterns

| | Autosomal Dominant | Autosomal Recessive | X-Linked Recessive | Mitochondrial |
|---|---|---|---|---|
| Definition | Heterozygosity for mutation of a single gene is sufficient to cause the condition. | Homozygosity for mutation of a single gene is necessary to cause the condition. Carriers usually have no clinical manifestations. | Mutation of a single gene on the X chromosome (also called sex-linked) | Mutation of a gene on the mitochondrial chromosome, following autosomal or X-linked patterns |
| Family distribution | Multiple generations affected | Only one generation | Multiple generations affected | Multiple generations affected |
| Parents of affected | Typically one or the other affected | Both carriers, neither affected | Mother often carrier, fathers of affected sons are never affected | Mothers almost always affected<br>Father never affected |
| Siblings of affected | 50% chance of being affected | 25% chance of being affected<br>50% chance of being a carrier | Brothers have 50% chance of being affected<br>Sisters have 50% chance of being a carrier | All are affected |
| Children of affected | 50% chance of being affected | All are carriers | Sons of affected fathers are never affected<br>Daughters of affected fathers are always carriers.<br>Sons of carrier mothers have 50% chance of being affected<br>Daughters of carrier mothers have 50% chance of being a carrier | All children of affected mothers are affected<br>No children of affected fathers are affected |
| Sex ratio | Males and females equally likely to be affected | Males and females equally likely to be affected | All affected patients are male | Males and females equally likely to be affected |

ii. Symptoms are due to development of thick secretions that block the airways and ductal system in other organs.
   1. Other organ systems involved include pancreatic and hepatic.
      (a) Can lead to malabsorption of fats, fat-soluble vitamins, and protein
   2. Many males with cystic fibrosis are infertile due to obstructive azoospermia.
iii. Airways are commonly infected with *Staphylococcus aureus* and *Haemophilus influenzae* as a child and *Pseudomonas aeruginosa* as adults.

**b. Clinical Manifestations**
   i. Common symptoms include chronic cough with sputum production and dyspnea.
      1. Newborns with cystic fibrosis present with intestinal obstruction and meconium ileus.
   ii. Physical examination reveals weight loss, wheezing, and a salty taste on the skin.
   iii. Patients typically have a history of recurrent pneumonia, sinusitis, or asthma.

**c. Diagnosis**
   i. Most specific test result for cystic fibrosis is elevated sweat chloride.
      1. Values greater than 60 mEq/L in children are abnormal.

ii. Pancreatic insufficiency is diagnosed by demonstrating fat malabsorption with a qualitative or quantitative fecal fat test.
iii. Diagnostic criteria.
   1. Clinical symptoms consistent with cystic fibrosis in at least one organ system or positive newborn screen or a sibling with cystic fibrosis AND
   2. Evidence of cystic fibrosis transmembrane conductance regulator via:
      (a) Elevated sweat chloride.
      (b) Presence of two disease-causing mutations in CFTR gene from each patient allele.
      (c) Abnormal nasal potential difference.

**d. Treatment**
   i. Maintenance therapy goal is to slow the progression of lung damage by improving mucus clearance, controlling infection, and controlling inflammation.
      1. Mucus clearance is improved with percussion and postural drainage.
   ii. Bronchodilators, corticosteroids, and NSAIDS reduce inflammation.
   ii. Pancreatic insufficiency is treated with pancreatic enzyme supplements.

iii. Antibiotic selection should include coverage for *Pseudomonas* with antipseudomonal beta-lactam agents and an aminoglycoside or ciprofloxacin.

iv. FTR corrector and potentiator drugs are indicated for about 90% of the variants carried by CF patients.

## IV. DOWN SYNDROME (TRISOMY 21)
### a. General
i. Most common autosomal chromosomal abnormality in humans with an incidence of 1 in 700 live births.

ii. Increased risk with advancing maternal age (>35 years of age).

### b. Clinical Manifestations
i. Common dysmorphic facial features include flat facial profile, upslanted palpebral fissures, flat nasal bridge with epicanthal folds, small mouth with protruding tongue, micrognathia, and short ears.

ii. Functional and structural abnormalities include sleep apnea, cardiac defects (septal), gastrointestinal (GI) anomalies (duodenal atresia and Hirschsprung's disease), developmental delay, and moderate intellectual disability.

iii. At increased risk for the development of leukemia, early onset of Alzheimer-like dementia, and hypothyroidism.

### c. Diagnosis
i. Chromosomal abnormalities are pathognomonic.
1. 95% of patients have 47 chromosomes with 3 number 21 chromosomes.
2. 4% have 46 chromosomes with translocation of chromosome 21 to another chromosome.
3. 1% have a chromosome mosaicism, with cells having a varying number of chromosomes.

### d. Treatment
i. Treatment focused on specific complications.

ii. Prenatal diagnosis with amniocentesis or chorionic villus sampling.

iii. Family genetic counseling is indicated.

## V. KLINEFELTER'S SYNDROME
### a. General
i. Autosomal recessive and due to an extra X chromosome.

ii. Affects 1 in 1000 newborn males.
1. 80% have 47, XXY karyotype; 20% are mosaic with one 46, XY and one 47, XXY cell line.

### b. Clinical Manifestations
i. Clinical manifestations typically appear at puberty.

ii. At puberty, patients present with incomplete masculinization, female body habitus, decreased body hair, gynecomastia, small phallus, and small soft testes.

iii. Infertility is common secondary to hypospermia or aspermia.

iv. Patients are typically taller than relatives, have wide arm span, and have mild intellectual disability.

### c. Diagnosis
i. Based on chromosomal analysis.

### d. Treatment
i. Testosterone may be helpful to improve secondary sexual characteristics.

## VI. TRISOMY 13 (PATAU SYNDROME)
### a. General
i. Autosomal chromosome disorder.
1. 75% have 47 chromosomes with three number 13 chromosomes.

ii. Increased risk with advancing maternal age.

iii. Occurs in 1 in 10,000 live births.

### b. Clinical Manifestations
i. Present with cleft lip and palate (60% to 80%), congenital heart disease (80%), microcephaly, sloping forehead, polydactyly, and overlapping fingers and toes.

ii. Will have developmental delays, as well as prenatal and postnatal growth restriction.

### c. Diagnosis
i. Based on clinical findings and chromosome analysis.

### d. Treatment
i. Treat clinical manifestations.

ii. Prognosis is poor: 50% die before reaching 1 month of age, and 90% die by 1 year of age.

## VII. TRISOMY 18 (EDWARDS SYNDROME)
### a. General
i. Autosomal chromosome disorder.
1. 80% of cases are a result of meiotic nondisjunction.
2. Meiotic nondisjunction is the failure of two members of a chromosome to separate during meiosis, both going to one daughter cell.

ii. Increased risk with advancing maternal age.

iii. Occurs in 1 in 8000 live births.

### b. Clinical Manifestations
i. Presents with cleft lip and palate, congenital heart disease, narrow nose and hypoplastic nasal alae, small and premature appearance, limited hip abduction, and overlapping fingers.

ii. Will have developmental delays and prenatal and postnatal growth restriction.

c. **Diagnosis**
    i. Based on clinical findings and chromosome analysis.
d. **Treatment**
    i. Treat clinical manifestations.
    ii. Prognosis is poor: 30% die before reaching 1 month of age, and 90% die by 1 year of age.

## VIII. TURNER'S SYNDROME

a. **General**
    i. Female sex chromosome abnormality with only one X chromosome.
        1. Mosaic chromosomal abnormality.
        2. 60% of cases have 45, XO phenotype; and 25% have 46, XX with deletion of the short arm of one of the X chromosomes.
    ii. Results from defective embryonic cell division after fertilization.
b. **Clinical Manifestations**
    i. Clinical manifestations include short stature, webbed neck, low hairline, lymphedema of hands and feet at birth, shield-shaped chest, and multiple pigmented nevi.
    ii. Renal anomalies, congenital heart disease, and learning disabilities are common.
    iii. Gonadal dysgenesis is present in all patients.
        1. Will have primary amenorrhea and lack of pubertal development.
        2. With rare exception, patients cannot become pregnant.
c. **Diagnosis**
    i. Based on clinical findings and chromosome analysis.
d. **Treatment**
    i. 98% die in utero.
    ii. Correct any anomalies.
    iii. Short stature can be treated with growth hormone and anabolic steroids.
    iv. Estrogen and progesterone used to develop secondary sexual characteristics.

# CARDIAC DISEASES

## I. GENERAL

a. **Fetal Circulation**
    i. Fig. 14.5 shows fetal circulation.
    ii. In fetal circulation, the right and left ventricles are in a parallel circuit, as opposed to the series circuit of the newborn or adult.
    iii. Three structures maintain this parallel circuit.
        1. Ductus venosus.
          (a) Connects the umbilical venous blood with the inferior vena cava, bypassing the liver.

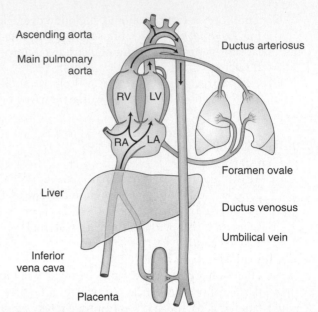

**Fig. 14.5** Fetal circulation. *LA*, Left atrium; *LV*, left ventricle; *RA*, right atrium; *RV*, right ventricle. *(From McCance KL: Pathophysiology: The Biologic Basis for Disease in Adults and Children, 5th ed. St. Louis: Elsevier Mosby, 2006:1150, Fig. 31.4.)*

          (b) Once the umbilical cord is tied, the ductus venosus evolves into the ligamentum venosum.
        2. Foramen ovale.
          (a) Allows passage of blood from the right atrium to the left atrium.
          (b) Increased pulmonary venous return and decreased inferior vena cava return cause functional closure of the foramen ovale.
          (c) Typically closes within the first year of life.
        3. Ductus arteriosus.
          (a) Allows passage of blood from the right ventricle to the descending aorta, bypassing the lungs.
          (b) An increase in oxygen saturation and a decrease in the amount of endogenous prostaglandins cause closure of the ductus arteriosus.
          (c) Closure occurs within 10 to 21 days after birth.
b. **Table 14.6 summarizes common congenital heart defects**
c. **Table 14.7 distinguishes between cardiac and pulmonary causes of cyanosis**

## II. CONGENITAL HEART DISEASE

a. **Atrial Septal Defect**
    i. General

**TABLE 14.6**

| Summary of Common Congenital Heart Defects | | |
| --- | --- | --- |
| **Defect** | **Cyanosis** | **Cardiovascular Findings** |
| Ventricular septal defect | No | Pansystolic murmur |
| Tetralogy of Fallot | Yes | Rough, systolic ejection murmur |
| Aortic stenosis | No | Systolic ejection murmur at right upper sternal border and systolic click at the apex |
| Atrial septal defect | No | Fixed split $S_2$ systolic ejection murmur at left sternal border
Mid-diastolic murmur at left sternal border, 4th intercostal space |
| Patent ductus arteriosus | No | Continuous machinelike murmur |
| Coarctation of aorta | No | Decreased femoral pulses |
| Transposition of great vessels | Yes | Vary depending on presence of ventricular septal defect |

**TABLE 14.7**

| Cardiac and Pulmonary Causes of Cyanosis | | |
| --- | --- | --- |
| | **Cardiac Cause** | **Pulmonary Cause** |
| Respiratory status | May be comfortably blue | Respiratory distress |
| Response to crying | Worsening cyanosis | Improved cyanosis |
| Response to oxygen | Minimal to no improvement | Improvement of cyanosis |

1. Defect in the atrial septum allowing shunting of blood between the atria.
2. Most common type is the ostium secundum defect noted in the midportion of the atrial septum.

ii. Clinical manifestations
1. Not typically associated with symptoms.
   (a) May have a history of slow weight gain and recurrent lower respiratory tract infections.
   (b) Large defects present with congestive heart failure and failure to thrive.
2. On physical examination, there is a right ventricular heave, wide and constantly split $S_2$, and a systolic ejection murmur in the pulmonic area and a mid-diastolic rumble in the lower right sternal border.
   (a) Murmurs and rumble are due to increased blood flow across the pulmonic and tricuspid valves.

3. Chest x-ray film reveals cardiomegaly and increased pulmonary vascularity.
4. Electrocardiogram (EKG) reveals right ventricular hypertrophy and right ventricular conduction delay.

iii. Diagnosis
1. Echocardiogram reveals an enlarged right ventricle and flow across the defect.

iv. Treatment
1. Spontaneous closure is likely to occur in most cases in the first year of life.
2. If symptomatic, the defect should be closed as soon as possible.
3. If asymptomatic, most patients undergo closure between ages 2 and 4 years.

b. **Coarctation of Aorta**
   i. General
   1. Male-to-female ratio is 2:1.
      (a) When occurs in a female, must consider presence of Turner's syndrome.
   2. Obstruction is in the descending aorta, at the insertion site of the ductus arteriosus.
   ii. Clinical manifestations
   1. Patients may present with or without cardiovascular symptoms.
      (a) Congestive heart failure may develop.
   2. On physical examination, note weak or absent femoral pulses and delayed femoral pulse when compared with upper extremities.
   3. Upper extremity hypertension.
   4. A systolic ejection murmur may be heard at the apex.
   5. Chest x-ray reveals an enlarged aortic knob.
      (a) Notching of the posterior one third of ribs 3 to 8 may be noted.
   6. EKG shows right ventricular hypertrophy (RVH) in the neonate and left ventricular hypertrophy (LVH) in older children.
   iii. Diagnosis
   1. Based on echocardiogram findings of the coarctation.
      (a) If the ductus arteriosus is still patent, the coarctation may not be seen.
   iv. Treatment
   1. Signs of heart failure must be treated aggressively.
   2. Prostaglandin $E_1$ can be used to dilate the patent ductus arteriosus (PDA).
   3. Repair via balloon angioplasty or surgical anastomosis.

c. **Patent Ductus Arteriosus**
   i. General
   1. Higher incidence in premature neonates (weighing <1500 g) with a female-to-male ratio of 2:1.

2. Increased incidence in children whose mothers contracted rubella in the first trimester.
3. Function of the ductus arteriosus is to connect the aorta and the left pulmonary artery.
   (a) If pulmonary resistance is above systemic resistance, a right-to-left shunt develops.
   (b) Typically closes spontaneously by 4 days of age.

ii. Clinical manifestations
1. Symptoms vary with degree of shunting.
   (a) Small defect causes no symptoms.
   (b) Patients with large defect may present with signs of congestive heart failure, slow growth, and recurrent lower respiratory tract infections.
      (i) Symptoms include shortness of breath, dyspnea on exertion, and cyanosis.
2. Physical examination in the patient with a large shunt reveals bounding pulses and a machinelike murmur.
   (a) Murmur starts after $S_1$, peaks at $S_2$, and softens during diastole.
   (b) Wide pulse pressure noted.
3. Chest x-ray film.
   (a) In a small PDA, x-ray is normal.
   (b) In a large PDA, cardiomegaly, left atrial and ventricular enlargement, and increased pulmonary congestion are noted.
4. EKG.
   (a) Normal EKG in patients with a small PDA.
   (b) Left or biventricular hypertrophy may be noted with a large PDA.

iii. Diagnosis
1. Echocardiogram confirms presence of PDA.

iv. Treatment
1. Indomethacin is often effective in closing PDA.
   (a) Works by decreasing prostaglandin $E_1$ levels.
2. Surgical ligation may be needed.

**d. Tetralogy of Fallot**
i. General
1. A cause of cyanotic congenital heart disease.
   (a) May be acyanotic at birth.
2. Cyanosis is due to right-to-left shunting and decreased pulmonary flow.
3. Are four defects.
   (a) Ventricular septal defect (VSD).

(b) Right ventricular outflow obstruction lesion.
(c) Right ventricular hypertrophy.
(d) Overriding large ascending aorta.
4. Other causes of cyanotic congenital heart disease.
   (a) Truncus arteriosus.
   (b) Transposition of the great vessels.
   (c) Tricuspid atresia.
   (d) Total anomalous pulmonary venous return.
   (e) Ebstein anomaly.

ii. Clinical manifestations
1. Degree of cyanosis is related to severity of right ventricular outflow obstruction.
2. Patients may assume a squatting position after exercise.
   (a) Squatting increases systemic vascular resistance and decreases right-to-left shunt.
3. Neonates present with cyanosis and agitation.
   (a) Episodes of cyanosis are called "tet spells."
      (i) May last minutes to hours.
4. On cardiac examination, a right ventricular heave is noted with a loud systolic ejection murmur at the upper left sternal border.
   (a) Clubbing of the fingers may be present in older children.
5. EKG reveals right ventricular enlargement and right axis deviation.
6. Chest x-ray film shows boot-shaped heart and decreased pulmonary vascularity.

iii. Diagnosis
1. Based on clinical findings and cardiac echocardiogram results.
   (a) Echocardiogram reveals thick right ventricular wall, overriding of the aorta, and a VSD.

iv. Treatment
1. Must decrease right-to-left shunting by increasing systemic vascular resistance and decreasing pulmonary vascular resistance.
   (a) Acute treatment options include vagal maneuvers, oxygen, vasoconstrictors, beta-blockers, morphine, and fluid administration.
   (b) Prostaglandin $E_1$ infusion to prevent ductal closure.
2. Surgical repair is performed during the first 4 to 12 months of life.

**e. Ventricular Septal Defect**
i. General
1. Most common congenital heart defect.
2. Has presence of a communication between the right and left ventricles.

3. Has increased pulmonary blood flow that may lead to pulmonary hypertension.
ii. Clinical manifestations
   1. Symptoms vary with size of defect and range from being asymptomatic to presenting signs of congestive heart failure.
      (a) Signs include tachypnea, tachycardia, poor weight gain, trouble feeding, and edema.
   2. Physical examination reveals a holosystolic murmur heard best at the middle to lower left sternal border.
      (a) The smaller the defect, the louder the murmur.
   3. Chest x-ray film may be normal in small defects and reveal cardiomegaly and increased pulmonary vascularity in large defects.
   4. EKG is normal in small defects and reveals left atrial, left ventricular, or biventricular hypertrophy.
iii. Diagnosis
   1. Echocardiogram confirms the presence of the defect.
iv. Treatment
   1. Most small VSDs close without intervention by age 10 years.
   2. Large VSDs will require surgical closure.

# EYES, EARS, NOSE, AND THROAT/PULMONARY

## I. ACUTE BRONCHIOLITIS
a. **General**
   i. Infection and inflammation of the smaller airways.
      1. Most common cause is respiratory syncytial virus (RSV).
         (a) May also be due to rhinovirus, parainfluenza, influenza, adenovirus, and *Mycoplasma*.
      2. Have accumulation of mucus and inflammatory cells in the small airways.
   ii. Typically presents between birth and 2 years of age.
   1. Peak incidence is at 6 months of age.
   iii. Increased risk with exposure to smoking and day-care attendance.
b. **Clinical Manifestations**
   i. Presents with diffuse wheezing, variable fever, cough, tachypnea, rhinorrhea, difficulty feeding, and cyanosis.
   ii. Physical examination reveals intercostal retractions, hyperinflation, crackles, nasal flaring, prolonged expiration, and wheezing.

c. **Diagnosis**
   i. Based on clinical findings and isolation of offending organism.
   ii. Chest x-ray film reveals hyperinflation and possible mild interstitial infiltrates.
   iii. Hypoxia is common.
d. **Treatment**
   i. Supportive care, IV hydration as needed, and oxygen as needed.
   ii. Bronchodilator can be used short-term in some patients.
   ii. Antiviral (ribavirin) is given by aerosolization for RSV in immunocompromised patients.
   iii. Some patients may develop wheezing later in life.
   iv. High-risk patients can be prophylactically treated with palivizumab on a monthly basis.
      1. Palivizumab is a monoclonal antibody and an RSV F-protein blocker.

## II. ACUTE EPIGLOTTITIS
a. **General**
   i. Rare condition; medical emergency secondary to possible airway obstruction.
      1. Inflammation of epiglottis and supraglottis.
   ii. Noted more frequently in adolescents and adults.
      1. Decreased frequency in children with development and use of the *H. influenzae* type B vaccine.
   iii. Etiologies include the following:
      1. *H. influenzae* type B (rare).
      2. *Streptococcus pneumoniae*.
      3. *S. aureus*.
      4. *Streptococcus pyogenes*.
      5. *H. influenzae*, non-typeable.
b. **Clinical Manifestations**
   i. On presentation, patient appears anxious and toxic.
   ii. Fever, muffled voice, and cyanosis may be noted.
   iii. Patients prefer the sitting position; children have the classic "sniffing" or "tripod" position.
      1. Sitting up with chin forward and neck slightly extended.
   iv. Late symptoms include stridor, drooling, and trouble handling secretions.
   v. Examination of the upper airway should be performed with caution.
      1. If patient is examined, the epiglottis is cherry red and swollen.
c. **Diagnosis**
   i. Based on clinical findings.
   ii. Lateral soft tissue neck x-ray film reveals an enlarged epiglottis and surrounding structures.

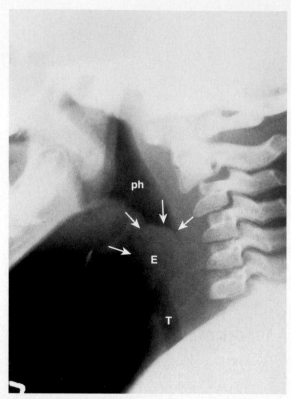

**Fig. 14.6** Acute epiglottitis. Lateral soft tissue x-ray of patient with epiglottitis. Note thumbprint sign *(arrows)*. *E*, Epiglottitis; *ph*, pharynx; *T*, trachea.

1. Thumbprint sign noted on lateral x-ray film (Fig. 14.6).
  iii. Blood cultures may be positive.
**d. Treatment**
  i. Airway management is key to treatment.
  ii. Humidified oxygen and intravenous (IV) fluids.
  iii. Antibiotic options include the following:
    1. Cefotaxime.
    2. Ceftriaxone.
    3. Ampicillin-sulbactam.
    4. Cefuroxime.
    5. Vancomycin added if concern about methicillin-resistant *S. aureus* (MRSA).

## III. CROUP (LARYNGOTRACHEITIS)
**a. General**
  i. Acute inflammatory disease of the larynx.
    1. Involves mainly the larynx and subglottic area.
  ii. Affects younger children (3 months to 3 years of age) in the fall and early winter.
  iii. Etiologies are typically viral and include the following:
    1. Parainfluenza types 1, 2, and 3.
    2. RSV.
    3. Adenovirus.
    4. Influenza.
**b. Clinical Manifestations**
  i. Prodrome of upper respiratory tract symptoms followed by a barking cough, inspiratory stridor, and hoarseness.
  ii. Fever is typically absent or low grade.
  iii. Rhinitis, pharyngitis, and wheezing may be noted.
**c. Diagnosis**
  i. Based on clinical findings.
  ii. Lateral neck x-ray film reveals narrowing of the subglottic area and normal epiglottis (steeple sign).
**d. Treatment**
  i. Supportive care, oral hydration, mist therapy, and minimal handling, for mild croup.
  ii. Patients with stridor are treated with active intervention.
    1. Oxygen.
    2. Nebulized epinephrine.
    3. Glucocorticoids.
  iii. Artificial airway may be needed in severe cases.

## IV. HYALINE MEMBRANE DISEASE (RESPIRATORY DISTRESS SYNDROME)
**a. General**
  i. Most common cause of respiratory failure in the first few days of life.
    1. A self-limiting disease.
  ii. Results from collapse of the alveoli and terminal bronchioles due to lack of adequate lung surfactant and immature state of alveolarization of the lung acini.
  iii. Can result in chronic lung disease that may persist for weeks to months.
  iv. Predisposing factors.
    1. Premature birth.
    2. Diabetic mother.
    3. Positive family history.
**b. Clinical Manifestations**
  i. Present with signs of increased inspiratory effort (accessory muscle use and chest wall retractions) and hypoxemia.
  ii. On physical examination, note tachypnea; grunting respirations; and diminished, harsh, tubular lung sounds.
**c. Diagnosis**
  i. Arterial blood gases reveal hypoxia that responds to oxygen.
  ii. Chest x-ray film reveals a diffuse reticulogranular pattern of uniform distribution (ground-glass appearance).
    1. Air bronchograms are noted.

iii. Lecithin–sphingomyelin ratio is used to predict risk for development of hyaline membrane disease.

**d. Treatment**

i. Adequate resuscitation and respiratory support (oxygen) should begin immediately with assisted ventilation or continuous positive end-expiratory pressure.

ii. Restrict fluids to avoid pulmonary edema.

iii. Surfactant replacement can be considered as prophylactic therapy or rescue therapy.

iv. 80% to 90% of patients survive, most with normal lungs, by 1 month of age.

v. Primary prevention consists of avoiding premature delivery and antenatal betamethasone.

   1. Complications include bronchopulmonary dysplasia.

## V. FOREIGN BODY ASPIRATION

**a. General**

i. Most cases of foreign body aspiration in children involve preschoolers.

ii. Most common location of obstruction is right main stem bronchus.

iii. About half of cases are caused by nuts or peanuts.

iv. Aspiration due to two factors.

   1. Children more likely to place things in their mouths.

   2. Lack of molar teeth development, making it impossible for small children to finely chew foods.

**b. Clinical Manifestations**

i. Most common symptom is cough.

ii. Acute aspiration presents with sudden onset of choking and coughing followed by wheezing, dyspnea, and stridor.

iii. Symptoms vary depending on where the aspirated material lodges.

   1. Table 14.8 lists common signs and symptoms.

**c. Diagnosis**

i. Sometimes delayed up to 1 month after aspiration.

ii. Diagnosis suggested based on history.

**TABLE 14.8**

| Most Common Signs and Symptoms of Foreign Body Obstruction | |
| --- | --- |
| **Bronchial** | **Laryngotracheal** |
| Cough | Cough |
| Decreased air entry | Cyanosis |
| Dyspnea | Dyspnea |
| Wheezing | Stridor |

iii. Chest x-ray film may reveal obstructive asymmetric hyperinflation.

**d. Treatment**

i. Varies with age of patient.

   1. Patients younger than 1 year of age are placed face down, and forceful back blows are given.

   2. Patients older than 1 year of age are treated with the Heimlich maneuver.

   3. Blind finger sweeps are to be avoided because the material could be pushed farther back.

ii. Bronchoscopy should be performed if material is beyond the oropharynx.

## VI. KAWASAKI'S DISEASE

**a. General**

i. A systemic vasculitis, mostly affecting medium-sized arteries, especially coronary arteries.

ii. Occurs most commonly in male infants and young children (most are younger than 5 years of age).

iii. Common cause of acquired heart disease and arthritis.

iv. Etiology unknown; possible infectious etiology.

**b. Clinical Manifestations**

i. Patient appears ill, with abdominal pain, carditis, and large joint pain.

ii. Diagnostic criteria.

   1. Acute onset fever (up to 105° F) for at least 5 days.

   2. Four of five of the following:

      (a) Bilateral nonexudative conjunctivitis.

      (b) Cervical lymphadenopathy.

      (c) Truncal polymorphous rash.

      (d) Oropharynx mucosal changes: bright red, swollen lips with fissures; strawberry tongue.

      (e) Peripheral extremity changes: edema, erythema, desquamation.

   3. Illness not explained by other disease process.

**c. Diagnosis**

i. Based on criteria noted in Clinical Manifestations.

ii. Present with elevated sedimentation rate, white blood cell (WBC) count, and C-reactive protein.

iii. Thrombocytosis is also noted.

iv. Presence of protein and WBCs in the urine.

**d. Treatment**

i. IV immunoglobulin reduces the initial inflammation and reduces incidence of complications.

ii. Low-dose aspirin to reduce inflammation.
   1. Corticosteroids are contraindicated, except in refractory disease.
iii. Complications include coronary vasculitis and aneurysm formation.
iv. Prognosis based on severity of complications.
   1. Fatal in less than 0.3% of cases.

## VII. MECONIUM ASPIRATION
### a. General
i. Caused by perinatal asphyxia of meconium-contaminated amniotic fluid.
   1. May lead to hypoxia and acidosis.
ii. Between 10% to 15% of newborns pass meconium, but only a small percent aspirate the meconium.
iii. Increased risk in postmature infants and neonates that suffer from intrauterine growth restriction.
### b. Clinical Manifestations
i. Patients present with signs of respiratory distress and aspiration pneumonitis.
   1. Hypoxia, tachypnea, and hypercapnia.
ii. Meconium present in trachea or amniotic fluid.
iii. Chest x-ray film reveals diffuse infiltrates with hyperinflation, increased anteroposterior (AP) diameter, and flattening of diaphragm.
   1. Pneumothorax may be present.
### c. Treatment
i. Most effective therapy is prevention.
ii. Suctioning of oropharynx.
iii. If respiratory distress, start oxygen and mechanical ventilation.
iv. Complications include persistent pulmonary hypertension of the newborn.

## VIII. ACUTE OTITIS MEDIA
### a. General
i. Due to inflammation that results in fluid collection in the middle ear.
ii. Risk factors include the following:
   1. Day-care attendance.
   2. Parental smoking.
   3. Drinking from a bottle while lying flat.
iii. Etiology.
   1. Most cases are viral (RSV, rhinovirus, influenza, and enterovirus).
   2. Bacterial causes include the following:
      (a) S. pneumoniae.
      (b) H. influenzae.
      (c) Moraxella catarrhalis.
      (d) S. Aureus.
      (e) Group A Streptococcus.
### b. Clinical Manifestations
i. Children present with irritability, crying, lethargy, and pulling at their ears.

ii. Physical examination reveals an erythematous tympanic membrane (TM).
   1. TM may be bulging, retracted, or perforated.
   2. An air-fluid level may be noted behind the TM, and mobility of the TM is diminished.
   3. Hearing may be decreased.
### c. Diagnosis
i. Based on history and physical examination.
ii. Culture, via tympanocentesis, is rarely done unless patient appears toxic or has recurrent infection.
### d. Treatment
i. Symptomatic treatment, mainly pain control, is required.
ii. Antibiotic treatment includes the following:
   1. Amoxicillin.
   2. Cefdinir.
   3. Amoxicillin-clavulanate.
   4. Cefpodoxime.
   5. Ceftriaxone.
iii. Most patients start to respond in 48 to 72 hours.
iv. Complications include chronic otitis media, mastoiditis, and intracranial extension.
v. Recurrent disease, ossicular erosion, cholesteatoma, and conductive hearing loss with chronic otitis media are indications for placement of tympanostomy tubes.
vi. Prevention with routine childhood vaccinations, eliminate household smoking, and do not allow infant to sleep with a bottle.

## IX. PHARYNGITIS
### a. General
i. Etiologies include viral and bacterial.
   1. Spread by close contact.
   2. Viral causes include rhinovirus, adenovirus, enterovirus, Epstein-Barr virus, and cytomegalovirus.
   3. Most common bacterial cause is group A beta-hemolytic streptococcus.
      (a) Mycoplasma can be the cause in young adults and adolescents.
### b. Clinical Manifestations
i. Bacterial infection.
   1. Rapid onset of sore throat, fever, headache, and GI symptoms such as abdominal pain and vomiting.
   2. Typically no cough.
   3. On physical examination, a red pharynx, swollen tonsils with yellow exudate, and cervical lymphadenopathy are noted.
ii. Viral infection.
   1. Gradual onset of rhinorrhea, cough, and diarrhea.

2. Conjunctivitis, coryza, and hoarseness also present.
3. On physical examination the pharynx is red and vesicles may be present; lymphadenopathy may also be noted.

c. **Diagnosis**
   i. Goal is to identify group A beta-hemolytic streptococcus via rapid strep screen or throat culture.

d. **Treatment**
   i. Treatment of streptococcal pharyngitis with antibiotics will hasten recovery by 12 to 24 hours.
      1. Treatment of choice is penicillin, or a macrolide for patients who are penicillin allergic.
   ii. Symptomatic treatment is used in viral pharyngitis.
   iii. Complications of bacterial pharyngitis include acute rheumatic fever and poststreptococcal glomerulonephritis.
      1. Antibiotics can prevent acute rheumatic fever but have no effect on the development of glomerulonephritis.

## X. PERTUSSIS

a. **General**
   i. Whooping cough is a highly communicable respiratory illness.
   ii. Most common in young children (younger than age 10) and in infants.
   iii. Etiology is *Bordetella pertussis*.
   iv. Incubation period is 7 to 10 days.

b. **Clinical Manifestations**
   i. Catarrhal stage (1 to 2 weeks).
      1. Present with sneezing, rhinorrhea, injected conjunctivae, and mild nocturnal cough.
      2. Resembles a simple upper respiratory tract infection.
   ii. Paroxysmal stage (2 to 4 weeks).
      1. Paroxysmal cough with a whooping sound.
      2. Physical examination may reveal scattered rhonchi.
   iii. Convalescent stage (1 to 2 weeks).
      1. Cough disappears.

c. **Diagnosis**
   i. Diagnosis based on clinical findings and whooping cough.
   ii. Lymphocytosis may be noted.
   iii. Gold standard is polymerase chain reaction (PCR) of nasopharyngeal aspirate.

d. **Treatment**
   i. Antibiotic options include erythromycin, azithromycin, or clarithromycin.
      1. Avoid erythromycin in infants younger than 1 month of age due to possible infantile hypertrophic pyloric stenosis.

2. Trimethoprim-sulfamethoxazole is an alternative agent in children over 2 months of age.
   ii. Prevention.
      1. Exposed susceptible individuals can be treated with a macrolide.
      2. Active immunization.
         (a) Diphtheria and tetanus toxoids and acellular pertussis (DTaP) vaccine is given at 2, 4, and 6 months of age.
         (b) A fourth dose is given at 15 to 18 months with a booster at 4 to 5 years of age.
         (c) Does not confer lifelong immunity.

## XI. SUDDEN INFANT DEATH SYNDROME

a. **General**
   i. Defined as the sudden death of an infant that is unexpected by history and unexplained by a postmortem examination, including a complete autopsy, investigation of the death, and review of the medical history.
   ii. Leading cause of infant mortality with an incidence rate of 0.5 in 1000 in infants between 1 month and 1 year of age.
   iii. The cause is unknown, most likely due to dysfunction of neural cardiorespiratory control mechanisms.

b. **Risk Factors**
   i. Black or Indigenous American.
   ii. Infant sleeping in the prone position.
   iii. Bed-sharing with parent/caregiver.
   iv. Low birth weight.
   v. Low socioeconomic status.
   vi. Male sex.
   vii. Maternal age <20 years.
   viii. Growth failure.

c. **Prevention**
   i. Infant should sleep in the supine position on a firm mattress.
   ii. Infant should sleep in own crib or bassinette.
   iii. Discontinue smoking during and after the pregnancy.
   iv. Home monitoring does not decrease risk.

# GASTROENTEROLOGY

## I. COLIC

a. **General**
   i. A benign condition with symptom complex of paroxysmal abdominal pain and severe crying.
   ii. Etiology unknown, but may be associated with the following:
      1. Hunger or swallowed air that has passed into the intestines.

2. High-carbohydrate–containing foods.

3. Food allergy.

  iii. Typically occurs in infants starting around age 10 weeks and rarely persists past the age of 3 to 4 months.

**b. Clinical Manifestations**

  i. Attacks begin suddenly with abdominal pain and continuous crying.

    1. Onset typically in the late afternoon or evening.

  ii. May persist for several hours.

  iii. Face may be flushed, abdomen distended, and legs drawn up to the abdomen.

  iv. Physical examination is normal and done to rule out intussusception, strangulated hernia, or other serious causes of abdominal pain.

**c. Treatment**

  i. Relief typically with passage of feces or flatus.

  ii. Holding infant upright or prone across the lap occasionally helps.

  iii. Attacks may be prevented with change in diet and improved feeding techniques.

  iv. Support of the parents is needed as well.

## II. DUODENAL ATRESIA

**a. General**

  i. Due to failure to recanalize lumen after solid phase of intestinal development.

  ii. A history of polyhydramnios (excessive amniotic fluid) is common.

  iii. Down syndrome seen in about one-fourth of the cases.

  iv. Associated with other anomalies such as malrotation, esophageal atresia, congenital heart disease, and anorectal malformation.

  v. Half of children with doudenal atresia are born premature.

**b. Clinical Manifestations**

  i. On first day of life, patient presents with bilious vomiting without abdominal distention.

**c. Diagnosis**

  i. X-ray film of abdomen reveals a double-bubble sign, distal bowel gas is absent.

  ii. See Fig. 14.7.

**d. Treatment**

  i. Decompression of GI tract and IV fluids.

  ii. Surgery (duodenoduodenostomy) is indicated.

## III. JAUNDICE

**a. General**

  i. Yellowing of the skin, mucous membranes, and sclera secondary to hyperbilirubinemia.

    1. Jaundice noted with bilirubin greater than 5 mg/dL in neonates and 2.5 mg/dL in children and adolescents.

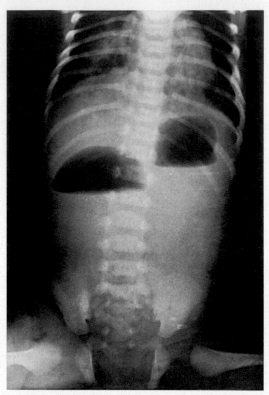

**Fig. 14.7** Duodenal atresia. Note the double-bubble sign. *(From Behrman RE. Nelson Textbook of Pediatrics, 17th ed. Philadelphia: WB Saunders, 2004:1233, Fig. 311-7.)*

  ii. Bilirubin is a bile pigment formed from the breakdown of heme that is derived from red blood cell breakdown and ineffective erythropoiesis.

  iii. Elevation in unconjugated (indirect) bilirubin can be physiologic or pathologic in origin.

    1. Having levels greater than 25 mg/dL in a full-term infant is neurotoxic and causes kernicterus.

  iv. Elevation in conjugated (direct) bilirubin is always pathologic.

  v. Differential diagnosis of hyperbilirubinemia (Table 14.9).

**b. Physiologic Jaundice**

  i. Most full-term and preterm neonates develop physiologic jaundice during the first week of life.

  ii. Begins after 24 hours of life, with a bilirubin peak of 12–15 mg/dL at 3 days of life; returns to normal by end of the first week.

  iii. Risk factors for developing more severe disease include: prematurity, maternal diabetes, drugs (vitamin K), and Asian or Native American ancestry.

**c. Clinical Manifestations**

  i. Can estimate bilirubin level based on progression of jaundice.

**TABLE 14.9**

| Differential Diagnosis of Hyperbilirubinemia | |
| --- | --- |
| **Unconjugated Hyperbilirubinemia** | **Conjugated Hyperbilirubinemia** |
| Physiologic jaundice | Extrahepatic obstruction |
| Hemolytic process | Persistent intrahepatic |
| Polycythemia | cholestasis |
| Extravascular blood loss | Acquired intrahepatic |
| Swallowed maternal blood | cholestasis |
| Increased enterohepatic | Dubin-Johnson syndrome |
| circulation | Rotor's syndrome |
| Breast-milk jaundice | Inborn errors of metabolism |
| Disorders of bilirubin metabolism | |
| Gilbert syndrome | |
| Crigler-Najjar syndrome | |
| Bacterial sepsis | |

    1. Face/Head equals bilirubin 5 mg/dL.
    2. Knees/Elbows equal 15 mg/dL.
    3. Midabdomen equals 9–15 mg/dL.
    4. Feet/Soles equal 20 mg/dL.
  **d. Treatment**
    i. Treatment goal is to avoid kernicterus or encephalopathy.
    ii. Two treatment options.
      1. Phototherapy.
      2. Exchange transfusion.
    iii. Breastfeeding must be discontinued for 1 to 2 days until bilirubin decreases to 2–8 mg/dL.
  **e. Kernicterus**
    i. General
      1. Due to elevation and deposition of unconjugated (indirect) bilirubin.
      2. Have yellow staining of the basal ganglia and hippocampus, which results in widespread cerebral dysfunction.
    ii. Clinical manifestations
      1. Develop lethargy and irritability, hypotonia, seizures, intellectual disability, poor sucking, and hearing loss.

## IV. INBORN ERRORS OF METABOLISM
  **a. Screening**
    i. All newborns should be screened for specific inborn errors of metabolism.
      1. Test must be completed between the ages of 24 hours and 7 days of life.
  **b. Biochemistry**
    i. Energy metabolism.
      1. Glucose is the energy source for the human body.
      (a) Glucose is converted to adenosine triphosphate (ATP) via acetyl coenzyme A (CoA) via the Krebs cycle.

      2. In fat metabolism, fat is converted from long-chain fatty acids to short-chain fatty acids and then acetyl CoA.
      3. In protein metabolism, protein is converted to amino acids, which are converted to acetyl CoA.
      (a) When conversion fails because of a genetic defect, the amino acid accumulates to toxic levels.
        (i) Cause of inborn errors of metabolism.
      4. Acetyl CoA is converted to energy (ATP) via glycolysis and the Krebs cycle.
  **c. General**
    i. Most are autosomal recessive disorders.
    ii. Due to enzyme defects that result in the accumulation of excess precursors, toxic metabolites, or deficiency of the product needed for normal metabolism.
    iii. Consider inborn errors of metabolism in the following:
      1. Critically ill newborns.
      2. Child with seizures.
      3. Reye's-like syndrome.
      4. Recurrent vomiting.
      5. Unusual odors.
      6. Unexplained acidosis.
      7. Hyperammonemia.
      8. Hypoglycemia.
  **d. Clinical Manifestations**
    i. Vary with different disorders but common findings include the following:
      1. Alopecia/abnormal hair.
      2. Retinal cherry-red spots.
      3. Cataracts/corneal opacity.
      4. Hepatomegaly/splenomegaly.
      5. Skeletal changes.
      6. Ataxia.
      7. Failure to thrive.
      8. Jaundice.
  **e. Disorders**
    i. Glycogen storage diseases.
      1. Result from deficiency of one of the enzymes involved with glycogen synthesis or breakdown.
      2. All are autosomal recessive disorders.
      3. Major types.
      (a) Type I: von Gierke's disease.
        (i) Affected enzyme is glucose-6-phosphatase.
        (ii) Patients present with hypoglycemia, lactic acidosis, hepatomegaly, slow growth, bleeding disorders, and hypertriglyceridemia.
        (iii) Early death from hypoglycemia.

(b) Type II: Pompe's disease.
  (i) Affected enzyme is lysosomal glucosidase.
  (ii) Patients present with symmetric profound muscle weakness, cardiomegaly, and heart failure.
  (iii) Prognosis is very poor; most die within first year.
(c) Type V: McArdle's disease.
  (i) Affected enzyme is muscle phosphorylase.
  (ii) Patients present with muscle fatigue beginning in adolescence.
  (iii) Prognosis is good with sedentary lifestyle.

ii. Galactosemia.
  1. Incidence is 1 in 60,000, and it is the most common error of carbohydrate metabolism.
  2. Due to almost total deficiency of galactose-1-phosphate uridyltransferase.
  3. Onset with jaundice, liver failure, vomiting, abnormal renal function, hepatomegaly, and poor growth.
    (a) Cataracts and learning difficulties may be noted.
  4. Laboratory findings include increased bilirubin, aspartate aminotransferase (AST), alanine aminotransferase (ALT), prothrombin time (PT), and hypoglycemia.
  5. Treatment is removing galactose from the diet.
    (a) Death in weeks if not treated.

iii. Disorders of amino acid metabolism.
  1. Phenylketonuria.
    (a) Autosomal recessive and secondary to decreased activity of phenylalanine hydroxylase.
      (i) Occurs in 1 in 14,000 live births.
    (b) Clinical manifestations.
      (i) Noted in childhood if untreated and includes intellectual disability, hypertonicity, tremors, and behavioral problems.
      (ii) Hypopigmentation may be noted due to decreased production of melanin.
      (iii) Urine has a musty, wet mouse–like odor.
      (iv) Elevated serum levels of phenylalanine and low tyrosine level.
    (c) Treatment.
      (i) Restrict the intake of phenylalanine.
  2. Homocystinuria.

(a) Autosomal recessive and secondary to deficiency in cystathionine synthetase.
  (i) Noted in 1 in 100,000 live births.
(b) Clinical manifestations.
  (i) No symptoms in infancy.
  (ii) In childhood, develop a Marfan's body habitus, dislocated eye lens, mild- to-moderate intellectual disability, and vascular thromboses.
  (iii) Increased risk of childhood stroke or myocardial infarction (MI).
(c) Treatment
  (i) Dietary management is difficult.
  (ii) High-dose vitamin $B_6$ may be helpful.

iv. Table 14.10 summarizes defects in lipidoses lysosomal storage diseases.

## V. INTUSSUSCEPTION
a. General
  i. Defined as an invagination or telescoping of one part of the bowel into itself.
    1. May lead to impaired blood supply and necrosis.
  ii. The most frequent cause of intestinal obstruction during the first 2 years of life.
  iii. More common in males (3:1) than in females.
  iv. Most common cause is idiopathic.
  v. Most common location is ileocolic.
    1. Commonly follows adenovirus or rotavirus infection.

**TABLE 14.10**

| Defects in Lipidoses Lysosomal Storage Diseases | | |
|---|---|---|
| **Disorder** | **Genetics** | **Clinical Manifestations** |
| Hurler syndrome | Autosomal recessive | Intellectual disability Hepatosplenomegaly Coarse facies Corneal clouding Severe heart disease |
| Niemann-Pick disease | Autosomal recessive | Hepatosplenomegaly Developmental delay Macular cherry-red spot |
| Gaucher disease | Autosomal recessive (common in Ashkenazi Jewish population) | Acute and chronic forms Hepatosplenomegaly Developmental delay Osteolytic bone lesions Macular cherry-red spot |
| Tay-Sachs disease | Autosomal recessive (common in Ashkenazi Jewish population) | Hypotonia Hyperacusis Developmental delay Macular cherry-red spot |

**b. Clinical Manifestations**
  i. Develops paroxysmal colicky abdominal pain followed by vomiting and diarrhea.
  ii. Diarrhea becomes bloody with mucus (currant jelly stool).
  iii. On examination, abdomen is noted to be distended and tender.
    1. On palpation, a sausage-shaped mass is noted in the upper midabdomen.
    2. Infants often draw legs up to abdomen.
  iv. Some patients may show signs of fever, altered consciousness, lethargy, and seizures.

**c. Diagnosis**
  i. Abdominal film shows a lack of bowel gas.
  ii. Ultrasound reveals a single or hypoechoic ring with hyperechoic center (target or donut sign).
  iii. Air enema is diagnostic and therapeutic.
    1. Will reveal the intussusception as an inverted cap and possible obstruction.
    2. Contraindicated with free air present in the abdomen.

**d. Treatment**
  i. Decompression of the intestine.
  ii. Correct dehydration if present.
  iii. Surgery may be indicated if reduction is not possible or not successful.

## VI. PYLORIC STENOSIS
**a. General**
  i. Hypertrophy of pyloric circular muscle.
  ii. Most common etiology is idiopathic.
  iii. There is male predominance (4:1) and a positive family history in 10% to 15%.

**b. Clinical Manifestations**
  i. Onset at about 3 weeks of age, but may be as late as 5 months.
  ii. Projectile nonbilious vomiting.
    1. Vomitus may be blood tinged.
  iii. A palpable olive-shaped mass noted in the midepigastrium.

**c. Diagnosis**
  i. Ultrasound reveals elongated pyloric channel and thickened pyloric wall.
  ii. Radiographic contrast studies.
    1. String sign: from elongated pyloric channel.
    2. Shoulder sign: bulge of pyloric muscle into the antrum.
  iii. Laboratory tests may reveal a hypochloremic metabolic alkalosis with hypokalemia.

**d. Treatment**
  i. Surgery (pyloromyotomy) is curative.

## VII. VOLVULUS (MALROTATION)
**a. General**
  i. Due to incomplete rotation of the intestine during fetal development.
    1. Axis for rotation is the superior mesenteric artery.
  ii. Typically present at younger than 1 month of age.

**b. Clinical Manifestations**
  i. Resembles an acute abdomen.
  ii. Present with recurrent bile-stained vomiting.
  iii. Will note distended, rigid abdomen, irritability, vomiting, and decreased stool volume and frequency.
    1. Secondary to obstruction.

**c. Diagnosis**
  i. Abdominal x-ray film reveals a double-bubble sign.
  ii. Ultrasound reveals inversion of the superior mesenteric artery and vein.
  iii. Upper GI reveals malposition of the ligament of Treitz.

**d. Treatment**
  i. Surgical intervention is required.

# MUSCULOSKELETAL

## I. DEVELOPMENTAL HIP DYSPLASIA
**a. General**
  i. Abnormal development of the acetabulum and proximal femur, as well as mechanical instability of the hip joint.
  ii. Incidence is 1 to 2 per 1000 children.
  iii. Risk factors.
    1. Female sex.
    2. Breech presentation.
    3. Positive family history.
    4. Swaddling.

**b. Clinical**
  i. Presentation varies with patient age and severity of disease.
  ii. Asymmetric gait noted in toddlers.

**c. Diagnosis**
  i. Physical examination reveals a positive Ortolani's and Barlow's maneuvers in children younger than 3 months of age.
  ii. Older than 3 months, note limited abduction and thigh-length discrepancy.
  iii. In walking age children, note weakness of hip abductors, a positive Trendelenburg pelvic tile test, and a Trendelenburg lurch when walking.
  iv. Ultrasound of hip x-ray may be helpful.

**d. Treatment**
  i. Depends on severity of disease and patient age.
    1. Options include surgery or Pavlik harness.

## II. JUVENILE RHEUMATOID ARTHRITIS
### a. General
   i. Characterized by chronic synovitis.
     1. Also note villous hypertrophy, hyperplasia of the synovial lining, edema, hyperemia, and increased lymphocytes and plasma cells.
   ii. More common in girls, with age of onset younger than 16 years of age.
   iii. Risk factors include a positive family history or other rheumatologic disorders.

### b. Clinical Manifestations
   i. May present polyarticular, oligoarthritic, or systemic.
   ii. Specific symptoms include morning stiffness, night pain, refusal to bear weight, and joint deformity.
   iii. Systemic symptoms include fatigue, anorexia, low-grade fever, rash (macular, salmon-pink), and hepatosplenomegaly.
   iv. Laboratory results reveal anemia and leukocytosis.
     1. Positive rheumatoid factor indicates poor prognostic outcome.
     2. Positive antinuclear antibodies (ANA) noted in 50% to 85% of patients.
   v. Examination of the synovial fluid reveals an elevated WBC count.

### c. Diagnosis
   i. Based on specific criteria.
     1. Age of onset younger than 16 years.
       (a) Many are affected between the ages of 1 and 3 years of age.
     2. Arthritis in one or more joints.
       (a) Note swelling or effusion with two or more of the following:
         (i) Limitation of range of motion.
         (ii) Tenderness.
         (iii) Pain on motion.
         (iv) Increased heat.
     3. Duration of disease 6 weeks or longer.
     4. Exclusion of other disorders.

### d. Treatment
   i. Control of inflammation with nonsteroidal antiinflammatory drugs (NSAIDs), immunosuppressive drugs (methotrexate), and steroids.
   ii. Physical therapy is vital to maintaining joint function.

## III. OSGOOD-SCHLATTER DISEASE
### a. General
   i. Microfracture at location of patellar tendon insertion into the tibia tubercle.
   ii. More common in boys 12 to 15 years of age and in girls 11 to 13 years of age.
     1. During periods of rapid growth.

### b. Clinical Manifestations
   i. Pain may limit normal activities.
   ii. Physical examination reveals swelling, tenderness, and increased prominence of the tibia tubercle.

### c. Diagnosis
   i. Based on history and physical examination.
   ii. X-ray film is often needed to rule out other possible disorders.
     1. May note irregularities of the tubercle contour.

### d. Treatment
   i. Rest; restriction of activities; and, at times, immobilization arc nccded.
   ii. Complete healing occurs in 12 to 24 months.
   iii. Casting may be required in severe cases.
     1. Antiinflammatory medications typically are not helpful.

## IV. SLIPPED CAPITAL FEMORAL EPIPHYSIS
### a. General
   i. Separation of the proximal femoral epiphysis through the growth plate.
   ii. Femoral head is typically displaced medially and posteriorly relative to the femoral neck.
   iii. More common in Black patients than White.

### b. Clinical Manifestations
   i. Noted most commonly in obese adolescent males.
     1. Also noted in thin patients with recent growth spurt.
   ii. Cause is unknown.
     1. Trauma is not a cause.
   iii. Patients note pain referred to the thigh and to the medial side of the knee, as well as a limp.
     1. Any child with knee pain should have hip pathology ruled out.
   iv. On physical examination, internal rotation of the hip is limited; hip flexion contracture and local tenderness around the hip are noted.

### c. Diagnosis
   i. Based on clinical findings and x-ray film.
     1. X-ray views include AP and Lauenstein (frog) lateral views that show epiphyseal displacement.

### d. Treatment
   i. Surgical repair with pinning.
   ii. Long-term complications include avascular necrosis and chondrolysis.

# NEUROLOGY

## I. CEREBRAL PALSY
### a. General
   i. A nonprogressive disorder of movement and posture that results from a lesion of the immature brain.

ii. Most common movement disorder of children.
    1. Will note delay in motor milestones.
iii. Risk factors include premature birth, birth asphyxia, intrauterine growth restriction, infection, or trauma.

**b. Clinical Manifestations**
   i. Presentation varies, with infants being initially hypotonic and older patients divided into two groups.
     1. Pyramidal (spastic).
       (a) Tone remains constant despite activity, with primitive and pathologic reflexes present; note significant hyperreflexia.
       (b) Four types.
          (i) Diplegia: bilateral lower extremity spasticity.
          (ii) Quadriplegia: all limbs severely involved, lower extremities more than upper.
          (iii) Hemiplegia: one side involved, upper extremity more than lower.
          (iv) Bilateral hemiplegia: all limbs severely involved, upper extremities more than lower.
     2. Extrapyramidal.
       (a) Tone is variable depending on level of arousal, primitive reflexes noted, and hyperreflexia may or may not be present.
       (b) Three types.
          (i) Ataxic: have difficulty coordinating purposeful movements.
          (ii) Choreoathetoid: rapid, irregular, unpredictable contractions of muscles.
          (iii) Dystonic have uncontrollable jerking, writhing, and posturing movements.
   ii. Associated neurologic deficits are common.
     1. Seizures, intellectual disability, hearing and vision problems are common.

**c. Diagnosis**
   i. Based on clinical presentation.

**d. Treatment**
   i. A multidisciplinary approach is needed to maximize function and to minimize impairment.
   ii. No cure is available.

## II. COMA

**a. Table 14.11 lists common causes of coma in infants and children**

## III. NEUROBLASTOMA

**a. General**
   i. Embryonal cancer of the peripheral sympathetic nervous system.

**TABLE 14.11**

| Common Causes of Coma in Infants and Children | |
| --- | --- |
| **Etiology** | **Note** |
| Alcohol | Oral intake or absorbed through the skin |
| Cardiovascular | May be due to shock or stroke |
| Epilepsy | Postictal state may be confused with coma |
| Hypoglycemia or hyperglycemia | Check blood sugar in all comatose children |
| Infection | Most common cause of change in mental status |
| Intussusception | Vacant blank stare often noted in children with intussusception |
| Overdose | Intentional or accidental |
| Trauma | Retinal hemorrhages in shaken baby syndrome |
| Uremia | Renal failure or other metabolic causes |

ii. Third most common pediatric cancer; makes up 8% of childhood malignancies.
iii. Median age at diagnosis is 2 years of age; 90% are diagnosed by age 5.
iv. Triggering event is unknown.
    1. Increased incidence with maternal and paternal occupational chemical exposure, work in farming, and work related to electronics
    2. Folate deficiency linked to increased risk.

**b. Clinical Manifestations**
   i. Clinical signs and symptoms reflect site of the tumor.
     1. Can present with ataxia or opsomyoclonus.
   ii. Most cases arise in the abdomen; in the adrenal gland or retroperitoneal sympathetic ganglia.
   iii. Palpate a firm, nodular mass in the flank or midline of the abdomen.
   iv. May have hypertension and diarrhea.

**c. Diagnosis**
   i. Computed tomography (CT) scan or abdominal x-ray film may reveal calcification and hemorrhage in the tumor.
   ii. Wilms' tumor, which also presents as a mass in the flank, does not show calcification.
   iii. Homovanillic acid and vanillylmandelic acid are elevated in the urine.

**d. Treatment**
   i. Surgery, chemotherapy, or radiation therapy depending on stage of disease.

## IV. SEIZURES

**a. Table 14.12 lists common causes of seizures by age group**

**TABLE 14.12**

| Common Causes of Seizures by Age Group | |
| --- | --- |
| **Age Group** | **Etiologies** |
| First day of life | Hypoxia |
| | Drugs |
| | Trauma |
| | Infection |
| | Hyperglycemia |
| | Hypoglycemia |
| | Vitamin B$_6$ deficiency |
| Days 2–3 of life | Infection |
| | Hypoglycemia |
| | Hypocalcemia |
| | Developmental malformations |
| | Intracranial hemorrhage |
| | Inborn error of metabolism |
| | Hyponatremia |
| | Hypernatremia |
| 1 week to 6 months of life | Infection |
| | Hypocalcemia |
| | Developmental malformations |
| | Hyponatremia |
| | Inborn error of metabolism |
| 6 months to 3 years of age | Febrile seizures |
| | Birth injury |
| | Infection |
| | Toxin |
| | Trauma |
| | Metabolic disorder |
| Older than 3 years of age | Idiopathic |
| | Infection |
| | Trauma |
| | Cerebral degenerative disease |

**TABLE 14.13**

| Hyperactivity-Impulsivity and Inattention Symptoms | |
| --- | --- |
| **Hyperactivity/Impulsivity** | **Inattention** |
| Excessive fidgetiness | Failure to provide close attention to detail; careless mistakes |
| Difficulty remaining seated when sitting is required | Difficulty maintaining attention in play, school, or home activities |
| In younger children, feelings of restlessness, inappropriate running around, or climbing | Seems to not listen, even when directly addressed |
| Difficulty playing quietly | Fails to follow through: homework, chores |
| Difficult to keep up with, seeming always on the go | Difficulty organizing tasks, activities, and belongings |
| Excessive talking | Avoids tasks that require consistent mental effort |
| Difficulty waiting turns | Loses objects required for tasks or activities |
| Blurting out answers too quickly | Easily distracted by irrelevant stimuli |
| Interruption or intrusion of others | Forgets routine activities: homework, chores |

# PSYCHIATRY

## I. ATTENTION-DEFICIT DISORDER

a. **General**
   i. Disorder runs in families.
   ii. Concurrent psychiatric disorders are common.
   iii. More common in boys than in girls.
   iv. Etiology is unknown.

b. **Clinical Manifestations**
   i. Frequently noted when child enters school.
      1. Child presents with discipline difficulties, incomplete chores and projects, forgetting assignments, and poor impulse control.
   ii. Symptoms must be present before 12 years of age.
   iii. Criteria for diagnosis include the following:
      1. Either six or more inattention or six or more hyperactivity-impulsivity symptoms must be noted.
         (a) Table 14.13 lists symptoms.
      2. Some impairment occurs in at least two or more settings.

3. Must be evidence of clinically significant impairment in social, academic, or occupational functioning.
4. Symptoms do not occur due to some other psychiatric disorder.

c. **Treatment**
   i. Treatment includes behavioral management, such as positive reinforcement, firm limit setting, and reduction in stimulation.
   ii. Medications include psychostimulants, such as methylphenidate or dextroamphetamine.
      1. Side effects with long-term use of these medications may include weight loss and diminished body growth.

## II. AUTISM SPECTRUM DISORDER

a. **General**
   i. A very rare familial disorder with a male-to-female ratio of 4:1.
   ii. A number of patients with autistic spectrum disorder have fragile X chromosome and tuberous sclerosis.
   iii. One-fourth of patients with autistic spectrum disorder have seizures, and three-fourths have some form of intellectual disability.
   iv. Four disorders integrated into the autism spectrum disorders.
      1. Autistic disorder.
      2. Asperger's syndrome.
      3. Childhood disintegrative disorder.
      4. Pervasive developmental disorder—not otherwise specified (PDD-NOS).

**b. Clinical Manifestations**

    i. Typically note abnormal development shortly after birth.

      1. Deficits in social communication and interaction.

        (a) Deficits in social interaction: lack of reciprocity in conversation.

        (b) Problems with nonverbal communication: lack of eye contact; body language.

        (c) Difficulty understanding relationships: creating, maintaining, and understanding nuances in behavior.

      2. Restricted repetitive behaviors, interests, and activities.

        (a) Repetitive motor movement: head banging, flapping, rocking.

        (b) Ritualized behaviors: verbal and nonverbal.

        (c) Unusually strong interests in unusual objects or perseveration.

        (d) Heightened sensitivity to sensory stimulation: pain, sound, smell, touch.

**c. Treatment**

    i. A chronic lifelong disorder.

    ii. Behavioral management techniques are used to reduce the rigid behaviors and improve social functioning.

    iii. Antiseizure medications are used in patients with seizure disorder.

    iv. Neuroleptics, such as haloperidol, are used to help decrease aggressive behaviors.

## III. CHILD ABUSE

**a. General**

    i. Occurs at all levels of society.

      1. Increased incidence in families in which alcohol is abused.

    ii. Child abuse is defined as a nonaccidental serious physical injury, sexual exploitation or misuse, neglect, or serious mental injury in a child younger than 18 years old, as a result of commission or omission by a parent, guardian, or caregiver.

    iii. There are four categories.

      1. Physical abuse: refers to serious bodily injury.

      2. Sexual abuse: includes exposure or involvement of children to sexual material or acts.

      3. Neglect: result of failure to provide for the basic needs of a child.

      4. Emotional abuse: is a coercive, demeaning behavior toward a child that interferes with normal development.

**b. Clinical Manifestations**

    i. Diagnosis of abuse relies on physical evidence of abuse.

      1. Includes multiple skin lesions in various stages of healing, subdural and subarachnoid bleeding, retinal hemorrhages, long bone (spiral fractures) and rib fractures, pattern burns, and spinal injuries.

        (a) Retinal hemorrhages are commonly noted in shaken baby syndrome.

**c. Treatment**

    i. All possible cases of abuse must be investigated.

    ii. Strategies to improve the environment and reduce caregiver stress should be incorporated.

    iii. Family counseling and family support to resolve family dysfunction is beneficial.

# GENITOURINARY

## I. CRYPTORCHIDISM

**a. General**

    i. Unilateral or bilateral undescended testis.

    ii. In most cases, the testes descend by the fourth month.

    iii. Increased risk for infertility and testicular malignancy.

**b. Clinical Manifestations**

    i. Lack of testes on testicular examination.

**c. Diagnosis**

    i. Testosterone level after human chorionic gonadotropin (hCG) stimulation to confirm presence or absence of abdominal testes.

    ii. Ultrasound or CT scan can be utilized.

**d. Treatment**

    i. Surgical orchidopexy by 1 year of age.

## II. HYDROCELE

**a. General**

    i. Accumulation of fluid in the tunica vaginalis surrounding testes.

    ii. Typically is noncommunicating type.

      1. In noncommunicating type, the processus vaginalis was obliterated during development.

      2. Will usually disappear by 1 year of age.

      3. Communicating hydrocele may develop into an inguinal hernia.

    iii. Etiology also includes testicular torsion, epididymitis, or tumor.

**b. Clinical Manifestations**

    i. Mass is smooth and nontender.

**c. Diagnosis**

    i. Transillumination of the scrotum confirms a fluid-filled mass.

d. **Treatment**
  i. Typically resolves spontaneously.
  ii. Surgery may be needed if mass lasts past age 18 months.

## III. WILMS' TUMOR (NEPHROBLASTOMA)
a. **General**
  i. Occurs most commonly between the ages of 2 and 5 years.
  ii. Frequently associated with other malformations and cytogenetic disorders.
b. **Clinical Manifestations**
  i. Patients present with increasing abdominal mass.
    1. Mass is smooth, firm, and well demarcated.
  ii. Microscopic hematuria is often noted, but gross hematuria is uncommon.
c. **Diagnosis**
  i. Intrarenal mass noted on ultrasound or CT scan of the abdomen.
d. **Treatment**
  i. Surgical resection of the tumor.
  ii. Chemotherapy is used in all cases.
  iii. Advanced cases also treated with radiation therapy.

# DERMATOLOGY

## I. DIAPER DERMATITIS
a. **General**
  i. Includes a large group of conditions causing red, scaly rashes in the diaper region.
  ii. Decrease incidence with frequent diaper changes.
  iii. Can be due to an irritant or *Candida albicans*.
b. **Clinical Manifestations**
  i. Irritant diaper dermatitis presents with red, scaly, eroded, painful plaques.
    1. The creases are spared.
  ii. *Candida* diaper dermatitis presents with bright, beefy red plaques in the inguinal or gluteal folds.
    1. Satellite pustules are common.
c. **Diagnosis**
  i. Based on history and clinical findings.
  ii. Potassium hydroxide (KOH) prep will reveal pseudohyphae and spores if due to *Candida*.
d. **Treatment**
  i. Treatment should be directed at decreasing wetness.
  ii. Barrier ointments can be used for prophylaxis along with frequent changes of diapers.
  iii. *Candida* infections can be treated with imidazole cream. Oral nystatin if coexisting oral candidiasis.

# QUESTIONS

### QUESTION 1
A 2-year-old presents with fever and drooling. The patient appears toxic and is sitting up with chin forward. Thumbprint sign is noted on lateral neck x-ray film. Which of the following is the treatment of choice for this patient?
A Ampicillin
B Prednisone
C Artificial airway
D Nebulized albuterol
E Racemic epinephrine

### QUESTION 2
Which of the following is the pathophysiologic mechanism of hyaline membrane disease?
A Surfactant deficiency
B Meconium aspiration
C Congenital diaphragmatic hernia
D High pulmonary vascular resistance
E Slow absorption of fetal lung fluid

### QUESTION 3
Which of the following is the treatment of choice for Kawasaki's disease?
A Methotrexate
B Prednisone
C Penicillin
D Ibuprofen
E Aspirin

### QUESTION 4
Which of the following increases the risk of sudden infant death syndrome?
A Macrosomia
B Pacifier use
C Immunizations
D Prone sleeping
E Upper respiratory tract infection

# QUESTIONS—cont'd

## QUESTION 5

A 1-day-old patient develops bilious vomiting without abdominal distention. Abdominal x-ray reveals a double-bubble sign. Which of following is the intervention of choice for this patient?

A Duodenoduodenostomy

B IV glucocorticosteroids

C Pyloromyotomy

D Barium enema

E Sigmoidoscopy

## QUESTION 6

Which of the following results from the deposition of unconjugated bilirubin in the brain?

A Kernicterus

B Rett's syndrome

C Neurocysticercosis

D Sturge-Weber syndrome

E Ehlers-Danlos syndrome

## QUESTION 7

Which of the following is the treatment of choice for homocystinuria?

A Vitamin B$_6$

B Riboflavin

C Niacin

D Folate

E Iron

## QUESTION 8

An 18-month-old patient presents with abdominal pain and bloody diarrhea. On physical examination a sausage-shaped mass is noted in the upper midabdominal region. Which of the following is the most likely diagnosis?

A Pyloric stenosis

B Intussusception

C Duodenal atresia

D Meckel diverticulum

E Hirschsprung's disease

## QUESTION 9

Which of the following is a common side effect of psychostimulants?

A Tardive dyskinesia

B Visual hallucinations

C Weight loss

D Headache

E Tinnitus

## QUESTION 10

A 6-month-old male presents with a scrotal mass. The scrotum is swollen, and the testicles are nontender. The scrotum does transilluminate. Which of the following is the treatment of choice?

A Orchidopexy

B Varicocelectomy

C Radical orchiectomy

D Dextranomer/hyaluronic acid copolymer

E No treatment is needed at this time.

# ANSWERS

## 1. C

EXPLANATION: Acute epiglottitis is a medical emergency, and immediate treatment with an artificial airway in a controlled environment is indicated. Steroids, racemic epinephrine, and albuterol are ineffective and not indicated. The antibiotic of choice is ceftriaxone or cefotaxime. Ampicillin is not considered first line due to increased resistance of *H. influenzae* to ampicillin. ***Topic: Eyes, Ears, Nose, and Throat/Pulmonary: acute epiglottitis***

☐ Correct ☐ Incorrect

## 2. A

EXPLANATION: Hyaline membrane disease (respiratory distress syndrome) results from alveoli collapse due to lack of adequate lung surfactant and immature lungs. ***Topic: Eyes, Ears, Nose, and Throat/Pulmonary: hyaline membrane disease***

☐ Correct ☐ Incorrect

*Continued*

## ANSWERS—cont'd

**3. E**

EXPLANATION: Patients with Kawasaki's disease present with fever, bilateral conjunctival injection, pharyngeal erythema, edema of the hands and feet, rash, and lymphadenopathy. Treatment of choice is high-dose aspirin and IV immunoglobulin. *Topic: Eyes, Ears, Nose, and Throat/Pulmonary: Kawasaki's disease*

□ Correct   □ Incorrect

**4. D**

EXPLANATION: The risk of sudden infant death syndrome is increased with infants sleeping prone, exposure to cigarette smoking, low birth weight, and preterm birth. *Topic: Eyes, Ears, Nose, and Throat/Pulmonary: sudden infant death syndrome*

□ Correct   □ Incorrect

**5. A**

EXPLANATION: Duodenal atresia presents within the first day of life with bilious vomiting without abdominal distention. A double-bubble sign is noted on abdominal x-ray film. Treatment of choice is a duodenoduodenostomy. *Topic: Gastroenterology: duodenal atresia*

□ Correct   □ Incorrect

**6. A**

EXPLANATION: Kernicterus results from the deposition of unconjugated bilirubin in the basal ganglia and brainstem. Rett's syndrome is a neurodegenerative disorder of unknown cause. Neurocysticercosis is caused by infection with a tapeworm. Sturge-Weber syndrome is caused by abnormal development of meningeal vasculature. Ehlers-Danlos syndrome is a connective tissue disorder. *Topic: Gastroenterology: jaundice*

□ Correct   □ Incorrect

**7. A**

EXPLANATION: Homocystinuria is a disorder of amino acid metabolism and is best treated with high doses of vitamin $B_6$. *Topic: Gastroenterology: inborn errors of metabolism*

□ Correct   □ Incorrect

**8. B**

EXPLANATION: Intussusception, telescoping of proximal bowel into distal bowel, is most common in children younger than age 2, who present with abdominal pain and bloody "currant jelly" stool. On physical examination a sausage-shaped mass is noted in the midabdomen. Patients with pyloric stenosis present with vomiting and an olive-size mass in the midabdomen. Those with Hirschsprung's disease present with vomiting and abdominal distention. Duodenal atresia is noted in the first day of life, with vomiting without abdominal distention. Meckel diverticulum presents with intermittent painless rectal bleeding. *Topic: Gastroenterology: intussusception*

□ Correct   □ Incorrect

**9. C**

EXPLANATION: The side effects of the psychostimulants, such as Ritalin, include appetite suppression, weight loss, and sleep disturbances. *Topic: Psychiatry: attention deficit disorder*

□ Correct   □ Incorrect

**10. E**

EXPLANATION: A hydrocele presents with a swollen, nontender scrotum. Due to the scrotum being filled with fluid, the mass will transilluminate. No treatment is required unless the hydrocele persists after the age of 2 years. *Topic: Genitourinary: hydrocele*

□ Correct   □ Incorrect

## EXAMINATION BLUEPRINT TOPICS

### PHARMACOKINETICS

Absorption

Distribution

Metabolism

Excretion

### PHARMACODYNAMICS

Dose–response relationships

Sites of drug action

### ANALGESICS

Acetaminophen

Nonsteroidal Antiinflammatory Drugs (NSAIDs)

COX-2s

Tramadol (Ultram)

Opioids

### MIGRAINE ABORTIVE THERAPY

Basic and combination medications

Ergotamine alkaloids

$5\text{-HT}_{1B/1D}$ agonists (triptans)

### ANTIBIOTICS

Beta-lactam antibiotics

Protein synthesis inhibitors

Fluoroquinolones

Antifolate drugs

Metronidazole

Nitrofurantoin

### ANTITUBERCULOSIS DRUGS

Isoniazid

Rifampin

Pyrazinamide

Ethambutol

### ANTIVIRAL RESPIRATORY AGENTS

Zanamivir (Relenza)

Oseltamivir (Tamiflu)

Ribavirin (Virazole)

### HUMAN IMMUNODEFICIENCY VIRUS (HIV) DRUGS

Nucleoside reverse transcriptase inhibitors (NRTIs)

Nonnucleoside reverse transcriptase inhibitors (NNRTIs)

Protease inhibitors

### CARDIAC DRUGS

Diuretics

Angiotensin-converting enzyme (ACE) inhibitors

Angiotensin II receptor blockers (ARBS)

Beta-blockers

Alpha-blockers

Calcium channel blockers (CCBs)

Direct vasodilators

Centrally acting agents

Nitroglycerin/Nitrates

Antiarrhythmics

Digitalis (Digoxin)

### ENDOCRINE DRUGS

Insulin

Biguanides

Sulfonylureas

Thiazolidinediones

Alpha-glucosidase inhibitors

Glucagon-like peptide-1 receptor agonist

Sodium-glucose co-transporter 2 inhibitors

### LIPID-LOWERING AGENTS

Bile acid–binding resins

HMG-CoA reductase inhibitors

Fibric-acid inhibitors

Nicotinic acids

Summary of lipid-lowering agents

### GASTROINTESTINAL (GI) MEDICATIONS

Antacids

Histamine$_2$ receptor antagonists

Proton-pump inhibitors

Sucralfate (Carafate)

Bismuth subsalicylate (BSS) (Pepto-Bismol)

Metoclopramide

Antidiarrheals

Laxatives

Antiemetics

Butyrophenone antiemetics (Droperidol)

Serotonin ($5\text{-HT}_3$) antagonists (Ondansetron, granisetron, dolasetron)

### PSYCHIATRIC MEDICATIONS

Benzodiazepines

Antidepressants: selective serotonin reuptake inhibitors (SSRIs)

Antidepressants: serotonin–norepinephrine reuptake inhibitors (SNRIs)

Antidepressants: tricyclic antidepressants (TCAs)

Antidepressants: monoamine oxidase inhibitors (MAOIs)

Bupropion (Wellbutrin, Zyban)

Mirtazapine (Remeron)

Buspirone (Buspar)

Lithium (Eskalith)

Antipsychotics

Stimulants

### OTHER

Cholinesterase inhibitors

Anticoagulants

Antigout

Anticonvulsants

Chemotherapy

# PHARMACOKINETICS

## I. ABSORPTION
a. Ability of the drug to cross body membranes and enter the bloodstream
b. Mechanisms
   i. Passive diffusion requires no energy and is the method used by most drugs.
   ii. Active transport requires energy and is carrier dependent, and competition may limit transport.
   iii. Facilitated diffusion requires a carrier, but no energy is required.
c. Influencing Factors
   i. Routes of administration: inhalation, intramuscular (IM), oral (PO), rectal, and topical.
   ii. Drug concentration.
   iii. Properties of the drug.
   iv. Patient physiologic factors.
   v. Metabolism before reaching circulation.
      1. First-pass effect is the metabolism, in the intestines and liver, which occurs with PO medications before reaching the systemic circulation.

## II. DISTRIBUTION
a. The extent that the drug spreads throughout the body
b. Influencing Factors
   i. Physiologic.
   ii. Protein binding.
   iii. Tissue binding.
c. Volume of distribution is the amount of drug in the body related to plasma concentration

## III. METABOLISM
a. Is the process of alteration for the drug to make the drug inactive or to increase solubility to increase renal elimination
b. Liver is the major site of metabolism via the cytochrome P (CYP) 450 system
   i. Other sites of metabolism include the lungs and gastrointestinal (GI) tract.

## IV. EXCRETION
a. The removal of the drug and its metabolites from the body
b. The kidney is the primary site of excretion
   i. Other sites include lungs and skin (sweat).
c. Influencing Factors
   i. Chemical properties of the drug.
   ii. Body physiologic factors.
   iii. Drug interactions.

# PHARMACODYNAMICS

## I. DOSE–RESPONSE RELATIONSHIPS
a. The relationship between the dose of the drug and resultant effect

## II. SITES OF DRUG ACTION
a. Channels
   i. Drugs that prevent channels from opening (e.g., calcium channel blockers).
b. Enzymes
   i. Are both inhibitors and activators.
   ii. Inhibitor drugs are drugs that inhibit the activity of the enzyme (e.g., angiotensin-converting enzyme [ACE] inhibitor).
   iii. Activators are drugs that block receptors and prevent binding of neurotransmitters (e.g., beta-blockers).
c. Receptors
   i. Agonists are drugs that bind to a receptor and increase the effects of the endogenous neurotransmitter.
   ii. Antagonists are drugs that block receptors and prevent binding of neurotransmitters.

# ANALGESICS

## I. ACETAMINOPHEN
a. Mechanism of Action
   i. Inhibits synthesis of prostaglandins in the central nervous system (CNS) and peripherally blocks brain-impulse generation.
   ii. Onset of action is 30 to 60 minutes.
   iii. Duration of action is 4 hours.
      1. Analgesic and antipyretic effects.
      2. No antiinflammatory or antiplatelet effects.
b. Metabolism
   i. Maximum dose 4 g/day (3 g/day for chronic use).
c. Metabolized in Liver; Excreted in Urine
   i. Hepatic impairment limited to 2 g/day.
   ii. With severe renal insufficiency (CrCl <10 mL/minute), decrease frequency.
d. Side Effects
   i. Well-tolerated without common toxicities expected with nonsteroidal antiinflammatory drugs (NSAIDs).
   ii. Hepatotoxicity when combined with carbamazepine, ethanol, isoniazid (INH).
   iii. Preferred analgesic during pregnancy and breastfeeding.
   iv. Overdose treated with N-acetylcysteine (Mucomyst).

## II. NONSTEROIDAL ANTIINFLAMMATORY DRUGS (NSAIDs)

a. **Mechanism of Action**
   i. Inhibit cyclooxygenase (COX) enzyme that releases prostaglandin (PG) known to sensitize or activate peripheral nociceptors in producing pain.
   ii. Analgesic, antipyretic, and antiinflammatory effects.
      1. Low dose: analgesic (used for mild to moderate pain).
      2. High dose: antiinflammatory.
   iii. Produces synergy with opioids.

b. **Medications**
   i. Aspirin.
      1. Risk of Reye's syndrome in patients with viral infection.
         (a) Inhibits fatty acid metabolism and damage to cellular mitochondria.
         (b) Leads to liver failure and brain damage.
      2. Contraindicated in pregnancy.
      3. Stop drug 1 week prior to surgery.
   ii. Diclofenac (Voltaren).
   iii. Ibuprofen (Motrin).
   iv. Naproxen (Anaprox, Naprosyn).
   v. Indomethacin (Indocin).
      1. Used in treatment of patent ductus arteriosus.
   vi. Ketorolac (Toradol).
      1. Intravenous (IV) and IM routes.
      2. Can be as effective as morphine, no euphoria.
      3. Limit duration of use to 5 days because of increased risk of ulcers.

c. **Side Effects and Limitations**
   i. NSAID-induced gastropathy.
   ii. Antiplatelet effect.
   iii. May increase risk of thrombosis, stroke, and myocardial infarction (MI).
   iv. Increased risk of hypersensitivity in patients with aspirin receptors.
      1. Bronchial asthma, aspirin intolerance, rhinitis.
   v. Renal toxicity.
      1. Can compromise existing renal function.

d. **Drug Interactions**
   i. Enhances effect of heparin, warfarin, digoxin, and lithium.
   ii. Decreases effects of ACE inhibitors and angiotensin receptor blockers, beta-blockers, and diuretics.

## III. COX-2s

a. **Mechanism of Action**
   i. Inhibits cyclooxygenase-2 (COX-2), which inhibits prostaglandin synthesis, which results in decreased formation of prostaglandin precursors.
   ii. Does not appear to block COX-1, decreasing GI toxicity.

b. **Indications**
   i. Used in patients where an NSAID is indicated with the following:
      1. History of GI ulcers.
      2. Elderly.
      3. Low platelet count (<50 K) because it does not inhibit platelet aggregation.
      4. Receiving anticoagulation.
      5. Receiving corticosteroids.
      6. Coagulopathy.
      7. Prior intolerance to nonselective NSAID.

c. **Medications**
   i. Celecoxib (Celebrex).
      1. Used for acute and chronic pain.
         (a) Osteoarthritis (OA), rheumatoid arthritis (RA), dysmenorrhea.
      2. Used in familial adenomatous polyposis.
      3. Many drug interactions that should be watched (warfarin, CYP 450).
      4. Use with caution in patients with sulfonamide allergy.
      5. Use with caution in patients with congestive heart failure (CHF), fluid retention, and hypertension (HTN).
      6. Avoid in renal insufficiency, severe heart disease, dehydration, and liver failure.
      7. Can increase the cardiovascular risk of thrombosis, stroke, and MI.

## IV. TRAMADOL (ULTRAM)

a. **Mechanism of Action**
   i. Binds to mu-opiate receptors but also binds to norepinephrine.
      1. Modifies the ascending pain pathway.

b. **Needs to be adjusted in renal dysfunction (CrCl < 30 mL/minute) and hepatic dysfunction**

c. **Side Effects**
   i. Use limited by nausea and vomiting, constipation, and dizziness.
      1. May lower seizure threshold.
   ii. Concurrent use of quinidine will increase drug level.
   iii. Risk of serotonin syndrome when used with monoamine oxidase inhibitors (MAOIs), tricyclic antidepressants (TCAs), and selective serotonin reuptake inhibitors (SSRIs).

## V. OPIOIDS

a. **General**
  i. Major class of analgesics in the management of moderate to severe pain.
  ii. Act as a mu-opiate receptor agonist, altering perception and response to pain, centrally and peripherally.
  iii. Have a well-established efficacy with doses easily titrated.
  iv. Common toxicities are generally easily managed or prevented.
  v. Overdose can be treated with naloxone (Narcan).

b. **Opioid Classes**
  i. Phenanthrenes.
    1. Morphine.
    2. Codeine.
    3. Hydrocodone.
    4. Oxycodone.
    5. Oxymorphone.
  ii. Phenylpiperidines.
    1. Fentanyl.
  iii. Diphenylheptanes.
    1. Methadone.
    2. Propoxyphene.

c. **Opioid Equivalence (Table 15.1)**

d. **Medications**
  i. Morphine.
    1. Is the gold standard for cancer pain management.
    2. Has an active metabolite: morphine-6-glucuronide.
    3. Is well-tolerated, may have some flushing due to release of histamine.
    4. Inexpensive and has multiple formulations.
    5. May increase intracranial pressure in head trauma patients.
  ii. Hydromorphone.
    1. Multiple dosage forms.
    2. Used in moderate to severe pain.
    3. Multiple drug interactions.
    4. Side effects include hallucinations, respiratory and CNS depression, sedation.
  iii. Oxycodone.
    1. Slightly more potent than morphine.
    2. Fewer dosage forms.
      (a) Oral.
      (b) Multiple combination products with acetaminophen and ibuprofen.
    3. Milder side-effect profile relative to morphine.
    4. May be less sedating in the elderly.
  iv. Fentanyl.
    1. One hundred times as potent as morphine.
      (a) 1 mg IV morphine = 10 mcg fentanyl.
    2. Unique dosage forms including IV, transdermal, and lozenge.
    3. Least likely to induce histamine release.
    4. Not known whether dose requires adjustment for renal or hepatic failure.
      (a) Is eliminated by the kidneys and is metabolized in the liver.
  v. Meperidine.
    1. Only recommended for pain management unless no other options.
    2. Has a short duration of action.
    3. The drug metabolite—normeperidine—is toxic.
    4. CNS toxic symptoms include seizures.
    5. Useful for post-anesthesia and amphotericin B–related rigors.
  vi. Methadone.
    1. Opioid agonist and N-Methyl-D-aspartate (NMDA) antagonist.
      (a) Used in detoxification of opiate addiction.
    2. Long half-life can lead to accumulation and toxicity.
    3. Many drug interactions.
    4. Increased toxicity (sedation and respiratory depression) with CYP 3A4 inhibitors (fluvoxamine and other antidepressants).
    5. May prolong QT interval and lead to torsades de pointes.

e. **Major Adverse Effects of Opioids**
  i. CNS effects include mood changes, somnolence/CNS excitation, and meiosis.
  ii. Respiratory system depression.
  iii. Urinary retention.
  iv. Cardiovascular effects include hypotension and bradycardia.
  v. Constipation.

**TABLE 15.1**

| Opioid Equivalence | | |
| --- | --- | --- |
| Oral (mg) | Agent | Parenteral (mg) |
| 100 | Codeine | 50 |
| NA | Fentanyl | 0.05 |
| 15 | Hydrocodone | NA |
| 4 | Hydromorphone | 1 |
| 15 | Morphine | 5 |
| 10 | Oxycodone | NA |
| 5 | Oxymorphone | 0.5 |

*NA*, Not available.

# MIGRAINE ABORTIVE THERAPY

## I. BASIC AND COMBINATION MEDICATIONS
### a. Aspirin
  i. Appropriate, if tolerated, due to potent antiinflammatory effect.
  ii. Combination products with caffeine and butalbital (Fiorinal) are no more effective than aspirin alone.
  iii. Excedrin Migraine consists of aspirin, acetaminophen, and caffeine.
### b. NSAIDs
  i. See page 353 for mechanism of action.
  ii. Recommend short-acting NSAIDs (ibuprofen, naproxen sodium) for faster onset.
### c. Acetaminophen if aspirin or NSAIDs not tolerated
### d. Midrin is a combination product
  i. Not much more effective than simple analgesics.
  ii. Contains isometheptene (vasoconstrictor), dichloralphenazone (antinausea properties), and acetaminophen (analgesic).

## II. ERGOTAMINE ALKALOIDS
### a. Direct vasoconstrictor of smooth muscle in cranial vessels/nonselective 5-HT agonist
### b. Dosage Forms
  i. Tablets/Suppositories: Cafergot in combination with caffeine.
  ii. Nasal spray: Migranal (D.H.E. dihydroergotamine).
  iii. Injectable: D.H.E. for IM or IV use.
### c. Adverse effects are mainly from vasoconstrictor effects
  i. Most common are nausea/vomiting and abdominal pain. These can be prevented by concomitant use of antiemetics.
  ii. Ergotism: abdominal cramps, nausea/vomiting, diarrhea, vertigo, distal paresthesias.
  iii. Large doses have potential for angina and MI.
### d. Contraindicated in angina, history of MI, peripheral arterial disease, pregnancy, and uncontrolled HTN

## III. 5-HT$_{1B/1D}$ AGONISTS (TRIPTANS)
### a. 5-HT$_{1B}$ receptors are in meningeal arteries, and stimulation produces vasoconstriction
### b. 5-HT$_{1D}$ receptors are in trigeminal nerves; and stimulation interrupts nociceptive transmission and neuropeptide release, therefore decreasing transmission
### c. Multiple Dosage Forms
  i. Tablets: sumatriptan (Imitrex); naratriptan (Amerge); rizatriptan (Maxalt, Maxalt XLT); zolmitriptan (Zomig, Zomig ZMT); frovatriptan (Frova); eletriptan (Relpax); almotriptan (Axert).
  ii. Injectable: sumatriptan (Imitrex).
  iii. Nasal spray: sumatriptan (Imitrex); zolmitriptan (Zomig).
### d. Adverse reactions are due to vasoconstriction properties
  i. Cardiovascular reactions include arrhythmias, chest pain, angina, and MI in patients with a history of coronary artery disease.
  ii. Other adverse reactions include tingling, flushing, nausea, and dizziness.
  iii. Injection adverse reactions include a warm, tingling sensation; feeling of chest heaviness; and irritation at the injection site.
### e. Drug Interactions
  i. Ergotamine derivatives increase vasoconstriction.
  ii. SSRIs may increase risk of serotonin syndrome.
    1. Serotonin syndrome symptoms include myoclonus, hyperreflexia, tremors.
  iii. MAOIs inhibit metabolism of triptans, markedly increasing levels and leading to dangerous vasoconstrictor effects, except with naratriptan.
### f. Contraindications
  i. Coronary artery disease.
  ii. Uncontrolled HTN.
  iii. Ischemic heart disease.
  iv. Concurrent MAOI therapy or within 2 weeks of discontinuing MAOIs.
  v. Use of ergotamine within previous 24 hours.

# ANTIBIOTICS

## I. BETA-LACTAM ANTIBIOTICS
### a. General
  i. Mechanism of action.
    1. Inhibit the transpeptidase enzyme (penicillin-binding proteins) and prevent cross-linking of peptidoglycan chains, inhibiting bacterial cell wall.
  ii. Resistance.
    1. Develops by production of beta-lactamase that cleaves the beta-lactam ring to inactivate the metabolite.
    2. Alteration in penicillin-binding proteins.
      (a) Decreases penetrability of the cell wall.

iii. Side effects.
1. Type 1 hypersensitivity reaction.
2. Nausea, vomiting, diarrhea, and rash.

**b. Medications**
i. Natural penicillins.
1. Penicillin G (IM) and penicillin V (PO).
(a) Penicillin V is acid stable.
(b) Renally excreted. The addition of probenecid decreases renal secretion and increases blood levels.
(c) Crosses blood–brain barrier with inflammation.
2. Spectrum of activity.
(a) Gram-positive.
(i) Nonresistant *Staphylococcus* and *Streptococcus*, anthrax.
(ii) Enterococcus coverage with aminoglycoside addition.
(b) Gram-negative: *Neisseria meningitidis.*
(c) Anaerobes: *Clostridium* (not *Bacteroides fragilis*).
(d) Spirochetes: *Treponema.*
ii. Anti-staphylococcal penicillinase resistant.
1. Methicillin (IV), nafcillin (IV), oxacillin (IV), dicloxacillin (PO).
(a) Resistant to breakdown by beta-lactamase.
2. Spectrum of activity.
(a) Beta-lactamase–producing *Staphylococcus.*
(b) Not effective against gram-negative organisms.
(c) For methicillin-resistant *Staphylococcus aureus* (MRSA), treat with vancomycin.
3. Side effects.
(a) Type 1 hypersensitivity reaction.
(b) Nausea, vomiting, diarrhea, and rash.
(c) Methicillin can cause interstitial nephritis and is not used clinically.
iii. Extended-spectrum penicillins.
1. Ampicillin (PO, IV), amoxicillin (PO).
2. Spectrum of activity.
(a) Cover *Streptococcus* and have some gram-negative coverage.
(i) *Haemophilus influenzae.*
(ii) *Escherichia coli.*
(iii) *Listeria monocytogenes.*
(iv) *Proteus mirabilis.*
(v) *Salmonella.*
(vi) *Neisseria.*
3. Beta-lactam inhibitors will extend the spectrum of activity.
(a) Clavulanate plus amoxicillin is Augmentin.
(b) Sulbactam plus ampicillin is Unasyn.

4. Side effects.
(a) Ampicillin can lead to diarrhea and pseudomembranous colitis.
(b) Ampicillin rash is noted in patients with infectious mononucleosis taking ampicillin.
(c) Other side effects as noted with other penicillins.
iv. Antipseudomonal penicillin.
1. Ticarcillin (IV), piperacillin (IV).
2. Spectrum of activity.
(a) Cover *Pseudomonas* and some aerobic and anaerobic gram-negative rods.
(i) *E. coli, Proteus, Enterobacter, Citrobacter, Serratia,* and *Klebsiella.*
3. Side effects.
(a) GI disturbances.
(b) Prolonged bleeding time due to platelet dysfunction.
v. Beta-lactamase inhibitors will add additional *Staphylococcus* coverage.
1. Clavulanate plus ticarcillin is Timentin.
2. Tazobactam plus piperacillin is Zosyn.
vi. Monobactams.
1. Aztreonam (IV).
(a) Spectrum of activity.
(i) Active against gram-negative rods, including *Pseudomonas.*
(ii) No activity against gram-positive rods or anaerobes.
(b) Side effects.
(i) While it is a beta-lactam, it is not contraindicated in patients allergic to penicillin or cephalosporins.
(ii) Note GI upset, vertigo, and headache.
vii. Cephalosporins: first generation.
1. Cefazolin (Ancef) (IV); cephalexin (Keflex) (PO); cephalothin (Keflin) (IV); cefadroxil (Duricef) (PO).
2. Spectrum of activity.
(a) Oral cavity anaerobes except *B. fragilis.*
(b) Cover some gram-negatives (use in urinary tract infection [UTI]) such as *E. coli.*
(c) Cover *Streptococcus pneumoniae* and *H. influenzae* but not as well as later generations of cephalosporins.
(i) Avoid first-generation cephalosporins in treating upper respiratory tract infections.
(d) Cover *Staphylococcus* but not MRSA.
(e) Cefazolin is regularly used in surgical prophylaxis.
3. Side effects.

(a) Diarrhea.

(b) Hypersensitivity reactions.

(c) Fever.

(d) Increased liver function tests (LFTs), neutropenia, and thrombocytopenia are seen but are uncommon.

(e) Avoid alcohol as it may cause a disulfiram-like reaction.

viii. Cephalosporins: second generation.

1. Cefaclor (Ceclor) (PO); loracarbef (Lorabid) (PO); cefoxitin (Mefoxin) (IV); cefuroxime (Zinacef, IV) (Ceftin, PO); cefotetan (Cefotan) (IV); cefprozil (Cefzil) (PO).

2. Spectrum of activity.

(a) Increased activity against *S. pneumoniae* and *H. influenzae*.

(i) Cefuroxime is the best for upper respiratory infection/sinusitis.

(b) Active against anaerobic infection, including *B. fragilis*.

(i) Cefoxitin and cefotetan provide the best coverage and are used in pelvic inflammatory disease (PID).

(c) Covers same gram-negatives as first generation plus *H. influenzae*, *Enterobacter*, *Klebsiella*, *Proteus*, and *Neisseria* species.

3. Side effects are the same as first generation.

ix. Cephalosporins: third generation.

1. Ceftriaxone (Rocephin) (IV); cefixime (Suprax) (PO); ceftizoxime (Cefizox) (IV); ceftazidime (Fortaz) (IV); cefpodoxime (Vantin) (PO).

2. Spectrum of activity.

(a) Activity against *S. pneumoniae* and *H. influenzae*.

(b) Good penetration of CNS so used to treat meningitis.

(c) Ceftriaxone is used to treat *Neisseria gonorrhoeae*.

(d) Cover *Pseudomonas* with ceftazidime and cefepime.

(e) Activity against methicillin-sensitive *S. aureus*.

3. Side effects.

(a) Same as first and second generations.

(b) Increased risk of enterococcal superinfection.

(c) Ceftriaxone can lead to gallstones with long-term use.

x. Cephalosporins: fourth and fifth generations.

1. Cefepime (Maxipime) (IV) is a fourth-generation cephalosporin.

(a) Spectrum of activity.

(i) Gram-negative bacilli including *Pseudomonas*.

(ii) *S. pneumoniae*.

(b) Side effects.

(c) Same as other groups.

2. Ceftaroline fosamil (Teflaro) (IV) is a fifth-generation cephalosporin.

(a) Active against MRSA and *S. pneumoniae*.

xi. Carbapenems.

1. Imipenem plus cilastatin (IV); meropenem (IV).

(a) Cilastatin inhibits breakdown of imipenem in the kidney.

(b) Imipenem used for urinary tract infections, pneumonia, intra-abdominal infections, and skin infections.

(c) Meropenem used intra-abdominal infections, skin infections, and meningitis.

2. Spectrum of activity.

(a) Are very broad spectrum covering most gram-positive, gram-negative, and anaerobes.

(i) Covers 90% of clinically important bacteria.

(b) Meropenem has increased activity against *Pseudomonas*.

3. Side effects.

(a) Can cause seizures and GI upset

xii. Vancomycin

1. Mechanism of action.

(a) Is a glycoprotein that binds to portion of cell wall precursors, D-alanyl-D-alanine, preventing elongation of peptidoglycan strands and halting cell wall synthesis.

(b) Is bactericidal against most bacteria, except *Enterococcus*.

2. Spectrum of activity.

(a) Covers *S. aureus* (including MRSA), *Staphylococcus epidermidis*, *Streptococcus*, *Corynebacterium diphtheriae*, and *Clostridium* species.

(b) Used in the treatment of endocarditis, osteomyelitis, and necrotizing fasciitis.

(c) PO vancomycin used in the treatment of pseudomembranous colitis.

(i) PO vancomycin not absorbed systemically, so no side effects.

(d) No coverage against gram-negative organisms.

3. Side effects.

(a) Red man syndrome.

(i) Rash, flushing, tachycardia, hypotension.

(ii) Is due to histamine release.

(iii) No problem if drug is given slowly.

(b) Ototoxicity, which can be permanent.

(c) Nephrotoxicity, which can be increased with other nephrotoxic drugs.

(d) Bone marrow suppression can occur but is rare.

## II. PROTEIN SYNTHESIS INHIBITORS

### a. Chloramphenicol
i. Mechanism of action.
1. Bacteriostatic and binds to 50S ribosomal subunit.
2. Metabolized in the liver and enters CNS.
(a) Good choice for brain abscess.
ii. Spectrum of activity.
1. Kills most gram-positive, gram-negative, and anaerobes.
2. Effective against *Rickettsia* infections, such as Rocky Mountain spotted fever.
iii. Side effects.
1. Major side effect is bone marrow suppression and aplastic anemia.
2. Gray baby syndrome may develop and is due to inability to metabolize drug to inactive metabolite.
(a) Present with shock, abdominal distention, and cyanosis.
3. Use of medication has decreased due to severe side effects.

### b. Tetracycline
i. Are short-acting and long-acting agents.
1. Tetracycline is short acting with a half-life of 6 to 12 hours.
2. Doxycycline and minocycline are long acting with half-lives of 16 to 18 hours.
ii. Mechanism of action.
1. Bacteriostatic and reversibly bind to 30S ribosomal subunit.
2. Crosses the placenta and is noted in breast milk.
3. Binds to calcium and antacids.
(a) Inhibits absorption of the drug.
4. Renal excretion.
(a) Doxycycline eliminated non-renally, so safe in renal failure.
iii. Spectrum of activity.
1. Covers gram-positive and gram-negative, but not drug of choice due to increased resistance.
2. Covers the following:
(a) Rickettsial infections.
(b) Spirochete infections (Lyme disease).
(c) *Mycoplasma pneumoniae*.
(d) Chlamydial infection.
(e) Minocycline used for acne.
iv. Side effects.

1. Hepatotoxicity.
2. GI upset including diarrhea, nausea, and vomiting.
3. Phototoxic dermatitis.
4. Discolored teeth and decreased bone growth.
(a) Drug contraindicated in children under age 8 and in pregnant women.
5. Use of outdated or expired drug can lead to Fanconi's syndrome.
(a) Disease of the proximal renal tubules in which substances are passed in the urine instead of being reabsorbed.

### c. Macrolides
i. Medications.
1. Erythromycin (E-Mycin).
2. Clarithromycin (Biaxin).
3. Azithromycin (Zithromax).
4. Fidaxomicin (Dificid).
ii. Mechanism of action.
1. Bacteriostatic; bind to 50S ribosomal subunit.
2. Metabolized in the liver.
3. Azithromycin concentrates in tissue and releases slowly over prolonged period.
(a) This gives azithromycin a very long half-life, about 72 hours, and only needs to be given for 5 days instead of 7 days.
iii. Spectrum of activity.
1. Group A *Streptococcus*, *S. pneumoniae*, *Chlamydia*, *Mycoplasma*, *Haemophilus*, and *Legionella*.
2. Clarithromycin or azithromycin also used in the treatment of *Mycobacterium avium* complex.
3. Fidaxomicin used in treatment of *Clostridium difficile*.
iv. Side effects.
1. GI side effects include nausea, diarrhea, and cholestatic hepatitis.
2. Erythromycin and clarithromycin inhibit CYP 450.
(a) Can lead to an increase in other drug levels if metabolized in liver, such as theophylline, warfarin, and digoxin.
3. Can develop acute ergot toxicity when combined with ergot derivatives.
4. Can prolong QTc interval leading to arrhythmia.

### d. Aminoglycosides
i. Medications include the following:
1. Gentamicin.
2. Tobramycin.
3. Amikacin.
4. Streptomycin.

5. Neomycin combined with polymyxin for topical use in superficial infections.

ii. Mechanism of action.

1. Are bactericidal; bind to 30S ribosomal subunit and inhibit bacterial protein synthesis, resulting in cell death.

2. Antibiotic enters bacteria by oxygen-dependent active transport.

   (a) Are not effective against anaerobes.

3. Due to poor PO absorption, drugs not given PO.

4. Eliminated by the kidneys.

iii. Spectrum of activity.

1. Aerobic gram-negative.

   (a) Tobramycin more active against *Pseudomonas*.

      (i) Used as inhaled drug in cystic fibrosis.

2. Amikacin reserved for the most serious infections.

3. Endocarditis due to *Enterococcus*, in combination with a penicillin.

   (a) Must combine with cell wall inhibitor to be effective against gram-positives.

4. Streptomycin used to treat tuberculosis, mycobacterium avium, brucellosis, plague, tularemia, and rat bite fever.

iv. Side effects.

1. Ototoxicity.

2. Hearing loss (usually irreversible), tinnitus, vertigo, ataxia.

3. Nephrotoxicity.

4. Acute tubular necrosis.

   (a) Monitor serum creatinine while on medication, and adjust dose as needed.

e. **Clindamycin**

i. Can be given via multiple routes: PO, IV, topically.

ii. Mechanism of action.

1. Is bacteriostatic; binds to 50S ribosomal subunit to inhibit bacterial protein synthesis.

iii. Spectrum of activity.

1. Gram-positive and anaerobic bacteria.

2. Anaerobes above the diaphragm.

3. MRSA (most strains).

4. Will cover *Streptococcus pyogenes*.

5. Treatment of pneumocystis pneumonia and toxoplasmosis.

6. Alternative agent to penicillin and cephalosporin in penicillin-allergic patients.

iv. Side effects.

1. Abdominal pain, nausea, vomiting, rash, pruritus.

2. Pseudomembranous colitis due to infection with *C. difficile*.

f. **Linezolid**

i. Mechanism of action.

1. Inhibits protein synthesis by binding to the 50S subunit.

ii. Spectrum of activity.

1. MRSA, vancomycin-resistant *Enterococcus*, *Corynebacterium*, *Listeria*.

iii. Side effects.

1. GI upset, diarrhea, headache, rash, thrombocytopenia.

## III. FLUOROQUINOLONES

a. **Medications**

i. Levofloxacin (Levaquin).

ii. Moxifloxacin (Avelox).

iii. Ciprofloxacin (Cipro).

b. **Mechanism of Action**

i. Are bactericidal; bind to and inhibit bacterial enzyme DNA gyrase (topoisomerase II), resulting in inability of bacterial DNA to supercoil; and inhibit DNA replication and RNA transcription.

ii. Undergo hepatic biotransformation and are excreted unchanged in the urine.

iii. Moxifloxacin is not eliminated by the kidneys.

iv. PO absorption is decreased with ingestion of dairy products and antacids.

c. **Spectrum of Activity**

i. Broad spectrum.

1. Aerobic gram-positive and gram-negative bacteria.

ii. Urinary tract infections/prostatitis.

1. Due to gram-negative rods plus *Pseudomonas*.

iii. Anaerobic infections use moxifloxacin.

iv. Traveler's diarrhea.

1. Due to *Shigella*, *Salmonella*, *E. coli* or *Campylobacter*.

v. Upper respiratory tract infections.

1. Due to pneumococci, *Chlamydia*, *Mycoplasma*, *Haemophilus*, *Legionella*.

vi. Some coverage of *Mycobacterium*.

vii. Treatment of anthrax.

d. **Side Effects**

i. Nausea, headache, dizziness, hepatitis.

ii. Photosensitivity, prolonged QTc interval, can lead to ventricular tachycardia.

iii. Damage to growing cartilage.

1. Contraindicated in children (<18 years of age) and during pregnancy.

iv. Except for ciprofloxacin used to treat anthrax and pneumonia in children with cystic fibrosis.

v. Multiple drug interactions including theophylline, phenytoin, and warfarin.

## IV. ANTIFOLATE DRUGS
  **a. Medications**
    i. Sulfacetamide (Sulamyd) (topical).
    ii. Sulfadiazine (PO or topical).
    iii. Sulfamethoxazole (PO).
    iv. Folate reductase inhibitors.
      1. Trimethoprim (PO).
      2. Trimethoprim-sulfamethoxazole (Bactrim) (PO, IV).
  **b. Mechanism of Action**
    i. Decreased production of essential cofactors for the synthesis of DNA, RNA, and proteins through the blockage of tetrahydrofolic acid production.
      1. Folate reductase inhibitors inhibit dihydrofolate reductase.
    ii. Sulfonamides compete with para-aminobenzoic acid in folate synthesis.
  **c. Spectrum of Activity**
    i. Gram-positive: *S. pneumoniae*.
      1. Gram-negative: *H. influenzae, E. coli, Shigella,* and *Salmonella*.
    ii. Other: *Pneumocystis, Toxoplasmosis*.
  **d. Side Effects**
    i. Allergic skin rash and possible Stevens-Johnson syndrome.
    ii. Kernicterus.
      1. Displacement of bilirubin, which then penetrates the CNS.
    iii. Trimethoprim-sulfamethoxazole can cause GI upset, nausea, vomiting, bone marrow suppression.
    iv. Avoid during pregnancy due to fetotoxicity.
    v. Multiple drug interactions.
      1. Use with thiazides can lead to thrombocytopenia and bruising.
      2. Use with PO hypoglycemic agents can potentiate hypoglycemia.

## V. METRONIDAZOLE
  **a. Mechanism of Action**
    i. Is bactericidal; drug reduced to toxic agents that bind intracellular macromolecules.
    ii. Is metabolized in the liver.
  **b. Spectrum of Activity**
    i. Active against nearly all anaerobic and microaerophilic bacteria, including *B. fragilis*.
    ii. Used in treatment of *C. difficile* colitis.
    iii. Antiparasitic coverage including *Entamoeba, Giardia,* and *Trichomonas*.
  **c. Side Effects**
    i. Disulfiram reaction.
      1. Nausea and vomiting when used with alcohol.
    ii. Carcinogenic potential.

    iii. Metallic taste.
    iv. Pancreatitis.

## VI. NITROFURANTOIN
  **a. Medications**
    i. Macrobid.
    ii. Macrodantin.
  **b. Mechanism of Action**
    i. Inhibits several bacterial enzyme systems interfering with metabolism and possibly cell wall synthesis.
      1. Rapidly excreted in the urine.
  **c. Spectrum of Activity**
    i. Treats UTIs due to *E. coli, Enterococcus,* and *Staphylococcus saprophyticus*.
    ii. Safe in pregnancy except at term.
      1. May cause hemolytic disease of the newborn.
  **d. Side Effects**
    i. Nausea and vomiting, hemolytic anemia in patients with G-6-PD deficiency, pulmonary and hepatic toxicity, and lupus like syndrome.

# ANTITUBERCULOSIS DRUGS

## I. ISONIAZID
  **a. Mechanism of Action**
    i. Is bactericidal; inhibits synthesis of mycolic acid in the mycobacterial cell wall.
  **b. Side Effects**
    i. Hepatic impairment.
      1. Can lead to hepatitis. Need to monitor AST/ALT.
    ii. Peripheral neuropathy.
      1. Rare at standard doses.
      2. Minimize with administration of pyridoxine (B6).
    iii. Abdominal pain, nausea, and vomiting.
    iv. Drug-induced lupus.
    v. Increases toxicity from phenytoin and theophylline when used in combination.

## II. RIFAMPIN
  **a. Mechanism of Action**
    i. Bactericidal; inhibits DNA-dependent RNA polymerase.
      1. Also used to treat carriers of *N. meningitidis*.
  **b. Side Effects**
    i. Nausea, vomiting, and elevated LFTs.
      1. Increased risk when combined with INH.
    ii. Induces CYP 450 and increases metabolism of many drugs, including warfarin, birth control pills (BCP), phenytoin, beta-blockers, and digoxin.

iii. Can cause orange discoloration of body fluids.

iv. Can lead to pseudomembranous colitis.

### III. PYRAZINAMIDE

a. **Mechanism of Action**

   i. Bactericidal; unknown mechanism.

   ii. Works best in the acid environment.

b. **Side Effects**

   i. Liver toxic and can cause hyperuricemia.

   ii. Along with streptomycin, not used in pregnancy.

### IV. ETHAMBUTOL

a. **Mechanism of Action**

   i. Bacteriostatic; inhibits the enzyme involved in synthesis of cell wall.

   ii. Eliminated mainly by the kidneys.

b. **Side Effects**

   i. Optic neuropathy with diminished visual acuity and loss of color vision.

## ANTIVIRAL RESPIRATORY AGENTS

### I. ZANAMIVIR (RELENZA)

a. **Used in the treatment of influenza A and B**

b. **Competes with viral enzyme neuraminidase, which is needed to release the virus**

c. **No Major Side Effects**

   i. Some risk of bronchospasm.

### II. OSELTAMIVIR (TAMIFLU)

a. **Similar to zanamivir, used to treat influenza A and B**

   i. Same mechanism of action.

b. **Side effects include mild nausea and vomiting**

### III. RIBAVIRIN (VIRAZOLE)

a. **Inhibits viral messenger RNA formation**

b. **Used in the treatment of influenza A and B, respiratory syncytial virus, and hepatitis A, B, and C**

c. **Side Effects**

   i. Hemolytic anemia, headache, nausea.

   ii. Is teratogenetic and mutagenetic.

     1. Contraindicated in pregnancy.

## HUMAN IMMUNODEFICIENCY VIRUS (HIV) DRUGS

### I. NUCLEOSIDE REVERSE TRANSCRIPTASE INHIBITORS (NRTIs)

a. **Mechanism of Action**

   i. Inhibit reverse transcriptase and are incorporated into viral DNA causing chain termination.

     1. This class of medication is part of most HIV drug regimens.

     2. Are used together with protease inhibitors (PIs).

   ii. Highly active antiretroviral therapy (HAART) often results in decreased viral load, increases in CD4 cell count, and decreased opportunistic infections.

b. **Medications**

   i. Zidovudine (AZT).

   ii. Lamivudine (3TC).

   iii. Didanosine (DDI).

   iv. Abacavir (ABC).

   v. Stavudine (D4T).

   vi. Tenofovir (TDF).

c. **Side Effects**

   i. Bone marrow suppression (AZT).

   ii. Headache (AZT).

   iii. Pancreatitis (DDI).

   iv. Peripheral neuropathy (DDI).

### II. NONNUCLEOSIDE REVERSE TRANSCRIPTASE INHIBITORS (NNRTIs)

a. **Mechanism of Action**

   i. Inhibits reverse transcriptase and also incorporated into viral DNA causing chain termination.

     1. Bind to a different site than NRTIs.

   ii. Do not require metabolic activation.

b. **Medications**

   i. Nevirapine.

   ii. Efavirenz.

     1. Is the preferred agent.

   iii. Etravirine.

   iv. Delavirdine.

   v. Rilpivirine (RPV)

   vi. Doravirine (DOR)

c. **Side Effects**

   i. All cause a rash.

   ii. Efavirenz causes vivid dreams.

   iii. Are not myelosuppressant.

### III. PROTEASE INHIBITORS

a. **Mechanism of Action**

   i. Bind to the enzyme aspartate protease inhibiting this enzyme and limiting protein formation in the mature virus core.

   ii. Resistance occurs via specific point mutations.

b. **Medications**

   i. Atazanavir.

   ii. Saquinavir.

   iii. Ritonavir.

   iv. Fosamprenavir.

   v. Nelfinavir.

   vi. Indinavir.

vii. Darunavir (DRV).

viii. Tipranavir (TPV).

c. **Side Effects**

i. All cause nausea, vomiting, and diarrhea.

ii. Lipodystrophy and hyperlipidemia.

iii. Ritonavir has multiple drug interactions.

iv. Indinavir leads to crystalluria.

# CARDIAC DRUGS

## I. DIURETICS

a. **General**

i. Lower blood pressure primarily by depleting body of sodium and reducing blood volume.

1. Will see a 10 to 15 mm Hg reduction in blood pressure in most patients.

ii. Most effective in low-renin or volume-expanded forms of HTN.

b. **Classes**

i. Thiazides.

ii. Loops.

iii. Potassium-sparing/aldosterone antagonists (AA).

c. **Thiazide Diuretics**

i. Mechanism of action.

1. Bind to $Na^+/Cl^-$ cotransporter in distal tubules and inhibit the reabsorption of $Na^+$ and $Cl^-$, which result in increased urinary excretion of $Na^+$, $Cl^-$ and $H_2O$.

2. Have direct arteriolar vasodilatory effect.

3. Not effective in renal dysfunction (CrCl <30 mL/min).

(a) Except in combination with loop diuretics.

ii. Benefits.

1. Provides diuresis generally within 4 to 6 hours.

iii. Indications.

1. Used in the treatment of HTN, mild heart failure, and lithium-induced diabetes insipidus.

iv. Medications.

1. Chlorothiazide (Diuril).

2. Chlorthalidone.

3. Hydrochlorothiazide (HCTZ).

4. Indapamide (Lozol).

5. Metolazone (Zaroxolyn).

v. Adverse effects.

1. Electrolyte disturbances.

(a) Decreases in potassium, sodium, and magnesium.

(b) Increases calcium and uric acid.

(i) Use is contraindicated in patients with gout.

2. Dehydration.

3. Sexual dysfunction.

4. Induction of new-onset diabetes with long-term use.

5. Hyperlipidemia

d. **Loop Diuretics**

i. Mechanism of action.

1. Inhibit apical $Na^+$-$K^+$-$Cl^-$ cotransporter in thick ascending loop of Henle, thereby increasing their excretion, results in loss of concentrating ability of the kidneys.

2. Loss of electrostatic driving force also increases excretion of calcium, magnesium, and ammonium.

3. Powerful with rapid onset.

(a) Diuresis noted in 30 to 60 minutes.

ii. Use in HTN only as an adjunct agent.

iii. Generally used only in severe HTN, when multiple drugs with sodium-retaining properties are used, in renal insufficiency (GFR <30–40), and/or CHF exacerbations.

iv. Medications.

1. Bumetanide (Bumex).

2. Furosemide (Lasix).

(a) Note: Furosemide 40 mg PO is equal to Bumetanide 1 mg PO. With IV, the ratio is 20:1.

3. Torsemide (Demadex).

4. Ethacrynic acid (Edecrin).

v. Adverse effects.

1. Hypokalemia.

2. Hypomagnesemia.

3. Chronic dilutional hyponatremia.

4. Metabolic alkalosis.

5. Hyperuricemia.

6. Ototoxicity.

e. **Potassium Sparing/Aldosterone Antagonist (AA) Diuretics**

i. Mechanism of action.

1. Potassium-sparing diuretics block apical $Na^+$ channel in principal cells of the cortical collecting duct.

2. Blockade of $Na^+$ entry causes drop in apical membrane potential (less negative), which is driving force for $K^+$ secretion.

3. AA prevent conversion of the receptor to the active form, thereby preventing the action of aldosterone.

4. Can be used in combination with other diuretics to prevent $K^+$ loss.

5. Do not use together (e.g., triamterene + spironolactone) and use with caution with angiotensin-converting enzyme inhibitors (ACEIs)/angiotensin II receptor blockers (ARBs).

6. AAs are good choice for patients with CHF and post-MI.
    (a) AAs are also androgen blockers used to treat hirsutism in polycystic ovarian syndrome.
ii. Medications.
    1. Potassium-sparing.
        (a) Amiloride (Midamor).
        (b) Triamterene (Dyrenium).
    2. AA.
        (a) Eplerenone (Inspra).
        (b) Spironolactone (Aldactone).
iii. Adverse effects.
    1. Hyperkalemia.
    2. Antiandrogen-like effects such as gynecomastia with spironolactone.
    3. GI disturbances and diarrhea.
    4. Leg cramps.

## II. ANGIOTENSIN-CONVERTING ENZYME (ACE) INHIBITORS

**a. Mechanism of Action**
i. Inhibition of angiotensin II formation from angiotensin I, thereby reducing vasoconstriction, sodium retention, and cell proliferation and remodeling.
ii. Most effective in high-renin HTN.

**b. Indications**
i. Drugs of choice in patients with HTN and diabetes mellitus.
ii. Also used in the treatment of CHF, arrhythmias, post MI, and chronic kidney disease.
iii. Most lower blood pressure less than 10 mm Hg. However, these drugs do have important long-term benefits in preventing or reducing renal disease in patients with diabetes mellitus and in reduction of heart failure.

**c. Medications**
i. Benazepril (Lotensin).
ii. Captopril (Capoten).
iii. Enalapril (Vasotec).
iv. Fosinopril (Monopril).
v. Lisinopril (Prinivil, Zestril).
vi. Moexipril (Univasc).
vii. Perindopril (Aceon).
viii. Quinapril (Accupril).
ix. Ramipril (Altace).
x. Trandolapril (Mavik).

**d. Adverse Effects**
i. Cough.
    1. Due to production of bradykinins.
ii. Renal insufficiency in renal artery stenosis.
iii. Hyperkalemia.
iv. Taste alterations, angioedema, and rash.

v. Are contraindicated in pregnancy.
vi. Eliminated by kidneys, except fosinopril and moexipril.
    1. Reduce dose with renal insufficiency.

## III. ANGIOTENSIN II RECEPTOR BLOCKERS (ARBs)

**a. Mechanism of Action**
i. Competitive inhibition of angiotensin II receptors, thereby reducing vasoconstriction and aldosterone effects.
ii. Lack bradykinin effects, so no cough side effect.

**b. Indications**
i. Similar place in therapy to ACEIs.
ii. Benefit in CHF and chronic kidney disease.
iii. Used in patients who cannot tolerate ACEI due to cough.

**c. Medications**
i. Candesartan (Atacand).
ii. Eprosartan (Teveten).
iii. Irbesartan (Avapro).
iv. Losartan (Cozaar).
v. Olmesartan (Benicar).
vi. Telmisartan (Micardis).
vii. Valsartan (Diovan).

**d. Adverse Effects**
i. Teratogenic.
ii. Dizziness.
iii. GI side effects.
iv. Hyperkalemia.
v. Angioedema.

## IV. BETA-BLOCKERS

**a. Mechanism of Action**
i. Beta-adrenoceptor antagonism.
    1. $\beta_1$ receptors are located in the heart and kidneys.
        (a) Blockade decreases force, rate, conduction, and automaticity of heart and decreases renin release from juxtaglomerular cells of kidneys.
    2. $\beta_2$ receptors are located in the lungs, liver, GI tract, and smooth muscle.
        (a) Blockade enhances bronchoconstriction and decreases glycogenolysis and gluconeogenesis.

**b. Indications**
i. Most effective in high-renin HTN.
ii. Indicated in patients with CHF and post MI.
iii. Arrhythmias.
iv. Also used in the treatment of migraine, essential tremor, and anxiety disorders.

**c. Medications**
i. Propranolol (Inderal).

ii. Atenolol (Tenormin).

iii. Carvedilol (Coreg).

iv. Esmolol (Brevibloc).

v. Labetalol (Normodyne).

vi. Metoprolol (Lopressor, Toprol).

vii. Nadolol (Corgard).

viii. Pindolol (Visken).

ix. Timolol (Blocadren).

d. **Adverse Effects**

i. Bronchospasm.

ii. Hypotension.

iii. Heart block.

iv. Hypoglycemia.

v. Lipid abnormalities.

vi. Fatigue.

vii. Sexual dysfunction.

viii. Insomnia.

ix. Depression.

e. **Special Indications**

i. Nonselective affects $\beta_1$ and $\beta_2$ receptors.

1. Propranolol, nadolol, carteolol, timolol.

2. Avoid in patients with asthma, diabetes, or peripheral vascular disease.

ii. Cardioselective affects only $\beta_1$ receptors.

1. Metoprolol, atenolol, nebivolol, betaxolol, bisoprolol, esmolol.

2. Atenolol is hydrophilic so may produce fewer CNS effects.

3. No effects on lungs, GI tract, or diabetes.

iii. Drugs with intrinsic sympathomimetic activity (ISA).

1. Pindolol, acebutolol, penbutolol.

2. Have low-level agonist activity at $\beta$-adrenergic receptor.

3. May be useful in patients with excessive bradyarrhythmias or peripheral vascular disease (PVD).

iv. Drugs with vasodilating effects.

1. Labetalol and carvedilol due to $\alpha_1$ effects; nebivolol due to effects on nitric oxide release.

v. Parenterally available.

1. Labetalol, esmolol, atenolol, metoprolol, propranolol.

2. Labetalol given as needed (PRN) IV boluses to treat hypertensive emergencies.

3. Esmolol has short half-life so given via continuous infusion for perioperative HTN and hypertensive emergencies.

4. Metoprolol has long half-life so is not generally given IV to treat HTN, but rather for heart rate (HR) control.

vi. Mortality benefit in CHF.

1. Metoprolol succinate, carvedilol, bisoprolol, and nebivolol benefit patients with CHF.

## V. ALPHA-BLOCKERS

a. **Mechanism of Action**

i. Blockade of vascular alpha-adrenoceptor.

1. Prevent sympathetic vasoconstriction and lead to dilation of both peripheral arterioles and veins.

2. Also relax smooth muscles in the prostate and bladder neck.

ii. $\alpha_1$ receptors located in blood vessels, GI sphincters, and male sex organs.

iii. $\alpha_2$ receptors located in blood vessels, GI smooth muscle, and adrenergic nerve terminals.

b. **Selective $\alpha_1$ Blockers**

i. Medications.

1. Prazosin (Minipress).

2. Terazosin (Hytrin).

3. Doxazosin (Cardura).

ii. Indications.

1. Monotherapy or adjunctive therapy in HTN.

2. More commonly used to treat benign prostatic hypertrophy.

iii. Adverse effects.

1. First dose for hypotension and syncope, tachycardia, dizziness, dry mouth, salt and water retention when used without a diuretic.

c. **Nonselective Alpha-Blockers**

i. Medications.

1. Phentolamine, phenoxybenzamine.

ii. Indications.

1. Used to treat hypertensive crisis in pheochromocytoma.

iii. Adverse effects.

1. Postural hypotension, reflex tachycardia, fluid retention, and diarrhea.

2. Contraindicated in patients with decreased coronary perfusion.

## VI. CALCIUM CHANNEL BLOCKERS (CCBs)

a. **Mechanism of Action**

i. Block "L" type calcium channels located in cardiac and smooth muscle.

ii. Effects on vascular smooth muscle leads to coronary and peripheral vascular relaxation which leads to decreased blood pressure and reduced cardiac afterload.

iii. Effects on cardiac muscle cells lead to decreased contractility.

1. Certain CCBs also decrease heart rate (HR) (nondihydropyridines).

b. **Indications**

i. Most effective in low-renin HTN.

c. **Nondihydropyridine**

i. Have vasodilatory, negative chronotropic, and negative inotropic effects.

ii. Often used to treat angina and arrhythmias.
    1. Avoid use in acute MI and heart failure.

iii. Adverse effects.
    1. Constipation, flushing.
    2. Atrioventricular (AV) block, may worsen heart failure, hypotension, and bradycardia with IV formulations.

iv. Medications.
    1. Verapamil (Calan, Isoptin, Verelan).
      (a) Least selective CCB.
      (b) Avoid use with beta-blockers.
    2. Diltiazem (Cardizem).
      (a) Less pronounced negative inotropic effect than verapamil.
      (b) More favorable side-effect profile.

d. **Dihydropyridine CCBs**

i. Medications.
    1. Amlodipine (Norvasc).
    2. Felodipine (Plendil).
    3. Isradipine (DynaCirc).
    4. Nicardipine (Cardene).
    5. Nifedipine (Adalat, Procardia).
    6. Nisoldipine (Sular).
    7. Clevidipine (Cleviprex).

ii. Indications.
    1. More selective vasodilators.
    2. Decrease afterload and increase reflex in sympathetic stimulation of heart.
    3. Increase contractility and HR, increasing cardiac output.

iii. Adverse effects.
    1. Peripheral edema, flushing, headache, nausea, reflex tachycardia, dizziness, and constipation.

## VII. DIRECT VASODILATORS

a. **Hydralazine**

i. Mechanism of action.
    1. Release of nitric oxide from endothelial cells.
    2. Dilation of arteries and arterioles. Leads to decreased peripheral vascular resistance.
    3. Use in combination with other agents (beta-blockers, diuretics, and nitrates) in heart failure.

ii. Adverse effects.
    1. Tachycardia with palpitations.
    2. Hypotension.
    3. Dry mouth, headache, nausea, edema.
    4. Drug-induced lupus-like syndrome with prolonged use or high doses.

b. **Minoxidil**

i. Mechanism of action.

    1. Opening of $K^+$ channels in smooth muscle stabilizes membrane, making contraction less likely; affects arterioles.

ii. Used in severe HTN as add-on agent.

iii. Adverse effects
    1. Tachycardia, angina, edema.
    2. Headache, edema.
    3. Hypertrichosis.

c. **Sodium Nitroprusside**

i. Used IV only in hypertensive emergencies and severe heart failure.

ii. Mechanism of action.
    1. Dilation of arterial and venous vessels due to activation of guanylyl cyclase via nitric oxide release.
    2. Increased intracellular cyclic guanosine monophosphate (cGMP), causing vascular relaxation.
    3. Short acting.

iii. Adverse effects.
    1. Tachycardia, sweating, nausea.
    2. Psychosis.
    3. Cyanide toxicity from metabolite.
      (a) If used for prolonged periods or high doses.

d. **Diazoxide**

i. Used IV only.

ii. Mechanism of action.
    1. Similar to minoxidil.

iii. Adverse effects.
    1. Excessive hypotension and reflex sympathetic response.
      (a) Avoid in ischemic heart disease.

## VIII. CENTRALLY ACTING AGENTS

a. **Alpha-Methyldopa (Aldomet)**

i. Mechanism of action.
    1. Prodrug taken up by central adrenergic neurons; converted to $\alpha_2$ adrenoceptor agonist, alpha-methylnorepinephrine.
    2. Reduced adrenergic outflow from CNS leads to reduction in peripheral vascular resistance.

ii. Indications.
    1. HTN during pregnancy.
    2. Patients with renal insufficiency.
      (a) Does not reduce blood flow to kidneys.

iii. Adverse effects.
    1. Sedation, depression.
    2. Lactation due to increased prolactin.
    3. Positive direct Coombs' test.

b. **Clonidine (Catapres)**

i. Mechanism of action.
    1. Central $\alpha_2$ agonist.

2. $\alpha_2$ stimulation in the brain stem reduces sympathetic tone, causing centrally mediated vasodilation, reduction in HR, and reduction in blood pressure.
 ii. Typically an adjunctive agent.
  1. Good in patients with renal insufficiency.
  2. Also available as weekly patch (Catapres-TTS).
 iii. Adverse effects.
  1. Dry mouth, sedation, depression, vivid dreams.
  2. Abrupt withdrawal can lead to a hypertensive crisis.
   (a) Dose must be tapered.
  3. Skin reactions with the patch.
 iv. Other indications.
  1. Used in opioid withdrawal.
   (a) Decreases sympathetic tone.
  2. Migraine prophylaxis
  3. Restless leg syndrome.

## IX. NITROGLYCERIN/NITRATES

a. **Mechanism of Action**
 i. Formation of nitric oxide leads to activation of guanylyl cyclase, which increases cGMP. This in turn decreases cytosolic free calcium ion and causes vascular smooth muscle relaxation.
 ii. Reduces preload and afterload and dilates coronary arteries.

b. **Absorption**
 i. PO.
  1. Undergoes first-pass effect so bioavailability is low (<10% to 20%).
 ii. Sublingual.
  1. Avoids first-pass effect but has a short duration of action, only 15 to 30 minutes.
 iii. Contraindicated in patients with previous hypersensitivity.

c. **Side Effects**
 i. Headache, flushing.
 ii. Hypotension. (Do not use if systolic blood pressure less than 80–90 mm Hg.)
 iii. Reflex tachycardia.
 iv. Reflex increase in contractility.
 v. Drug interaction with phosphodiesterase inhibitors.
  1. May result in severe hypotension and death.

## X. ANTIARRHYTHMICS

a. **Class 1**
 i. Sodium channel blockers.
 ii. Have varying speed of channel blocking.

b. **Class 2**
 i. Beta-blockers.
  1. Decrease HR and slow phase 4 depolarization.

  2. Good for atrial arrhythmias and tachycardias.

c. **Class 3**
 i. Potassium channel blockers.
  1. Prolong phase 3 repolarization and may have some beta-blocking effects.
  2. Good for atrial arrhythmias and ventricular reentrant arrhythmias.
  3. Can cause torsades de pointes.

d. **Class 4**
 i. Calcium channel blockers.
 ii. Good for atrial arrhythmia and ventricular tachycardia.

e. **See Table 15.2**

## XI. DIGITALIS (DIGOXIN)

a. **Mechanism of Action**
 i. Influences sodium and calcium ion flow in cardiac muscle, increasing contraction of atrial and ventricular myocardium and ejection fraction, and has a positive inotropic effect.

b. **Used in treatment of left-sided heart failure**
 i. Not indicated in right-sided heart failure.
 ii. Used in patients with heart failure and atrial fibrillation.

c. **Side Effects**
 i. Arrhythmia by slowing AV conduction.
 ii. Anorexia, nausea, and vomiting.
 iii. Headache and alteration in color perception.

d. **Increased toxicity noted with hypokalemia, quinidine, verapamil, amiodarone, and hypothyroidism, as well as in patients with renal failure**

# ENDOCRINE DRUGS

## I. INSULIN

a. **Mechanism of Action**
 i. Released from the beta cells of the pancreas.
 ii. Lowers glucose by stimulating peripheral glucose uptake in the skeletal muscles and fat, and by inhibiting hepatic glucose production.

b. **Indications**
 i. Used in the treatment of diabetes mellitus types I and II and diabetic ketoacidosis (Table 15.3).

c. **Side Effects**
 i. Hypoglycemia, edema, and lipoatrophy.

## II. BIGUANIDES

a. **Mechanism of Action**
 i. Decrease hepatic glucose production and intestinal absorption of glucose and improve insulin sensitivity.

**TABLE 15.2**

| Antiarrhythmia Agents | | | | |
| --- | --- | --- | --- | --- |
| Class | Mechanism | Agents | EKG Effect | Indications |
| I | Sodium channel blockers | | | |
| IA | Intermediate kinetics | Disopyramide<br>Quinidine<br>Procainamide | Increased QRS interval<br>Increased QT interval | Atrial fibrillation<br>Atrial flutter<br>Ventricular tachycardia |
| IB | Rapid kinetics | Lidocaine<br>Tocainide<br>Mexiletine<br>Phenytoin | Decreased QT interval | Ventricular tachycardia |
| IC | Slow kinetics | Moricizine<br>Flecainide<br>Propafenone | Increased QRS interval | Atrial fibrillation<br>Atrial flutter<br>Ventricular tachycardia<br>AV nodal reentrant tachycardia |
| II | Beta-blockers | Propranolol<br>Esmolol<br>Timolol<br>Metoprolol<br>Atenolol | Decreased heart rate<br>Increased PR interval | Sinus tachycardia<br>SA and AV nodal reentrant tachy-<br>cardia |
| III | Potassium channel blockers | Amiodarone<br>Bretylium<br>Dofetilide<br>Ibutilide<br>Sotalol | Increased QT interval | Ventricular tachycardia<br>Atrial fibrillation<br>Atrial flutter<br>AV nodal reentrant tachycardia |
| IV | Calcium channel blockers | Verapamil<br>Diltiazem | Decreased heart rate<br>Increased PR interval | SA and AV nodal reentrant tachy-<br>cardia |

*AV*, Atrioventricular; *EKG*, electrocardiogram; *SA*, sinoatrial.

**TABLE 15.3**

| Insulin | | | | |
| --- | --- | --- | --- | --- |
| Type | | Onset (hour) | Peak (hour) | Duration (hour) |
| Aspart<br>Glulisine<br>Lispro | Rapid-acting | 0.25–0.50 | 0.5–2 | 3–4 |
| Regular | Short-acting | 0.5–1 | 2–3 | 3–6 |
| NPH | Intermediate | 2–4 | 6–10 | 10–16 |
| Lente | Intermediate | 1.5–3 | 7–15 | 16–24 |
| Ultralente | Long-acting | 3–4 | 9–15 | 22–28 |
| Glargine | Long-acting | 4 | No peak | 24–36 |

   b. **Indications**
      i. Drug of choice for initial therapy.
   c. **Side Effects**
      i. Include diarrhea, vomiting, and weight loss.
      ii. Contraindicated in renal disease (creatinine >1.5 mg/dL), active liver disease, decompensated heart failure, metabolic acidosis.
      iii. Hold in patients undergoing a radiologic procedure involving contrast media.
   d. **Medications**
      i. Glucophage (Metformin)

### III. SULFONYLUREAS
   a. **Mechanism of Action**
      i. Lowers glucose by stimulating insulin release from the beta cells of the islet cells of the pancreas.
      ii. Use cautiously in patients with renal and hepatic impairment.
      iii. Start with low doses and titrate upward according to patient response.
      iv. Lowers hemoglobin A1c by 1% to 2%.
   b. **Medications**
      i. Glimepiride (Amaryl).
      ii. Glipizide (Glucotrol).
      iii. Glyburide (Micronase).
         1. Can be used in pregnancy.
      iv. Chlorpropamide (Diabinese).
         1. Has a very long half-life.
      v. Tolazamide (Tolinase).
      vi. Tolbutamide (Orinase).
         1. Safe in renal dysfunction.

### IV. THIAZOLIDINEDIONES
   a. **Mechanism of Action**
      i. Decrease insulin resistance by enhancing insulin receptor sensitivity.
      ii. Typically used in combination therapy.

iii. Reduces hemoglobin A1c by 1% to 1.5%.
b. Side Effects
  i. Hypoglycemia, weight gain, edema,
  ii. Contraindicated in heart failure and liver failure.
c. Medications
  i. Pioglitazone (Actos).
  ii. Rosiglitazone (Avandia).
d. Side Effects
  i. Use increases risk of MI, so use with caution in patients with previous MI.

## V. ALPHA-GLUCOSIDASE INHIBITORS
a. Medications
  i. Acarbose (Precose).
b. Mechanism of Action
  i. Delays postprandial digestion of sugars.
c. Side Effects
  i. Nausea and diarrhea.

## VI. GLUCAGON-LIKE PEPTIDE-1 RECEPTOR AGONIST
a. Medications
  i. Exenatide (Byetta).
b. Mechanism of Action
  i. Enhances glucose-dependent insulin secretion by the pancreatic beta-cell.
c. Side Effects
  i. Thyroid cancer, pancreatitis, renal impairment.

## VII. SODIUM-GLUCOSE CO-TRANSPORTER 2 INHIBITORS
a. Medications.
  i. Empagliflozin (Jardiance), dapagliflozin (Farxiga), canagliflozin (Invokana).
  ii. Not considered first line therapy.
  iii. Consider in diabetes with cardiovascular disease or heart failure.
b. Mechanism of action.
  i. Reduce blood glucose by increasing urinary glucose excretion.
c. Side effects.
  i. Includes genitourinary tract infection, bladder cancer, hypotension, acute kidney injury, and bone fracture.

# LIPID-LOWERING AGENTS

## I. BILE ACID–BINDING RESINS
a. Mechanism of Action
  i. Form compounds with bile acids in intestine.
b. Side Effects
  i. GI distress, constipation.
c. Contraindication
  i. Bowel obstruction.

## II. HMG-COA REDUCTASE INHIBITORS
a. Mechanism of Action
  i. Limit cholesterol synthesis.
b. Side Effects
  i. Myositis, elevated LFTs.
c. Contraindications
  i. Pregnancy, active liver disease.

## III. FIBRIC-ACID INHIBITORS
a. Mechanism of Action
  i. Reduce hepatic triglyceride production and increase HDL synthesis.
b. Side Effects
  i. Cholelithiasis, dyspepsia.
c. Contraindications
  i. Severe hepatic or renal disease.

## IV. NICOTINIC ACIDS
a. Mechanism of Action
  i. Very-low-density lipoprotein (VLDL) secretion inhibitors.
b. Side Effects
  i. Flushing, hepatotoxicity, hyperglycemia.
c. Contraindications
  i. Severe peptic ulcer disease, chronic liver disease, severe gout.

## V. SUMMARY OF LIPID-LOWERING AGENTS (TABLE 15.4)

# GASTROINTESTINAL (GI) MEDICATIONS

## I. ANTACIDS
a. Mechanism of Action
  i. Neutralize acid secretions and raise gastric pH to greater than 4.
  ii. Inactivate pepsin and bile salts.
  iii. Increase lower esophageal sphincter (LES) tone.
b. High and frequent dosing needed for maximal effectiveness
c. Many drug interactions including those with tetracyclines, fluoroquinolones, ketoconazole, itraconazole, and warfarin
d. Medications
  i. Aluminum-containing (Amphojel, Alterna-GEL).
  ii. Magnesium-containing (milk of magnesia).
  iii. Aluminum/magnesium combination (Maalox).
  iv. Calcium-containing (Tums, Rolaids).
  v. Simethicone-containing (Mylanta, Gelusil).
    1. Antiflatulent agent added.

## II. HISTAMINE$_2$ RECEPTOR ANTAGONISTS
a. Mechanism of Action

**TABLE 15.4**

| Hyperlipidemia Drugs | | | | |
| --- | --- | --- | --- | --- |
| **Drug Class** | **Generic** | **Lipid Effects** | **Side Effects** | **Contraindications** |
| Statins | Lovastatin<br>Pravastatin<br>Simvastatin<br>Atorvastatin<br>Rosuvastatin | Decrease LDL<br>Increase HDL<br>Decrease triglycerides | Rhabdomyolysis<br>Myolysis<br>Increased LFTS | Acute liver disease<br>Chronic liver disease |
| Bile acid–binding resins | Cholestyramine<br>Colestipol | Decrease LDL<br>Increase HDL<br>Increase triglycerides | GI distress<br>Constipation<br>Decrease drug absorption | Triglycerides >400 mg/dL |
| Niacin and nicotinic acids | Niacin | Decrease LDL<br>Increase HDL<br>Decrease triglycerides | Flushing<br>Hyperglycemia<br>Liver damage<br>Increased uric acid | Chronic liver disease<br>Gout |
| Fibric acids | Fenofibrate<br>Gemfibrozil | Decrease LDL<br>Increase HDL<br>Decrease triglycerides | Gallstones<br>Myopathy | Severe renal disease<br>Severe liver disease |
| Omega-3 ethyl esters | | Decrease LDL<br>Increase HDL<br>Decrease triglycerides | | |

*HDL*, High-density lipoprotein; *LDL*, low-density lipoprotein; *LFT*, liver function tests.

i. Competitively and reversibly bind to $H_2$ receptor on parietal cell, decreasing histamine-stimulated gastric acid production by 90% to 95%.

ii Well-absorbed PO.

iii. Dose adjustment needed in renal impairment.

iv. Drug interactions can occur via hepatic enzyme inhibition (CYP 450 3A4), mainly seen with cimetidine.

b. **Medications**

i. Cimetidine (Tagamet).

ii. Ranitidine (Zantac).

iii. Famotidine (Pepcid).

iv. Nizatidine (Axid).

c. **Indications**

i. Healing and maintenance of duodenal and gastric ulcers.

ii. Gastroesophageal reflux disease (GERD) and erosive esophagitis.

iii. Prevention of stress ulcer.

iv. Hypersecretory conditions.

d. **Side Effects**

i. CNS disturbances.

1. Dizziness, headache, confusion, hallucinations.

ii. Hematologic effects.

1. Thrombocytopenia, leukopenia, anemia.

iii. Gynecomastia.

1. Noted with cimetidine.

## III. PROTON-PUMP INHIBITORS

a. **Mechanism of Action**

i. Bind *irreversibly* to $H^+/K^+$-ATPase enzyme needed to pump $H^+$ ions and acid secretions.

ii. Inhibit basal and stimulated gastric acid secretion almost completely (99%).

b. **Medications**

i. Omeprazole (Prilosec).

ii. Lansoprazole (Prevacid).

iii. Rabeprazole (AcipHex).

iv. Pantoprazole (Protonix).

v. Esomeprazole (Nexium).

c. **Indications**

i. Healing of duodenal and gastric ulcers.

ii. GERD and erosive esophagitis.

iii. Prevention/Treatment of NSAID-induced ulcers.

iv. *Helicobacter pylori* eradication.

v. Hypersecretory conditions.

d. **Side Effects**

i. Nausea.

ii. Diarrhea.

iii. Headache.

iv. Long-term use can lead to osteoporosis and vitamin $B_{12}$ deficiency.

## IV. SUCRALFATE (CARAFATE)

a. **Mechanism of Action**

i. Aluminum hydroxide and sucrose sulfate dissolve in stomach acid and release aluminum, forming a viscous gel.

ii. Gel binds to ulcers, creating a barrier to irritants.

b. **Indications**

i. Maintenance and healing of gastric and duodenal ulcers.

ii. Must be taken on empty stomach and requires multiple daily doses.

iii. Administer separately from meals and from interacting medications.

c. Adverse Effects
   i. Constipation.
   ii. Nausea.
   iii. Metallic taste.

## VI. BISMUTH SUBSALICYLATE (BSS) (PEPTO-BISMOL)

a. Mechanism of Action
   i. In presence of pH less than 3.5, reacts with acid to form bismuth oxide and salicylic acid.
   ii. Disrupts *H. pylori* integrity and the ability to adhere to epithelial surface.
   iii. Salicylate provides antisecretory effects.

b. Adverse Effects
   i. Black stools, tongue.

## VII. METOCLOPRAMIDE

a. A Prokinetic Agent

b. Mechanism of Action
   i. Blocks dopamine receptors in the chemoreceptor zone and enhances response to acetylcholine in the upper GI tract, causing increased motility and accelerating gastric emptying.

c. Indications
   i. Used to treat diabetes gastroparesis, nausea and vomiting, GERD, and postpyloric placement of enteral feeding tube.

d. Side Effects
   i. Extrapyramidal reactions.
   ii. Dizziness.
   iii. Headache.

iv. Fatigue.

v. Patients can develop neuroleptic malignant syndrome and tardive dyskinesia.

## VIII. ANTIDIARRHEALS (TABLE 15.5)

## IX. LAXATIVES (TABLE 15.6)

## X. ANTIEMETICS

a. Antihistamine Antiemetics (Diphenhydramine, dimenhydrinate, meclizine)
   i. Mechanism of action.
      1. Antihistamine and anticholinergic effect on vestibular apparatus.
   ii. Indications.
      1. Treatment of simple nausea and vomiting.
      2. Adjunctive treatment in complex nausea and vomiting.
   iii. Adverse effects.
      1. Sedation.
      2. Dry mouth.
      3. Urinary retention.

b. Phenothiazine Antiemetics (Chlorpromazine, prochlorperazine)
   i. Mechanism of action.
      1. Block dopamine receptors primarily in chemotactic trigger zone (CTZ).
   ii. Indications.
      1. Treatment of simple nausea and vomiting.
      2. Treatment and prevention of mildly emetogenic chemo-induced nausea and vomiting.
   iii. Adverse effects.
      1. Drowsiness.
      2. Extrapyramidal reactions.
      3. Sedation.

**TABLE 15.5**

### Antidiarrheal Agents

| Antidiarrheal | Brand | Mechanism | Comments |
|---|---|---|---|
| **Antimotility** | | | |
| Diphenoxylate/Atropine Loperamide | Lomotil Imodium AD | Decrease GI motility and propulsion | For short-term use only |
| **Absorbent** | | | |
| Polycarbophil | FiberCon | Absorbs water and decreases stool liquidity | Nonspecific in action; affect absorption of drugs and nutrients |
| **Antisecretory** | | | |
| Bismuth subsalicylate | Pepto-Bismol Kaopectate | Blocks secretory flow | High doses can lead to salicylate toxicity |
| **Enzymes** | | | |
| Lactase | Lactaid | Hydrolyzes lactose into digestive sugars | |
| **Bacterial Replacement** | | | |
| Lactobacillus acidophilus | Lactinex | Replaces colonic bacterial microflora | |

**TABLE 15.6**

## Laxatives

| Laxative | Brand | Comments |
| --- | --- | --- |
| **Agents that Cause Softening of Stool in 1–3 days** | | |
| *Bulk-forming* | | |
| Polycarbophil | FiberCon | Work by absorbing water and expanding the stool content, leading to intestinal distention and peristalsis |
| Psyllium | Metamucil | |
| Methylcellulose | Citrucel | |
| *Emollients* | | |
| Docusate sodium | Colace | Promote water permeation of stool; typically used in prevention of constipation |
| Docusate calcium | Kaopectate | |
| *Hyperosmotic* | | |
| Lactulose | Cephulac | Attract water into the intestines leading to fluid accumulation, peristalsis, and bowel evacuation |
| Sorbitol | MiraLAX | |
| Polyethylene glycol | | |
| *Lubricant* | | |
| Mineral oil | | Coats stool surface and retains water |
| **Agents that Result in Soft or Semifluid Stool in 6–12 hours (Acute Use Only)** | | |
| *Stimulant* | | |
| Bisacodyl (PO) | Dulcolax | Mechanism of action unknown but may increase peristalsis by direct irritant effect on intestinal smooth muscle |
| Senna | Senokot | |
| Cascara sagrada | | |
| **Agents that Result in Watery Evacuation in 1–6 hours (Acute Use Only)** | | |
| *Saline Laxatives* | | |
| Magnesium citrate | Citroma | Highly osmotic ions draw water into the gut, leading to increased intestinal motility; usually reserved for complete bowel evacuation |
| Sodium phosphate | Fleet Phospho Soda | |
| Polyethylene glycol-electrolyte preps | GoLYTELY | |
| | CoLyte | |
| *Stimulants* | | |
| Bisacodyl (rectal) | Dulcolax | Used in pediatrics |
| Glycerin | | |

*PO*, Orally.

4. Bone marrow suppression.
   (a) Rare side effect.

## XI. BUTYROPHENONE ANTIEMETICS (Droperidol)
a. **Mechanism of Action**
   i. Block dopamine receptors in CTZ.
b. **Indications**
   i. Postoperative nausea and vomiting.
c. **Adverse Effects**
   i. Sedation.
   ii. Dystonic reactions.
   iii. Prolong QT interval.

## XII. SEROTONIN (5-HT₃) ANTAGONISTS (Ondansetron, granisetron, dolasetron)
a. **Mechanism of Action**
   i. Block serotonin in the CTZ and possibly the GI tract.

b. **Indications**
   i. Prevention and treatment of chemotherapy-induced nausea and vomiting.
   ii. Postoperative nausea and vomiting.
c. **Adverse Effects**
   i. Constipation.
   ii. Drowsiness.
   iii. Headache.
   iv. Prolong QT interval.

# PSYCHIATRIC MEDICATIONS

## I. BENZODIAZEPINES
a. **Mechanism of Action**
   i. Work by augmenting γ-aminobutyric acid (GABA) function in the limbic system.
   1. Rapid onset of action.

b. **Indications**
   i. Used in anxiety, agitation, and insomnia and as an anticonvulsant.
      1. Do not reduce depressive symptoms.
c. **Safety**
   i. Ability to overdose, high abuse potential.
   ii. Dependence can occur even in the absence of abuse.
   iii. If used long term, must taper the dose gradually to avoid rebound, relapse, or withdrawal symptoms.
d. **Side Effects**
   i. Drowsiness.
   ii. Respiratory depression.
   iii. Memory impairment.
e. **Medications (Table 15.7)**

## II. ANTIDEPRESSANTS: SELECTIVE SEROTONIN REUPTAKE INHIBITORS (SSRIs)

a. **Mechanism of Action**
   i. Bind to presynaptic serotonin reuptake proteins, inhibiting reuptake.
   ii. Onset of effect in about 6 weeks.
b. **Indications**
   i. Used in depression and anxiety disorders.
c. **Side Effects**
   i. Nausea.
   ii. Headache.
   iii. Insomnia and sedation.
   iv. Sexual dysfunction.
   v. Withdrawal delirium.
   vi. Increased suicide risk.

**TABLE 15.7**

| Benzodiazepines | | | |
|---|---|---|---|
| **Drug** | **Trade** | **Onset** | **Indications** |
| Alprazolam | Xanax | Intermediate | Anxiety, panic, phobias |
| Chlordiazepoxide | Librium | Intermediate | Anxiety, acute alcohol withdrawal |
| Clonazepam | Klonopin | Intermediate | Anxiety, panic, seizures |
| Diazepam | Valium | Fast | Anxiety, preoperative sedation, muscle relaxation |
| Lorazepam | Ativan | Intermediate | Anxiety, preoperative sedation, status epilepticus |
| Midazolam | Versed | Fast | Preoperative sedation, IV anesthesia |
| Oxazepam | Serax | Slow | Sleep disorders, anxiety |
| Temazepam | Restoril | Intermediate | Sleep disorders |
| Triazolam | Halcion | Fast | Sleep disorders |

vii. Risk of serotonin syndrome.
d. **Medications**
   i. Citalopram (Celexa).
   ii. Escitalopram (Lexapro).
   iii. Fluoxetine (Prozac).
   iv. Fluvoxamine (Luvox).
   v. Paroxetine (Paxil).
   vi. Sertraline (Zoloft).

## III. ANTIDEPRESSANTS: SEROTONIN-NOREPINEPHRINE REUPTAKE INHIBITORS (SNRIS)

a. **Mechanism of Action**
   i. Inhibit reuptake of serotonin and norepinephrine.
   ii. Used in treatment of major depression, mood disorders, attention-deficit hyperactivity disorder (ADHD), and obsessive-compulsive disorder (OCD).
   iii. Use with caution in HTN.
b. **Side Effects**
   i. Loss of appetite, weight, and sleep; diminished libido; and syndrome of inappropriate antidiuretic hormone (SIADH).
   ii. Increased suicide risk.
   iii. Discontinuation syndrome occurs with abrupt-withdrawal anxiety.
c. **Medications**
   i. Venlafaxine (Effexor).
   ii. Desvenlafaxine (Pristiq).
   iii. Duloxetine (Cymbalta).
      1. Can lead to hepatic failure.

## IV. ANTIDEPRESSANTS: TRICYCLIC ANTIDEPRESSANTS (TCAs)

a. **Mechanism of Action**
   i. Block uptake of serotonin and norepinephrine.
   ii. Potentially fatal in high doses.
   iii. Onset of effects takes 1 to 6 weeks.
b. **Side Effects**
   i. Dry mouth.
   ii. Blurred vision.
   iii. Drowsiness.
   iv. Arrhythmia.
   v. Hypotension.
   vi. See Table 15.8.

## V. ANTIDEPRESSANTS: MONOAMINE OXIDASE INHIBITORS (MAOIs)

a. **Mechanism of Action**
   i. Inhibit presynaptic monoamine oxidase, which catabolizes norepinephrine, dopamine, and serotonin.
   ii. Foods high in tyramine (e.g., aged cheeses, cured meats, beer, and red wine) should be avoided.
      1. Can lead to hypertensive crisis.

**TABLE 15.8**

| Side Effects of Tricyclic Antidepressants | | | | |
| --- | --- | --- | --- | --- |
| Name | Anticholinergic | Arrhythmia | Sedation | Weight Gain |
| Nortriptyline (Pamelor) | ++ | ++ | ++ | +++ |
| Imipramine (Tofranil) | +++ | +++ | +++ | ++++ |
| Desipramine (Norpramin) | ++ | ++ | ++ | ++ |
| Amitriptyline (Elavil) | ++++ | +++ | ++++ | ++++ |
| Doxepin (Sinequan) | ++++ | ++ | ++ | +++ |

+, Low; ++, medium; +++, high; ++++, very high.

**b. Side Effects**
  i. Insomnia, agitation, sedation.
  ii. Sexual dysfunction.
  iii. Orthostatic hypotension.
**c. Medications**
  i. Isocarboxazid (Marplan).
  ii. Phenelzine (Nardil).
  iii. Selegiline (Emsam).
  iv. Tranylcypromine (Parnate).

## VI. BUPROPION (WELLBUTRIN, ZYBAN)
**a. Mechanism of Action**
  i. Inhibits uptake of dopamine and norepinephrine.
**b. Indications**
  i. Effective in depression and smoking cessation.
**c. Side Effects**
  i. Headache, insomnia, weight loss.
  ii. Seizures.
    1. Contraindicated in patients with seizure risk.
  iii. Low incidence of sexual side effects or sedation.

## VII. MIRTAZAPINE (REMERON)
**a. Mechanism of Action**
  i. Central presynaptic $\alpha_2$ adrenergic antagonist, leads to increased release of serotonin and norepinephrine.
**b. Indications**
  i. Used in depression.
**c. Side Effects**
  i. Sedation.
  ii. Weight gain.
  iii. Sexual side effects are rare.
  iv. No CYP 450 inhibition.

## VIII. BUSPIRONE (BUSPAR)
**a. Mechanism of Action**
  i. Agonist of serotonin receptors and antagonist of dopamine receptors.
**b. Indications**
  i. A nonbenzodiazepine antianxiety agent.
  ii. Used in the treatment of generalized anxiety disorder.
    1. May take several weeks to note improvement in symptoms.

**c. Side Effects**
  i. Dizziness.
  ii. Nervousness.
  iii. Nausea.
  iv. Restless leg syndrome.
  v. Extrapyramidal symptoms.

## IX. LITHIUM (ESKALITH)
**a. Mechanism of Action**
  i. Not well determined; possibly alters reuptake of serotonin and/or norepinephrine by altering cation transport across cell membrane.
**b. Indications**
  i. Mood stabilizer, mainstay in treatment of bipolar disease/mania.
  ii. Must monitor lithium levels on a regular basis.
**c. Side Effects**
  i. Minor side effects include tremor, weight gain, polyuria, GI distress, acne.
  ii. Major side effects include ataxia, confusion, course tremor, coma, sinus arrhythmia, teratogenicity, death.
  iii. Contraindicated in severe renal function decline, cardiac disease, and pregnancy.

## X. ANTIPSYCHOTICS
**a. Mechanism of Action**
  i. Block dopamine receptors (first and second generation) and block serotonin (second generation).
  ii. Effective in treating positive psychotic symptoms.
**b. Side Effects**
  i. Neurologic side effects including restlessness, neuroleptic malignant syndrome, extrapyramidal symptoms, and reduced seizure threshold.
  ii. Weight gain.
  iii. Anticholinergic side effects including dry mouth, constipation, and urinary retention.
  iv. Hypotension is common with risperidone.
  v. Agranulocytosis is noted with clozapine.
  vi. Increased QT prolongation.
  vii. Elevated prolactin.
**c. Antipsychotics (Table 15.9)**

**TABLE 15.9**

| Antipsychotics | | | | |
| --- | --- | --- | --- | --- |
| **Drug** | **EPS** | **Sedation** | **Alpha Block** | **Other** |
| **Typicals** | | | | |
| Chlorpromazine | + + | + + + | + + + | |
| Thioridazine | + | + + + | + + + | Cardiotoxicity: torsades de pointes |
| Fluphenazine | + + + + | + | + | |
| Haloperidol | + + + + | + | + | Most likely to cause NMS and TD |
| **Atypicals** | | | | |
| Clozapine | ± | + | + + + | Agranulocytosis, seizures, increased salivation |
| Olanzapine | ± | + | + + | Improves negative symptoms |
| Risperidone | + | + + | + + | Improves negative symptoms |
| Aripiprazole | + | ± | ± | |

*EPS*, Extrapyramidal symptoms; *NMS*, neuroleptic malignant syndrome; *TD*, tardive dyskinesia; ±, none/low; +, low; + +, medium; + + +, high; + + + +, very high.

## XI. STIMULANTS

a. **Mechanism of Action**
   i. Mediate CNS stimulation through the release of norepinephrine and dopamine and by blocking their uptake.
   ii. Used in the treatment of ADHD, narcolepsy, and excessive daytime sleepiness.
   iii. Have a black box warning for abuse and addiction potential and for serious cardiac events.

b. **Side Effects**
   i. Insomnia, headache, weight loss, loss of appetite.
   ii. Long-term use can suppress growth in children.

c. **Medications**
   i. Amphetamine/dextroamphetamine (Adderall).
   ii. Methylphenidate (Ritalin, Concerta).
   iii. Lisdexamfetamine (Vyvanse).
   iv. Modafinil (Provigil).

# OTHER

## I. CHOLINESTERASE INHIBITORS

a. **Mechanism of Action**
   i. Inhibit acetylcholinesterase and increase the amount of acetylcholine at the synapse.

b. **Indications**
   i. Used in the treatment of Alzheimer's dementia, dementia associated with Parkinson's disease, and Lewy body dementia.
   ii. Are not cures but may reduce symptoms.

c. **Medications**
   i. Donepezil (Aricept).
   ii. Rivastigmine (Exelon).

d. **Side Effects**
   i. Nausea and vomiting, diarrhea, bradycardia, HTN, and insomnia.
   ii. Concurrent use of ginkgo biloba may worsen side effects with donepezil.

## II. ANTICOAGULANTS

a. **Heparin**
   i. Mechanism of action.
      1. Binds to antithrombin and increases inhibition of factors IXa, Xa, XIa, XIIa, and IIa.
   ii. Indications.
      1. Used in the treatment of deep venous thrombosis, pulmonary embolism, peripheral arterial embolism, disseminated intravascular coagulation, and deep venous thrombosis prophylaxis.
   iii. Side effects.
      1. Bleeding, thrombocytopenia.
      2. Osteoporosis noted with long-term use.
      3. Multiple drug interactions.
   iv. Monitor levels with activated partial thromboplastin time (aPTT).
   v. Overdose.
      1. Very short half-life, about 1 hour, holding drug will decrease levels quickly.
      2. Protamine sulfate is antidote.

b. **Low-Molecular-Weight Heparin**
   i. Mechanism of action.
      1. Inhibit factors Xa and IIa.
   ii. Indications.
      1. Used in the treatment of deep venous thrombosis, pulmonary embolism, peripheral arterial embolism, and deep venous thrombosis prophylaxis.
   iii. Medications.
      1. Dalteparin (Fragmin).
      2. Enoxaparin (Lovenox).
   iv. Anti-Xa levels can be used to monitor low-molecular-weight heparin (LMWH) levels.

c. **Warfarin (Coumadin)**
   i. Mechanism of action.
      1. Inhibits the carboxylation (activation) of vitamin K–dependent factors (II, VII, IX, and X) and increases clotting time.

ii. Indications.
  1. Used in the treatment of deep venous thrombosis, pulmonary embolism, peripheral arterial embolism, atrial fibrillation, and deep venous thrombosis prophylaxis.
iii. Multiple drug interactions; avoid foods high in vitamin K.
iv. Side effects.
  1. Bleeding and skin necrosis.
  2. Contraindicated in pregnancy.
v. Levels monitored with prothrombin time and international normalized ratio (INR).
vi. Vitamin K is the antidote.
vii. Drug effects with warfarin (Table 15.10).

## III. ANTIGOUT
### a. Colchicine
i. Mechanism of action.
  1. Unknown, possibly preventing activation and migration of neutrophils associated with mediating some gout symptoms.
ii. Indications.
  1. Used in the treatment and prophylaxis of acute gout, also used in pericarditis and primary biliary cirrhosis
iii. Side effects.
  1. Diarrhea, nausea and vomiting.
  2. Myelosuppression and aplastic anemia.
  3. Hepatotoxicity.
  4. Dose adjustment in hepatic and renal failure.
### b. Allopurinol
i. Mechanism of action.
  1. Decreases production of uric acid by blocking xanthine oxidase.
    (a) Xanthine oxidase converts hypoxanthine to xanthine and then to uric acid.
ii. Indications.
  1. Used to prevent gout attacks, treatment and prevention of tumor lysis syndrome, and prevent recurrent calcium oxalate calculi.

iii. Side effects.
  1. Include maculopapular rash and pruritus.
  2. Rare side effects include Stevens-Johnson syndrome and toxic epidermal necrolysis.
  3. Reduce dose in renal failure.

## IV. ANTICONVULSANTS
### a. General
i. Medications decrease neuronal discharge within the CNS and therefore inhibit seizure activity.
ii. Therapeutic drug monitoring may be needed.
iii. Medication selection is based on type of seizure (Table 15.11).
### b. Medications
i. Carbamazepine (Tegretol).
  1. Mechanism of action
    (a) Decreases axonal conduction by preventing sodium ion influx through fast sodium channels.
  2. Side effects.
    (a) CNS depression, ataxia, aplastic anemia, osteomalacia, exfoliative dermatitis, and increased ADH secretion.
  3. Monitor.
    (a) Complete blood count (CBC), LFTs, and renal function.
    (b) Contraindicated in patients with bone marrow suppression, and hypersensitivity to tricyclic antidepressants and MAOIs.
  4. Also used in the treatment of trigeminal neuralgia.
ii. Ethosuximide (Zarontin).
  1. Mechanism of action.
    (a) Decreases presynaptic calcium ion influx through type-T channels in thalamic neurons.

**TABLE 15.10**

| Drug Interactions with Warfarin | |
| --- | --- |
| **Increase INR** | **Decrease INR** |
| Amiodarone | Carbamazepine |
| Fluconazole | Rifampin |
| Metronidazole | Alcohol (chronic) |
| Ciprofloxacin | Propylthiouracil |
| Erythromycin | |
| Prednisone | |
| TMP/Sulfa | |
| Cimetidine | |
| Alcohol (acute) | |

*INR*, International normalized ratio; *TMP/Sulfa*, trimethoprim-sulfamethoxazole.

**TABLE 15.11**

| Anticonvulsant Selection | |
| --- | --- |
| **Seizure Type** | **Effective Medications** |
| Partial | Carbamazepine |
| Simple or complex | Gabapentin: adjunctive therapy |
| | Lamotrigine |
| | Phenytoin |
| | Valproic acid |
| General: Tonic-clonic | Carbamazepine |
| | Lamotrigine |
| | Phenytoin |
| | Valproic acid |
| General: Absence | Ethosuximide |
| | Valproic acid |
| Status epilepticus | Diazepam |
| | Lorazepam |
| | Phenytoin/fosphenytoin |

2. Side effects.
   (a) Drowsiness, ataxia, headache, GI complaints, and pancytopenia.
3. Monitor.
   (a) CBC.
iii. Felbamate (Felbatol).
   1. Mechanism of action.
      (a) Decreases excitatory effects of glutamic acid.
   2. Side effects.
      (a) Hepatotoxicity and aplastic anemia.
   3. Monitor.
      (a) CBC and LFTs.
      (b) Contraindication in patients with renal or hepatic failure.
iv. Gabapentin (Neurontin).
   1. Mechanism of action.
      (a) Unknown, but may be by decreasing axonal conduction by preventing sodium ion influx through fast sodium channels.
   2. Side effects.
      (a) CNS depression, fatigue, ataxia, and peripheral edema.
   3. Monitor.
      (a) Renal function.
         (i) Dosage must be adjusted.
   4. Also used in the treatment of neuropathic pain, diabetic peripheral neuropathy, and restless leg syndrome.
v. Lamotrigine (Lamictal).
   1. Mechanism of action
      (a) Decreases excitatory effects of glutamic acid.
   2. Side effects.
      (a) Headache, dizziness, blurry vision, and Stevens-Johnson syndrome.
   3. Monitor.
      (a) Drug levels will decrease in patients on oral contraceptives.
vi. Phenobarbital.
   1. Mechanism of action.

(a) Increases inhibitory tone by facilitation of GABA-mediated hyperpolarization.
2. Side effects.
   (a) CNS and respiratory depression, hepatotoxicity, acute intermittent porphyria, and Stevens-Johnson syndrome.
3. Monitor.
   (a) LFTs.
vii. Phenytoin (Dilantin).
   1. Mechanism of action
      (a) Decreases axonal conduction by preventing sodium ion influx through fast sodium channels.
   2. Side effects.
      (a) Nystagmus, gingival hyperplasia, CNS depression, hirsutism, osteomalacia, and aplastic anemia.
         (i) Nystagmus is an initial side effect of toxicity.
      (b) IV phenytoin can cause hypotension.
   3. Monitor.
      (a) CBC and urinalysis.
      (b) There are many drug interactions with phenytoin.
viii. Valproic acid (Depakene).
   1. Mechanism of action.
      (a) Decreases presynaptic calcium ion influx through type-T channels in thalamic neurons.
   2. Side effects.
      (a) Hepatotoxicity, thrombocytopenia, pancreatitis, and alopecia.
   3. Monitor.
      (a) CBC and LFTs.
      (b) Contraindicated in patients with hepatic dysfunction.

## V.  CHEMOTHERAPY
a. **See Table 15.12 for chemotherapy medications and mechanisms of action**
b. **See Table 15.13 for side effects of chemotherapy**

**TABLE 15.12**

### Chemotherapy Mechanisms of Action

| Drug Class | Medications | Mechanism of Action |
| --- | --- | --- |
| Alkylating agent | Cyclophosphamide | Forms strong covalent bonds with DNA inhibiting replication and causing bond breaks and cell death |
| Anthracyclines | Doxorubicin Bleomycin | Inhibit DNA and RNA synthesis by intercalation of DNA base pairs and inhibition of DNA repair by topoisomers |
| Antimetabolites | Cytarabine 5-Fluorouracil Methotrexate | Inhibit DNA synthesis or incorporate themselves into DNA, causing apoptosis |
| Aromatase inhibitor | Letrozole | Inhibits aromatase that converts androgens to estrogens |
| Monoclonal antibodies | Rituximab Trastuzumab | Bind to receptors on tumor cells, stopping cell growth and spread |

**TABLE 15.12**

| Chemotherapy Mechanisms of Action—cont'd | | |
| --- | --- | --- |
| **Drug Class** | **Medications** | **Mechanism of Action** |
| Platinum compounds | Carboplatin Cisplatin | Form covalent bonds with DNA, inhibiting replication and causing cell death |
| Vinca alkaloids | Vincristine | Prevent microtubule assembly, preventing cell mitosis |
| Tyrosine kinase inhibitors | Imatinib | Block signaling pathway and slowing or stopping cell proliferation |
| Hormone regulators | Tamoxifen | Compete with estrogen for binding sites in target tissues, decreasing the effects of estrogen |
| Taxanes | Paclitaxel | Stabilize microtubule bundles by promoting assembly and preventing depolymerization, thereby inhibiting cell replication |

**TABLE 15.13**

| Side Effects of Chemotherapy | |
| --- | --- |
| **Medication** | **Side Effects** |
| Cyclophosphamide (Cytoxan) | BMS, hemorrhagic cystitis |
| Doxorubicin (Adriamycin) | BMS, cardiomyopathy |
| Bleomycin (Blenoxane) | Pneumonitis, pulmonary fibrosis |
| Cytarabine (ARA-C) | BMS, mucositis, diarrhea, N/V |
| 5-Fluorouracil (5-FU) | BMS, mucositis, palmar erythema |
| Methotrexate (Rheumatrex) | BMS, hepatotoxicity, N/V |
| Letrozole (Femara) | Hot flashes, night sweats, edema |
| Rituximab (Rituxan) | Lymphopenia, tumor lysis syndrome, rash |
| Trastuzumab (Herceptin) | Rash, nausea, cardiotoxicity, pulmonary toxicity |
| Carboplatin (Paraplatin-AQ) | BMS, ototoxicity, peripheral neuropathy |
| Cisplatin (Platinol) | N/V, peripheral neuropathy, nephrotoxicity |
| Vincristine (Oncovin) | Peripheral neuropathy, constipation, depression |
| Imatinib (Gleevec) | BMS, fluid retention, rash, hepatotoxicity |
| Tamoxifen (Nolvadex) | Hot flashes, mood changes, vaginal bleeding, endometrial hyperplasia, blood clots |
| Paclitaxel (Taxol) | BMS, peripheral neuropathy |

*BMS*, Bone marrow suppression; *N/V*, nausea and vomiting.

# QUESTIONS

### QUESTION 1
Which of the following is the mechanism of action of enalapril (Vasotec)?
A  Inhibition of angiotensin-converting enzyme
B  Direct smooth muscle relaxation
C  Inhibition of phosphodiesterase
D  Blocking of beta receptors
E  Inhibition of alpha receptors

### QUESTION 2
Which of the following chemotherapy agents is most likely to lead to pulmonary fibrosis?
A  Vincristine
B  Bleomycin
C  Cisplatin
D  Tamoxifen
E  Methotrexate

### QUESTION 3
Which of the following medications irreversibly inhibits the $H^+/K^+$-ATPase pump in the parietal cells?
A  Sucralfate (Carafate)
B  Omeprazole (Prilosec)
C  Cimetidine (Tagamet)
D  Amantadine (Symmetrel)
E  Metoclopramide (Reglan)

### QUESTION 4
A man with prostatic hyperplasia is placed on prazosin (Minipress). To which of the following classes of medications does this drug belong?
A  Gonadotropin-releasing hormone inhibitor
B  Direct testosterone antagonist
C  5-Alpha reductase inhibitor
D  Antimuscarinic
E  Alpha-blocker

*Continued*

## QUESTIONS—cont'd

### QUESTION 5

Which of the following is a major side effect of the long-term use of nitrofurantoin in the elderly?

A  Pulmonary fibrosis
B  Renal insufficiency
C  Macrocytic anemia
D  Cardiomyopathy
E  Neuropathy

### QUESTION 6

Which of the following is the most effective treatment for *M. pneumoniae*?

A  Cephalexin
B  Amoxicillin
C  Vancomycin
D  Azithromycin
E  Streptomycin

### QUESTION 7

Which of the following inhibits xanthine oxidase and is used in the treatment of chronic gout to prevent recurrence?

A  Indomethacin
B  Probenecid
C  Prednisone
D  Febuxostat
E  Colchicine

### QUESTION 8

Which of the following is an opioid antagonist?

A  Hydromorphone (Dilaudid)
B  Buprenorphine (Buprenex)
C  Flumazenil (Romazicon)
D  Butorphanol (Stadol)
E  Naloxone (Narcan)

### QUESTION 9

Which of the following classes of medications should be avoided in patients with tyramine in their diet?

A  Selective-serotonin reuptake inhibitors
B  Second-generation antipsychotics
C  Monoamine oxidase inhibitors
D  Tricyclic antidepressants
E  Benzodiazepines

### QUESTION 10

Which of the following is used in the treatment of hirsutism secondary to polycystic ovarian syndrome?

A  Acarbose (Precose)
B  Pioglitazone (Actos)
C  Subcutaneous insulin
D  Metformin (Glucophage)
E  Spironolactone (Aldactone)

## ANSWERS

**1. A**
EXPLANATION: Enalapril is an ACE inhibitor that works by inhibiting the ACE that converts angiotensin I to angiotensin II. *Topic: Angiotensin-converting enzyme inhibitors*
☐ Correct   ☐ Incorrect

**2. B**
EXPLANATION: The major side effects noted with the use of bleomycin include pulmonary fibrosis and pneumonitis. Vincristine can cause peripheral neuropathy, cisplatin can cause peripheral neuropathy and nephrotoxicity, tamoxifen can lead to vaginal bleeding and endometrial hyperplasia, and methotrexate can lead to hepatotoxicity. *Topic: Chemotherapy*
☐ Correct   ☐ Incorrect

**3. B**
EXPLANATION: Omeprazole is used in the treatment of peptic ulcer disease and works by irreversibly inhibiting the $H^+/K^+-$ ATPase pump in the parietal cells. Sucralfate works by dissolving in stomach acid and releasing aluminum, forming a viscous gel covering the ulcer surface. Cimetidine competitively and reversibly binds to $H_2$ receptors on parietal cells, decreasing histamine-stimulated gastric acid production. Amantadine is an antiviral agent that inhibits viral uncoating. Metoclopramide is a motility agent and an antiemetic that works as a dopamine antagonist. *Topic: Proton-pump inhibitors*
☐ Correct   ☐ Incorrect

**4. E**
EXPLANATION: Prazosin and terazosin are alpha-blockers. *Topic: Alpha-blockers*
☐ Correct   ☐ Incorrect

**5. A**
EXPLANATION: Nitrofurantoin is an antibiotic that works by inhibiting several bacterial enzyme systems interfering with metabolism and possibly cell wall synthesis. Side effects noted with long-term usage include pulmonary fibrosis, hemolytic anemia, nausea and vomiting, hepatic toxicity, and lupus like syndrome. *Topic: Nitrofurantoin*
☐ Correct   ☐ Incorrect

**6. D**
EXPLANATION: *M. pneumoniae* is a common cause of atypical pneumonia and is best treated with the macrolides, such as azithromycin. *Topic: Protein synthesis inhibitor*
☐ Correct   ☐ Incorrect

**7. D**
EXPLANATION: Febuxostat and allopurinol are xanthine oxidase inhibitors and are used in the treatment of gout. *Topic: Antigout*
☐ Correct   ☐ Incorrect

## ANSWERS—cont'd

**8.  E**

EXPLANATION: Naloxone is an opioid antagonist and is used in the treatment of opioid overdoses. Hydromorphone, buprenorphine and butorphanol are opioid drugs. Flumazenil inhibits the activity of benzodiazepines. ***Topic: Benzodiazepines***

☐ Correct    ☐ Incorrect

**9.  C**

EXPLANATION: Patients taking monoamine oxidase inhibitors for depression should be instructed to avoid foods high in tyramine (e.g., aged cheeses, cured meats, red wine, and beer). ***Topic: Antidepressants: MAOI***

☐ Correct    ☐ Incorrect

**10.  E**

EXPLANATION: Hirsutism is a common finding in polycystic ovarian syndrome. It is best treated with an androgen blocker, such as spironolactone. ***Topic: Diuretics***

☐ Correct    ☐ Incorrect

# CHAPTER 16
# LABORATORY MEDICINE

## EXAMINATION BLUEPRINT TOPICS

**GENERAL**
Specificity
Sensitivity
Predictive values
Normal ranges (Reference ranges)
Profiles
**COMPLETE BLOOD COUNT**
White blood cell (WBC) count
Hemoglobin/Hematocrit
Red blood cell (RBC) indices
Platelet count
**COAGULATION TESTING**
Prothrombin time (PT)/Partial thromboplastin time (PTT)
Bleeding time
Fibrinogen/Fibrin degradation products (FDP)

D-dimer
Platelet aggregation studies
**CHEMISTRY TESTING**
General
Electrolytes
Liver function tests
Renal tests
Lipid profile
Proteins
Calcium/Phosphorus
Amylase/Lipase
Other
**URINALYSIS**
Macroscopic
Microscopic

**THYROID TESTING**
Triiodothyronine ($T_3$)
Thyroxine ($T_4$)
Thyroid-stimulating hormone (TSH)
**RHEUMATOLOGY TESTING**
Antinuclear antibodies (ANA)
Autoantibodies
Erythrocyte sedimentation rate
Rheumatoid factor
C-reactive protein (CRP)
**MICROBIOLOGY**
Gram stain

## GENERAL

### I. SPECIFICITY
a. **The ability of a test to correctly identify those without the disease or the proportion of patients without the disease who test negative**
   i. Calculation.
      1. Specificity = True negatives / (False positives + True negatives).

### II. SENSITIVITY
a. **The ability of a test to correctly identify those with the disease or the proportion of patients with the disease who test positive**
   i. Calculation.
      1. Sensitivity = True positives / (True positives + False negatives).
b. **Accuracy and precision are different from sensitivity and specificity**
   i. Accuracy is how closely the measurement approaches the true value of the substance being measured.

   ii. Precision is how closely together repeat measurements of the same substance in the same sample fall.
      1. Is the same as reproducibility.

### III. PREDICTIVE VALUES
a. **Positive Predictive Value**
   i. Defined as the possibility of disease among patients with a positive test.
   ii. Calculations.
      1. Positive predictive value = True positives / (True positives + False positives)
b. **Negative Predictive Value**
   i. Defined as the probability of no disease among patients with a negative test.
   ii. Calculation.
      1. Negative predictive value = True negatives / (True negatives + False negatives).

### IV. NORMAL RANGES (REFERENCE RANGES)
a. **Performed on a large number of normal persons with values plotted in a distribution graph**

b. Mean and standard deviation (SD) are calculated with normal ranges being determined by values falling within ±2 SD of the mean

c. Many factors, including smoking, alcohol consumption, exercise, and the patient's position can have an effect on normal ranges

d. Normal ranges for common laboratory tests are located in Appendix 6

## V. PROFILES

a. Many laboratory tests can be done as a group or a profile. The chemistry profile can be used to determine which organ system is involved in the disease process by looking at which test is abnormal

b. Table 16.1 summarizes common chemistry tests and typical organ systems evaluated

# COMPLETE BLOOD COUNT

## I. WHITE BLOOD CELL (WBC) COUNT

a. Normal Maturation Sequence (Fig. 16.1)

b. Measure of total WBC count and may include a differential that breaks down the various types of WBCs

c. Total WBC count may be elevated in the following:

    i. Inflammation.

    ii. Leukemia.

    iii. Bacterial infection.

    iv. Uremia.

    v. Pregnancy.

d. Total WBC count may be decreased in the following:

    i. Viral infection.

    ii. Hypersplenism.

    iii. Bone marrow suppression.

e. Elevation in specific WBC types can also indicate a possible diagnosis

    i. Neutrophilia.

      1. Secondary to infection, inflammation, myeloproliferative disorders, stress, metabolic disorders, steroid therapy, and splenectomy.

        (a) In infection may also note toxic granulation or Döhle bodies.

    ii. Eosinophilia.

      1. Secondary to allergic disorders, asthma, parasitic infection, sarcoidosis, psoriasis, and malignancies.

    iii. Basophilia.

      1. Secondary to myeloproliferative disorders (such as chronic myelogenous leukemia), hypersensitivity reactions, ulcerative colitis, hypothyroidism, and varicella or smallpox infection.

    iv. Monocytosis.

      1. Secondary to acute infection (bacterial, disseminated tuberculosis [TB], subacute bacterial endocarditis [SBE], or syphilis), collagen vascular disease, or chronic ulcerative colitis.

    v. Lymphocytosis.

      1. Secondary to viral infection, drug sensitivity, autoimmune disorders, Addison's disease, and leukemia.

**TABLE 16.1**

| Organ Systems Evaluated by Common Chemistry Tests | | | |
|---|---|---|---|
| **Test** | **Organ System** | **Test** | **Organ System** |
| Albumin | Nutrition<br>Liver<br>Kidney | Creatinine | Kidney<br>Fluid balance |
| ALP | Liver<br>Bone | Glucose | Fluid balance<br>Pancreas |
| ALT | Liver<br>Muscle | LDH | Liver<br>Muscle |
| AST | Liver | Phosphorus | Kidney<br>Bone |
| Bicarbonate | Kidney<br>Fluid balance | Potassium | Kidney<br>Fluid balance |
| Bilirubin | Liver | Sodium | Kidney<br>Fluid balance |
| BUN | Kidney<br>Liver<br>Fluid balance | Triglycerides | Nutrition<br>Cardiac risk |
| Calcium | Bone<br>Fluid balance | Total protein | Nutrition<br>Liver |
| Chloride | Kidney<br>Fluid balance | Uric acid | Kidney |
| Cholesterol | Nutrition<br>Cardiac risk | | |

*ALP,* Alkaline phosphatase; *ALT,* alanine aminotransferase; *AST,* aspartate aminotransferase; *BUN,* blood urea nitrogen; *LDH,* lactate dehydrogenase.

**Myelopoiesis**

Myeloblast → Promyelocyte → Myelocyte → Metamyelocyte → Band → Segmented neutrophil

Monoblast → Promonocyte → Monocyte

**Lymphopoiesis**

Lymphoblast → Prolymphocyte → Lymphocyte

**Erythropoiesis**

Proerythroblast → Basophilic erythroblast → Polychromatophilic erythroblast → Orthochromic erythroblast → Polychromatophilic erythrocyte (reticulocyte) → Erythrocyte

**Fig. 16.1** Normal blood cell maturation sequence.

## II. HEMOGLOBIN/HEMATOCRIT

a. Decreased in anemia, hemorrhage, or fluid overload

b. Elevated in polycythemia, living at a high altitude, smoking, chronic obstructive pulmonary disease (COPD), and dehydration

## III. RED BLOOD CELL (RBC) INDICES

a. General

  i. Used in the diagnosis of the various causes of anemia.

b. Mean Cell Volume (MCV)

  i. Detects an increase or decrease in RBC size.

  ii. May be in error secondary to RBC agglutination or marked increase in the number of WBCs.

  iii. Used to determine if a cell is microcytic (low MCV), normocytic (normal MCV), or macrocytic (elevated MCV).

c. Mean Cell Hemoglobin (MCH)

  i. Used to measure the average amount of hemoglobin in each red blood cell.

  ii. Used to determine if an RBC is hypochromic (decreased MCH) or normochromic (normal MCH).

d. Mean Cell Hemoglobin Concentration (MCHC)

  i. Used to measure the relative concentration of intracellular hemoglobin.

  ii. Decreased in anemia and elevated in the presence of cold agglutinins or hereditary spherocytosis.

e. RBC Distribution Width (RDW)

  i. Used to measure anisocytosis (variation in cell size).

  ii. Used to separate out the common causes of microcytic anemia, thalassemia, and anemia of chronic disease from iron-deficiency anemia.

   1. Normal or slightly elevated in thalassemia and anemia of chronic disease and very elevated in iron-deficiency anemia.

f. Anemia Flowchart (Fig. 16.2)

## IV. PLATELET COUNT

a. General

  i. Platelets are important in the first steps of coagulation and in the formation of the platelet plug.

  ii. Surgical bleeding typically does not occur until platelet count is below 50,000/mm$^3$.

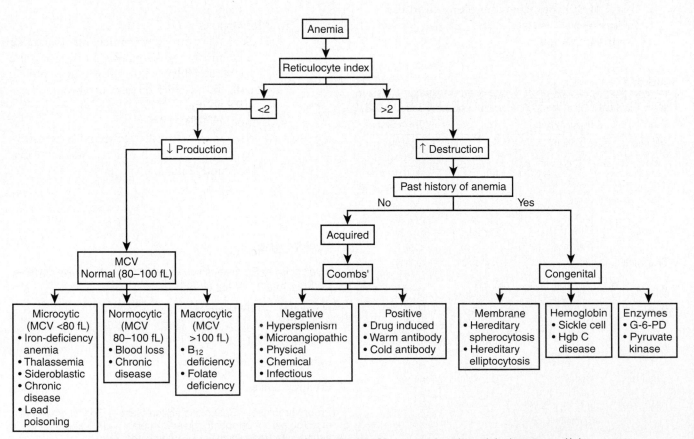

**Fig. 16.2** Evaluation of the patient with anemia. *G-6-PD*, Glucose-6-phosphate dehydrogenase; *Hgb*, hemoglobin; *MCV*, mean cell volume.

iii. Severe spontaneous bleeding most likely with platelet count below 10,000/mm$^3$.

b. **Thrombocytosis**

   i. Etiologies include the following:

     1. Primary thrombocytosis due to essential thrombocytosis, chronic myelogenous leukemia, polycythemia vera, and myelofibrosis.

     2. Secondary thrombocytosis due to inflammation, surgery, hyposplenism, and iron-deficiency anemia.

c. **Thrombocytopenia**

   i. Mechanisms include the following:

     1. Decreased production secondary to vitamin B$_{12}$ or folate deficiency, leukemia, infection, Bernard-Soulier syndrome, May-Hegglin anomaly, and Alport's syndrome.

     2. Increased destruction secondary to idiopathic thrombocytopenic purpura, thrombotic thrombocytopenic purpura, hemolytic uremic syndrome, disseminated intravascular coagulation (DIC), paroxysmal nocturnal hemoglobinuria, lupus, hypersplenism, and human immunodeficiency virus (HIV).

     3. Medication induced secondary to valproic acid, methotrexate, carboplatin, and other chemotherapy drugs.

       (a) May also be secondary to heparin, heparin-induced thrombocytopenia (HIT).

       (b) Aspirin does not decrease the number of platelets but does decrease the function of the platelets.

# COAGULATION TESTING

## I. PROTHROMBIN TIME (PT)/PARTIAL THROMBOPLASTIN TIME (PTT)

a. **PT**

   i. A measure of the activity of the extrinsic and common coagulation pathways.

     1. Fig. 16.3 shows coagulation pathways.

   ii. Measures activity of factors II (prothrombin), V, VII, and X, as well as fibrinogen.

   iii. Test standardized using the international normalized ratio (INR).

   iv. Used to monitor warfarin therapy.

   v. Prolonged also in vitamin K deficiency, liver disease, DIC, and deficiencies in factors II, V, VII, X and fibrinogen.

b. **PTT**

   i. A measure of the activity of the intrinsic and common coagulation pathways.

     1. See Fig. 16.3.

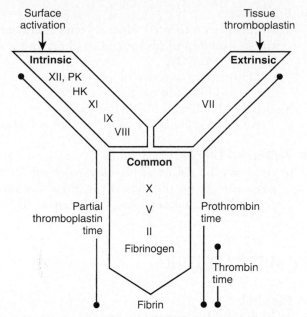

**Fig. 16.3** Coagulation pathways. *(From McPherson RA, Pincus MR: Henry's Clinical Diagnosis and Management by Laboratory Methods, 21st ed. Fig. 38-7.)*

   ii. Measures activity of factors prekallikrein (PK), HMW kininogen (HK), V, VIII, IX, X, XI, XII, II (prothrombin), and fibrinogen.

   iii. Used to monitor heparin therapy.

   iv. Prolonged also in deficiencies of the above factors and von Willebrand's disease.

     1. Anti-Xa heparin assay can also be used to monitor standard or unfractionated heparin therapy.

## II. BLEEDING TIME

a. **Is a measure of the efficiency of the vascular and platelet phases of clotting**

   i. Normal range is 3 to 9 minutes.

b. **Can be used as a screening test for inherited disorders of platelet function**

## III. FIBRINOGEN/FIBRIN DEGRADATION PRODUCTS (FDP)

a. **Fibrinogen**

   i. Thrombin converts fibrinogen to fibrin, which is used to stabilize the platelet plug.

     1. Fibrin monomers with activated factor XIII leads to cross-linking of the fibrin and stabilization of the clot.

   ii. Used to diagnose fibrinogen disorders or inhibitors of thrombin.

   iii. Fibrinogen level will be decreased in DIC.

b. **FDP**

   i. Measure of the plasmin cleaved fibrinogen by-products.

   ii. Normal range is 0 to 5 μg/mL.

   iii. Increased in DIC or fibrinogenolysis.

## IV. D-DIMER

a. **A neoantigen formed when thrombin initiates the conversion of fibrinogen to fibrin and activates factor XIII**

   i. Formed as a result of plasmin digestion of cross-linked fibrin.

b. **Is a test for fibrinolysis (clot lysing)**

c. **Elevated levels in DIC and pulmonary embolism**

## V. PLATELET AGGREGATION STUDIES

a. **Assesses the ability of platelets to clump in response to the addition of various activators (eg, collagen, epinephrine, ADP, ristocetin).**

# CHEMISTRY TESTING

## I. GENERAL

a. **Body Fluid Compartments**

   i. Intracellular.

   1. 66% of total body volume.

   2. Major intracellular ions include potassium, magnesium, phosphate, and proteins.

   ii. Extracellular.

   1. 33% of total body volume.

   (a) Made up of interstitial fluid (75% of the extracellular volume) and intravascular fluid (25% of the extracellular volume).

   2. Major extracellular ions include sodium, chloride, and bicarbonate.

   iii. Osmolality.

   1. Is a measure of the number of particles dissolved in a fluid.

   2. Determines the distribution of water between the intracellular and extracellular compartments.

   3. Calculation.

   (a) Calculated osmolality = 2 (Sodium [mEq/L]) + Glucose (mg/dL)/18 + Blood urea nitrogen (mg/dL)/2.8 + Alcohol (mg/dL)/4.6.

   (i) Alcohol added to formula in cases with elevated alcohol levels.

   4. Osmolal gap.

   (a) Difference between the measured serum osmolality and the calculated serum osmolality.

   (b) If osmolal gap is greater than 10, consider accumulation of abnormal substances. Includes the following:

   (i) Methanol.

   (ii) Ethylene glycol.

   (iii) Isopropyl alcohol.

   (iv) Acetone.

## II. ELECTROLYTES

a. **Sodium**

   i. Is the major extracellular cation.

   ii. Is responsible for maintenance of normal water distribution and osmotic pressure.

   iii. Excretion is by the kidneys and is controlled by aldosterone.

   iv. Mechanisms of hypernatremia include excessive hypertonic salt solutions, hyperaldosteronism, Cushing's syndrome, water deprivation, and water loss.

   v. Mechanisms of hyponatremia include inadequate intake, hypoaldosteronism, excessive diuretic therapy, and excessive water intake.

   vi. Table 16.2 summarizes the causes of hypernatremia and hyponatremia.

   1. Pseudohyponatremia may be noted secondary to hyperlipidemia and paraproteinemia.

b. **Potassium**

   i. Is the major intracellular cation.

   1. Readily obtained in the diet.

   ii. Excreted by the kidneys without a threshold.

   iii. Is responsible for the resting membrane potential of cells.

   iv. Serum potassium levels change with change in blood pH.

   1. Acidosis leads to an elevated potassium level, and alkalosis leads to a decreased potassium level.

   v. Hyperkalemia occurs with tissue destruction and renal failure.

   vi. Hypokalemia occurs with decreased dietary intake, loss in the urine with diabetes mellitus and diuretic therapy, vomiting, and diarrhea.

   1. In diabetes mellitus, treatment with insulin will cause movement of potassium into the cells with glucose leading to hypokalemia.

   vii. Table 16.3 summarizes causes of hypokalemia and hyperkalemia.

   1. Pseudohyperkalemia is noted with RBC hemolysis, leukocytosis, and thrombocytosis.

c. **Chloride**

   i. Is the major extracellular anion.

**TABLE 16.2**

| Causes of Hypernatremia and Hyponatremia | |
| --- | --- |
| **Hypernatremia** | **Hyponatremia** |
| Cushing's syndrome | Cardiac failure |
| Diabetes insipidus | Cirrhosis |
| Diarrhea | Hypoaldosteronism |
| Excessive diaphoresis | Inadequate water intake |
| Hyperaldosteronism | IV hypotonic saline |
| IV hypertonic saline | Nephrotic syndrome |
| Water deprivation | Syndrome of inappropriate antidiuretic hormone (SIADH) |

**TABLE 16.3**

| Causes of Hypokalemia and Hyperkalemia | |
|---|---|
| **Hypokalemia** | **Hyperkalemia** |
| Albuterol | ACE inhibitors |
| Amphotericin B | Addison's disease |
| Decreased water intake | Crush injuries |
| Diuretics | Heparin |
| Hypomagnesemia | K+-sparing diuretics |
| | Oliguric renal failure |

    ii. Obtained in the diet and excreted by the kidneys.

    iii. Assists in maintaining proper water distribution and osmotic pressure.

    iv. Hypochloridemia is noted with prolonged vomiting, nasogastric suctioning, anion-gap metabolic acidosis, and hyponatremia.

    v. Hyperchloridemia is noted in dehydration, renal tubular acidosis, respiratory alkalosis, and bromism.

  **d. Bicarbonate**

    i. Second major extracellular anion.

    ii. Most of the carbon dioxide in the body is in the form of bicarbonate.

      1. Bicarbonate serves as a buffer of hydrogen ions.

## III. LIVER FUNCTION TESTS

  **a. Alkaline Phosphatase (ALP)**

    i. Found in liver, bone, intestine, and placenta.

    ii. Increased in obstructive hepatobiliary disease, osteomalacia, osteosarcoma, bone metastases, Paget's disease, hyperparathyroidism, pregnancy, hepatotoxic drugs, and physiologic bone growth.

      1. Used to measure extent of bone metastases in prostate cancer.

      2. Increase secondary to gallstones may take several hours to occur.

    iii. Levels normal in osteoporosis.

    iv. γ-Glutamyltransferase (GGT) and 5'-nucleotidase can be used to separate elevated ALP due to liver disease versus bone source.

      1. GGT and 5'-nucleotidase will be elevated in liver disease and will be normal in bone disease.

  **b. Alanine Aminotransferase (ALT)**

    i. Intracellular enzyme involved in amino acid metabolism.

    ii. Present in liver, kidney, skeletal muscle, and heart.

      1. Released with tissue damage.

    iii. Increased in acute viral hepatitis, biliary tract obstruction, alcoholic hepatitis, cirrhosis, liver abscess, liver cancer, and right heart failure.

    iv. ALT is preferred over aspartate aminotransferase (AST) to evaluate liver injury.

      1. ALT greater than AST in acute viral hepatitis.

      2. Levels greater than 300 IU/L are rare in alcoholic liver disease.

  **c. Aspartate Aminotransferase (AST)**

    i. Intracellular enzyme involved in amino acid metabolism.

    ii. Present in liver, skeletal muscle, brain, red blood cells, and heart.

      1. Released with tissue injury.

    iii. Increased in acute viral hepatitis, biliary tract obstruction, alcoholic hepatitis, cirrhosis, liver abscess, liver cancer, and right heart failure.

      1. AST greater than ALT in alcoholic hepatitis and cirrhosis.

  **d. γ-Glutamyltransferase (GGT)**

    i. Enzyme present in liver, kidney, and pancreas.

    ii. Increased with liver disease, biliary obstruction, liver neoplasm, and medications.

      1. Medications include phenytoin and phenobarbital.

    iii. Increased levels noted with alcohol usage.

      1. May be helpful in screening for alcohol use disorder.

      2. Increased levels indicate three or more drinks (>15 g) per day.

    iv. Used to confirm hepatic origin of elevated serum ALP.

  **e. Bilirubin**

    i. Bilirubin is a product of hemoglobin metabolism.

    ii. Conjugated in the liver and secreted in the bile.

    iii. Jaundice noted when bilirubin greater than 2.5 mg/dL.

      1. Table 16.4 lists laboratory findings in the various etiologies of jaundice.

    iv. Elevated levels noted in liver disease, biliary obstruction, and hemolysis.

      1. Only conjugated (direct) bilirubin appears in the urine and indicates liver disease.

      2. Increased unconjugated (indirect) bilirubin is noted with hemolysis.

    v. Isolated increase in bilirubin without other elevation in liver function tests indicates familial cause or hemolysis.

      1. Familial causes include the following:

        (a) Gilbert's syndrome: elevation in indirect bilirubin.

        (b) Dubin-Johnson syndrome: elevation in direct bilirubin.

        (c) Rotor's syndrome: elevation in direct bilirubin.

          (i) Dubin-Johnson syndrome is separated from Rotor's syndrome in

**TABLE 16.4**

| Laboratory Findings in the Various Etiologies of Jaundice | | | | | | | |
|---|---|---|---|---|---|---|---|
| | Blood | | | | | Urine | |
| Disease | Indirect Bilirubin | Direct Bilirubin | ALP | AST/ALT | Stool Color | Bilirubin | Urobilinogen |
| Hemolytic | ↑↑ | Normal | Normal | Normal | Normal | None | ↑ |
| Gilbert's syndrome | ↑ | Normal | Normal | Normal | Normal | None | Normal or ↓ |
| Hepatocellular damage | ↑ | ↑ | Normal or ↑ | ↑↑ | Normal | ↑ | ↑ |
| Intrahepatic cholestasis | Normal | ↑ | ↑ | Normal | Pale | ↑ | ↓ |
| Extrahepatic biliary obstruction | Normal | ↑↑ | ↑↑ | Normal or ↑ | Pale | ↑ | ↓ |

*ALP,* Alkaline phosphatase; *AST/ALT,* aspartate aminotransferase/alanine aminotransferase.

that Dubin-Johnson syndrome has dense pigmentation on liver biopsy and has normal urine coproporphyrin. Elevated urine coproporphyrin is noted in Rotor's syndrome.

vi. Table 16.5 summarizes liver function tests.

## IV. RENAL TESTS

a. **Blood Urea Nitrogen (BUN)**
   i. Urea is formed in the liver and is the final product of protein metabolism.
   ii. BUN is used as an index of glomerular function.
      1. Is freely filtered across the glomerular membrane, with 25% of urea reabsorbed into the extracellular fluid (ECF) from the tubules.
      2. Amount excreted varies depending on dietary protein intake, fever, diabetes, and increased adrenal gland activity.
      3. Doubling of the BUN equals a decrease in the glomerular filtration rate (GFR) by 50%.
   iii. Is increased in chronic renal failure, urinary tract obstruction, gastrointestinal (GI) hemorrhage,

diabetes mellitus with ketoacidosis, congestive heart failure (CHF), dehydration, shock, and increasing age.
      1. If BUN is elevated and the serum creatinine is normal, consider a nonrenal cause of the elevated BUN.
   iv. Is decreased in liver failure, malnutrition, anabolic steroid use, nephrotic syndrome, and syndrome of inappropriate antidiuretic hormone (SIADH).

b. **Creatinine**
   i. Is a by-product of the breakdown of muscle creatine phosphate resulting from energy metabolism.
      1. Produced at a constant rate depending on muscle mass.
   ii. Removed from the body via the kidneys and is a measure of glomerular filtration or renal function.
      1. Becomes significantly elevated when GFR decreases by 40% to 60%.
   iii. Creatinine is decreased in patients with decreased muscle mass, advanced liver disease, and pregnancy.
   iv. Creatinine is increased in impaired renal function, urinary tract obstruction, muscle disease, CHF, dehydration, shock, and rhabdomyolysis.

c. **BUN:Creatinine Ratio**
   i. Normal ratio is 10–20:1.
   ii. Ratio is increased in prerenal causes (e.g., dehydration and hypotension) and postrenal causes (e.g., obstruction).
   iii. Ratio is decreased in intrinsic renal disease, such as acute tubular necrosis.
   iv. Table 16.6 lists laboratory findings in renal failure.

## V. LIPID PROFILE

a. **Cholesterol**
   i. Produced in the liver or consumed in the diet.

**TABLE 16.5**

**Summary of Liver Function Tests**

**Measures of Hepatocellular Damage**
Alanine aminotransferase
Aspartate aminotransferase

**Measures of Biliary Obstruction**
Alkaline phosphatase
Bilirubin
γ-Glutamyltransferase

**Measures of Liver Function (Synthesis)**
Albumin
Ammonia
Prothrombin time

**TABLE 16.6**

## Laboratory Findings in Renal Failure

| Site | Serum BUN:Crt Ratio | Urine Na (mEq/L) | Urine Osmolality (mOsm/kg) | Proteinuria | Urinary Sediment |
|---|---|---|---|---|---|
| Prerenal | >20:1 | <20 | >500 | Trace | Benign or few hyaline casts |
| **Intrarenal** | | | | | |
| Acute glomerulonephritis | <10:1 | <20 | Variable | 4+ | RBC casts, WBC casts, fatty casts, dysmorphic RBCs |
| Acute tubular necrosis | <10:1 | >20 | 250-300 | 2+ | Renal tubular cells, pigmented granular casts |
| Acute interstitial nephritis | <10:1 | Variable | Variable | 2+ | RBCs, WBCs, WBC casts, granular casts, renal tubular cells, eosinophils |
| Postrenal | >20:1 | Variable | <400 | Trace | Benign or crystals |

*BUN*, Bun urea nitrogen; *RBC*, red blood cell; *WBC*, white blood cell.

1. Used as the building block for cell membranes and steroid hormones.
2. Levels influenced by heredity, diet, and endocrine organ function.
   ii. Lipid profile typically includes total cholesterol, triglycerides, low-density lipoprotein–cholesterol (LDL-C), and high-density lipoprotein–cholesterol (HDL-C).
   iii. Primary causes of elevation include polygenic hypercholesterolemia and familial hypercholesterolemia.
   iv. Secondary causes of elevation include hypothyroidism, nephrotic syndrome, biliary obstruction, Cushing's syndrome, and use of corticosteroids.
   v. Decreased in severe liver disease, hyperthyroidism, acute or chronic illness, malnutrition, and malabsorption.

b. **High-Density Lipoprotein (HDL)**
   i. A lipoprotein used to transport cholesterol or triglycerides in the blood.
      1. Smallest lipoprotein particle, but the densest.
   ii. 30% of blood cholesterol is carried by HDL.
   iii. Can remove cholesterol from an atheroma and transport it back to the liver.
      1. Called the "good" cholesterol.
   iv. Optimal level is greater than 60 mg/dL.

c. **Low-Density Lipoprotein (LDL)**
   i. Lipoprotein that transports cholesterol and triglycerides from the liver to the peripheral tissue.
      1. Called the "bad" cholesterol.
   ii. Calculated by the following:
      1. LDL-C = Total cholesterol (mg/dL) − HDL-C (mg/dL) − (0.20 × Triglyceride [mg/dL]).
   iii. Optimal level is less than 100 mg/dL.

d. **Triglycerides**
   i. Fat is hydrolyzed in the small intestine, absorbed and resynthesized by mucosal cells, and secreted into lacteals.
   ii. Triglycerides are in chylomicrons and are cleared from the blood by lipase.
      1. Endogenous triglycerides are produced in the liver.
   iii. Elevated levels are risk factors for coronary artery disease and pancreatitis.
      1. If serum is clear, triglycerides are less than 350 mg/dL.
   iv. Increased level in hypertriglyceridemia, hypothyroidism, diabetes mellitus, fatty liver, biliary tract obstruction, obesity, metabolic syndrome, cirrhosis, and pancreatitis.
      1. Levels may increase with the use of beta-blockers, cholestyramine, corticosteroids, estrogens, and diuretics.
   v. Decreased levels in malnutrition, malabsorption, hyperthyroidism, and parenchymal liver disease.
   vi. Optimal level is less than 165 mg/dL.

## VI. PROTEINS

a. **Total Protein**
   i. Plasma protein concentration determines the colloidal osmotic pressure.
   ii. Plasma protein concentration is determined by nutritional status, liver function, renal function, hydration, and various disease states.
   iii. Total protein consists primarily of albumin and globulin.
   iv. Increased levels noted in gammopathies, dehydration, and the use of anabolic steroids, androgens, and corticosteroids.
   v. Decreased levels noted in protein-losing enteropathies, burns, nephrotic syndrome,

dietary deficiency, malabsorption, and chronic liver disease.

**b. Albumin**
　i. The major component of the plasma proteins.
　　1. Levels influenced by nutritional state, liver function, renal function, and various disease states.
　　2. Functions as carrier of a variety of substances.
　ii. Increased levels noted in dehydration, shock, and hemoconcentration.
　iii. Decreased levels due to decreased liver synthesis (liver disease, malnutrition, malabsorption), increased losses (nephrotic syndrome, burns, trauma, hemorrhage, glomerulonephritis), or hemodilution (pregnancy, CHF).

**c. Serum Protein Electrophoresis**
　i. Electrophoresis separates out the various types of proteins.
　ii. Used to diagnose monoclonal gammopathy.
　　1. If Bence Jones proteins (light chains) are suspected, a urine protein electrophoresis is indicated.
　iii. Table 16.7 interprets serum protein electrophoresis.

## VII. CALCIUM/PHOSPHORUS
　**a. Calcium**

**TABLE 16.7**

| Interpretation of Serum Protein Electrophoresis | | |
| --- | --- | --- |
| **Band** | **Contents** | **Disease States** |
| Albumin | Albumin | Increased: dehydration, shock<br>Decreased: nephrotic syndrome, liver disease, glomerulonephritis |
| Alpha 1 | Alpha-1 antitrypsin<br>Alpha-1 lipoprotein<br>Alpha-1 acid glycoprotein | Increased: inflammatory states, pregnancy<br>Decreased: alpha-1-antitrypsin deficiency |
| Alpha 2 | Alpha-2 macro-globulin<br>Haptoglobin<br>Ceruloplasmin | Increased: nephrotic syndrome, inflammatory states, oral contraceptives, steroid therapy, hyperthyroidism<br>Decreased: hemolysis, liver disease |
| Beta | Transferrin<br>Hemopexin<br>Complement C3<br>Beta-lipoproteins | Increased: hyperlipidemia, hemoglobinemia, iron-deficiency anemia<br>Decreased: hypobetalipoprotein-emias |
| Gamma | Immunoglobulins G, A, D, E, and M | Increased: gammopathies, liver disease, chronic infections, multiple myeloma, Waldenström's macroglobulinemia<br>Decreased: immunodeficiency |

　i. Is necessary in bone structure, blood coagulation, muscle contraction, and nerve impulse transmission.
　ii. Calcium levels are controlled by various substances.
　　1. Vitamin D is required for absorption of calcium in the intestine.
　　2. Parathyroid hormone (PTH) causes calcium to be released from the bone into the serum and increases calcium reabsorption in the kidney.
　　3. Calcitonin, which originates in the thyroid, inhibits osteoblast activity, and lowers calcium by inhibiting PTH and vitamin D.
　iii. Calcium distribution.
　　1. 50% is bound to albumin.
　　　(a) Total calcium should be corrected in the presence of low albumin.
　　　(b) For each 1 g drop in albumin from a normal of 4.0 g/dL, add 0.8 mg/dL to the total calcium.
　　2. 47% is free or ionized.
　　3. 3% is bound to phosphate, citrate, lactate, or bicarbonate.
　iv. Hypocalcemia is noted in hypoparathyroidism, chronic renal disease, and hypomagnesemia.
　v. Hypercalcemia is noted in primary hyperparathyroidism, malignancy, sarcoidosis, and vitamin D excess.

**b. Phosphorus**
　i. Important in the regulation of cellular enzymes, as a substrate for adenosine triphosphate (ATP) synthesis, and the bone-building process.
　ii. Levels are controlled by acid-base status, vitamin D (will increase serum phosphate level), and PTH (will decrease serum phosphate level).
　iii. Calcium and phosphorus are reciprocals of each other, as one goes up the other goes down.
　iv. Hyperphosphatemia is noted in renal failure, hypoparathyroidism, chemotherapy, and rhabdomyolysis.
　v. Hypophosphatemia is noted in renal tubular defects, hyperparathyroidism, and the use of diuretics.

## VIII. AMYLASE/LIPASE
　**a. Amylase**
　　i. Used to hydrolyze complex carbohydrates.
　　ii. Derived from the pancreas and salivary glands.
　　　1. Other tissues with some amylase activity include the ovaries and intestines.
　　iii. Levels increased in acute pancreatitis, pancreatic duct obstruction, bowel obstruction

or infarct, mumps, diabetic ketoacidosis (DKA), peritonitis, and ruptured ectopic pregnancy.

    1. In acute pancreatitis the amylase level will increase in 6 to 24 hours, remain elevated for a few days, and return to normal in 2 to 7 days.

b. **Lipase**

    i. Responsible for the hydrolysis of the glycerol esters of long-chain fatty acids to produce fatty acids and glycerol.

    ii. Found almost exclusively in the pancreas.

    iii. Increased in acute pancreatitis, peritonitis, diabetes mellitus with DKA, cystic fibrosis, and inflammatory bowel disease.

        1. May be normal in chronic pancreatitis and pancreatic malignancy.

## IX. OTHER

a. **Ammonia**

    i. Is an end product of protein metabolism.

        1. Formed by bacteria in the intestine.

        2. Liver removes most of the ammonia via the portal vein circulation and converts it to urea.

        3. Is excreted by the kidneys.

    ii. Is increased in Reye's syndrome, liver disease (cirrhosis), hepatic encephalopathy, GI bleed, renal disease, shock, and certain inborn errors of metabolism.

b. **Lactate Dehydrogenase (LDH)**

    i. Enzyme that catalyzes the interconversion of lactate and pyruvate in the presence of NAD/NADH.

    ii. Found in all body cells and fluids.

        1. High concentration in red blood cells, so may be falsely elevated in hemolyzed samples.

    iii. Values used as prognostic factor in patients with lymphoma, chronic lymphocytic leukemia, and metastatic melanoma.

    iv. LDH isoenzymes are not clinically useful.

    v. Levels are increased in tissue necrosis, pneumocystis pneumonia, hemolytic anemias, vitamin $B_{12}$ and folate deficiency, hepatitis, cirrhosis, renal disease, CHF, and hepatotoxicity (due to acetaminophen).

        1. May be decreased in patients on clofibrate.

c. **Magnesium**

    i. Is essential as an activator of more than 300 enzymes.

        1. Found in green vegetables, meat, grain, and seafood.

    ii. Hypermagnesemia develops with intake of magnesium-containing antacids.

    iii. Hypomagnesemia is noted with diarrhea, diuretics, diabetes, alcohol consumption, and medications such as cyclosporine, gentamicin, and cisplatin.

d. **Uric Acid**

    i. Is the end product of purine (adenosine and guanosine) metabolism via xanthine oxidase.

        1. Metabolism occurs primarily in the liver and intestinal mucosa.

    ii. Excreted via the kidneys.

    iii. Hyperuricemia noted in chronic renal disease (most common), leukemia, chemotherapy, polycythemia vera, thiazide diuretics, eclampsia, and hyperparathyroidism.

    iv. Hypouricemia noted in severe liver disease, use of allopurinol, and Fanconi's syndrome.

## URINALYSIS

## I. MACROSCOPIC

a. **Color/Odor**

    i. Color may indicate disease states.

        1. Cloudy: pyuria, lipiduria, and hyperoxaluria.

        2. Brown: bile pigments, myoglobin.

        3. Orange: bile pigments.

        4. Red: hematuria, hemoglobin, and myoglobin.

        5. Yellow: concentrated urine.

        6. Dark yellow: bilirubin.

    ii. Odor.

        1. Foul smelling: infection.

        2. Maple sugar: maple syrup disease.

        3. Musty: phenylketonuria.

        4. Acetone: diabetes mellitus.

b. **Specific Gravity**

    i. Measure of the kidney's ability to concentrate the urine.

    ii. Normal range is 1.005 to 1.025.

    iii. Typically the specific gravity varies inversely with amount of urine excreted.

        1. Exceptions include diabetes and hypertension.

    iv. Elevated specific gravity noted in glycosuria, fever, dehydration, diarrhea, and SIADH.

    v. Decreased specific gravity in diabetes insipidus, adrenal insufficiency, acute renal failure, and diuretic use.

c. **Glucose**

    i. Glucose may be elevated in diabetes mellitus and stress.

    ii. Renal threshold for glucose is 180 to 200 mg/dL before it is lost in the urine.

    iii. Routine glucose test does not detect reducing sugars.

        1. Clinitest used to test for reducing sugars such as galactose, fructose, and lactose.

            (a) Clinitest used in infants to detect possible inborn errors of metabolism.

d. **Protein**
  i. Single most important indicator of renal disease.
    1. Protein is not filtered by the glomeruli in normal kidney function.
  ii. Transient proteinuria noted with exercise, postural, pregnancy, or emotional stress.
  iii. Persistent proteinuria noted with CHF, multiple myeloma, toxemia of pregnancy, and primary renal disease.
  iv. Mechanisms include glomerular damage or decreased tubular reabsorption.
    1. Glomerular damage noted in glomerulonephritis, systemic lupus erythematosus (SLE), malignant hypertension, amyloidosis, and diabetes mellitus.
    2. Decreased tubular reabsorption noted in renal tubular acidosis, pyelonephritis, interstitial nephritis, and Wilson's disease.
  v. Routine protein test detects only albumin.
    1. Bence Jones, immunoglobulins, or microalbumin are not detected.

e. **Blood**
  i. Present due to glomerular injury.
  ii. Hematuria, presence of intact RBCs, is secondary to trauma, kidney stones, tumors, and acute glomerulonephritis.
  iii. Hemoglobinuria, presence of free hemoglobin, noted with transfusion reactions and hemolytic anemias.
    1. Myoglobin will cause a false-positive test.

f. **Ketones**
  i. Develop because of fat metabolism.
  ii. There are three ketone bodies:
    1. Acetone.
    2. Beta-hydroxybutyric acid.
    3. Acetoacetic acid.
  iii. Are present in diabetes mellitus, starvation, high-fat diets, prolonged vomiting, anorexia, fever, and hyperthyroidism.

g. **Bilirubin**
  i. Product of RBC breakdown.
  ii. Detects presence of water soluble or conjugated bilirubin.
  iii. Positive in liver inflammation and biliary obstruction.
  iv. Negative in hemolytic anemia.
    1. Unconjugated bilirubin noted in hemolytic anemia and is not water soluble.

h. **Urobilinogen**
  i. End product of conjugated bilirubin.
  ii. Small amount filtered by the glomerulus and excreted in the urine.
  iii. Increased levels noted in hemolytic anemia and liver damage.

i. **Nitrite**
  i. Several bacteria convert nitrate to nitrite.
    1. Most common in gram-negative rods, such as *Escherichia coli*.
  ii. Used in combination with the leukocyte esterase to diagnose urinary tract infections.

j. **Leukocyte Esterase**
  i. The enzyme, leukocyte esterase, is found in neutrophils.
    1. Will also detect disintegrated neutrophils.
  ii. Used in combination with the nitrite test to diagnose urinary tract infections.

II. **MICROSCOPIC**
  a. **Table 16.8 lists common urinalysis microscopic findings**

# THYROID TESTING

I. **TRIIODOTHYRONINE ($T_3$)**
  a. **$T_3$ reflects the metabolically active thyroid hormone**
    i. Influenced by thyroid hormone–binding activity.
  b. **Increased in hyperthyroidism and decreased in hypothyroidism and in the use of amiodarone**
    i. Check $T_3$ in patients with low TSH and normal thyroxine ($T_4$) to evaluate for $T_3$ toxicosis.

**TABLE 16.8**

| Common Urinalysis Microscopic Findings | |
| --- | --- |
| **Substance** | **Disease States** |
| White blood cells | Renal/urinary tract infections<br>Glomerulonephritis<br>Interstitial nephritis (eosinophils) |
| Red blood cells | Damage to glomerular membrane<br>Vascular injury<br>Exercise<br>Trauma<br>Tumor |
| Squamous epithelial | Normal finding that may represent vaginal contamination |
| Renal tubular cells | Tubular necrosis |
| Transitional cells | Normal in small number |
| Hyaline casts | Normal in small number<br>Increased in glomerulonephritis, pyelonephritis, fever, and exercise |
| WBC casts | Pyelonephritis (most common)<br>Acute glomerulonephritis<br>Interstitial nephritis<br>Lupus nephritis |
| RBC casts | Glomerulonephritis<br>Renal infarction<br>Goodpasture's disease |
| Waxy casts | Chronic renal failure<br>Nephrotic syndrome |

## II. THYROXINE (T$_4$)

a. Measure of thyroid gland secretion of T$_4$, bound and free, and is influenced by serum thyroid–binding activity

   i. Free T$_4$ level is a more exact measure of biologically active hormone.

     1. Free T$_4$ best used to diagnose central hypothyroidism.

b. Elevated in hyperthyroidism, use of amiodarone, and pregnancy; decreased in hypothyroidism and use of phenytoin, carbamazepine, and androgens

## III. THYROID-STIMULATING HORMONE (TSH)

a. An anterior pituitary hormone that stimulates the thyroid gland to produce thyroid hormone

b. Secretion stimulated by thyrotropin-releasing hormone (TRH) from the hypothalamus

   i. Negative feedback of TSH secretion by circulating thyroid hormone.

c. Increased levels in hypothyroidism and decreased in hyperthyroidism and acute medical or surgical disease

d. TSH is best test for screening of thyroid disease and for monitoring thyroid hormone replacement therapy

## RHEUMATOLOGY TESTING

## I. ANTINUCLEAR ANTIBODIES (ANA)

a. Heterogeneous antibodies to nuclear antigens

b. Elevated in the following conditions:

   i. SLE.

   ii. Drug-induced lupus.

   iii. Sjögren's syndrome.

   iv. Rheumatoid arthritis.

   v. Scleroderma.

   vi. Mixed connective tissue disease.

c. Not useful as a screening test, should be used when clinical evidence of connective tissue disease is present

## II. AUTOANTIBODIES

a. Table 16.9 summarizes autoantibodies in disease

## III. ERYTHROCYTE SEDIMENTATION RATE

a. Result of the aggregation of red blood cells due to presence of plasma proteins (acute phase reactants)—in particular fibrinogen

b. Elevated in infections (osteomyelitis and pelvic inflammatory disease [PID]), inflammatory disease (temporal arteritis and polymyalgia rheumatica), neoplasms, inflammatory bowel disease, and endocarditis

**TABLE 16.9**

### Summary of Autoantibodies in Disease

| Autoantibody | Diseases |
|---|---|
| Anti-Smith (Sm) | Systemic lupus erythematosus |
| ds DNA | Systemic lupus erythematosus |
| Scl-70 | Scleroderma |
| Smooth muscle antibodies | Autoimmune chronic active hepatitis<br>Primary biliary cirrhosis |
| SS-A/Ro antibody | Sjögren's syndrome<br>Systemic lupus erythematosus |
| SS-B/La antibody | Sjögren's syndrome |
| Anti-centromere | Limited scleroderma |
| Anti-histone | Drug-induced lupus |
| Anti-RNP | Mixed connective tissue disease |

c. Decreased in sickle cell anemia, polycythemia, CHF, and high-dose corticosteroids

d. Should not be used to screen asymptomatic patients for disease

e. Used to monitor response to therapy in temporal arteritis and polymyalgia rheumatica

## IV. RHEUMATOID FACTOR

a. IgM autoantibody that reacts against the Fc region of IgG

b. Positive in rheumatoid arthritis, Sjögren's syndrome, scleroderma, SLE, and Waldenström's macroglobulinemia

   i. Low titers in viral infections and chronic bacterial infections.

c. Should not be used as a screening test for rheumatoid arthritis in asymptomatic patient population

## V. C-REACTIVE PROTEIN (CRP)

a. An acute-phase reactant

b. Produced in response to inflammatory cytokines and not affected by hormones

c. Rapid increase noted with infection, inflammation, trauma, tissue necrosis, and autoimmune disorders

   i. Levels increase within 2 hours, peak in 24 to 48 hours, and then start to decline.

   ii. Patients with rheumatoid arthritis will have consistently elevated levels during active disease and decreased levels during remissions.

d. Elevated high sensitivity CRP is a risk factor for atherosclerotic disease

## MICROBIOLOGY

## I. GRAM STAIN

a. Table 16.10 summarizes common Gram stain results

**TABLE 16.10**

| Common Gram Stain Results | | | |
| --- | --- | --- | --- |
| **Gram-Positive Cocci** | **Gram-Positive Rods** | **Gram-Negative Cocci** | **Gram-Negative Rods** |
| Peptostreptococcus | Bacillus | Neisseria | Enterobacter |
| Staphylococcus | Corynebacterium | | Escherichia |
| Streptococcus | Bordetella | | Haemophilus |
| | Erysipelothrix | | Klebsiella |
| | Lactobacillus | | Moraxella |
| | Listeria | | Proteus |
| | Propionibacterium | | Pseudomonas |
| | | | Salmonella |
| | | | Serratia |
| | | | Shigella |

# QUESTIONS

## QUESTION 1
Which of the following findings is noted in patients with iron-deficiency anemia?

A  Elevated MCV

B  Elevated MCHC

C  Decreased RDW

D  Decreased MCH

E  Increased reticulocyte count

## QUESTION 2
Which of the following is used to monitor heparin therapy?

A  PT

B  PTT

C  D-dimer

D  Bleeding time

E  Ristocetin cofactor assay

## QUESTION 3
Which of the following is responsible for the maintenance of normal water distribution?

A  Potassium

B  Creatinine

C  D-xylose

D  Sodium

E  BUN

## QUESTION 4
In which of the following conditions is the alkaline phosphatase level normal?

A  Obstructive liver disease

B  Hyperparathyroidism

C  Paget's disease

D  Osteoporosis

E  Pregnancy

## QUESTION 5
Which of the following laboratory abnormalities is noted in patients with recent alcohol use?

A  Elevated GGT

B  Elevated bilirubin

C  Decreased RBC count

D  Decreased MCV

E  Decreased AST

## QUESTION 6
Which of the following is a primary source of amylase?

A  Liver

B  Spleen

C  Testicles

D  Small intestine

E  Salivary glands

## QUESTION 7
A patient presents for her annual physical examination. Physical examination is normal. Laboratory tests are normal except for an elevated indirect bilirubin. Which of the following is the most likely diagnosis?

A  Hepatitis A

B  Rotor's syndrome

C  Gilbert's syndrome

D  Dubin-Johnson syndrome

E  Biliary tract obstruction

## QUESTION 8
A 24-year-old female presents with joint pain and a facial rash. Laboratory testing reveals a negative RF and positive ANA. Which of the following autoantibodies is most likely to be positive in this patient?

A  SS-B

B  Scl-70

C  Ro antibody

D  Anti-ds DNA

E  Anti-histone

## QUESTIONS—cont'd

### QUESTION 9
Which of the following organisms is a gram-positive rod?
A  *Giardia lamblia*
B  *Serratia marcescens*
C  *Neisseria meningitidis*
D  *Haemophilus influenzae*
E  *Corynebacterium diphtheriae*

### QUESTION 10
Which of the following is the Gram stain result of *Clostridium tetani?*
A  Gram-positive rod
B  Gram-positive cocci
C  Gram-negative rod
D  Gram-negative cocci
E  Organism does not Gram stain

## ANSWERS

**1.  D**
EXPLANATION: Iron-deficiency anemia presents with decreased MCH, MCV, and reticulocyte count, with normal MCHC, and with increased RDW. *Topic: Complete blood count*
☐ Correct   ☐ Incorrect

**2.  B**
EXPLANATION: PTT is used to monitor heparin therapy. PT is used to monitor warfarin therapy. D-dimer is used in the diagnosis of pulmonary embolism. Bleeding time is used to monitor platelet function. Ristocetin cofactor assay is used to test the function of von Willebrand's factor (vWF). *Topic: Coagulation testing*
☐ Correct   ☐ Incorrect

**3.  D**
EXPLANATION: Sodium is responsible for maintaining water distribution and osmotic pressure. *Topic: Chemistry testing: electrolytes*
☐ Correct   ☐ Incorrect

**4.  D**
EXPLANATION: Alkaline phosphatase is normal in osteoporosis and is elevated in hyperthyroidism, Paget's disease, obstructive liver disease, and pregnancy. *Topic: Chemistry testing: liver function tests*
☐ Correct   ☐ Incorrect

**5.  A**
EXPLANATION: Recent use of alcohol will cause an elevation in GGT and MCV. Elevated bilirubin is noted in liver disease, and decreased RBC count and MCV are noted in anemia. *Topic: Chemistry testing: liver function tests*
☐ Correct   ☐ Incorrect

**6.  E**
EXPLANATION: Amylase is primarily found in the pancreas and the salivary glands. *Topic: Chemistry testing: amylase/lipase*
☐ Correct   ☐ Incorrect

**7.  C**
EXPLANATION: Patients with Gilbert's syndrome present with an isolated elevation in indirect bilirubin. Patients with Rotor's syndrome and Dubin-Johnson syndrome present with isolated elevation in direct bilirubin. Patients with hepatitis A present with elevations in AST, ALT, and both direct and indirect bilirubin. Patients with biliary tract obstruction present with an elevated alkaline phosphatase, AST/ALT, and bilirubin. *Topic: Chemistry testing: liver function tests*
☐ Correct   ☐ Incorrect

**8.  D**
EXPLANATION: Patients with lupus present with joint pain and malar rash. ANA will be positive. Anti-ds DNA and Anti-Sm are specific autoantibodies for lupus. *Topic: Rheumatology testing: antinuclear antibodies (ANA)*
☐ Correct   ☐ Incorrect

**9.  E**
EXPLANATION: *Corynebacterium diphtheriae* is a gram-positive rod. *Giardia lamblia* is a parasite and does not Gram stain. *Serratia marcescens* is a gram-negative rod. *Neisseria meningitidis* is a gram-negative coccus. *Haemophilus influenzae* is a tiny gram-negative rod. *Topic: Microbiology: Gram stain*
☐ Correct   ☐ Incorrect

**10.  A**
EXPLANATION: *C. tetani* is a gram-positive rod. *Topic: Microbiology: Gram stain*
☐ Correct   ☐ Incorrect

# CHAPTER 17
# PROFESSIONAL ISSUES

**ADDITIONAL EXAM CONTENT:**
**PROFESSIONAL PRACTICE**

Legal/medical ethics

Medical informatics

Patient care and communication

Physician/PA relationship

Professional development

Public health (population/society)

Risk management

## ADDITIONAL EXAM CONTENT: PROFESSIONAL PRACTICE

The Physician Assistant National Certifying Exam (PANCE) and Physician Assistant National Recertifying Exam (PANRE) now include a new task category labeled *Professional Practice*. This category includes questions related to professional behaviors and practice of medicine as a physician assistant, and knowledge and skills essential for entry into practice and throughout the careers of PAs. This required knowledge makes up to 5% of questions on the PANCE and 2% of questions on the PANRE.

The professional practice task area is by the National Commission on Certification of Physician Assistants (NCCPA).

### I. LEGAL/MEDICAL ETHICS

This area assesses the test taker's knowledge of religious and cultural beliefs related to health care, informed consent and refusal process, living wills, advance directives, organ donation, code status, do not resuscitate, do not intubate, medical power of attorney, medicolegal issues, patient/provider rights and responsibilities, and privacy, security, and responsibilities related to medical record documentation and management. It also assesses skills in caring for patients with cognitive impairment.

### II. MEDICAL INFORMATICS

This area assesses the test taker's knowledge of billing and coding for accuracy and completeness for reimbursement as well as skill in appropriate medical documentation and using appropriate sources for medical informatics.

### III. PATIENT CARE AND COMMUNICATION

This area assesses the test taker's knowledge of cultural and religious diversity, stewardship of community and patient resources, and providing patient-specific effective and affordable health-care. It also assesses skills related to applying patient/provider rights and responsibilities, patient satisfaction, and providing advice and education related to informed consent and refusal as well as end-of-life decisions.

### IV. PHYSICIAN/PA RELATIONSHIP

This area assesses the test taker's knowledge of scope of practice, professional and clinical limitations, and supervision parameters, including malpractice, mandated reporting, conflict of interest, and impaired provider. It also assesses skills in communicating and consulting with the supervising physician and other specialists or consultants.

### V. PROFESSIONAL DEVELOPMENT

This area assesses the test taker's knowledge of continuing medical education resources and skills including analyzing evidence-based medicine, interpreting data from medical informatics sources, identifying appropriate references, and using epidemiologic techniques to evaluate the spread of disease.

### VI. PUBLIC HEALTH (POPULATION/SOCIETY)

This area assesses the test taker's knowledge of disaster preparedness, infection control measures, occupational health issues in health-care and non-health-care workers, population health, travel health, and epidemiology of disease states. It also includes skills in protecting vulnerable populations and recognizing disparities in access and provision of health care.

### VII. RISK MANAGEMENT

This area assesses the test taker's knowledge of quality improvement and patient safety as well as resource stewardship. It also assesses skills in ensuring patient safety and avoiding medical errors.

# QUESTIONS

## QUESTION 1

A 14-year-old patient is being evaluated for atopic dermatitis that has been refractory to treatment in the past. She is an ideal candidate for participation in a clinical research trial for her condition, for which you are a sub investigator. Which of the following is true regarding ethical considerations for clinical trials?

A Compensation should be commensurate with possible complications

B This patient falls into the category of a "vulnerable population" for clinical trials

C Participants may only discontinue the trial before starting the course of treatment

D Risks and benefits of the treatment should be discussed, but alternative options are unnecessary because the patient has been refractory to these treatments in the past

E A written consent document given to the patient and her parent or guardian is a sufficient method of obtaining informed consent for the patient

## QUESTION 2

You work as an urgent care physician assistant and a friend calls you on Sunday night. He has been suffering from a cold for the past week and believes he now has an ear infection. He is wondering if you will write him a prescription, so he won't have to miss work tomorrow for an appointment. How do you proceed with this situation?

A Call in one dose of medication for tonight and instruct the patient to follow up at a local clinic in the morning

B Discuss the patient's medical history over the phone prior to calling in the prescription to the nearest pharmacy

C Create a chart for the patient, and document the phone call using your office's electronic medical record system before sending the full prescription to the nearest pharmacy

D Encourage the patient to schedule an appointment at his primary care office or urgent care clinic tomorrow

E Instruct the patient to get an appointment at the local clinic tomorrow as it is illegal to prescribe medications for a close friend or family member

## QUESTION 3

You are caring for a patient who has been placed on airborne precautions. Which of the following is the appropriate order for putting on the necessary personal protective equipment (PPE)?

A Eye protection, respirator, gown, gloves

B Eye protection, gloves, respirator, gown

C Gloves, eye protection, gown, respirator

D Gown, eye protection, gloves, respirator

E Gown, respirator, eye protection, gloves

## QUESTION 4

A 42-year-old patient presents for cholecystectomy. Which of the following actions may increase the risk of surgical site infections?

A Positive pressure ventilation in the operating room

B Smoking cessation by the patient 4–6 weeks prior to surgery

C Hair removal at the operative site performed in the operating room

D Using 70% isopropyl alcohol for skin preparation in the operating room

E Target blood glucose levels of surgical patients less than or equal to 200 mg/dL

## QUESTION 5

While walking through the hallway at the hospital, you see your patient who has just been discharged. She states she had forgotten to ask earlier but was wondering about your opinion on CBD (cannabidiol) gummies for her anxiety. Which of the following is the most appropriate course of action?

A Tell the patient that they should discuss this with their primary care provider at their follow-up appointment

B Discuss the lack of research and regulation of CBD gummies for anxiety and document the conversation in her chart

C Suggest that the patient reach out to a local CBD retailer for more information about CBD gummies and add a note in the patient's chart

D Advise the patient against using CBD gummies, no further action is necessary as this conversation occurred outside of the patient's hospital stay

E Warn the patient of the variability in purity and dosage with unregulated products such as CBD gummies and instruct her to bring it up at her follow-up appointment so the conversation can be documented

# ANSWERS

### 1.  B

EXPLANATION: Minors are seen as a vulnerable population in clinical trials as they may not fully comprehend or evaluate the risks and benefits, they may be persuaded by compensation, and may be vulnerable to outside pressure (from providers or parents). *Topic: Legal/medical ethics*

☐ Correct    ☐ Incorrect

### 2.  D

EXPLANATION: Ethics committees generally agree that medical providers should not treat themselves, family members, or close friends. Exceptions, however, include times of emergency, when treatment would not only be warranted but expected, and for short-term, minor problems where an unbiased complete history and physical exam can be performed. *Topic: Legal/medical ethics*

☐ Correct    ☐ Incorrect

### 3.  E

EXPLANATION: Per the Centers for Disease Control and Prevention (CDC), the proper sequence for donning, or putting on, PPE is gown, mask or respirator, goggles or face shield, gloves. The proper sequence for doffing, or removing, PPE is gloves, goggles or face shield, gown, mask or respirator. *Topic: Public health (population/society)*

☐ Correct    ☐ Incorrect

### 4.  C

EXPLANATION: Hair removal prior to surgery may be necessary, but certain practices have been demonstrated to reduce the risk of surgical site infection. This includes avoiding hair removal unless necessary, removing hair with clippers rather than razors, and removing hair before entering the operating room. *Topic: Risk management*

☐ Correct    ☐ Incorrect

### 5.  B

EXPLANATION: Currently, there is limited data regarding the medical benefits or risks associated with CBD products, thus providers should use caution in recommending their use to patients. As patients may use CBD products regardless, it is important to warn them that there may be unreliability of the purity and dosage of CBD among products and manufacturers. Conversations of this type, even outside the patient's appointment, should always be documented in the patient's chart. *Topics: Medical informatics, and Risk management*

☐ Correct    ☐ Incorrect

# CHAPTER 18

# TEST-TAKING STRATEGIES

## CHAPTER OUTLINE

**THE EXAMINATION**
The PANCE
The PANRE

**TEST-TAKING STRATEGIES**
Before the examination
Day of the examination
Test-anxiety strategies

General tips
During the examination
After the examination

## THE EXAMINATION

The Physician Assistant National Certifying Exam (PANCE) and Physician Assistant National Recertifying Exam (PANRE) are developed by the National Commission on the Certification of Physician Assistants (NCCPA). The examination questions are developed by committees comprised of physician assistants (PAs) and physicians. The committee members are selected based on their areas of expertise, geographic locations, and test-writing skills. Each test item goes through multiple levels of review before being placed on the examination. The exam will include scored questions as well as rare questions that are under review; there is no way to distinguish which type of question is which. A number of different versions of the examination are used during each examination block.

When the examination is scored, candidates are given one point for every correct answer and zero points for every incorrect answer to produce the raw examination score. Therefore, you should answer every question; there is no penalty for guessing. After the raw score has been calculated by two different computer systems, the raw score is used to calculate the examinee's proficiency measure. The proficiency measure is based on item difficulty and on the number of correct responses. This process ensures that all proficiency measures are calculated as if each student took the same examination. This proficiency measure is then converted to a scaled score so that results can be compared over time and between different groups of examinees. Scores are in the range of 200 to 800.

## THE PANCE

The PANCE has the following breakdown of tasks, which make up the corresponding percentage of the total examination questions.

| Task | PANCE |
| --- | --- |
| History taking and performing physical examination | 17% |
| Using laboratory and diagnostic studies | 12% |
| Formulating the most likely diagnosis | 18% |
| Health maintenance, patient education, preventative measures | 10% |
| Clinical intervention | 14% |
| Pharmaceutical therapeutics | 14% |
| Applying basic science concepts | 10% |
| Professional practice | 5% |

The majority of the exam (95%) is made up of medical content and coded to one of the task areas. Questions related to professional practice issues make up 5% of the exam. Up to 20% of the exam questions may be questions related to general surgery topics.

Each of the task areas is defined by the NCCPA. The "history taking and performing physical examination" area assesses the test taker's knowledge in the areas of pertinent historical information; signs, symptoms, and physical examination findings associated with medical conditions; risk factors for selected medical conditions; and physical examination techniques.

The "using laboratory and diagnostic studies" area assesses the test taker's knowledge in the areas of indications for initial and subsequent diagnostic and laboratory studies, relevance of common screening tests, diagnostic studies and procedural risk factors, and selection and interpretation of appropriate diagnostic and laboratory studies.

The "formulating the most likely diagnosis" area assesses the test taker's knowledge in the areas of the significance of history, physical examination findings, and diagnostic and laboratory studies as they relate to formulating a diagnosis.

The "health maintenance, patient education, and preventative measures" area assesses the test taker's knowledge in the areas of epidemiology of selected medical conditions, early detection and prevention of selected medical conditions, patient education, prevention of communicable diseases, immunizations, human sexuality, and barriers to care.

The "clinical intervention" area assesses the test taker's knowledge in the areas of management and treatment of selected medical conditions; follow-up and monitoring of therapeutic regimens; indications, contraindications, complications, risks, and benefits of selected procedures; end-of-life issues; and risks and benefits of alternative medicine.

The "pharmaceutical therapeutics" area assesses the test taker's knowledge in the areas of mechanisms of action, indications for use, contraindications, side effects, adverse reactions, drug interactions, drug toxicity, and selection of appropriate pharmacologic therapy for selected medical conditions.

The "applying basic science concepts" area assesses the test taker's knowledge in the areas of human anatomy, physiology, pathophysiology, microbiology, and biochemistry.

The "professional practice" area assesses the test taker's knowledge in the areas of legal and medical ethics, risk management, public health, documentation and billing, patient care and communication, PA and physician relationship, and professional development.

The approximate percentage of questions based on each organ system is noted in the following table.

| Organ System | PANCE Percentage of the Exam | PANRE Percentage of the Exam |
|---|---|---|
| Cardiovascular | 13% | 12% |
| Pulmonary | 10% | 10% |
| Gastrointestinal/ Nutritional | 9% | 10% |
| Musculoskeletal | 8% | 8% |
| Eyes, ears, nose, and throat | 7% | 8% |
| Reproductive | 7% | 5% |
| Endocrine | 7% | 8% |
| Genitourinary | 5% | 5% |
| Neurologic system | 7% | 5% |
| Psychiatry/ Behavioral | 6% | 7% |
| Dermatologic | 5% | 5% |
| Hematologic | 5% | 4% |
| Infectious disease | 6% | 7% |
| Renal | 5% | 4% |

See the NCCPA website (www.nccpa.net) for complete details on task areas and organ-system information related to the examination.

## THE PANRE

The recertification exam tests core medical knowledge deemed relevant to a practicing PA regardless of medical specialty or practice setting. There are now two options for meeting requirements for recertification. The first option is the PANRE exam, which consists of 240 questions delivered in one session at a testing center. The second option is the PANRE-LA, which is administered quarterly over a 3-year period (beginning in the 7th year of the certification cycle). During this period, 25 questions are taken each quarter and a score is calculated after 8 quarters. The PANRE-LA questions can be taken on a personal device at your convenience each quarter.

A list of specific diseases and disorders within each content area that may be included on the PANRE can be found on the NCCPA website (www.nccpa.net). Also provided is the level at which each disease and disorder will be assessed:

Level 1: Recognize the most likely diagnosis based on signs, symptoms, and risks; make appropriate referrals.

Level 2: Use signs, symptoms, risk factors, and diagnostic studies to make an appropriate diagnosis and have knowledge of the first-line treatment.

Level 3: Use signs, symptoms, risk factors, and diagnostic studies to make an appropriate diagnosis and have knowledge of the first-line treatment. In addition, demonstrate the knowledge required to manage well-known comorbid conditions, as well as contraindications and complications.

In addition to covering the topics listed in each category, up to 2% of the questions on PANRE may cover emergent issues (Legal, Ethical, DEI).

## TEST-TAKING STRATEGIES

You have been preparing for this examination since the start of PA school and through all the years of clinical practice. Now is the time to focus on the examination.

### BEFORE THE EXAMINATION

- Take a refresher course that offers sample testing. See the American Association of Physicians Assistants (AAPA) Web site (www.aapa.org) for a list of current board review courses.
- Set up a schedule to study for the examination.
- Design your review schedule to follow the organ systems as noted in the table.
- Remember that the examination is focused on primary care.
- Review the NCCPA website to see sample questions and familiarize yourself with the examination format.

- It is better to study 1 to 2 hours per day for 1 month prior to the examination than to try to study 12 hours per day just a few days prior to the examination.
- See Table 18.1 for a sample 90-day studying schedule; see Table 18.2 for a 31-day studying schedule; and see Table 18.3 for a 15-day studying schedule. Adjust the hours per day based on your availability and studying needs.
- If time is limited, review and study for the systems that make up the largest parts of the examination.

**TABLE 18.1**

## 90-Day Sample Study Schedule

| | | | | | | |
|---|---|---|---|---|---|---|
| **Day 1**<br>Take sample test | **Day 2**<br>Cardiology review—2 hours | **Day 3**<br>Cardiology review—2 hours | **Day 4**<br>Cardiology review—2 hours | **Day 5**<br>Cardiology review—2 hours | **Day 6**<br>Cardiology review—2 hours | **Day 7**<br>Take day off |
| **Day 8**<br>Cardiology review—2 hours | **Day 9**<br>Cardiology review—2 hours | **Day 10**<br>Cardiology review—2 hours | **Day 11**<br>Cardiology review—2 hours | **Day 12**<br>Pulmonary review—2 hours | **Day 13**<br>Pulmonary review—2 hours | **Day 14**<br>Take day off |
| **Day 15**<br>Pulmonary review—2 hours | **Day 16**<br>Pulmonary review—2 hours | **Day 17**<br>Pulmonary review—2 hours | **Day 18**<br>Pulmonary review—2 hours | **Day 19**<br>Gastrointestinal review—2 hours | **Day 20**<br>Gastrointestinal review—2 hours | **Day 21**<br>Take day off |
| **Day 22**<br>Gastrointestinal review—2 hours | **Day 23**<br>Gastrointestinal review—2 hours | **Day 24**<br>Gastrointestinal review—2 hours | **Day 25**<br>Gastrointestinal review—2 hours | **Day 26**<br>Musculoskeletal review—2 hours | **Day 27**<br>Musculoskeletal review—2 hours | **Day 28**<br>Take day off |
| **Day 29**<br>Musculoskeletal review—2 hours | **Day 30**<br>Musculoskeletal review—2 hours | **Day 31**<br>Musculoskeletal review—2 hours | **Day 32**<br>Eyes, ears, nose, and throat review—2 hours | **Day 33**<br>Eyes, ears, nose, and throat review—2 hours | **Day 34**<br>Eyes, ears, nose, and throat review—2 hours | **Day 35**<br>Take day off |
| **Day 36**<br>Eyes, ears, nose, and throat review—1 hours | **Day 37**<br>Eyes, ears, nose, and throat review—2 hours | **Day 38**<br>Reproductive review—2 hours | **Day 39**<br>Reproductive review—2 hours | **Day 40**<br>Reproductive review—2 hours | **Day 41**<br>Reproductive review—2 hours | **Day 42**<br>Take day off |
| **Day 43**<br>Reproductive review—2 hours | **Day 44**<br>Endocrine review—2 hours | **Day 45**<br>Endocrine review—2 hours | **Day 46**<br>Endocrine review—2 hours | **Day 47**<br>Endocrine review—2 hours | **Day 48**<br>Endocrine review—2 hours | **Day 49**<br>Take day off |
| **Day 50**<br>Genitourinary review—2 hours | **Day 51**<br>Genitourinary review—2 hours | **Day 52**<br>Genitourinary review—2 hours | **Day 53**<br>Renal review— 2 hours | **Day 54**<br>Renal review— 2 hours | **Day 55**<br>Renal review— 2 hours | **Day 56**<br>Take day off |
| **Day 57**<br>Neurology review—2 hours | **Day 58**<br>Neurology review—2 hours | **Day 59**<br>Neurology review—2 hours | **Day 60**<br>Neurology review—2 hours | **Day 61**<br>Psychiatry review—2 hours | **Day 62**<br>Psychiatry review—2 hours | **Day 63**<br>Take day off |
| **Day 64**<br>Psychiatry review—2 hours | **Day 65**<br>Psychiatry review—2 hours | **Day 66**<br>Dermatology review—2 hours | **Day 67**<br>Dermatology review—2 hours | **Day 68**<br>Dermatology review—2 hours | **Day 69**<br>Hematology review—2 hours | **Day 70**<br>Take day off |
| **Day 71**<br>Hematology review—2 hours | **Day 72**<br>Hematology review—2 hours | **Day 73**<br>Hematology review—2 hours | **Day 74**<br>Infectious disease review—2 hours | **Day 75**<br>Infectious disease review—2 hours | **Day 76**<br>Infectious disease review—2 hours | **Day 77**<br>Infectious disease review—2 hours |
| **Day 78**<br>Take day off | **Day 79**<br>Dermatology review—2 hours | **Day 80**<br>Psychiatry review—2 hours | **Day 81**<br>Neurology review—2 hours | **Day 82**<br>Genitourinary/ Renal review— 2 hours | **Day 83**<br>Endocrine review—2 hours | **Day 84**<br>Reproductive review—2 hours |
| **Day 85**<br>Eyes, ears, nose, and throat review—2 hours | **Day 86**<br>Musculoskeletal review—2 hours | **Day 87**<br>Gastrointestinal review—2 hours | **Day 88**<br>Pulmonary review—2 hours | **Day 89**<br>Cardiology review—2 hours | **Day 90**<br>Take sample test | |

**TABLE 18.2**

| 31-Day Sample Study Schedule | | | | | | |
|---|---|---|---|---|---|---|
| **Day 1**<br>Take sample test | **Day 2**<br>Cardiovascular review—4 hours | **Day 3**<br>Cardiovascular review—4 hours | **Day 4**<br>Cardiovascular review—4 hours | **Day 5**<br>Electrocardiogram review—2 hours | **Day 6**<br>Pulmonary review—4 hours | **Day 7**<br>Pulmonary review—4 hours |
| **Day 8**<br>Pulmonary review—4 hours | **Day 9**<br>Pulmonary review—4 hours | **Day 10**<br>Gastrointestinal review—4 hours | **Day 11**<br>Gastrointestinal review—4 hours | **Day 12**<br>Musculoskeletal review—4 hours | **Day 13**<br>Musculoskeletal review—4 hours | **Day 14**<br>Take day off |
| **Day 15**<br>Eyes, ears, nose, and throat review—4 hours | **Day 16**<br>Eyes, ears, nose, and throat review—4 hours | **Day 17**<br>Reproductive review—4 hours | **Day 18**<br>Reproductive review—4 hours | **Day 19**<br>Endocrine review—4 hours | **Day 20**<br>Endocrine review—4 hours | **Day 21**<br>Genitourinary review—4 hours |
| **Day 22**<br>Renal review—4 hours | **Day 23**<br>Take day off | **Day 24**<br>Neurology review—4 hours | **Day 25**<br>Neurology review—4 hours | **Day 26**<br>Psychiatry review—4 hours | **Day 27**<br>Psychiatry review—4 hours | **Day 28**<br>Dermatology review—4 hours |
| **Day 29**<br>Hematology review—4 hours | **Day 30**<br>Infectious disease review—4 hours | **Day 31**<br>Take sample test | | | | |

**TABLE 18.3**

| 15-Day Sample Study Schedule | | | | | | |
|---|---|---|---|---|---|---|
| **Day 1**<br>Take sample test | **Day 2**<br>Cardiology review—6 hours | **Day 3**<br>Pulmonary review—5 hours | **Day 4**<br>Gastrointestinal review—5 hours | **Day 5**<br>Musculoskeletal review—4 hours | **Day 6**<br>Eyes, ears, nose and throat review—4 hours | **Day 7**<br>Reproductive review—4 hours |
| **Day 8**<br>Endocrine review—4 hours | **Day 9**<br>Genitourinary & Renal review—5 hours | **Day 10**<br>Neurology review—4 hours | **Day 11**<br>Psychiatry review—3 hours | **Day 12**<br>Dermatology review—3 hours | **Day 13**<br>Hematology review—3 hours | **Day 14**<br>Infectious disease review—3 hours |
| **Day 15**<br>Take sample test | | | | | | |

- Practice as many sample questions as possible before the examination. Use questions that match the types seen on the examination. Consider taking the practice exams offered by the NCCPA to see how the questions are presented.
- Practice your pacing (use the timing of approximately 1 minute per question).
- Remember to register for the examination on time, to make sure you know the location of the testing center, materials to bring, and to arrive at the testing center at least 30 minutes prior to your examination time.
- Review the examination policies and procedures on the NCCPA Web site.

**DAY OF THE EXAMINATION**
- Get plenty of rest the night before.
- Eat before the examination, but not a large meal since a large meal may make you sleepy.
- Dress in layers so that you can adjust to the temperature in the room.
- Remember your admission card and forms of identification.

- Remember that no personal belongings are allowed in the testing room.
- Bring a snack or drink (to consume during a break if needed).

## TEST-ANXIETY STRATEGIES

- Being well prepared is the best way to reduce anxiety.
- Space out your studying and continually review material.
- Reduce stress by exercising or taking frequent breaks while preparing for the examination.
- Try to maintain a positive attitude while preparing for the examination.
- Stay relaxed. If you begin to get nervous, take a few deep breaths slowly to relax yourself.
- Focus on the question at hand; don't let your mind wander onto other things.

## GENERAL TIPS

- The PANCE examination is a 5-hour examination consisting of 300 multiple-choice questions. It is administered in five blocks of 60 questions with 60 minutes to complete each block.
- The PANRE examination is a 4-hour examination consisting of 240 multiple-choice questions. It is administered in four blocks of 60 questions with 60 minutes to complete each block.
- For both the PANCE and PANRE, each test taker has 45 minutes' worth of break time to use during the examination, between blocks or during the exam. Note that the examination clock does not stop if you take a break during a block of questions so if possible, take breaks between question blocks.

- Write down important formulas and facts on the laminated note board or paper supplied by the testing center prior to starting the examination.
- Do not worry about how fast others are completing the examination. They may not even be taking the PANCE or PANRE examinations.
- Most questions have five answer options.

## DURING THE EXAMINATION

- Read directions carefully and complete the computer tutorial.
- Pace yourself to avoid rushing at the end of the examination.
- Take a break after two or three question blocks to step away from the computer.
- Laboratory normal ranges are available during the examination; just click the button on the screen.
- Answer all items. Mark the questions you are not sure of to review once you have completed the examination, but do not leave any answers blank the first time through the examination.
- Do not change answers unless you are sure you marked the answer wrong.
- Remember, the examination is professionally written, and the test writers are not out to trick you.
- Read each question carefully and try to answer it before looking at the choices.
- Read all the choices before answering the question.
- Answer all questions; there is no penalty for guessing.

## AFTER THE EXAMINATION

Relax and celebrate.

# ADULT PREVENTIVE HEALTH GUIDELINES

| Screening Activity | | 18 | 25 | 30 | 35 | 40 | 45 | 50 | 55 | 60 | 65 and Over |
|---|---|---|---|---|---|---|---|---|---|---|---|
| **Exams** | Physical exam | Every 5 years | | | | Every 2 years | | Annually | | | |
| | Gynecological/Breast exam | Annually | | Every 1-2 years | | | | | | | |
| **Cardiovascular Health** | Blood pressure | Every 2 years or at every visit | | | | | | | | | |
| | Cholesterol | Those with cardiac risk[1] | | | Every 5 years: men from age 35, women from age 45 | | | | | | |
| | Fasting glucose | Those with cardiac risk[1] or diabetes | | | | Every 3 years | | | | | |
| | EKG | | | | | | | Consider if cardiac risk[1] | | | |
| | Aspirin therapy | | | | | Men age 45 and women age 55 if increased stroke/cardiac risk and low bleeding risk | | | | | |
| | AA Ultrasound | | | | | | | | | | Men who ever smoked |
| **Cancer Screening** | Mammogram | | | | | Test if + FH | | Every 2 years | | | |
| | Pap smear | Starting at age 21 every 3 years | | Every 3-5 years until age 65 | | | | | | | |
| | Colonoscopy | | | | | Every 5 years if high risk[2] | | Every 10 years | | | |
| | PSA | | | | | Test high risk[3] | | Discuss harms and benefits before testing | | | |
| **Bone** | Bone density test | | | | | | | | If high risk[4] | | All women |
| **Sexual Health** | Chlamydia test | Yearly if active | Women, as needed, if new partner or multiple partners | | | | | | | | |
| | HIV testing | Offer to all adults annually, if high risk[5] | | | | | | | | | |
| **Vaccinations** | Tetanus booster | Every 10 years | | | | | | | | | |
| | Pneumonia | For patients with chronic illness, 1-2 doses | | | | | | | | | Once |
| | Influenza | Annually for patients with a chronic illness and their household contacts, pregnant women, health-care workers, and parents of young children | | | | | | Annually | | | |
| | Shingles | | | | | | | | | | Once |
| | HPV | Both sexes, 3 doses | ▨ For all persons who meet age requirements | | | | | | ▢ For all persons who meet specified criteria | | |

*AA*, Abdominal aorta; *EKG*, electrocardiogram; *FH*, family history; *HIV*, human immunodeficiency virus; *HPV*, human papillomavirus; *PSA*, prostate-specific antigen.

1 Cardiac risk factors include smoking, hypertension, diabetes, strong family history of heart attack, obesity, and physical inactivity.
2 Colon cancer risks include family history of colon cancer in a relative before age 60, family history of polyps, and ulcerative colitis.
3 Prostate cancer risks include African-American race or family history of prostate cancer.
4 Osteoporosis risks include family history of osteoporosis, smoking, corticosteroid use, chronic alcohol use, and low BMI with FRAX score >9.3.
5 HIV risks include history of drug use, men who have sex with men, transfusion, multiple partners, and unprotected sex with an infected partner.

# U.S. Preventive Services Task Force Screening Guidelines for Common Diseases

| Disorder | Screening Guideline |
| --- | --- |
| Obesity | Offer or refer adults with a BMI of 30 or higher to intensive, multicomponent behavioral interventions |
| Hypercholesterolemia | Start screening at age 20 if increased risk of coronary artery disease, otherwise at age 35 in men and at age 45 in women if increased risk of coronary heart disease |
| Hypertension | Start screening for hypertension in adults 18 years or older with OBPM. Obtain blood pressure measurements outside of the clinical setting for diagnostic confirmation before starting treatment |
| Coronary artery disease | EKG or stress test not recommended in absence of cardiac risk factors or asymptomatic patient |
| Abdominal aortic aneurysm | One-time screening in men between ages 65 and 70 who have ever smoked. Offer screening to men aged 65–75 who have never smoked. Screening in women is not recommended |
| Diabetes mellitus type 2 | Recommend screening for prediabetes and type 2 diabetes in adults aged 35 to 70 years who have overweight or obesity. Clinicians should offer or refer patients with prediabetes to effective preventive interventions |
| Thyroid disease | Routine screening not recommended in nonpregnant, asymptomatic adults |
| Hearing | There is insufficient evidence to recommend for or against routine screening |
| Osteoporosis | Routine screening for women aged 65 or older and in younger women who are at increased risk of osteoporotic fractures |
| Hepatitis C | Screening recommended in adults aged 18 to 79 years |
| Depression | Recommend screening for depression in the general adult population, including pregnant and postpartum women |

*BMI*, Body mass index; *OBPM*, office blood pressure measurement; *EKG*, electrocardiogram.

| Cranial Nerve | Name | Function |
| --- | --- | --- |
| I | Olfactory | Sense of smell |
| II | Optic | Visual acuity |
| III | Oculomotor | Pupillary constriction<br>Elevation of upper eyelid<br>Most extraocular movements |
| IV | Trochlear | Downward, internal rotation of the eye |
| V | Trigeminal | Motor: temporal and masseter muscles; lateral movement of the jaw<br>Sensory: facial<br>    Three branches:<br>        Ophthalmic (V1)—sensory<br>        Maxillary (V2)—sensory<br>        Mandibular (V3)—sensory and motor |
| VI | Abducens | Lateral deviation of the eye |
| VII | Facial | Motor: muscles of the face<br>Sensory: taste, anterior two thirds of the tongue |
| VIII | Auditory | Hearing and balance |
| IX | Glossopharyngeal | Motor: pharynx<br>Sensory: posterior tongue, including taste |
| X | Vagus | Motor: palate, pharynx, and larynx<br>Sensory: pharynx and larynx |
| XI | Spinal accessory | Motor: sternomastoid and upper portion of trapezius |
| XII | Hypoglossal | Motor: tongue |

| Sign | Clinical Indication | Description |
| --- | --- | --- |
| Babinski's | Pyramidal tract involvement | Extension of great toe and abduction of other toes with plantar stimulation |
| Barlow's | Congenital hip dislocation | Click of femoral head with bringing hip into mid adduction with posterior and lateral pressure while infant supine and hips flexed 90 degrees |
| Battle's | Base of skull fracture | Postauricular ecchymosis |
| Biot's | Increased intracranial pressure | Abnormal breathing with periods of apnea and with periods of several breaths of similar volumes |
| Brudzinski's | Meningitis | Forced flexion of the neck elicits a reflex flexion of the hips |
| Bulge's | Knee joint effusion | Bulge in the medial hollow to the patella after milking the knee and pressing the knee behind the lateral margin of the patella |
| Chadwick's | Pregnancy | Bluish discoloration of the cervix and vagina |
| Chvostek's | Tetany | Spasm of the orbicular oculi or oris with tapping of the facial nerve |
| Courvoisier's | Pancreatic cancer | Palpable gallbladder in a jaundiced patient |
| Cullen's | Ruptured ectopic pregnancy Hemorrhagic pancreatitis | Periumbilical darkening of the skin from blood |
| Drawer | Cruciate ligament injury | Forward or backward sliding of the tibia under applied stress |
| Gowers' | Muscular dystrophy | Use of limb muscles to assume an upright sitting position |
| Grey Turner's | Hemorrhagic pancreatitis | Local areas of discoloration in the region of the loins |
| Hegar's | Early pregnancy | Softening and compressibility of the lower segment of the uterus |
| Homans' | Deep venous thrombosis | Pain in calf with dorsiflexion of the ankle with the knee bent |
| Impingement | Rotator cuff tendonitis | Pain with provocative physical examination maneuvers |
| Kernig's | Meningitis | Incomplete extension of the leg on the thigh when patient is supine and when the thigh is flexed to a right angle with the axis of the trunk |
| Lasègue's | Lumbar nerve irritation Sciatic nerve irritation | Pain or spasms in the posterior thigh with hip flexed, knee extended, and ankle dorsiflexed, while patient is supine |
| Lhermitte's | Multiple sclerosis Cervical spinal cord injury | Sudden electric-like shocks extending down spine when flexing the neck |
| McBurney's | Appendicitis | Tenderness at site two-thirds of the distance between umbilicus and anterior superior iliac spine |
| Murphy's | Acute cholecystitis | Pain on palpation in right upper quadrant with inspiration |
| Obturator | Appendicitis | Pain in right hypogastric region with flexion of right leg at the hip with the knee bent and internally rotated |
| Ortolani's | Congenital hip dysplasia | Snapping with relocation of a dislocated femoral hip |
| Phalen's | Carpal tunnel syndrome | Pain with wrist flexion |
| Psoas | Appendicitis | Pain with flexion of leg against resistance. |
| Romberg's | Cerebellar dysfunction | Unsteadiness in patient when closing eyes and standing with feet approximated |
| Rovsing's | Appendicitis | Pain at McBurney's point with pressure over descending colon |
| Russell's | Bulimia | Abrasions and scars on back of hands and fingers due to self-induced vomiting |
| Snellen | Graves' disease | Bruit heard on auscultation over the eye |
| String | Pyloric stenosis | Narrowed pyloric canal on abdominal x-ray |
| Tinel's | Carpal tunnel syndrome | Sensation of tingling with percussion over medial nerve |
| Trendelenburg's | Congenital hip dislocation Hip abductor weakness | Sagging of pelvis on the side opposite the affected side during single-leg stance on the affected side |
| Trousseau's | Tetany | Carpopedal spasm when upper arm is compressed |
| Westermark's | Pulmonary embolism | Decreased lung markings from oligemia |
| Wrist | Marfan syndrome | Overlapping of thumb and fifth finger when the wrist is gripped with the opposite hand |

# APPENDIX 5    POISONING ANTIDOTES

| Poison | Antidote |
| --- | --- |
| Acetaminophen | N-acetylcysteine |
| Anticholinergic drugs | Physostigmine |
| Arsenic | Penicillamine |
|  | Dimercaptosuccinic acid |
| Benzodiazepine | Flumazenil |
| Carbon monoxide | Oxygen |
| Cyanide | Amyl nitrite, thiosulfate |
| Digoxin | Digoxin Fab fragment |
| Ethylene glycol | Ethyl alcohol or fomepizole |
| Gold | Dimercaptosuccinic acid |
| Heparin | Protamine sulfate |
| Iron | Deferoxamine |
| Lead | Calcium disodium edetate |
| Mercury | Dimercaptosuccinic acid |
| Methyl alcohol | Ethyl alcohol |
| Nitrites | Methylene blue |
| Opiates | Naloxone |
| Organophosphates | Pralidoxime or atropine |
| Sulfonylurea drugs | Octreotide |
| Warfarin | Vitamin K |

| Hematology and Coagulation | |
|---|---|
| **Test** | **Normal Range** |
| Antithrombin III | 22–39 mg/dL |
| Bleeding time | 2–10 minutes |
| Complete blood count (CBC) | |
|    White blood cell count | $5.0–10.5 \times 10^3$/mL |
|    Red blood cell count | $4.5–5.5 \times 10^6$/mm³ |
|    Hemoglobin | Female 12–14 g/dL |
| | Male 14–16 g/dL |
|    Hematocrit | Female 36%–42% |
| | Male 42%–48% |
| Mean corpuscular volume (MCV) | 80–100 fL |
| Mean corpuscular hemoglobin (MCH) | 26–34 pg/cell |
| Mean corpuscular hemoglobin concentration (MCHC) | 31–36 g/dL |
| Platelet count | $150–450 \times 10^9$/L |
| Differential | |
|    Neutrophils | 40%–70% |
|    Bands | 1%–10% |
|    Lymphocytes | 25%–45% |
|    Monocytes | 4%–10% |
|    Eosinophils | 0%–8% |
|    Basophils | 0%–2% |
| D-dimer | <0.5 mg/L |
| Eosinophil count | 40–500/mL |
| Erythrocyte sedimentation rate | 0–20 mm/hour |
| Ferritin | 30–300 ng/mL |
| Fibrinogen degradation products | <2.5 mg/L |
| Fibrinogen | 150–400 mg/dL |
| Folate | 3.0–17.0 ng/mL |
| Haptoglobin | 15–200 mg/dL |
| Hemoglobin electrophoresis | |
|    Hemoglobin A | 95%–98% |
|    Hemoglobin $A_2$ | 1.5%–3.5% |
|    Hemoglobin F | 0%–2% |
|    Other | Absent |
| Iron | 30–160 mcg/dL |
| Iron binding capacity | 225–430 mcg/dL |
| Partial thromboplastin time | 22–35 seconds |
| Prothrombin time | 11–13 seconds |
| Reticulocyte count | 0.5%–1.5% of erythro-cytes |
| Sickle cell test | Negative |
| Thrombin time | 16–25 seconds |
| Transferrin | 190–375 mg/dL |
| Vitamin $B_{12}$ | 125–900 pg/mL |

### Immunology

| Test | Normal Range |
|---|---|
| Anti-ds DNA antibody | Negative at 1:10 |
| Antinuclear antibody | Negative at 1:40 |
| C-reactive protein | 0.08–3.0 mg/L |
| Immunoglobulins | |
|   IgA | 60–310 mg/dL |
|   IgE | 10–180 IU/mL |
|   IgG | 615–1300 mg/dL |
|   IgM | 55–330 mg/dL |
| Rheumatoid factor | <30 IU/mL |
| Serum protein electrophoresis | |
|   Albumin | 3.5–5.5 g/dL |
|   Globulin | 2.0–3.5 g/dL |
|   Alpha 1 | 0.2–0.4 g/dL |
|   Alpha 2 | 0.5–0.9 g/dL |
|   Gamma | 0.7–1.7 g/dL |

### Toxicology

| Test | Therapeutic Range | Toxic Range |
|---|---|---|
| Acetaminophen | 10–30 mcg/mL | >200 mcg/mL |
| Digoxin | 0.8–2.0 ng/mL | >2.5 ng/mL |
| Ethanol | — | >20 mg/dL |
| Lithium | 0.6–1.3 mEq/L | >2 mEq/L |
| Phenobarbital | 10–40 mcg/mL | >65 mcg/mL |
| Phenytoin | 10–20 mcg/mL | >20 mcg/mL |
| Salicylates | 150–300 mcg/mL | >300 mcg/mL |
| Theophylline | 8–20 mcg/mL | >20 mcg/mL |

### Lipid Classification

| Test | Interpretation |
|---|---|
| LDL CHOLESTEROL | |
| <100 | Optimal |
| 100–129 | Above normal |
| 130–159 | Borderline high |
| 160–189 | High |
| 190 | Very high |
| TOTAL CHOLESTEROL | |
| <200 | Desirable |
| 200–239 | Borderline high |
| 240 | High |
| HDL CHOLESTEROL | |
| <40 | Low |
| 60 | High |

### Chemistry

| Test | Normal Range |
|---|---|
| Acetoacetate | <1 mg/dL |
| Adrenocorticotropic hormone (ACTH) | 6.0–76.0 pg/mL |
| Albumin | 3.5–5.5 g/dL |

| Chemistry | |
|---|---|
| **Test** | **Normal Range** |
| Aldosterone | 2–9 ng/dL |
| Alkaline phosphatase | 30–120 U/L |
| Alpha-1-antitrypsin | 85–213 mg/dL |
| Alpha-fetoprotein | <15 ng/mL |
| Alanine aminotransferase (ALT) | 0–40 U/L |
| Ammonia | 10–80 mcg/dL |
| Amylase | 60–180 U/dL |
| Angiotensin-converting enzyme (ACE) | <40 U/L |
| Anion gap | 7–16 mmol/L |
| Arterial blood gases | |
|    pH | 7.35–7.45 |
|    $P_{CO_2}$ | 35–45 mm Hg |
|    $P_{O_2}$ | 80–100 mm Hg |
|    Bicarbonate | 21–30 mEq/L |
|    Oxygen saturation | >95% |
| Aspartate aminotransferase (AST) | 0–40 U/L |
| Beta-human chorionic gonadotropin | <5 mIU/mL |
| Beta-hydroxybutyrate | <3 mg/dL |
| Bilirubin | |
|    Total | 0.3–1.0 mg/dL |
|    Direct | 0.1–0.3 mg/dL |
|    Indirect | 0.2–0.7 mg/dL |
| Blood urea nitrogen (BUN) | 5–20 mg/dL |
| Brain natriuretic peptide (BNP) | <167 pg/mL |
| Calcium | 8.5–10 mg/dL |
| Calcium, ionized | 1.1–1.4 mmol/L |
| Carbon dioxide | 21–30 mEq/L |
| Carcinoembryonic antigen (CEA) | 0.0–3.4 ng/mL |
| Ceruloplasmin | 27–37 mg/dL |
| Chloride | 98–106 mEq/L |
| Cortisol | 5–25 mcg/dL |
| C-peptide | 0.5–2.0 ng/mL |
| Creatine kinase, total (CK) | 40–200 ng/mL |
| Creatinine kinase MB (CK-MB) isoenzyme | 0–7 ng/mL |
| Creatinine | 0.5–1.5 mg/dL |
| Creatinine clearance (CRCL) | 90–140 mL/min/1.73 m$^2$ BSA |
| Ferritin | 15–200 ng/mL |
| Follicle-stimulating hormone (FSH) | |
|    Female | |
|       Follicular phase | 3.0–20.0 U/L |
|       Ovulatory phase | 9.0–26.0 U/L |
|       Luteal phase | 1.0–12.0 U/L |
|       Postmenopausal | 18.0–153.0 U/L |
|    Male | 1.0–12.0 U/L |
| γ-Glutamyltransferase (GGT) | 5–95 U/L |
| Gastrin | <100 pg/mL |
| Glucose | 65–110 mg/dL |
| Growth hormone | 0.5–17.0 ng/mL |
| Hemoglobin A1c | 3.8%–6.4% |
| Insulin | 0–180 pmol/L |
| Iron | 30–160 mcg/dL |
| Iron binding capacity | 225–430 mcg/dL |
| Iron percent saturation | 20%–45% |

*Continued*

| Chemistry | |
|---|---|
| **Test** | **Normal Range** |
| Ketone (acetone) | Negative |
| Lactate | 5–15 mg/dL |
| Lactate dehydrogenase | 100–190 U/L |
| Lead | |
|    Children | <25 mcg/dL |
|    Adult | <40 mcg/dL |
| Lipase | 0–160 U/L |
| Luteinizing hormone (LH) | |
|    Female | |
|       Follicular phase | 2.0–15.0 U/L |
|       Ovulatory phase | 22.0–105.0 U/L |
|       Luteal phase | 0.6–19.0 U/L |
|       Postmenopausal | 16.0–64.0 U/L |
|    Male | 2.0–12.0 U/L |
| Magnesium | 1.8–3.0 mg/dL |
| Osmolality | |
|    Plasma | 285–295 mOsm/kg water |
|    Urine | 300–900 mOsm/kg water |
| Parathyroid hormone | 10–60 pg/mL |
| Phosphorus | 3.0–4.5 mg/dL |
| Potassium | 3.5–5.5 mEq/L |
| Progesterone | |
|    Female | |
|       Follicular phase | <1.0 ng/mL |
|       Mid-luteal phase | 3–20 ng/mL |
|    Male | <1.0 ng/mL |
| Prolactin | |
|    Female | 2.0–26 ng/mL |
|    Male | 1.6–23 ng/mL |
| Prostate-specific antigen (PSA) | |
|    Female | <0.5 ng/mL |
|    Male <40 years of age | 0.0–2.0 ng/mL |
|    Male >40 years of age | 0.0–4.0 ng/mL |
| Sodium | 135–145 mEq/L |
| Testosterone | |
|    Female | 5–85 ng/dL |
|    Male | 270–1050 ng/dL |
| Thyroid-stimulating hormone (TSH) | 0.5–4.5 mcU/mL |
| Thyroxine ($T_4$) | 4.5–10.5 mcg/dL |
| Thyroxine, free ($FT_4$) | 0.8–2.7 ng/dL |
| Triiodothyronine ($T_3$) | 60–180 ng/dL |
| Total protein | 5.5–8.0 g/dL |
| Transferrin | 190–375 mg/dL |
| Triglycerides | <160 mg/dL |
| Troponin I | 0.0–0.4 ng/mL |
| Uric acid | 1.5–7.0 mg/dL |

*BSA*, Body surface area.

Page numbers followed by an "f" indicate figures and by a "t" indicate tables.

## A

Abatacept, 108t
Abdomen pain, acute
  abdominal causes of, 67t
  nonabdominal causes of, 68t
Abdominal aortic aneurysm, screening for,
  403t
Abortion, 180
Abrasion, corneal, 136
Abruptio placentae, 180
Abscess
  breast, 175–176
  dental, 147
  lung, in pneumonia, 34
  peritonsillar, 149
Absorption, drug, 352
Abuse, 230–231
  child, 230–231, 347
  domestic violence, 231
  elder, 231
  sexual, 231
Acanthosis nigricans, 276–277
Acarbose, 118t
Accutane. see Isotretinoin
ACE inhibitors. see Angiotensin-converting
  enzyme (ACE) inhibitors
Acetaminophen, 352, 355
Achalasia, 54–55, 55f
Acid-base disorders, 316–318
  interpretation of, 316
  normal ranges for, 316t
  primary, 317t
Acidosis
  metabolic, 317
  respiratory, 317–318, 317t
ACL injury. see Anterior cruciate ligament
  (ACL) injury
Acne inversa, 277
Acne severity grading, 255t
Acne vulgaris, 254–255
  severity grading for, 255t
Acneiform eruptions, 254–256
  acne vulgaris, 254–255
  folliculitis, 255–256
  rosacea, 256
Acneiform lesions, 254–256
Acoustic neuroma, 139
Acquired hemolytic anemia, 287–288
Acral erythema, chemotherapy-induced, 271
Acromegaly, 121
Actinic keratosis (AK), 265–266
Activators, 352
Acute hepatitis, serology testing for, 61t
Acute lymphocytic leukemia (ALL), 290
Acute myelogenous leukemia (AML), 291
Acute otitis media, 338

Acute renal failure, 310–311
  causes of, 310t
  urine study results in, 311t
Acute respiratory distress syndrome, 50–51
Acute rheumatic fever, 206–208
Acute stress disorder, 248
Acute viral hepatitis, causes of, 61t
Adenocarcinoma, 56t. see also Carcinoma
Adenomyosis, 198
Adenosine, 27–29t
Adrenal crisis, 114–115
Adrenal disorders, 113–115
  acute corticoadrenal insufficiency, 114–115
  adrenocortical function, tests of, 113
  chronic corticoadrenal insufficiency, 114
  Cushing's syndrome, 113–114
  glucocorticoids, 115
  location/function, 113
  primary hyperaldosteronism, 115
Adrenal gland, cortex, 113t
Adrenocortical function, tests of, 113
Adriamycin. see Doxorubicin
Adult preventive health guidelines, 402t
Agonists, 352
AK. see Actinic keratosis (AK)
Alanine aminotransferase (ALT), 385
Albumin, 388
Albuterol, 41–42t
Alcohol, 375t
  abuse, 245
  delirium from, 246
  dependence, 245–246
  hallucination from, 246
  intoxication, 245
  rehabilitation from, 246
  withdrawal from, 246
Aldomet. see Alpha-methyldopa
Aldosterone, 113t
Alkaline phosphatase (ALP), 385
Alkalosis
  metabolic, 317, 317t
  respiratory, 318
ALL. see Acute lymphocytic leukemia (ALL)
Allergens, common, 269t
Allergic rhinitis, 144
  medications for, 145t
Allopurinol, 375
Alopecia
  androgenetic, 257–258
  areata, 257
ALP. see Alkaline phosphatase (ALP)
Alpha-1-antitrypsin deficiency, 63t
Alpha-blockers, 364
Alpha-glucosidase inhibitors, 368
Alpha-methyldopa, 365
Alpha-thalassemia, 284–285

Alprazolam, 81–82t, 249–251t, 372t
ALT. see Alanine aminotransferase (ALT)
Altered level of consciousness, 162–163
Alzheimer's disease, 163–164
  clinical manifestations, 163
  treatment of, 163–164
Amantadine, 161
Amaurosis fugax, 137
Amblyopia, 137
Amebiasis, 213
Amenorrhea, 190, 190t, 191t
  causes of, 190t
  lactational, 185
  primary, 190, 190t
  secondary, 190, 190t
Aminocaproic acid, 295
Aminoglycosides, 358–359
Aminophylline, 41–42t
Amiodarone, 27–29t, 271t, 367t, 375t
Amitriptyline, 373t
AML. see Acute myelogenous leukemia
  (AML)
Ammonia, 389
Amrinone, 27–29t
Amylase, 388–389
Amyotrophic lateral sclerosis, 160
ANA. see Antinuclear antibodies (ANA)
Anal fissure, in rectum, 75
Analgesics, 352–354
  acetaminophen, 352
  COX-2s, 353
  nonsteroidal antiinflammatory drugs, 353
  opioids, 354
  tramadol (Ultram), 353
Anaprox. see Naproxen
Androgenetic alopecia, 257–258
Anemia, 282–290. see also Hemolytic anemia
  anemia of chronic disease, 287
  aplastic, 289–290
  of chronic disease, 287
  classifications of, 283, 300
  clinical signs of, 282–283
  definition of, 282
  flowchart, 284f, 382f
  folate deficiency, 286
  general, 282–283
  hemolytic, 287–289
  iron-deficiency, 283–284
  sickle cell, 289
  sideroblastic, 285
  symptoms of, 282–283
  thalassemia, 284–285
  vitamin $B_{12}$ deficiency, 285–286
Aneurysm
  aortic, abdominal, screening for, 403t
  cerebral, 169

Angina pectoris, 16–17
  Prinzmetal's variant, 17
    clinical manifestations, 17
    diagnosis, 17
    general, 17
    treatment, 17
  stable, 16–17
    clinical manifestations, 16
    diagnosis, 17
    general, 16
    treatment, 17
  unstable, 17
    clinical manifestations, 17
    diagnosis, 17
    general, 17
    treatment, 17
Angiotensin-converting enzyme (ACE)
    inhibitors, 363
Angiotensin II receptor blockers (ARBs), 363
Angle-closure glaucoma, 137
Ankle
  disorders of, 96
  fractures of, 97–98
  sprains, 96
  strains, 96
Ankle/brachial index, 20t
Ankylosing spondylitis, 89–90, 90f
Ann Arbor staging, in Hodgkin's lymphoma,
    292
Anorectal abscess/fistula, 75–76
Anorexia nervosa, 237
Antacids, 58t, 368
Antagonists, 352
Anterior cruciate ligament (ACL) injury, 95–96
Antiarrhythmic drugs, 7t, 366, 367t
Antibiotics, 226–227t, 355–360
  antifolate drugs, 360
  beta-lactam, 355–358
  fluoroquinolones, 359
  metronidazole, 360
  nitrofurantoin, 360
  protein synthesis inhibitors, 358–359
Anticholinergic agents, 145t, 161
Anticoagulants, 374–375
Anticonvulsants, 375–376, 375t
Antidepressants, 249–251t
  monoamine oxidase inhibitors (MAOIs),
    372–373
  selective serotonin reuptake inhibitors
    (SSRIs), 372
  serotonin-norepinephrine reuptake
    inhibitors (SNRIs), 372
  tricyclic
    side effects of, 373t
  tricyclic antidepressants (TCAs), 372
Antidiabetic medications, oral, 118t
Antidiarrheal agents, 370, 370t
Antidotes, for poison, 406t
Antiemetics, 370–371
Antiepileptic agent selection, 167t
Antiepileptic medications, 168t
Antifolate drugs, 360
Antigout, 375
Antihistamines, 145t
  antiemetics, 370–371
Antimalarial agents, 271t

Antinuclear antibodies (ANA), 391
Antiplatelet therapy, for myocardial
    infarction (MI), 15–16
Antipseudomonal penicillin, 356
Antipsychotics, 249–251t, 373, 374t
Antirheumatic drugs, disease-modifying, 108t
Antisocial disorder, 240
Antithrombin III, normal values for, 407–410t
Antithrombin therapy, for myocardial
    infarction (MI), 16
Antituberculosis drugs, 360–361
  ethambutol, 361
  isoniazid, 360
  pyrazinamide, 361
  rifampin, 360–361
Antiviral respiratory agents, 361
  oseltamivir (Tamiflu), 361
  ribavirin (Virazole), 361
  zanamivir (Relenza), 361
Anxiety
  disorders, 231–233
    generalized, 231–232
    panic disorder, 232
    phobias, 233
  test-taking strategies for, 401
Anxiolytics, 249–251t
Aortic aneurysm, 18–19
  clinical manifestations, 18–19
  diagnosis, 19
  general, 18
  screening for, abdominal, 403t
  treatment, 19
Aortic dissection, 19
  clinical manifestations, 19
  diagnosis, 19
  general, 19
  treatment, 19
Aortic regurgitation, 22
  clinical manifestations, 22
  diagnosis, 22
  general, 22
  treatment, 22
Aortic stenosis, 21–22
  clinical manifestations, 21
  diagnosis, 21
  general, 21
  treatment, 22
Apgar scoring, 322–323, 328t
Aphthous ulcers, 147–148
Aplastic anemia, 289–290
Appendicitis, 67
ARBs. see Angiotensin II receptor blockers
    (ARBs)
Aripiprazole, 374t
Arterial blood gases, 407–410t
Arterial embolism/thrombosis
  clinical manifestations, 19
  diagnosis, 19
  general, 19
  treatment, 19
Arterial mesenteric ischemia, 72
Arterial occlusion, chronic/acute
  clinical manifestations, 19–20
  diagnosis, 20
  general, 19
  treatment, 20

Arteriovenous malformation, 168–169
Arthritis
  osteo-, 103
  rheumatoid, 107, 107f
  septic, 101
Ascariasis, 213
Aseptic necrosis, 93–94
Aspartate aminotransferase (AST), 385
Aspiration, 34t
  foreign body, 337
Aspirin, 353, 355
AST. see Aspartate aminotransferase (AST)
Asthma, 40
  classification of, 40t
  diagnosis of, 40
  medications for, 41–42t
  treatment of, 40
Atenolol, 27–29t, 367t
Ativan. see Lorazepam
Atopic dermatitis, 268
  seborrheic dermatitis versus, 268t
Atorvastatin, 369t
Atrial fibrillation, 2–3
  EKG findings, 2–3
  general, 2
  treatment, 3
Atrial flutter, 3
  EKG findings, 3
  general, 3
  treatment, 3
Atrial septal defect, 332–333
Atrioventricular (AV) block, 3–4
  EKG findings, 3–4
  general, 3
  treatment, 4
Atropine, 370t
Attention-deficit disorder, 240, 346
Atypical mycobacterial disease, 212
Atypical pneumonia, 35–36
Augmentation, of labor, 195
Autism spectrum disorder, 240, 346–347
Autoantibodies, 288, 391, 391t
AV block. see Atrioventricular (AV) block
Avoidant disorder, 240

**B**

Babinski's sign, 405t
Bacille Calmette-Guérin (BCG) vaccine, 37
Back
  sprain, 90–91
  strain, 90–91
Back/spine, disorders of, 89–93
  ankylosing spondylitis, 89–90, 90f
  back strain/sprain, 90–91
  cauda equina syndrome, 91
  herniated disk pulposus, 91
  kyphosis, 90
  low back pain, 92
  scoliosis, 92
  spinal stenosis, 92–93
  thoracic outlet syndrome, 93
  torticollis, 93
Bacteria
  causing diarrhea, 79t
  infections, of skin, 259–260

Bacteria (*Continued*)
  cellulitis, 259–260
    erysipelas (St. Anthony's fire), 260
    impetigo, 260
Bacterial disease, 206–211
  acute rheumatic fever, 206–208
  botulism, 208
  Campylobacter infection, 208
  *Chlamydia*, 208–209
  cholera, 209
  diphtheria, 209
  gonococcal infections, 209–210
  methicillin-resistant *Staphylococcus aureus*
    infection, 210
  Salmonellosis, 210–211
    *Salmonella* infections, 210–211
    typhoid fever, 210
  shigellosis, 211
  tetanus, 211
Bacterial endocarditis, 24
  clinical manifestations, 24–25
  diagnosis, 25
  general, 24
  treatment, 25
Bacterial meningitis, 158–159
  antibiotic choices for, 159t
  initial therapy for, 160t
Bacterial pneumonia, 33–35
Balanitis, 305
Barlow's sign, 405t
Barotrauma, 139–140
  external ear, 139–140
  middle ear, 139–140
Barrier method, of contraception, 185–186
Barriers, 58t
Barton's fracture, 97t
Basal cell carcinoma, 266
Basophilia, 381
Bats, exposure to, 34t
Battle's sign, 405t
BBB. *see* Bundle branch block (BBB)
BCG vaccine. *see* Bacille Calmette-Guérin
    (BCG) vaccine
Beclomethasone dipropionate, 41–42t
Behavioral science, 230–253
Bell-clapper deformity, 305
Bell's palsy, 154–155
Benign neoplasms, 162
Benign prostatic hypertrophy (BPH),
    302–303
Bennett's fracture, 97t
Benzodiazepines, 232, 371–372, 372t
Beta-blockers, 16, 363–364
Beta-lactam antibiotics, 355–358
Beta-lactamase inhibitors, 356
Beta-thalassemia, 285
Bethanechol, 81–82t
Bicarbonate, 385
Biguanides, 366–367
Bile acid–binding agents, 14
Bile acid–binding resins, 368
Biliary tract, 67t
Bilirubin, 340, 385–386
  metabolism of, disorders of, 64, 64t
  normal values for, 407–410t
  in urinalysis, 390

Biot's sign, 405t
Bipolar disorder, 233–234
Birds, exposure to, 34t
Bird's-beak deformity, 55, 55f
Bisacodyl (PO), 371t
Bisacodyl (rectal), 371t
Bishop scoring system, 195
Bismuth subsalicylate (BSS), 81–82t,
    370, 370t
Black widow spider, 258–259
Bladder carcinoma, 309
Bleeding time, 383
  norml values for, 407–410t
Blenoxane. *see* Bleomycin
Bleomycin, 271t, 376–377t, 377t
Blepharitis, 132
Blood, 390
  CBC, 407–410t
  test, in jaundice, 386t
  in urinalysis, 390
Blood cell maturation sequence, normal,
    381f
Blood urea nitrogen (BUN), 386
Blowout fracture, 135
BMI. *see* Body mass index (BMI)
Body dysmorphic disorder, 239–240
Body fluid compartments, 384
Body mass index (BMI), weight-associated
    health risks and, 238t
Bone
  density test, 104t
  tumors, 102
Borderline disorder, 240–241
Botulism, 208
Bowels
  inflammatory, 70–71
  irritable, 71–72
  obstruction of, 73–74
  small, bacterial overgrowth, 73
Boxer's fracture, 97t, 98, 98f
BPH. *see* Benign prostatic hypertrophy
    (BPH)
Breast, 175–178
  abscess in, 175–176
  cancer
    mammogram of, 176f
    noninvasive types of, 177t
    surgical treatment for, 193–194
  carcinoma of, 176–177
    risk factors for, 176
  fibroadenoma, 177
  fibrocystic disease, 177–178
  galactorrhea, 178
  gynecomastia, 178
  mastitis, 178
  self-examination of, 176
Bretylium, 27–29t, 367t
Brief psychotic disorder, 243
Bronchial carcinoma, 38f
Bronchiectasis, 41–43
Bronchiolitis, acute, 335
Bronchitis
  acute, 32
  chronic, 43
    emphysema, comparison of, 43t
    treatment of, 43

Bronchogenic carcinoma, 38–39
  clinical manifestations of, 38
  diagnosis of, 38–39
  treatment of, 39
Bronchopneumonia, 34
Brown recluse spider, 258–259
Brudzinski's sign, 405t
BSS. *see* Bismuth subsalicylate (BSS)
Budesonide, 41–42t
Bulge's sign, 405t
Bulimia nervosa, 237–238
Bullous impetigo, 260
Bumetanide, 27–29t
BUN. *see* Blood urea nitrogen (BUN)
Bundle branch block (BBB), 4–6
  EKG findings, 4
  general, 4
  treatment, 4–6
Bupropion, 248, 249–251t, 373
Burns, 273–275
  deep partial-thickness, 273
  estimating percentage of, 274f
  first-degree, 273
  fourth-degree, 273–274
  hospital care after, 274–275
  pain management after, 275
  second-degree, 273
  third-degree, 273
  wound assessment of, 274
Bursitis, 94
BuSpar. *see* Buspirone
Buspirone, 249–251t, 373
Butyrophenone antiemetics, 371

**C**

C-reactive protein (CRP), 391
Calcium, 388
Calcium channel blockers (CCBs), 364–365
Campylobacter infection, 208
Cancer
  colorectal, inherited, 75t
  endometrial, 197
  esophageal, 56t
  prevention of, 402t
Candidiasis, 204–205, 260–261
  oral, 148
CAP treatment. *see* Community-acquired
    pneumonia (CAP) treatment
Captopril, 27–29t
Carafate. *see* Sucralfate
Carbamazepine, 168t, 375, 375t
Carbapenems, 357
Carboplatin, 376–377t, 377t
Carboxyhemoglobin, 274
Carbuncle, 255
Carcinoid tumors, 39
Carcinoma, 178–179. *see also* Bronchogenic
    carcinoma
  adeno-, 56t
  breast, 176–177
  ovarian, 192, 192t
  squamous cell, 56t
Cardiac diseases
  causing cyanosis, 333t
  congenital heart disease, 332–335

Cardiac diseases, pediatrics, 332–335
  congenital heart disease, 332–335
  general, 332
Cardiac drugs, 362–366
  alpha-blockers, 364
  angiotensin-converting enzyme (ACE)
    inhibitors, 363
  angiotensin II receptor blockers (ARBs), 363
  antiarrhythmics, 366
  beta-blockers, 363–364
  calcium channel blockers (CCBs), 364–365
  centrally acting agents, 365–366
  digitalis, 366
  direct vasodilators, 365
  diuretics, 362–363
  nitroglycerin/nitrates, 366
Cardiac enzyme markers in acute myocardial
  infarction, 15t
Cardiac tamponade, 26
  clinical manifestations, 26
  diagnosis, 26
  general, 26
  treatment, 26
Cardiogenic shock, 12–13
  clinical manifestations, 12
  diagnosis, 12
  general, 12
  treatment, 13
Cardiology drugs, 27–29t
Cardiomyopathy
  dilated, 1–2
    clinical manifestations, 1
    diagnosis, 1
    general, 1
    treatment, 1–2
  hypertrophic, 2
    clinical manifestations, 2
    diagnosis, 2
    general, 2
    treatment, 2
  restrictive
    clinical manifestations, 2
    diagnosis, 2
    general, 2
    treatment, 2
Cardiovascular system, 1–31
Carpal tunnel syndrome, 88–89, 165–166
Cascara sagrada, 371t
Castor oil, 81–82t
Catapres. *see* Clonidine
Cataract, 130–131
Catechol-O-methyl transferase (COMT)
  inhibitors, 162
Cauda equina syndrome, 91
CBC. *see* Complete blood count (CBC)
CCBs. *see* Calcium channel blockers (CCBs)
Celebrex. *see* Celecoxib
Celecoxib, 353
Celexa. *see* Citalopram
Celiac disease, 68
Celiac sprue, 73
Cellulitis, 259–260
  orbital, 134
Central nervous system (CNS) stimulant use
  disorder, 247

Central vertigo, 141t
Centrally acting agents, 365–366
Cephalosporins, 226–227t, 352, 357
  fifth generation, 357
  first generation, 356–357
  fourth generation, 357
  second generation, 357
  third generation, 357
Cerebral aneurysm, 169
Cerebral palsy, 164, 344–345
Cerumen impaction, 138
Cervical cap, 186
Cervical disorders, 178–180
  carcinoma, 178–179
  cervicitis, 179
  dysplasia, 179
  incompetent cervix (cervical insufficiency),
    179–180
Cervical esophageal webs, 56
Cervical insufficiency, 179–180
Cervical position, 195
Cervicitis, 179
Cervix, incompetent, 179–180
Chadwick's sign, 405t
Chalazion, 132–133
Chemistry test, 384–389
  ammonia, 389
  amylase, 388–389
  calcium, 388
  electrolytes, 384–385
  general, 384
  lactate dehydrogenase (LDH), 389
  lipase, 389
  lipid profile, 386–387
  liver function tests, 385–386
  magnesium, 389
  normal values for, 407–410t
  phosphorus, 388
  proteins, 387–388
  renal tests, 386
  uric acid, 389
Chemotherapeutic agent toxicity, 295t
Chemotherapy, 376
  mechanism of action, 376–377t
  side effects of, 377t
Chemotherapy toxicity, 294
Cherry angioma, 275–276
Chest pain, etiologies of, 16t
Chest x-ray
  of congestive heart failure, 9f
  of pneumonia, 34f
  tuberculosis, 212f
Child abuse, 230–231, 347
*Chlamydia*, 208–209
  diseases caused by, 209t
Chloramphenicol, 358
Chlordiazepoxide, 249–251t, 372t
Chloride, 384–385
Chlorpromazine, 249–251t, 374t
Cholecystitis, acute, 59–60
Cholelithiasis, 60
Cholera, 209
Cholesteatoma, 141
Cholesterol, 386–387
Cholestyramine, 369t

Cholinesterase inhibitors, 374
Chorea, 18
Chronic hepatitis, diagnostic tests for, 62t
Chronic lymphocytic leukemia (CLL),
  290–291
Chronic myelogenous leukemia (CML), 291
Chronic renal failure, 311–312
  causes of, 311t
Chvostek's sign, 405t
Cimetidine, 81–82t, 375t
Ciprofloxacin, 375t
Cirrhosis, 59
  causes of, 63t
Cisplatin, 376–377t, 377t
Citalopram, 249–251t
Claudication, neurogenic/vascular, 93t
Clavicle, fracture of, 100
Clindamycin, 359
Clinical intervention, on examination, 398
CLL. *see* Chronic lymphocytic leukemia
  (CLL)
Clonazepam, 249–251t, 372t
Clonidine, 27–29t, 365–366
Closed head injuries, 154
  concussion, 154
Clozapine, 249–251t, 374t
Clozaril. *see* Clozapine
Clue cells, 201, 201f
Cluster headache, 156
CML. *see* Chronic myelogenous leukemia
  (CML)
CNS stimulant use disorder. *see* Central nervous
  system (CNS) stimulant use disorder
Coagulation
  cascade, 295f
  disorders, 294–299
    factor VIII, 294–295
    factor IX, 295
    factor XI, 296
    hemostasis, 294
    hypercoagulable states, 296
    thrombocytopenia, 296–298
  disseminated intravascular, 297–298
  normal values for, 407–410t
  pathways, 383f
  testing, 383–384
    bleeding time, 383
    D-dimer, 384
    fibrin degradation products (FDP), 383
    fibrinogen, 383
    partial thromboplastin (PTT), 383
    prothrombin time (PT), 383
Coagulation disorders, 294–299
  Factor VIII disorder, 294–295
  Factor IX disorder, 295
  Factor XI disorder, 296
  hemostasis, 294
  hypercoagulable states, 296
  thrombocytopenia, 296–298
  thrombocytosis, 298
Coarctation of aorta, 333
Coccidioidomycosis, 36
Codeine, 354t
Coitus interruptus, 185
Colchicine, 375

Colestipol, 369t
Colic, 339–340
Colitis
   ischemic, 72
   ulcerative, 70, 71t
Colles' fracture, 98–99, 99f
Colon, 67–75
   malabsorption of, 72–73
   neoplasms of, 73
Color, in urinalysis, 389
Colorectal cancer, inherited, 75t
Coma
   in infants and children, 345, 345t
   myxedema, 125
Comedones, 255
Community-acquired pneumonia (CAP)
      treatment, 35f
Compartment syndrome, 104
Complete blood count (CBC), 381–383
   hemoglobin/hematocrit, 382
   normal values for, 407–410t
   platelet count, 382–383
   red blood cell (RBC) indices, 382
   white blood cell (WBC) count, 381
Complex regional pain syndrome, 172
Complicated pregnancy, 180–185
COMT inhibitors. *see* Catechol-O-methyl
      transferase (COMT) inhibitors
Concomitant disease, with hypertension, 11t
Concussion, 154
   grading scale, 155t
Condom, 185–186
   female, 185–186
   male, 185–186
Conduct disorder, 235–236
Conduction disorders, 2–9
Conductive hearing loss, 142
Condyloma acuminatum (venereal warts),
      262–263
Confusional state, causes of, 163t
Congenital abnormalities, 306
   horseshoe kidney, 306
   penile abnormalities, 306
   renal agenesis, 306
   vesicoureteral reflux, 306
Congenital heart defects, 333t
Congenital heart disease, 332–335
Congenital hemolytic anemia, 288–289
Congenital hypothyroidism (cretinism), 329
Congestive heart failure, 9–10
   clinical manifestations, 9
   diagnosis, 9
   general, 9
   treatment, 10
Conjunctival disorders, 130
   conjunctivitis, 130
Conjunctivitis, 130
   bacterial, 130t
   chlamydial, 130t
   signs and symptoms of, 130t
Consciousness, delirium/altered level of,
      162–163
Constipation, 68–69
   causes of, 68t
   treatment of, 69

Contact dermatitis, 268–269
Contraceptive methods, 185–187
   barrier methods, 185–186
   emergency, 187
   hormonal, 186–187
   intrauterine devices (IUDs), 186
   natural methods, 185
   oral contraindications to, 187t
   spermicides, 186
   sterilization, 187
Contraceptive patch, 186–187
Contraction stress test (CST), 181
Coombs' test, 287
Cor pulmonale, 48
Cord prolapse, 180–181
Corneal abrasion, 136
Corneal disorders, 130–132
   cataract, 130–131
   corneal ulcer, 131
   infectious, 131
   keratitis, 131–132
   pterygium, 132
Corneal ulcer, 131
Coronary artery disease, screening for, 403t
Coronary atherosclerosis, risk factors for,
      14b
Corticoadrenal insufficiency
   acute, 114–115
   chronic, 114
Corticosteroids, 44
   for allergic rhinitis, 145t
   oral, 278t
Cortisol, 113t
   normal values for, 407–410t
   plasma, 113
   urine free, 113
Coumadin, 46t
Courvoisier's sign, 405t
COX-2s, 353
Cranial nerves
   dysfunction, 155t
   function of, 404t
Cranial nerve palsies, 154–155
   Bell's palsy, 154–155
Creatinine, 386
   ratio, in BUN, 386
Crigler-Najjar syndrome Type II, 64t
Crohn's disease, 70–71, 71t
   ulcerative colitis, comparison of, 71t
Cromolyn sodium, 41–42t
Croup, 336
CRP. *see* C-reactive protein (CRP)
Cryptococcosis, 205
Cryptorchidism, 347
CST. *see* Contraction stress test (CST)
Cullen's sign, 405t
Cushing's syndrome, 113–114
Cyanosis
   cardiac causes of, 333t
   pulmonary causes of, 333t
Cyclophosphamide, 376–377t, 377t
Cyclothymic disorder, 234
Cystic fibrosis, 329–331
   pneumonia related to, 34t
Cystitis, 306–307

Cystocele, of vagina, 199
Cysts, 255
   bone, 102
   ganglion, 102
   ovarian, 191–192
   pseudo-, 65
Cytarabine, 376–377t, 377t
Cytochromic classification, 283
Cytomegalovirus infections, 218
Cytoxan. *see* Cyclophosphamide

**D**
D-dimer, 384, 407–410t
Dacryoadenitis, 132
Dacryocystitis, 132
De Quervain's tenosynovitis, 89
Decongestants, 145t
Decubitus ulcers, stages of, 275t
Deep neck infection, 148
Deep partial-thickness burns, 273
Degenerative dementias, 163t
Delirium, causes of, 163t
Delirium/altered level of consciousness,
      162–163
Delivery, normal, 194–196
Delusional disorders, 242
   subtypes of, 243t
Dental abscess, 147
Depakene. *see* Valproate; Valproic acid
Dependent disorder, 241
Depersonalization-derealization disorder,
      237
Depo-Provera, 187
Depression, screening for, 403t
Depressive disorders, 234–235
   homicidal behaviors, 235
   major depressive disorder, 234
   persistent depressive disorder (dysthymia),
      234–235
   premenstrual dysphoric disorder,
      235
   suicidal behaviors, 235
Dermatitis
   atopic, 268, 268t
   comparison of, 268t
   contact, 268–269
   diaper, 348
   nummular eczematous, 269
   perioral, 269
   seborrheic, 268t, 269–270
   stasis, 275
Dermatologic disorders, 276–279
   acanthosis nigricans, 276–277
   epidermal inclusion cysts (epidermoid
      cysts), 277
   hidradenitis suppurative (acne inversa),
      277
   lipomas, 277
   photosensitivity reactions, 277–278
   pilonidal disease, 278
   urticaria (hives), 278–279
Dermatologic system, 254–281
   desquamation, 256–257
   fungal infections in, 260–261
   neoplasms of, 266–268

Dermatology, pediatrics, 348
  diaper dermatitis, 348
Dermatomyositis, 106
Dermis, of skin, 273
Desipramine, 249–251t, 373t
Desquamation, 256–257
  erythema multiforme, 256
  Stevens-Johnson syndrome, 256–257
  toxic epidermal necrolysis, 257
Desyrel. *see* Trazodone
Development, 322
Developmental hip dysplasia, 343
Developmental milestones, 322, 327t
  delays, screening for, 327t
Dexedrine. *see* Dextroamphetamine
Dextroamphetamine, 249–251t
Diabetes
  complications during pregnancy,
    182t
  gestational, 181–182
  insipidus, 123
  mellitus, 115–120
    complications of, 116t, 118t
    hypoglycemia, 118–119
    screening for, 403t
    type 1, 115–117, 119t
    type 2, 117, 119t
Diabetic ketoacidosis, 116–117
Diabetic peripheral neuropathy,
  166–167
Diaper dermatitis, 348
Diaphragm method, 186
Diarrhea
  infectious, 78–80
  inflammatory, noninflammatory, 78t
  nosocomial, 80
  traveler's, 78–80
  viral causes of, 79t
Diazepam, 249–251t, 372t, 375t
Diazoxide, 365
DIC. *see* Disseminated intravascular
  coagulation (DIC)
Diclofenac, 353
Diffuse esophageal spasm, 55
Digitalis. *see* Digoxin
Digoxin, 27–29t, 366
Dihydropyridine CCBs, 365
Dilantin. *see* Phenytoin
Diltiazem, 27–29t, 367t
Diphenoxylate, 81–82t, 370t
Diphtheria, 209
Direct vasodilators, 365
Disaccharidase deficiency, 73
Dislocations, 87–88
  ankle/foot, 96
  elbow, 87
  hand, 87–88
  hip, 94
  knee, 94–95
  shoulder, 85–86, 86f
Disopyramide, 27–29t, 367t
Disorders of the ankle/foot, 96
  dislocations, 96
  sprains/strains, 96
Disruptive mood dysregulation disorder
  (DMDD), 236

Disseminated intravascular coagulation
    (DIC), 297–298
  pathogenesis of, 297f
Dissociative disorders, 236–237
  depersonalization-derealization disorder,
    237
  dissociative amnesia, 236–237
  dissociative identity disorders, 236
Distress, fetal, 181
Distribution, 352
Diuretics, 362–363
  effects of, 319t
Diverticular disease, 69–70
  acute diverticulitis, 69
  diverticular hemorrhage, 70
  diverticulosis, 69
Diverticular hemorrhage, 70
Diverticulitis, acute, 69
Diverticulosis, 69
Diverticulum, Zenker's, 56
DMDD. *see* Disruptive mood dysregulation
    disorder (DMDD)
Dobutamine, 27–29t
Docusate calcium, 371t
Docusate sodium, 371t
Dofetilide, 367t
Domestic violence, 231
Domperidone, 81–82t
Dopamine agonist, 161
Dose–response relationships, 352
Down syndrome, 331
Doxepin, 373t
Doxorubicin, 376–377t, 377t
Drawer sign, 405t
Droperidol, 81–82t
Drug eruptions, 270–271
Drug-induced hemolytic anemia, 288t
Drug-induced hyperpigmentation, 270–271,
    271t
Drugs. *see also specific drugs*
  absorption of, 352
  action, sites of, 352
  analgesics, 352–354
  antiarrhythmic, 7t
  antibiotics, 355–360
  anticoagulants, 374–375
  anticonvulsants, 375–376
  antidiabetic, 118t
  antifolate, 360
  antigout, 375
  antirheumatic, disease-modifying, 108t
  antituberculosis, 360–361
  antiviral respiratory agents, 361
  cardiac drugs, 362–366
  cardiology, 27–29t
  chemotherapy, 376
  cholinesterase inhibitors, 374
  endocrine, 366–368
  eruptions from, 270–271
    fixed, 270
  in gastroenterology, 81–82t
  for gastroesophageal reflux disease
      (GERD), 58t
  gastrointestinal medications, 368–371
  for human immunodeficiency virus (HIV),
      361–362

Drugs *(Continued)*
  for hyperlipidemia, 369t
  lipid-lowering agents, 368
  migraine abortive therapy, 355
  pharmacodynamics, 352
  pharmacokinetics, 352
  psychiatric, 249–251t
  psychiatric medications, 371–374
  sedative/hypnotic/anxiolytic, 246–247,
    247t
  sites of action, 352
DSM5 panic attack specifier, 232t
DUB. *see* Dysfunctional uterine bleeding
    (DUB)
Dubin-Johnson syndrome, 64t
Ductus arteriosus, 332
Ductus venosus, 332
Duodenal atresia, 340, 340f
Duodenal ulcer, 59t
Dwarfism, 122
Dysfunctional uterine bleeding (DUB), 196–197
Dyshidrotic eczema, 270
Dysmenorrhea, 191
Dysplasia, 179
  hip, developmental, 343
Dystocia, shoulder, 181

**E**
Ear
  abnormalities, 142–143
    foreign body, 143
    mastoiditis, 142
    Meniere's disease, 143
    tinnitus, 143
  disorders, 138–147
  external, 138–139
    cerumen impaction, 138
    otitis externa, 138–139
    trauma, 139
  inner, 139–141
    acoustic neuroma, 139
    barotrauma, 139–140
    eustachian tube, dysfunction of, 140
    labyrinthitis, 140
    vertigo, 140–141
  middle, 141–142
    cholesteatoma, 141
    otitis media, 141
    tympanic membrane perforation, 142
  of newborns, 335–339
Eating disorders, 237–238
  anorexia nervosa, 237
  bulimia nervosa, 237–238
  medical complications of, 238t
  obesity, 238
Eclampsia, 184
Ectopic pregnancy, 67t, 181
Ectropion, 133
Eczema, 268
Eczematic and papulosquamous disorders,
    268–279
Eczematous disorders, 268–270
  contact dermatitis, 268–269
  dyshidrotic eczema (pompholyx), 270
  eczema, 268

Eczematous disorders *(Continued)*
　lichen simplex chronicus, 270
　nummular eczematous dermatitis, 269
　perioral dermatitis, 269
　seborrheic dermatitis, 269–270
　stasis dermatitis, 275
Edwards syndrome, 331–332
Effacement, 194
Effexor. *see* Venlafaxine
Elavil. *see* Amitriptyline
Elbow
　dislocations, 87
　nursemaid's, 88
　tennis, 89
Elder abuse, 231
Electrolyte and acid-base disorders, 314–318
　acid-base disorders, 316–318
　hypercalcemia, 316
　hyperkalemia, 315
　hypernatremia, 314–315
　hypocalcemia, 315–316
　hypokalemia, 315
　hypomagnesemia, 316
　hyponatremia, 314
　urinalysis, 318
　volume depletion, 318
　volume excess, 318
Electrolytes, 384–385
Elliptocytosis, hereditary, 288
Emergency contraception, 187
Emicizumab, 295
Emphysema, 43–44
　chronic bronchitis, comparison of, 43t
Enalapril, 27–29t
Encephalitis, 157–158
Encephalopathic disorders, 155–156
　Wernicke's encephalopathy, 155–156
Endocarditis, bacterial, 24–25
Endocrine background, 112
　feedback loops, 112
　hypothalamic function, 112
　information, 112
Endocrine drugs, 366–368
　alpha-glucosidase inhibitors, 368
　biguanides, 366–367
　glucagon-like peptide-1 receptor agonist, 368
　insulin, 366
　sodium-glucose co-transporter 2 inhibitors, 368
　sulfonylureas, 367
　thiazolidinediones, 367–368
Endocrine system, 112–128
　neoplastic disease of, 126
Endometrial cancer, 197
Endometriosis, 67t, 197–198
*Entamoeba histolytica*, 213f
Entropion, 133
Enzyme deficiency, 288–289
Eosinophilia, 381
Epicondyle fracture, 99
Epicondylitis, 89
Epidermal inclusion cysts (epidermoid cysts), 277
Epidermoid cysts, 277
Epididymitis, 307

Epidural hematoma, 170t
Epiglottitis, 148
　acute, 335–336
　　thumbprint sign, lateral x-ray, 336f
Epiphyseal fractures, 97
Epispadias, 306
Epistaxis, 143–144
Epstein-Barr virus infections, 218, 219t
Erb's palsy, 328
Erectile dysfunction, 303
Ergotamine alkaloids, 355
Erysipelas, 260
Erythema infectiosum, 218–219
Erythema marginatum, 18
Erythema multiforme, 256
Erythematous tympanic membrane, 338
Erythrocyte sedimentation rate, 391, 407–410t
Erythromycin, 375t
Erythropoiesis, 282, 381f
Escharotomy, 275
Eskalith. *see* Lithium
Esmolol, 27–29t, 367t
Esophageal cancer, risk factors for, 56t
Esophageal spasm, diffuse, 55
Esophagitis, 53–54
　infectious, 53–54
　medication-induced, 54
　radiation, 54
Esophagus, 53–57
　esophagitis, 53–54
　　infectious, 53–54
　　medication-induced, 54
　　radiation, 54
　Mallory-Weiss tear, 55–56
　motility disorders, 54–55
　　achalasia, 54–55, 55f
　　diffuse esophageal spasm, 55
　　general, 54
　neoplasms, 56
　strictures, 56
　varices, 56–57
Essential thrombocythemia, 298
Essential tremor, 160
Estrogen precursor, 113t
ESWL. *see* Extracorporeal shock wave lithotripsy (ESWL)
Etanercept, 108t
Ethambutol, 361
Ethosuximide, 168t, 375–376, 375t
Eustachian tube, dysfunction of, 140
Examination, 397–398
　before, 398–400
　during, 401
　15-day study schedule for, 400t
　31-day study schedule for, 400t
　90-day study schedule for, 399t
　after, 401
　basic science concepts on, 398
　clinical intervention on, 398
　day of the, 400–401
　formulating diagnosis on, 397
　health maintenance on, 398
　organ system on, 398t
　pharmaceutical therapeutics on, 398
　strategies for, 398–401
　task for, 397t

Examination *(Continued)*
　using laboratory/diagnostic studies on, 397
Exanthems, 259
　hand-foot-and-mouth disease, 259
Excoriation, 239
Excretion, 352
Extended-spectrum penicillins, 356
External auditory canal, foreign body, 143
External ear, 138–139
　cerumen impaction, 138
　otitis externa, 138–139
　trauma, 139
Extracorporeal shock wave lithotripsy (ESWL), 305
Extrapulmonary tuberculosis, 37t
Eyes
　disorders, 130–138
　foreign body, 135–136
　of newborns, 335–339

**F**
Factitious disorder, 245
Factor VIII disorder, 294–295
Factor IX disorder, 295
Factor XI disorder, 296
Familial adenomatous polyps, 75
Familial polyposis, 75t
Famotidine, 81–82t
FDP. *see* Fibrin degradation products (FDP)
Fecal impaction, 76
Feedback loops, 112
　negative, 113f
Feeding and eating disorders, 237–238
　anorexia nervosa, 237
　bulimia nervosa, 237–238
　obesity, 238
Felbamate, 376
Felbatol. *see* Felbamate
Female condom, 185–186
Female infertility, 188
　causes of, 188t
Femara. *see* Letrozole
Fenofibrate, 369t
Fentanyl, 354, 354t
Ferritin, normal values for, 407–410t
Ferrous sulfate, for iron deficiency anemia, 283
Fetal circulation, 332, 332f
Fetal distress, 181
Fetal heart monitoring, 195
Fetal monitoring, 195–196
Fetal scalp
　electrode, 195
　pH, 195
Fibric-acid inhibitors, 368
Fibrin degradation products (FDP), 383
Fibrinogen, 383
　normal values for, 407–410t
Fibrinogen degradation products, 383
　normal values for, 407–410t
Fibroadenoma, 177
Fibrocystic disease, 177–178
Fibromyalgia, 104–105
Finasteride (Propecia), for androgenetic alopecia, 258

Fingers sprains, 88
First-degree burns, 273
Fixed drug eruptions, 270
Flecainide, 27–29t, 367t
Fluconazole, 375t
Fluid resuscitation, 274–275
Flunisolide, 41–42t
Fluoroquinolones, 359
5-Fluorouracil (5-FU), 376–377t, 377t
Fluoxetine, 249–251t
Fluphenazine, 249–251t, 374t
Fluticasone propionate, 41–42t
Fluvoxamine, 249–251t
Focal neuropathy, 166
Folate
    deficiency of, 286
    normal values for, 407–410t
Follicle-stimulating hormone, normal levels
    of, 407–410t
Follicular phase, 189
Folliculitis, 255–256
Food allergies, 80–82
Foot fractures, 97–98
Foramen ovale, 332
Forearm
    disorders of, 87–89
    fractures, 98–99
Foreign body, 135–136
    aspiration, 337
    in ear, 143
    in eyes, 135–136
    in nose, 147
    obstruction, signs of, 337t
Fosphenytoin, 375t
Fracture, 96–100
    accompanying nerve injuries, 97
    ankle, 97–98
    Barton's, 97t
    Bennett's, 97t
    Boxer's, 97t, 98, 98f
    blowout, 135
    clavicle, 100
    Colles', 98–99, 99f
    definition, 96–97
    descriptors, 97
    epicondyle, 99
    epiphyseal, 97
    foot, 97–98
    forearm, 98–99
    Galeazzi's, 97t
    hand, 98–99
    Hangman's, 97t
    hip, 99
    humeral shaft, 99
    knee, 99–100
    March, 97t
    Monteggia's, 97t
    nerve injury associated, 98t
    Nightstick, 97t
    radial, 99, 100f
    scaphoid, 99
    scapula, 100
    shoulder, 100
    Smith's, 97t
    supracondylar, 99
    wrist, 98–99

Fredrickson phenotypes for hyperlipidemia,
    13t
5-FU. see 5-Fluorouracil (5-FU)
Functional neurological symptom disorder,
    244
Fungal disease, 204–206
    candidiasis, 204–205
    cryptococcosis, 205
    histoplasmosis, 205–206
    Pneumocystis, 206
    systemic fungal infections, 206
Fungal infections, of skin, 260–261
    candidiasis, 260–261
    tinea corporis, 261
    tinea pedis, 261
    tinea versicolor, 261
Fungal pneumonia, 36
Furosemide, 27–29t
Furuncle (boil), 255

G

G-6-PD deficiency. see Glucose-6-phosphate
    dehydrogenase (G-6-PD) deficiency
Gabapentin, 168t, 375t, 376
Galactorrhea, 178
Galactosemia, 342
Galant's reflex, 329
Galeazzi's fracture, 97t
Gallbladder, 59–60
    cholecystitis, acute, 59–60
    cholelithiasis of, 60
    primary sclerosing cholangitis, 60
Galveston formula, 274–275
Gamekeeper's thumb, 88
γ-Glutamyltransferase (GGT), 385
Ganglion cysts, 102
Gardnerella vaginalis, 200–201
Gardner's syndrome, 75t
Gastric ulcer, 59t
Gastritis
    pain from, 67t
    of stomach, 57–58
Gastroenterology, 339–343
    drugs used in, 81–82t
    pediatrics
        colic, 339–340
        duodenal atresia, 340, 340f
        inborn errors of metabolism, 341–342
        intussusception, 342–343
        jaundice, 340–341
        malrotation, 343
        pyloric stenosis, 343
        volvulus, 343
Gastroesophageal reflux disease (GERD), 57
    drug therapy in, 58t
    lifestyle medications for, 68t
    lifestyle modifications for, 57t
Gastrointestinal (GI) medications, 368–371
    antacids, 368
    antidiarrheals, 370
    antiemetics, 370–371
    bismuth subsalicylate (BSS), 370
    butyrophenone antiemetics, 371
    histamine2 receptor antagonists, 368–369
    laxatives, 370

Gastrointestinal (GI) medications (Continued)
    metoclopramide, 370
    proton-pump inhibitors, 369
    serotonin (5-HT3) antagonists, 371
    sucralfate, 369–370
Gemfibrozil, 369t
Generalized anxiety disorder, 231–232
Genetic disorders, of newborn, 329–332
    congenital hypothyroidism (cretinism), 329
    cystic fibrosis, 329–331
    Down syndrome (trisomy 21), 331
    general, 329
    Klinefelter's syndrome, 331
    trisomy 13 (Patau syndrome), 331
    trisomy 18 (Edwards syndrome), 331–332
    Turner's syndrome, 332
Genitourinary system, 302–321
    infectious conditions of, 306–309
    inflammatory conditions of, 306–309
    neoplastic diseases of, 309–310
Genitourinary system, of pediatrics, 347–348
    cryptorchidism, 347
    hydrocele, 347–348
    Wilms' tumor (nephroblastoma), 348
Genitourinary tract, benign conditions
    of, 302–306
    benign prostatic hypertrophy (BPH),
        302–303
    congenital abnormalities, 306
    erectile dysfunction, 303
    incontinence, 303–304
    nephrolithiasis, 304–305
    paraphimosis, 305
    phimosis, 305
    testicular torsion, 305
    urethral stricture, 305–306
    urethrocele, 306
    varicocele, 303
GERD. see Gastroesophageal reflux disease
    (GERD)
Gestational diabetes, 181–182
    complications of, 182t
    risk factors for, 181–182
Gestational trophoblastic disease, 182
GGT. see γ-Glutamyltransferase (GGT)
GI medications. see Gastrointestinal (GI)
    medications
Giant cell arteritis, 20
    clinical manifestations, 20
    diagnosis, 20
    general, 20
    treatment, 20
Giardia lamblia, 214f
Giardiasis, 213–214
Gigantism, 121
Gilbert's syndrome, 64t
Gingivitis, 147
Glaucoma, 137–138
    angle-closure, 137
    open-angle, 137
Gleevec. see Imatinib
Glimepiride, 118t
Glipizide, 118t
Globe rupture, 136
Glomerulonephritis, 312–313
    summary of, 312t

Glucagon-like peptide-1 receptor agonist, 368
Glucocorticoids, 115
  side effects of, 115t
Glucose, in urinalysis, 389
Glucose-6-phosphate dehydrogenase (G-6-PD) deficiency, 288–289
Glyburide, 118t
Glycerin, 371t
GnRH. *see* Gonadotropin-releasing hormone (GnRH)
Gonadotropin-releasing hormone (GnRH), 112
Gonococcal infections, 209–210
Gonococcal urethritis, 308, 309t
Gout, 105
  pseudo-, 105
Gowers' sign, 405t
Gram stain, 391
Gram stain results, common, 392t
Granisetron, 81–82t
Graves' disease, 124
Grey Turner's sign, 405t
Growth, 322
Guillain-Barré syndrome, 166
Gums, diseases of, 147
Gynecomastia, 178

**H**

H₂ receptor antagonists, 58t
Hair and nails, diseases/disorders of, 257–258
  alopecia areata, 257
  androgenetic alopecia, 257–258
  onychomycosis, 258
  paronychia, 258
Hairy cell leukemia, 291–292
Halcion. *see* Triazolam
Haldol. *see* Haloperidol
Haloperidol, 81–82t, 249–251t, 374t
Hand
  dislocations, 87–88
  disorders of, 87–89
  fractures, 98–99
Hand-foot-and-mouth disease, 224, 259
Hangman's fracture, 97t
Hansen's disease, 212–213
Haptoglobin, normal values for, 407–410t
Hashimoto's thyroiditis, 125
HDL. *see* High-density lipoprotein (HDL)
Head injuries, closed, 154
  concussion, 154
Headaches, 156–157
  cluster headache, 156
  migraine, 156–157
  tension headache, 157
  types of, 157t
Health maintenance, on examination, 398
Hearing
  impairment of, 142
  loss of
    conductive, 142
    sensorineural, 142
  screening for, 403t
Heart failure, functional classification of, 10t

Hegar's sign, 405t
*Helicobacter pylori* infection, treatment of, 59t
HELLP Syndrome, 184
Hematocrit, 382
  normal values for, 407–410t
Hematologic system, 282–301
  malignancies in, 290–294
Hematology, normal values for, 407–410t
Hematomas
  comparison of, 170t
  external ear, 138–139
Hemochromatosis, 63t, 299
Hemoglobin, 382. *see also* Mean cell hemoglobin (MCH); Mean cell hemoglobin concentration (MCHC)
  C disease, 289
  electrophoresis, normal values for, 407–410t
  SC disease, 289
Hemoglobinopathies, 289
Hemolytic anemia, 287–289
  acquired, 287–288
  congenital, 288–289
  drug-induced, 288t
  enzyme deficiency, 288–289
  microangiopathic, 287
Hemorrhage, diverticular, 70
Hemorrhagic stroke, 171
Hemorrhoids, on rectum, 76
Hemostasis, 294
Heparin, 46, 374
  and coumadin, 46t
Hepatic abscess, 67t
Hepatitis
  acute, 60–61
    serology testing for, 61t
  acute viral, causes of, 61t
  chronic, 61–62
    diagnostic tests for, 61t
  virus specific, 61
Hepatitis C, screening for, 403t
Herceptin. *see* Trastuzumab
Hereditary elliptocytosis, 288
Hereditary nonpolyposis syndrome (Lynch syndrome), 75
Hernia, 77–78
  hiatal, 77
  incisional (ventral), 77
  inguinal, 77
  umbilical, 77–78
Herniated disk pulposus, 91
Herpangina, 224
Herpes simplex, 148–149, 219, 263–264
  type 1, 263
  type 2, 263
Herpes zoster, 264
Hiatal hernia, 77
Hidradenitis suppurative, 277
High-density lipoprotein (HDL), 387
Hip
  aseptic necrosis (osteonecrosis), 93–94
  dislocations of, 94
  disorders of, 93–94
  dysplasia, developmental, 343
  fracture of, 99

Histamine2 receptor antagonists, 368–369
Histoplasmosis, 36, 205–206
Histrionic disorder, 241
HIV. *see* Human immunodeficiency virus (HIV)
Hives, 278–279
HMG-CoA reductase inhibitors, 14, 368
Hoarding disorder, 239
Hodgkin's lymphoma, 292
Homans' sign, 405t
Homicidal behaviors, 235
Homocystinuria, 342
Hookworms, 214
Hordeolum, 133
Hormonal contraceptives, 186–187
Hormones
  growth, 121t
  luteinizing, 121t, 407–410t
  pituitary, 121t
  thyroid-stimulating, 121t, 407–410t
Horner's syndrome, 38
Horseshoe kidney, 306
5-HT₁ᴮ/₁ᴰ agonists, 355
Human immunodeficiency virus (HIV)
  opportunistic infections in, 220t
  pneumonia related to, 36
  prophylaxis treatment of, 222t
  drugs for, 361–362
    nonnucleoside reverse transcriptase inhibitors (NNRTIs), 361
    nucleoside reverse transcriptase inhibitors (NRTIs), 361
    protease inhibitors, 361–362
  infection, 220
Human papillomavirus infections, 220–222
Humeral shaft fractures, 99
Huntington's disease, 160–161
Hyaline membrane disease, 336–337
Hydantoin, 271t
Hydatidiform moles, 182
Hydralazine, 27–29t, 365
Hydrocele, 347–348
Hydrocephalus, normal-pressure, 169
Hydrochlorothiazide, 27–29t
Hydrocodone, 354t
Hydrocortisone, 270
Hydromorphone, 354, 354t
Hydronephrosis, 313
Hydroxychloroquine, 108t
Hyperactivity-impulsivity, symptoms of, 346t
Hyperaldosteronism, primary, 115
Hyperbilirubinemia, differential diagnosis of, 341t
Hypercalcemia, 316
Hypercholesterolemia, 13–14
  clinical manifestations, 14
  diagnosis, 14
  general, 13
  screening for, 403t
  treatment, 14
Hypercoagulable states, 296
Hyperkalemia, 315, 384
  causes of, 385t
Hyperlipidemia
  drugs of, 369t
  Fredrickson phenotypes for, 13t

Hypernatremia, 314–315
  causes of, 384t
Hyperosmolar hyperglycemic state, 117
Hyperparathyroidism, 120
Hyperpigmentation, drug-induced, 271t
Hyperprolactinemia, 123–124
Hypertension, 10–12
  classification of, 10t
  essential, 10–11
    clinical manifestations, 10
    diagnosis, 10
    general, 10
    treatment, 10–11
  hypertensive emergencies, 12
    clinical manifestations, 12
    diagnosis, 12
    general, 12
    treatment, 12
  in patients with concomitant disease, 11t
  in pregnancy, 183–184
  screening for, 403t
  secondary, 11–12
    clinical manifestations, 11
    diagnosis, 12
    general, 11
    treatment, 12
Hyperthyroidism, 124–125
  signs and symptoms of, 124t
Hypertriglyceridemia, 14
  clinical manifestations, 14
  diagnosis, 14
  general, 14
  treatment, 14
Hyphema, 136
Hypocalcemia, 315–316
Hypoglycemia, 118–119
  etiologies of, 119t
Hypogondanism, 119
Hypokalemia, 315, 384
  causes of, 385t
Hypomagnesemia, 316
  causes of, 316t
Hyponatremia, 314
  causes of, 384t
  diagnosis of, 314f
Hypoparathyroidism, 120–121
Hypospadias, 306
Hypotension
  cardiogenic shock, 12–13
  orthostatic/postural, 12–13
Hypothalamic function, 112
Hypothyroidism, 125
  primary, 122
  signs and symptoms of, 125t

**I**

Ibuprofen, 353
Ibutilide, 367t
Idiopathic interstitial pneumonias, 49t
Idiopathic pulmonary fibrosis, 48–49, 49t
  medications used in, 49t
Idiopathic thrombocytopenic purpura (ITP), 296
Illness anxiety disorder, 244–245
Imatinib, 376–377t, 377t

Imipramine, 249–251t, 373t
Immunization, 322
  schedules of, 322, 323f, 324f
    for 0 through 18 years, 323f
    for 4 months through 18 years, 324f
Immunology test, normal values for, 407–410t
Impetigo, 260
Impingement sign, 405t
Inattention, symptoms of, 346t
Inborn errors of metabolism, 341–342
Incisional (ventral) hernia, 77
Incompetent cervix, 179–180
Incontinence, 303–304
  mixed, 303
  overflow, 304
  stress, 303
  urge, 303–304
Indocin. *see* Indomethacin
Indomethacin, 353
Induction, of labor, 195
Infectious diarrhea, 78–80
  acute, 78
  causes of, 79t
  inflammatory *versus* noninflammatory, 78t
  nosocomial diarrhea, 80
  traveler's diarrhea, 78–80
Infectious diseases, 259–268
  of musculoskeletal system, 100–101
    osteomyelitis, 100–101
    septic arthritis, 101
Infectious disorders, 32–38
  bronchitis, acute, 32
  cornea, 131
  influenza, 32–33
  of neurologic system, 157–159
    encephalitis, 157–158
    meningitis, bacterial, 158–159
  pneumonia, 33–36
    atypical, 35–36
    bacterial, 33–35
    fungal, 36
    human immunodeficiency virus (HIV), 36
  tuberculosis, 36–38
Infectious endocarditis, 25t
Infectious/inflammatory disorders, 147–150
  aphthous ulcers, 147–148
  deep neck infection, 148
  epiglottitis, 148
  in genitourinary system, 306–309
    cystitis, 306–307
    epididymitis, 307
    orchitis, 307
    prostatitis, 307–308
    pyelonephritis, 308
    urethritis, 308–309
  herpes simplex, 148–149
  laryngitis, 149
  oral candidiasis, 148
  peritonsillar abscess, 149
  pharyngitis, 149–150
Infertility, 187–188
  female, 188
    causes of, 188t
  general, 187
  male, 187–188, 188t

Inflammatory bowel disease, 69–70
  Crohn's disease, 70–71
  ulcerative colitis, 70
Inflammatory diarrhea, noninflammatory *v.*, 78t
Infliximab, 108t
Influenza, 32–33, 222
  clinical manifestations of, 32
  diagnosis of, 33
  general, 32
  treatment of, 33
Inguinal hernia, 77
Inheritance patterns, 330t
Inherited colorectal cancer syndromes, 75t
Inhibitor drugs, 352
Inner ear, 139–141
  acoustic neuroma, 139
  barotrauma, 139–140
  eustachian tube, dysfunction of, 140
  labyrinthitis, 140
  vertigo, 140–141
Insulin, 366, 367t
  preparations of, 117t
Interstitial pneumonia, 34
Intestinal obstruction, 67t
Intrauterine devices (IUDs), 186
Intrauterine pressure catheter, 195–196
Intussusception, 342–343
Iodine, radioactive, 124
Ipratropium bromide, 41–42t
Iron
  -deficiency anemia, 283–284
  normal levels of, 407–410t
  studies, 284t
Iron binding capacity, normal values for, 407–410t
Irritable bowel disease, 71–72
Irritants, common, 269t
Ischemic bowel disease, 72
  acute arterial mesenteric ischemia, 72
  general, 55
  ischemic colitis, 72
Ischemic colitis, 72
Ischemic heart disease, MI, 14–17
Ischemic stroke, 170
Isoniazid, 360
Isosorbide, 27–29t
Isotretinoin, 255
ITP. *see* Idiopathic thrombocytopenic purpura (ITP)
IUDs. *see* Intrauterine devices (IUDs)

**J**

Jaundice, 340–341
  blood test in, 386t
  physiologic, 340
  urine test in, 386t
Jones criteria for acute rheumatic fever, 18t
Juvenile rheumatoid arthritis, 344

**K**

Kaposi's sarcoma, 266–267
Kawasaki's disease, 337–338
Keratitis, 131–132
Keratotic disorders, 265–266
  actinic, 265–266
  seborrheic, 266

Kernicterus, 341
Kernig's sign, 405t
Ketoacidosis, diabetic, 116–117
Ketones, in urinalysis, 390
Ketorolac, 353
Kidney stones on abdominal x-ray film, 304f
Klinefelter's syndrome, 331
Klonopin. *see* Clonazepam
Knee
  bursitis, 94
  dislocations of, 94–95
  disorders of, 94–96
  fractures of, 99–100
  meniscal injuries in, 95
  sprains/strains, 95–96
Kyphosis, 90

**L**

Labetalol, 27–29t
Labor
  augmentation of, 195
  cervical examination during, 194
  descent during, 196
  engagement during, 196
  extension during, 196
  external rotation during, 196
  flexion during, 196
  induction of, 195
  internal rotation during, 196
  normal, 194–196
  obstetric examination during, 194
  progression of, 196
  stages of, 196
Laboratory findings
  in meningitis, 159t
  in renal failure, 386t
Laboratory medicine, 380–393
  normal values in, 407–410t
  profiles in, 381
Labyrinthitis, 140
Lacrimal disorders, 132
  dacryoadenitis/dacryocystitis, 132
Lactase, 370t
Lactate dehydrogenase (LDH), 389
Lactational amenorrhea, 185
Lactobacillus acidophilus, 370t
Lactulose, 81–82t, 371t
Lamictal. *see* Lamotrigine
Lamotrigine, 168t, 249–251t, 375t, 376
Lansoprazole, 81–82t
Large intestine, obstruction, 74
Laryngitis, 149
Laryngotracheitis, 336
Lasègue's sign, 405t
Lateral collateral ligament injury, 95
Laxatives, 370, 371t
LDH. *see* Lactate dehydrogenase (LDH)
LDL. *see* Low-density lipoprotein (LDL)
Legal/medical ethics, 394
Leiomyoma, 198
Leprosy (Hansen's disease), 212–213
Lesions
  acne vulgaris, 254–255
  acneiform, 254–256
  nodular, in pneumonia, 34–35

Letrozole, 376–377t, 377t
Leukocyte esterase, in urinalysis, 390
Leukoplakia, 150–151
Leukotriene modifiers, 145t
Levodopa plus carbidopa, 161
Levothyroxine, 125
Lhermitte's sign, 405t
Librium. *see* Chlordiazepoxide
Lice, 262
Lichen planus, 271
Lichen simplex chronicus, 270
Lid disorders, 132–133
  blepharitis, 132
  chalazion, 132–133
  ectropion, 133
  entropion, 133
  hordeolum, 133
Lidocaine, 27–29t, 367t
Linezolid, 359
Lipase, 389
Lipid
  classification, normal values for, 407–410t
  disorders, 13–14
    hypercholesterolemia, 13–14
    hypertriglyceridemia, 14
  profile, 386–387
Lipid-lowering agents, 368
  bile acid–binding resins, 368
  fibric-acid inhibitors, 368
  HMG-COA reductase inhibitors, 368
  nicotinic acids, 368
Lipidoses lysosomal storage diseases, 342t
Lipomas, 277
Lisinopril, 27–29t
Lithium, 249–251t, 373
Liver, 60–64
  acute hepatitis, 60–61
  chronic hepatitis, 61–62
  cirrhosis of, 59
  disorders of bilirubin metabolism, 64t
  function tests, 385–386, 386t
  metabolic diseases of, 63t
  neoplasms of, 62
Liver function tests, 63t
Lobar pneumonia, 34
Loop diuretics, 362
Loperamide, 81–82t
Lorazepam, 81–82t, 249–251t, 372t, 375t
Losartan, 27–29t
Lou Gehrig's disease, 160
Lovastatin, 369t
Low back pain, 92
Low-density lipoprotein (LDL), 387
Low-molecular-weight heparin, 374
Lower esophageal ring, 56
Lumbar radiculopathies, 91t
Lungs
  abscess of, in pneumonia, 34
  of newborn, 327
Luteal phase, 191
Luteinizing hormone, normal levels of, 407–410t
Luvox. *see* Fluvoxamine
Lyme disease, 216
  treatment of, 216t

Lymphocytic leukemia
  acute, 290
  chronic, 290–291
Lymphocytosis, 381
Lymphoma, 292
  Hodgkin's, 292
  non-Hodgkin's, 292
Lymphopoiesis, 381f
Lynch syndrome, 75

**M**

Macrolides, 358
Macroscopic urinalysis, 389–390
  bilirubin, 390
  blood, 390
  color/odor, 389
  glucose, 389
  ketones, 390
  leukocyte esterase, 390
  nitrite, 390
  protein, 390
  specific gravity, 389
  urobilinogen, 390
Macular degeneration, 134
Magnesium, 389
Magnesium citrate, 371t
Major depression, criteria for, 234t
Major depressive disorder, 234
Malabsorption, 72–73
Malaria, 214–215
Male condom, 185–186
Male infertility, 187–188
  etiologies of, 188t
Malignancies, 290–294
  acute lymphocytic leukemia (ALL), 290
  acute myelogenous leukemia (AML), 291
  chronic lymphocytic leukemia (CLL), 290–291
  chronic myelogenous leukemia, (CML), 291
  hairy cell leukemia, 291–292
  lymphoma, 292
  melanoma, 267t
  multiple myeloma, 292–293
  myelodysplastic syndrome, 293
  oncologic emergencies, 294
  polycythemia vera, 293–294
Malignant neoplasms, 162
Malingering, 245
Mallory-Weiss tear, 55–56
Malrotation, 343
Mammogram of breast cancer, 176f
Manic episode, criteria for, 233t
MAOIs. *see* Monoamine oxidase inhibitors (MAOIs)
March fracture, 97t
Mast-cell stabilizers, 145t
Mastitis, 178
Mastoiditis, 142
McArdle's disease, 342
McBurney's sign, 405t
MCH. *see* Mean cell hemoglobin (MCH)
MCHC. *see* Mean cell hemoglobin concentration (MCHC)
McRoberts maneuver, 181
MCV. *see* Mean cell volume (MCV)

Mean cell hemoglobin (MCH), 382
Mean cell hemoglobin concentration (MCHC), 382
Mean cell volume (MCV), 382
Meconium aspiration, 338
Medial collateral ligament injury, 95
Medical informatics, 394
Medication-induced esophagitis, 54
Medroxyprogesterone acetate, 187
Melanoma, 267, 267t
Melasma, 272
Mellaril. *see* Thioridazine
Menarche, 189
Meniere's disease, 143
Meningitis
    bacterial, 158–159
        antibiotic choices for, 159t
        initial therapy for, 160t
    etiology of, age-based, 158t
    laboratory findings in, 159t
    *Staphylococcus aureus*, 158
Meniscal injuries, 95
Menopause, 188–189
    clinical manifestations, 188–189
    diagnosis, 189
    general, 188
    treatment, 189
Menstrual cycle, 189–190, 189f
    normal, 189f
Menstrual disorders, 190–191
    amenorrhea, 190, 190t, 191t
    dysmenorrhea, 191
    premenstrual syndrome (PMS), 191
Meperidine, 354
Mepolizumab, 41–42t
Mesenteric thrombus, 67t
Metabolic acidosis, etiology of, 317t
Metabolic alkalosis, etiology of, 317t
Metabolism, 352
    of bilirubin, disorders of, 64, 64t
    inborn errors of, 341–342
Metastatic tumors, 39
Metformin, 118t
Methadone, 354
Methicillin-resistant *Staphylococcus aureus* infection, 210
Methylcellulose, 371t
Methylmalonic acid (MMA), 286
Methylphenidate, 249–251t
Methylprednisolone, 41–42t
Metoclopramide, 81–82t, 370
Metoprolol, 27–29t, 367t
Metritis, 198
Metronidazole, 360, 375t
Mexiletine, 27–29t, 367t
MI. *see* Myocardial infarction (MI)
Microangiopathic hemolytic anemia, 287
Microbiology, 391
    gram stain, 391
Microscopic urinalysis, 390
Midazolam, 372t
Middle ear, 141–142
    cholesteatoma, 141
    otitis media, 141
    tympanic membrane perforation, 142

Midrin, 355
Miglitol, 118t
Migraine abortive therapy, 355
    5-HT$_{1B/1D}$ agonists (triptans), 355
    basic and combination medications, 355
    ergotamine alkaloids, 355
Migraine headaches, 156–157, 156t
Mineral oil, 81–82t, 371t
Minocycline, 271t
Minoxidil, 27–29t, 365
    for androgenetic alopecia, 257–258
Mirtazapine, 249–251t, 373
Misoprostol, 81–82t
Mitochondrial patterns, 330t
Mitral regurgitation, 22–23
    clinical manifestations, 22
    diagnosis, 23
    general, 22
    treatment, 23
Mitral stenosis, 22
    clinical manifestations, 22
    diagnosis, 22
    general, 22
    treatment, 22
Mitral valve prolapse, 23
    clinical manifestations, 23
    diagnosis, 23
    general, 23
    treatment, 23
Mixed incontinence, 303
MMA. *see* Methylmalonic acid (MMA)
Mobitz type I block, 4
Mobitz type II block, 4
Molar pregnancy, 182
Molluscum contagiosum, 264
Monoamine oxidase inhibitors (MAOIs), 232, 372–373
Monobactams, 356
Monocytosis, 381
Monozygotic twins, 183
Monteggia's fracture, 97t
Montelukast, 41–42t
Mood disorders, 233–234
    bipolar disorder, 233–234
    cyclothymic disorder, 234
Mood stabilizers, 234, 249–251t
Morbilliform eruptions, 270
Moricizine, 367t
Moro's reflex, 328
Morphine, 354, 354t
Motility disorders, 54–55
    achalasia, 54–55, 55f
    diffuse esophageal spasm, 55
    general, 54
Motor neuron disease, signs of, 160t
Motrin. *see* Ibuprofen
Movement disorders, 160–162
    amyotrophic lateral sclerosis, 160
    essential tremor, 160
    Huntington's disease, 160–161
    Parkinson's disease, 161–162
    Tourette's syndrome, 162
Multifocal atrial tachycardia, 3
    EKG findings, 3
    general, 3
    treatment, 3

Multiple endocrine neoplasia, 120
Multiple gestation, 183
Multiple myeloma, 292–293
    skull x-ray of, 293f
Multiple sclerosis, 164–165
Mumps, 222–223
Murmurs, maneuver effects on, 24t
Murphy's sign, 405t
Musculoskeletal diseases, of pediatrics, 343–344
    developmental hip dysplasia, 343
    juvenile rheumatoid arthritis, 344
    Osgood-Schlatter disease, 344
    slipped capital femoral epiphysis, 344
Musculoskeletal system, 85–111
    infectious diseases of, 100–101
    neoplastic disease of, 102–103
Myasthenia gravis, 165
Mycobacterial disease, 211–213
    atypical mycobacterial disease, 212
    leprosy (Hansen's disease), 212–213
    tuberculosis, 211–212
Myelodysplastic syndrome, 293
Myelogenous leukemia
    acute, 291
    chronic, 291
Myeloma, multiple, 292–293
Myelopoiesis, 381f
Myocardial damage, 15t
Myocardial infarction (MI)
    acute, 14–16
        clinical manifestations, 14–15
        diagnosis, 15
        general, 14
        treatment, 15–16
Myxedema coma, 125

**N**
Nägele's rule, 193
Nails, diseases/disorders of. *see* Hair and nails, diseases/disorders of
Naprosyn. *see* Naproxen
Naproxen, 353
Narcissistic disorder, 241
Narcolepsy, 243–244
Nardil. *see* Phenelzine
Nasal polyps, 144
National Commission on the Certification of Physician Assistants (NCCPA), 394, 397
Natural penicillins, 356
NCCPA. *see* National Commission on the Certification of Physician Assistants (NCCPA)
Nebivolol, 27–29t
Nedocromil sodium, 41–42t
Nefazodone, 249–251t
Negative feedback loop, 113f
Neoplasms, 119–120, 151, 162, 199
    benign, 162
    of colon, 73
    of dermatologic system, 266–268
        basal cell carcinoma, 266
        Kaposi's sarcoma, 266–267
        melanoma, 267
        squamous cell carcinoma, 267–268

Neoplasms *(Continued)*
  of esophagus, 56
  of liver, 62
  malignant, 162
  multiple endocrine neoplasia, 120
  oral cancer, 151
  of ovaries, 192
  of pancreas, 66
  pheochromocytoma, 123
  of rectum, 76
  of stomach, 58
  vaginal, 199
  vulva, 199
Neoplastic disease, 126
  of genitourinary system, 309–310
    bladder carcinoma, 309
    prostate carcinoma, 309–310
    renal cell carcinoma, 310
    testicular carcinoma, 310
  of musculoskeletal system, 102–103
    bone cysts, 102
    bone tumors, 102
    ganglion cysts, 102
    osteosarcoma, 102–103
  of pulmonary system, 38–40
    bronchogenic carcinoma, 38–39
    carcinoid tumors, 39
    metastatic tumors, 39
    pulmonary nodules, 39–40
Nephroblastoma, 348
Nephrolithiasis, 304–305
Nephrotic syndrome, 313
Nerves. *see also* Cranial nerves
  injuries, associated with fractures, 97
  peripheral, diseases of, 165–167
Neuritis, optic, 133
Neuro-ophthalmologic disorders, 133–134
  nystagmus, 133
  optic neuritis, 133
  papilledema, 133–134
Neuroblastoma, 345
Neurocognitive disorders, 162–163
  Alzheimer's disease, 163–164
  delirium/altered level of consciousness,
    162–163
Neurodevelopmntal disorders, 240
  attention-deficit/hyperactivity disorder,
    240
  autism spectrum disorder, 240
Neurogenic claudication, 93t
Neurologic system, 154–174
  infectious disorders of, 157–159
Neurology
  of pediatrics, 344–345
    cerebral palsy, 344–345
    coma, 345, 345t
    neuroblastoma, 345
    seizures, 345, 346t
Neuroma, acoustic, 139
Neuromuscular disorders, 164–165
  cerebral palsy, 164
  multiple sclerosis, 164–165
  myasthenia gravis, 165
Neurontin. *see* Gabapentin
Neuropathy
  diabetic peripheral, 166–167

Neuropathy *(Continued)*
  focal, 166
  pain control in, 166–167
  sensorimotor poly-, 166
Neutrophilia, 381
Newborn, 322–329
  abdomen of, 327
  biochemistry of, 341
  cardiac disease in, 332–335
  chest of, 327
  coma in, 345, 345t
  congenital heart disease in, 332–335
  congenital skin conditions in, 324
  cystic fibrosis in, 329–331
  dermatology in, 348
  ductus arteriosus, 332
  ears of, 327
  evaluation of, 322–329
  examination of, 323–329
  extremities of, 328
  eyes of, 325–327
  gastroenterology in, 339–343
  genetic disorders of, 329–332
  genitalia of, 327–328
  genitourinary disorders in, 347–348
  head of, 324–325
  heart of, 350
  hip examination in, 328
  lungs of, 327
  musculoskeletal disorders of, 343–344
  neck of, 327
  neurologic system of, 328–329
  neurology of, 344–345
  nutrition for, 329
  reflexes of, 328–329
  skin of, 323–324
  throat/mouth of, 327
  vitals of, 344
Niacin, 80t, 369t
Nicotine, 248
Nicotinic acids, 14, 368
Nifedipine, 27–29t
Nightstick fracture, 97t
Nitrates, 16, 352
Nitrite, in urinalysis, 390
Nitrofurantoin, 360
Nitroglycerin, 27–29t, 366
Nizatidine, 81–82t
NNRTIs. *see* Nonnucleoside reverse
    transcriptase inhibitors (NNRTIs)
Nodules, 255
Nolvadex. *see* Tamoxifen
Non-Hodgkin's lymphoma, 292
Nonbullous impetigo, 260
Nondihydropyridine, 364–365
Nongonococcal urethritis, 309t
Noninvasive breast cancer, types of, 177t
Nonnucleoside reverse transcriptase
    inhibitors (NNRTIs), 361
Nonselective alpha-blockers, 364
Nonsteroidal antiinflammatory drugs
    (NSAIDs), 353, 355
  for dysmenorrhea, 191
Nonstress test (NST), 181
Normal labor/delivery, 194–196
Normal-pressure hydrocephalus, 169

Normal ranges (reference ranges), 380–381
Norpramin. *see* Desipramine
Nortriptyline, 249–251t, 373t
Nose, 143–147
  acute sinusitis, 145–146
  chronic sinusitis, 146–147
  epistaxis, 143–144
  foreign body in, 147
  nasal polyps, 144
  of newborns, 335–339
  rhinitis, 144–145
  trauma, 147
Nosocomial diarrhea, 80
NRTIs. *see* Nucleoside reverse transcriptase
    inhibitors (NRTIs)
NSAIDs. *see* Nonsteroidal antiinflammatory
    drugs (NSAIDs)
NST. *see* Nonstress test (NST)
Nucleoside reverse transcriptase inhibitors
    (NRTIs), 361
Nummular eczematous dermatitis, 269
Nursemaid's elbow, 88
Nursing home residence, 34t
Nutritional deficiencies, 80, 80t
Nystagmus, 133

**O**
Obesity, 238
  screening for, 403t
Obsessive-compulsive disorder (OCD),
    238–242
  body dysmorphic disorder, 239–240
  excoriation, 239
  hoarding disorder, 239
  trichotillomania, 239
Obstruction, 73–74
  large intestine, 74
  small intestine, 73–74
Obstructive pulmonary disease, 40–44
  asthma, 40
  bronchiectasis, 41–43
  chronic bronchitis, 43
  emphysema, 43–44
  status asthmaticus, 40–41
Obturator sign, 405t
OCD. *see* Obsessive-compulsive disorder
    (OCD)
Odor, in urinalysis, 389
OGTT. *see* Oral glucose tolerance testing
    (OGTT)
Olanzapine, 249–251t, 374t
Omalizumab, 41–42t
Omeprazole, 81–82t
Oncologic emergencies, 294
  chemotherapy toxicity, 294
  spinal cord compression, 294
  superior vena cava syndrome, 294
  tumor lysis syndrome, 294
Oncovin. *see* Vincristine
Ondansetron, 81–82t
Onychomycosis, 258
Open-angle glaucoma, 137
Ophthalmic zoster, 265
Opiate withdrawal, symptoms of, 247t
Opioid equivalence, 354t

Opioid use disorder, 247
Opioids, 354
  equivalence, 354t
Optic neuritis, 133
Oral cancer, 151
Oral candidiasis, 148
Oral contraceptives, 186–187
  contraindications to, 187t
Oral corticosteroids, comparison of, 278t
Oral glucose tolerance testing (OGTT), 194
Orbital cellulitis, 134
Orbital disorders, 134
  orbital cellulitis, 134
Orchitis, 307
Organ systems, chemistry tests of, 381t
Oropharyngeal disorders, 147–151
  leukoplakia, 150–151
Orthostatic/postural hypotension
  clinical manifestations, 13
  diagnosis, 13
  general, 13
  treatment, 13
Ortolani's maneuver, 328f
Ortolani's sign, 405t
Oseltamivir, 33, 361
Osgood-Schlatter disease, 344
Osmolal gap, 384
Osmolality, 384
  normal values for, 407–410t
Osteoarthritis, 103
Osteomyelitis, 100–101
  treatment of, 101t
Osteonecrosis, 93–94
Osteoporosis, 103–104
  screening for, 104, 403t
Osteosarcoma, 102–103
Otitis externa, 138–139
Otitis media
  acute
    of newborn, 338
Ottawa Ankle Rules, 98t
Ovarian carcinoma, 192t
Ovaries, 191–193
  cysts on, 191–192
  neoplasms of, 192
  torsion, 193
Overflow incontinence, 304
Oxazepam, 249–251t, 372t
Oxycodone, 354, 354t
Oxymorphone, 354t


**P**

PA relationship. *see* Physician/physician
    assistant (PA) relationship
Paclitaxel, 376–377t, 377t
Paget's disease, 92
Pain
  abdominal, acute, 67t
  from burn, 275
  in gallbladder, 67t
  from gastritis, 67t
  from hepatitis, 67t
Pain syndrome, complex regional, 172
Palm method, for burns, 274
Palmar grasp, 328

Pamelor. *see* Nortriptyline
PANCE. *see* Physician Assistant National
    Certifying Exam (PANCE)
Pancoast's syndrome, 38
Pancreas, 64–66
  acute, 64–65
  chronic, 65–66
  neoplasms, 66
Pancreatic necrosis, 65
Pancreatitis, acute, 64–65
Panic disorder, 232
PANRE. *see* Physician Assistant National
    Recertifying Exam (PANRE)
Papilledema, 133–134
Papules, 255
Papulosquamous disorders, 270–272
  drug eruptions, 270–271
  lichen planus, 271
  pityriasis rosea, 271
  psoriasis, 271–272
Parachute reaction, 328
Paranoid disorder, 242
Paraphimosis/phimosis, 305
Paraplatin-AQ. *see* Carboplatin
Parasitic disease, 213–216, 262
  amebiasis, 213
  ascariasis, 213
  giardiasis, 213–214
  hookworms, 214
  lice, 262
  malaria, 214–215
  pinworms, 215
  scabies, 262
  tapeworms, 215
  toxoplasmosis, 215–216
Parasomnias, 244
Parathyroid disorders, 120–121
  hyperparathyroidism, 120
  hypoparathyroidism, 120–121
Parkinson's disease, 161–162
Parkland formula, 274
Parnate. *see* Tranylcypromine
Paronychia, 258
Parotitis, 150
Paroxetine, 249–251t
Paroxysmal supraventricular tachycardia, 6–7
  EKG findings, 7
  general, 6–7
  treatment, 7
Partial thromboplastin time (PTT), 383,
    383f
  normal values for, 407–410t
Patau syndrome, 331
Patent ductus arteriosus, 333–334
Patient care and communication, 394
Paxil. *see* Paroxetine
Pediatrics
  cardiac diseases, 332–335
  dermatology, 348
  developmental milestones, 322, 327t
  eyes, ears, nose, and throat/pulmonary,
    335–339
  gastroenterology, 339–343
  genetic disorders, 329–332
  genitourinary, 347–348
  growth and development, 322

Pediatrics (*Continued*)
  immunizations, 322, 323f, 324f
  musculoskeletal, 343–344
  neurology, 344–345
  newborn infant, 322–329
  psychiatry, 346–347
  tanner stages, 322, 325t, 326f
Pelvic inflammatory disease (PID), 193
  clinical manifestations, 193
  complications, 193
  diagnosis, 193
  general, 193
  treatment, 193
Pemphigoid, 276
Pemphigus, 276
Penicillins, 226–227t
  natural, 356
Penile abnormalities, 306
Peptic ulcer disease, 58–59, 67t
Pepto-Bismol, 370
Percutaneous nephrolithotomy, 305
Perennial allergic rhinitis, 144
Pericardial effusion, 26–29
  clinical manifestations, 26
  diagnosis, 26
  general, 26
  treatment, 26–29
Pericarditis
  acute, 25–26
    clinical manifestations, 26
    diagnosis, 26
    general, 25–26
    treatment, 26
  and tamponade, comparison of, 26t
Periodic abstinence, 185
Perioral dermatitis, 269
Peripheral nerve disorders, 165–167
  carpal tunnel syndrome, 165–166
  complex regional pain syndrome, 172
  diabetic peripheral neuropathy, 166–167
  Guillain-Barré syndrome, 166
Peripheral nerves, diseases of
  autonomic, 166
Peripheral vertigo, 141t
Peritonitis, 67t
Peritonsillar abscess, 149
Perphenazine, 249–251t
Persistent depressive disorder, 234–235
Personality disorders, 240–242
  classification of, 240t
  general, 240
  types, 240–242
Pertussis, 339
Peutz-Jeghers syndrome, 75
Phalen's sign, 405t
Pharmacodynamics, 352
  dose–response relationships, 352
  sites of drug action, 352
Pharmacokinetics, 352
  absorption, 352
  distribution, 352
  excretion, 352
  metabolism, 352
Pharmacology, 351–379
Pharyngitis, 149–150, 338–339
Phenelzine, 249–251t

Phenobarbital, 168t, 376
Phenothiazine antiemetics, 370–371
Phenylketonuria, 342
Phenytoin, 168t, 367t, 375t, 376
Pheochromocytoma, 123
Phimosis, 305
Phlebitis/thrombophlebitis, 20
    clinical manifestations, 20
    diagnosis, 20
    general, 20
    treatment, 20
Phobias, 233
Phosphorus, 388
Photosensitivity reactions, 277–278
Physician Assistant National Certifying
        Exam (PANCE), 394, 397–398, 401
Physician Assistant National Recertifying
        Exam (PANRE), 394, 397, 398, 401
Physician/physician assistant (PA) relation-
        ship, 394
Pica syndrome, 283
PID. see Pelvic inflammatory disease (PID)
Pigment disorders, 272–273
    melasma, 272
    vitiligo, 272–273
Pilonidal disease, 76, 278
Pinworms, 215
Pioglitazone, 118t
Pirbuterol, 41–42t
Pituitary disorders, 121–124
    acromegaly, 121
    diabetes insipidus, 123
    dwarfism, 122
    gigantism, 121
    hyperprolactinemia, 123–124
    short stature, 122
    syndrome of inappropriate antidiuretic
        hormone secretion (SIADH),
        122–123
Pituitary hormones, 121t
Pityriasis rosea, 271
Placenta previa, 183
Placing (stepping) response, 346
Platelet count, 382–383
Platinol. see Cisplatin
Pleural diseases, 44–45
    pleural effusion, 44–45
    pneumothorax, 45
Pleural effusion, 44–45
    diagnosis of, 44
PMS. see Premenstrual syndrome (PMS)
Pneumoconiosis, 49–50
    comparison of, 49t
Pneumocystis, 206
Pneumonia, 33–36
    atypical, 35–36
    bacterial, 33–35
    causes of, 33t
    chest x-ray of, 34f
    clinical manifestations of, 36
    cystic fibrosis related to, 34t
    empiric treatment of, 35t
    etiologies of, 34t
    fungal, 36
    HIV/AIDS related to, 34t
    human immunodeficiency virus (HIV), 36

Pneumonia (Continued)
    lung abscess in, 34
    nodular lesions in, 34–35
Pneumothorax, 45
    tension, with mediastinal shift, 45f
Poison, antidotes for, 406t
Polyarteritis nodosa, 105–106
Polyarthritis, 18
Polycarbophil, 370t, 371t
Polycystic kidney disease, 313
Polycythemia vera, 293–294
Polyethylene glycol, 81–82t, 371t
Polyethylene glycol-electrolyte preps, 371t
Polymyalgia rheumatica, 106
Polymyositis, 106
Polyps, 75, 76–77
    familial adenomatous polyps, 75
    Gardner syndrome, 75
    hereditary nonpolyposis syndrome
        (Lynch syndrome), 75
    nasal, 144
    Peutz-Jeghers syndrome, 75
Pompe's disease, 342
Pompholyx, 270
Posterior cruciate ligament injury, 96
Postherpetic neuralgia, 265
Postpartum bleeding, causes of, 183t
Postpartum hemorrhage, 183
    causes of, 182t
Posttraumatic stress disorder, 248–251
Potassium, 384
Potassium sparing diuretics, 362
PPIs. see Proton-pump inhibitors (PPIs)
Pravastatin, 369t
Prazosin, 27–29t
Predictive values, 380
    negative predictive value, 380
    positive predictive value, 380
Prednisone, 41–42t, 375t
Preeclampsia, 184
    manifestations of, 184t
Pregnancy
    complicated, 180–185
        abortion, 180
        abruptio placentae, 180
        cord prolapse, 180–181
        dystocia, shoulder, 181
        ectopic pregnancy, 181
        fetal distress, 181
        gestational diabetes, 181–182
        gestational trophoblastic disease, 182
        hypertension disorders in pregnancy,
            183–184
        molar pregnancy (hydatidiform moles), 182
        multiple gestation, 183
        placenta previa, 183
        postpartum hemorrhage, 183
        premature rupture of membranes, 184–185
        Rh incompatibility, 185
    diabetes during, 182t
    ectopic, 67t, 181
    hypertension disorders in, 183–184
    molar, 182
    uncomplicated, 193–196
        normal labor/delivery, 194–196
        prenatal diagnosis/care, 193–194

Premature atrial contractions, 7
    EKG findings, 7
    general, 7
    treatment, 7
Premature beats, 7
Premature rupture, of membranes, during
        pregnancy, 184–185
Premature ventricular contractions (PVCs),
        7, 7f
    EKG findings, 7
    general, 7
    treatment, 7
Premenstrual dysphoric disorder, 235
Premenstrual syndrome (PMS), 191
Prenatal care, 194
Prenatal diagnosis/care, 193–194
Presbycusis, 142
Pressure ulcers, 275
Preventive health guidelines, adult, 402t
Primary sclerosing cholangitis, 60
Prinzmetal's variant, 17
    clinical manifestations, 17
    diagnosis, 17
    general, 17
    treatment, 17
Procainamide, 27–29t, 367t
Prochlorperazine, 81–82t
Professional development, 394
Professional practice, 394
    legal/medical ethics, 394
    medical informatics, 394
    patient care and communication, 394
    physician/physician assistant (PA)
        relationship, 394
    professional development, 394
    public health (population/society), 394
    risk management, 394
Profiles, in laboratory medicine, 381
Progesterone, normal levels of, 407–410t
Prokinetics, 58t
Prolactin, 407–410t
Prolapse, uterine, 198–199
Prolixin. see Fluphenazine
Propafenone, 367t
Propecia. see Finasteride (Propecia)
Propranolol, 27–29t, 124, 367t
Propylthiouracil, 375t
Prostate. see also Benign prostatic
        hypertrophy (BPH)
    -specific antigen (PSA), 407–410t
        for prostate cancer, 302
    carcinoma, 309–310
Prostatitis, 307–308
    causes of, 307t
    comparison of, 308t
Protease inhibitors, 361–362
Protein synthesis inhibitors, 358–359
Proteins, 387–388, 390
    in urinalysis, 387–388
Prothrombin time (PT), 383, 383f
    normal values for, 407–410t
Proton-pump inhibitors (PPIs), 58t, 369
Prozac. see Fluoxetine
Pseudocysts, 65
Pseudogout, 105
Psoas sign, 405t

Psoriasis, 271–272
Psychiatric drugs, 249–251t
Psychiatric medications, 371–374
  antipsychotics, 373
  benzodiazepines, 371–372
  bupropion, 373
  buspirone, 373
  lithium, 373
  mirtazapine, 373
  monoamine oxidase inhibitors (MAOIs),
    372–373
  selective serotonin reuptake inhibitors
    (SSRIs), 372
  serotonin-norepinephrine reuptake
    inhibitors (SNRIs), 372
  stimulants, 374
  tricyclic antidepressants (TCAs), 372
Psychiatry science, 230–253
Psychiatry, pediatrics, 346–347
  attention-deficit disorder, 346
  autism spectrum disorder, 346–347
  child abuse, 347
Psychostimulants, 249–251t
Psychotic disorder, 242–243
Psyllium, 371t
PT. *see* Prothrombin time (PT)
Pterygium, 132
PTT. *see* Partial thromboplastin time (PTT)
Public health (population/society), 394
Pulmonary circulation, 45–48
  cor pulmonale, 48
  pulmonary embolism (PE), 45–46
  pulmonary hypertension, 47–48
Pulmonary diseases, of newborns, 335–339
Pulmonary hypertension, 47t
  angiography results in, 47t
Pulmonary nodules, 39–40
Pulmonary regurgitation, 23
  clinical manifestations, 23
  diagnosis, 23
  general, 23
  treatment, 23
Pulmonary stenosis, 23
  clinical manifestations, 23
  diagnosis, 23
  general, 23
  treatment, 23
Pulmonary system, 32–52
Pustules, 262–265
PVCs. *see* Premature ventricular contractions
  (PVCs)
Pyelonephritis, 308
Pyloric stenosis, 343
Pyrazinamide, 361
Pyruvate kinase deficiency, 289

**Q**

Quetiapine, 249–251t
Quinidine, 27–29t, 367t

**R**

Rabies, 223
Radial fracture, 99, 100f
Radial head, subluxation of, 88
Radiculopathies, cervical/lumbar, 91t

Radioactive iodine, 124
Ramipril, 27–29t
Ranitidine, 81–82t
Ranson's criteria, 65t
RBC indices. *see* Red blood cell (RBC)
  indices
RDW. *see* Red blood cell distribution width
  (RDW)
Reactive thrombocytosis, 298
Recanalization therapy, for myocardial
  infarction (MI), 15
Rectocele, vaginal, 200
Rectum, 75–77
  anal fissure, 75
  anorectal abscess/fistula, 75–76
  fecal impaction, 76
  hemorrhoids, 76
  neoplasms, 76
  pilonidal disease, 76
  polyps, 76–77
Red blood cell (RBC) indices, 382
Red blood cell distribution width (RDW),
  382
Red eye, 131t
  etiologies of, 131t
5-α-Reductase inhibitors, for benign
  prostatic hypertrophy, 302–303
Reed-Sternberg cells, 292
Reference ranges, 380–381
Reflexes
  Galant's, 329
  Moro's, 328
  of newborn, 328–329
  startle, 328
Reiter's syndrome, 106–107
Relenza. *see* Zanamivir
Remeron. *see* Mirtazapine
Renal agenesis, 306
Renal cell carcinoma, 310
Renal diseases, 310–313
  glomerulonephritis, 312–313
  hydronephrosis, 313
  nephrotic syndrome, 313
  polycystic kidney disease, 313
  renal vascular disease, 313
Renal failure
  acute, 310–311
    causes of, 310t
    urine study results in, 311t
  chronic, 311–312
    causes of, 311t
  laboratory findings in, 387t
Renal stone, 67t
Renal tests, 386
Renal vascular disease, 313
Repaglinide, 118t
Reproductive system, 175–203
Reslizumab, 41–42t
Respiratory acidosis, 317–318
  etiology of, 317t
Respiratory alkalosis, 318
Respiratory distress syndrome, 336–337
  acute, 50–51
Restoril. *see* Temazepam
Restrictive pulmonary disease, 48–50
  idiopathic pulmonary fibrosis, 48–49, 49t

Restrictive pulmonary disease *(Continued)*
  pneumoconiosis, 49–50
  sarcoidosis, 50, 50f
Reticulocyte index, 282
  formula for, 283f
Retinal detachment, 134–135
Retinal disorders, 134–135
  macular degeneration, 134
  retinal detachment, 134–135
  retinopathy, 135
Retinal vascular occlusion, 136–137
Retinopathy, 135
  hypertensive, 135
Rh incompatibility, 185
Rheumatic diseases, serology test used in, 109t
Rheumatic fever, acute, 18
  clinical manifestations, 18
  diagnosis, 18
  general, 18
  Jones criteria for, 18t
  treatment, 18
Rheumatoid arthritis, 107, 107f
  juvenile, 344
Rheumatoid factor, 391
Rheumatologic conditions, 104–109
  fibromyalgia, 104–105
  gout, 105
  polyarteritis nodosa, 105–106
  polymyalgia rheumatica, 106
  polymyositis/dermatomyositis, 106
  pseudogout, 105
  Reiter's syndrome, 106–107
  rheumatoid arthritis, 107, 107f
  Sjögren's syndrome, 109
  systemic lupus erythematosus, 107–108
  systemic sclerosis, 108–109
Rheumatology testing, 391
  antinuclear antibodies (ANA), 391
  autoantibodies, 391
  C-reactive protein (CRP), 391
  erythrocyte sedimentation rate, 391
  rheumatoid factor, 391
Rheumatrex. *see* Methotrexate
Rhinitis, 144–145
Rhythm identification flow chart, 5t
Rhythm method, 185
Ribavirin, 361
Riboflavin, 80t
Rifampin, 360–361, 375t
Rinne test, 142
Risk factors
  for breast carcinoma, 176
  for coronary atherosclerosis, 14b
  for endometrial cancer, 197
  for esophageal cancer, 56t
  for gestational diabetes, 181–182
  for stroke, 170
Risk management, 394
Risperdal. *see* Risperidone
Risperidone, 249–251t, 374t
Ritalin. *see* Methylphenidate
Rituxan. *see* Rituximab
Rituximab, 108t, 376–377t, 377t
Rocky mountain spotted fever, 216–217
Romberg's sign, 405t
Rooting response, 328

Rosacea, 256
Roseola, 223
Rosiglitazone, 118t
Rosuvastatin, 369t
Rotator cuff disorders, 86–87
    clinical manifestations, 86
    general, 86
Rovsing's sign, 405t
Rubella, 223–224
Rubeola (measles), 224
Rule of nines, for burns, 274, 274f
Russell's sign, 405t

**S**

Salivary disorders, 150
    parotitis, 150
    sialadenitis, 150
Salmeterol, 41–42t
*Salmonella* infections, 210–211
Salmonellosis, 210–211
    *Salmonella* infections, 210–211
    typhoid fever, 210
Salpingitis, 67t
Salter-Harris classification, 97
Sarcoidosis, 50, 50f
    stage I, 50f
Scabies, 262
Scaphoid fracture, 99
Scapula, fracture of, 100
Schatzki's ring, 56
Schilling test, 286, 286t
Schizoaffective disorder, 243
Schizoid, 242
Schizophrenia, 242–243
    brief psychotic disorder, 243
    delusional disorder disorders, 242
    schizoaffective disorder, 243
Schizotypal, 242
Scleritis, 138
Scoliosis, 92
Seasonal allergic rhinitis, 144
Seborrheic dermatitis, 269–270
    atopic dermatitis *versus*, 268t
Seborrheic keratosis, 266
Second-degree burns, 273
Sedative/hypnotic/anxiolytic drugs,
        withdrawal from, 247t
Sedative/hypnotic/anxiolytic use disorders,
        246–247
Seizures, 345
    causes of, by age, 346t
    disorders
    disorders, 167–168
        absence, 167
        atonic, 167
        febrile, 167
        generalized, 167
        myoclonic, 167
        partial, 167
        tonic-clonic, 167
Selective α$_1$ blockers, 364
Selective serotonin reuptake inhibitors
        (SSRIs), 372
Selegiline, 161–162
Senna, 81–82t, 371t

Sensitivity, 380
Sensorimotor polyneuropathy, 167
Sensorineural hearing loss, 142
Separations, in shoulders, 87
Sepsis, 225–226
Septic arthritis, 101
Serax. *see* Oxazepam
Serology test
    for acute hepatitis, 61t
    for rheumatic diseases, 109t
Seroquel. *see* Quetiapine
Serotonin (5-HT3) antagonists, 371
Serotonin-norepinephrine reuptake
        inhibitors (SNRIs), 372
Sertraline, 249–251t
Serum protein electrophoresis, 388
    interpretation of, 388t
Serzone. *see* Nefazodone
Sexual abuse, 231
Shigellosis, 211
Short stature, 122
    causes of, 122t
Shoulder, 85–87
    dislocations of, 85–86, 86f
        clinical manifestations of, 85
        diagnosis of, 85–86
    disorders of, 85–87
    dystocia, 181
    fracture of, 96–100
    rotator cuff disorders, 86–87
    separations in, 87
SIADH. *see* Syndrome of inappropriate
        antidiuretic hormone secretion
        (SIADH)
Sialadenitis, 150
Sick sinus syndrome, 7–8
    diagnosis, 8
    etiologies, 8
    general, 7
    symptoms, 8
    treatment, 8
Sickle cell anemia, 289
Sickle cell test, normal values for, 407–410t
Sickle cell trait, 289
Side effects, of glucocorticoids, 115
Sideroblastic anemia, 285
Sildenafil, for erectile dysfunction, 303
Simvastatin, 369t
Sinequan. *see* Doxepin
Sinus disorders, 143–147
    acute sinusitis, 145–146
    chronic sinusitis, 146–147
    epistaxis, 143–144
    foreign body in nose, 147
    nasal polyps, 144
    rhinitis, 144–145
    trauma, 147
Sinus infection x-ray, 146f
Sinusitis
    acute, 145–146
    chronic, 146–147
Sjögren's syndrome, 109
Skin
    bacteria infections of, 259–260
    fungal infections of, 260–261
    tuberculin, test, 37, 37t

Skin integrity, 273–275
    burns, 273–275
    pressure ulcers, 275
    stasis dermatitis, 275
SLE. *see* Systemic lupus erythematosus (SLE)
Sleep-wake disorders, 243–244
    narcolepsy, 243–244
    parasomnias, 244
Slipped capital femoral epiphysis, 344
Small bowel obstruction, 74f
Small intestine, 67–75
    appendicitis, 67
    celiac disease, 68
    constipation, 68–69
    diverticular disease, 69–70
        acute diverticulitis, 69
        diverticular hemorrhage, 70
        diverticulosis, 69
    inflammatory bowel disease, 69–70
        Crohn's disease, 70–71
        ulcerative colitis, 70
    irritable bowel disease, 71–72
    ischemic bowel disease, 72
        acute arterial mesenteric ischemia, 72
        general, 55
        ischemic colitis, 72
    malabsorption, 72–73
    neoplasms, 73
    obstruction, 73–74
        large intestine, 74
        small intestine, 73–74
    polyps, 75
        familial adenomatous polyps, 75
        Gardner syndrome, 75
        hereditary nonpolyposis syndrome
            (Lynch syndrome), 75
        Peutz-Jeghers syndrome, 75
    toxic megacolon, 75
Smith's fracture, 97t
Smoking, 34t
Snellen's sign, 405t
SNRIs. *see* Serotonin-norepinephrine
        reuptake inhibitors (SNRIs)
Sodium, 384
    nitroprusside, 27–29t, 365
    phosphate, 81–82t, 371t
Sodium-glucose co-transporter 2 inhibitors,
        368
Soft-tissue x-ray, 149f
Somatic symptoms disorders, 244–245
    factitious disorder, 245
    functional neurological symptom disorder,
        244
    illness anxiety disorder, 244–245
    malingering, 245
Sorbitol, 371t
Sotalol, 27–29t, 367t
Specific gravity, in urinalysis, 389
Specificity, 380
Spermicides, 186
Spider
    bites, 258
    black widow, 258–259
    brown recluse, 258–259
Spinal cord compression, 294
Spinal stenosis, 92–93

Spine, disorders of, 89–93
Spirochetal disease, 216–218
  Lyme disease, 216
  rocky mountain spotted fever, 216–217
  syphilis, 217–218
Spironolactone, 27–29t
Splenic rupture, 67t
Sprains, 95–96
  ankle, 96
  anterior cruciate ligament (ACL) injury,
    95–96
  back, 89–91
  fingers, 88
  lateral collateral ligament injury, 95
  medial collateral ligament injury, 95
  posterior cruciate ligament injury, 96
Sprains (fingers), 88
Squamous cell carcinoma, 56t, 267–268
SSRIs. see Selective serotonin reuptake
    inhibitors (SSRIs)
St. Anthony's fire. see Erysipelas
Stasis dermatitis, 275
Station, 195
Status asthmaticus, 40–41
Status epilepticus, 167–168
Stelazine. see Trifluoperazine
Sterilization, tubal, 187
Steroids, 278t. see also Corticosteroids
  topical, 278t
Stevens-Johnson syndrome, 256–257
Stimulants, 374
Stomach, 57–59
  gastritis, 57–58
  gastroesophageal reflux disease, 57
  neoplasms, 58
  peptic ulcer disease, 58–59
Strabismus, 138
Strains, 95–96
  ankle, 96
  anterior cruciate ligament (ACL) injury,
    95–96
  back, 90–91
  lateral collateral ligament injury, 95
  medial collateral ligament injury, 95
  posterior cruciate ligament injury, 96
Stress incontinence, 303
Strictures, 56
String sign, 405t
Stroke, 170–171
  clinical manifestations of, 171t
  hemorrhagic, 170
  risk factors for, 170
  small vessel, 170
  thrombolytic therapy for, 171
Subarachnoid hematoma, 170t
Subarachnoid hemorrhage, 169–170
Subcutaneous nodules, 18
Subcutaneous tissue, of skin, 273
Subdural hematoma, 170t
Substance use disorders, 245–248
  alcohol dependence, 245–246
  alcohol intoxication, 245
  drug use, 246–247
    central nervous system (CNS) stimulant
      use disorder, 247
    opioid use disorder, 247

Substance use disorders (Continued)
    sedative/hypnotic/anxiolytic use
      disorders, 246–247
  general, 245
  tobacco use, 247–248
Sucralfate, 81–82t, 369–370
Sudden infant death syndrome, 339
Suicidal behaviors, 235
Sulfasalazine, 108t
Sulfonylureas, 367
Superior vena cava syndrome, 38, 294
Supracondylar fractures, 99
Syncope, 171–172
Syndrome of inappropriate antidiuretic
    hormone secretion (SIADH), 122–123
Syphilis, 217–218
Systemic fungal infections, 206
Systemic fungal organisms, 207t
Systemic lupus erythematosus (SLE), 107–108
Systemic sclerosis, 108–109

T
Tamiflu. see Oseltamivir
Tamoxifen, 376–377t, 377t
Tanner stages, 322, 325t, 326f
Tapeworms, 215, 215t
Task force screening, guidelines for common
    diseases, 403t
Taxol. see Paclitaxel
TCAs. see Tricyclic antidepressants (TCAs)
Tear
  Mallory-Weiss, 55–56
  in shoulder, 86
    diagnosis of, 87
    treatment of, 87
Teeth/gums, diseases of, 147
  dental abscess, 147
  gingivitis, 147
Tegretol. see Carbamazepine
Telangiectasia, 276
Temazepam, 249–251t, 372t
Tendinitis, 86
  diagnosis of, 87
  treatment of, 87
Tennis elbow, 89
Tenosynovitis, 88–89
  carpal tunnel syndrome, 88–89
  de Quervain's, 89
  epicondylitis, 89
Tension headache, 157
Terbutaline, 41–42t
Test-taking strategies
  15-day study schedule for, 400t
  31-day study schedule for, 400t
  90-day study schedule for, 399t
  after the examination, 401
  anxiety, 401
  day of the examination, 400–401
    test-anxiety strategies, 401
  examination, 397–401
    PANCE, 397–398
    PANRE, 398
  before the examination, 398–400
  during the examination, 401
  general tips, 401
Testicular carcinoma, 310

Testicular torsion, 305
Testosterone, 407–410t
Tetanus, 211
Tetracycline, 358
Tetralogy of Fallot, 334
Thalassemia, 284–285
Theophylline, 41–42t, 43, 44
Thiamine, 80t
Thiazide diuretics, 362
Thiazolidinediones, 367–368
Thioridazine, 249–251t, 374t
Thiourea, 124
Thoracic outlet syndrome, 93
Thorazine. see Chlorpromazine
Throat, of newborns, 335–339
Thrombin time, normal values for, 407–410t
Thrombocytopenia, 296–298, 381
  disseminated intravascular coagulation
    (DIC), 297–298
  idiopathic thrombocytopenic purpura
    (ITP), 296
  thrombotic thrombocytopenic purpura
    (TTP), 296–297
  von Willebrand's disease, 297
Thrombocytosis, 298, 383
  essential thrombocythemia, 298
  reactive thrombocytosis, 298
Thrombolytic therapy
  contraindications to, 16t
  for MI, 15
  for stroke, 171
Thrombotic thrombocytopenic purpura
    (TTP), 296–297
Thyroid disorders, 124–126
  hyperthyroidism, 124–125
  hypothyroidism, 125
  neoplastic disease, 126
  thyroiditis, 125–126
Thyroid function test, 125t
Thyroid gland
  screening for thyroid disease, 403t
  storm, 124–125
Thyroid-stimulating hormone (TSH), 391
  level of, 125t
  normal levels of, 407–410t
Thyroid testing, 390–391
  thyroid-stimulating hormone (TSH), 391
  thyroxine ($T_4$), 391
  triiodothyronine ($T_3$), 390
Thyroiditis, 125–126
  Hashimoto's, 125
  subacute, 125
Thyrotropin-releasing hormone (TRH), 112
Thyroxine ($T_4$), 391
Timolol, 27–29t, 367t
Tinea corporis, 261
Tinea infections, 262t
Tinea pedis, 261
Tinea versicolor, 261
Tinel's sign, 405t
Tinnitus, 143
TMP/Sulfa, 375t
Tobacco use, 247–248
Tocainide, 367t
Tofranil. see Imipramine
Tonic-clonic seizure, 166

Tooth avulsion, 150
Topical steroids, 278t
Toradol. *see* Ketorolac
Torticollis, 93
Total protein, 387–388
Tourette's syndrome, 162
Toxic epidermal necrolysis, 257
Toxic megacolon, 75
Toxicity, chemotherapeutic agent, 295t
Toxicology test, normal values for, 407–410t
Toxoplasmosis, 215–216
Tramadol, 353
Transferrin, normal values for, 407–410t
Transfusion reactions, 298–299
Transurethral prostatectomy (TURP), for
    benign prostatic hypertrophy, 303
Tranylcypromine, 249–251t
Trastuzumab, 376–377t, 377t
Trauma, 147, 150
Trauma and stressor-related disorders, 248–251
  acute stress disorder, 248
  adjustment, 248
  posttraumatic stress disorder, 248–251
Traumatic disorders, 135–136
  blowout fracture, 135
  corneal abrasion, 136
  foreign body, 135–136
  globe rupture, 136
  hyphema, 136
Traveler's diarrhea, 78–80
Trazodone, 249–251t
Tremor, essential, 160
Trendelenburg's sign, 405t
TRH. *see* Thyrotropin-releasing hormone
    (TRH)
Triamcinolone, 41–42t
Triamterene, 27–29t
Triazolam, 249–251t, 377t
*Trichomonas vaginalis*, 200, 200f
Trichotillomania, 239
Tricuspid regurgitation, 23
  clinical manifestations, 23
  diagnosis, 23
  general, 23
  treatment, 23
Tricuspid stenosis, 23
  clinical manifestations, 23
  diagnosis, 23
  general, 23
  treatment, 23
Tricyclic antidepressants (TCAs), 372
  inhibitor, 232
  side effects of, 373t
Trifluoperazine, 249–251t
Triglycerides, 387
Triiodothyronine (T3), 390
Trilafon. *see* Perphenazine
Triptans, 355
Trisomy 13 (Patau syndrome), 331
Trisomy 18 (Edwards syndrome), 331–332
Trisomy 21, 331
Trousseau's sign, 405t
TSH. *see* Thyroid-stimulating hormone
    (TSH)
TTP. *see* Thrombotic thrombocytopenic
    purpura (TTP)

Tubal sterilization, 187
Tuberculin skin test, interpretation of, 37t
Tuberculosis, 36–38, 211–212
  chest x-ray, 212f
  extrapulmonary, 37t
Tumor lysis syndrome, 294
Tumors
  bone, 102
  carcinoid, 39
  metastatic, 39
  Wilms', 348
Turner's syndrome, 332
TURP. *see* Transurethral prostatectomy (TURP)
Tympanic membrane perforation, 142
Typhoid fever, 210

**U**

Ulcerative colitis, 70
  Crohn's disease *versus*, 71t
Ulcers
  aphthous, 147–148
  decubitus, 275t
  duodenal, 59t
  gastric, 59t
  peptic, 67t
Ultram. *see* Tramadol
Umbilical hernia, 77–78
Uncomplicated pregnancy, 193–196
  normal labor/delivery, 194–196
  prenatal diagnosis/care, 193–194
Upper and lower motor neuron disease, 160t
Uremia, symptoms of, 311t
Urethral stricture, 305–306
Urethritis, 308–309
  comparison of, 309t
  gonococcal, 308, 309t
  nongonococcal, 308, 309t
Urethrocele, 306
Urge incontinence, 303–304
Uric acid, 389
Urinalysis, 389–390
  common findings on, 319t
  for infection, 318
  macroscopic, 389–390
  microscopic, 390, 390t
  findings
Urine
  free cortisol, 113
  test, in jaundice, 386t
Urobilinogen, in urinalysis, 390
Urticaria, 278–279
  drug reactions in, 270
U.S. Preventive Services Task Force Screen-
    ing Guidelines, 403t
Uterine disorders, 196–199
  adenomyosis, 198
  dysfunctional uterine bleeding (DUB),
    196–197
  endometrial cancer, 197
  endometriosis, 197–198
  leiomyoma (uterine fibroids), 198
  metritis, 198
  uterine prolapse, 198–199
Uterine fibroids, 198
Uterine prolapse, 198–199
Uterus, prolapse of, 198–199

**V**

Vagina, 199–201
  cystocele, 199
  neoplasms of, 199
  rectocele of, 200
  vaginitis, 200–201
Vaginitis, 200–201
  *Gardnerella vaginalis*, 200–201
  *Trichomonas vaginalis*, 200
  yeast infection, 200
Valium. *see* Diazepam
Valproate, 249–251t
Valproic acid, 168t, 375t, 376
Valvular disease, 21–23
  aortic regurgitation, 22
  aortic stenosis, 21–22
  major, summary of, 24t
  mitral regurgitation, 22–23
  mitral stenosis, 22
  mitral valve prolapse, 23
  pulmonary regurgitation, 23
  pulmonary stenosis, 23
  tricuspid regurgitation, 23
  tricuspid stenosis, 23
Vancomycin, 357–358
Varenicline, 248
Varicella-zoster virus infections, 224, 264–265
Varices, of esophagus, 56–57
Varicocele, 303
Varicocelectomy, for varicocele, 303
Varicose veins, 21
  clinical manifestations, 21
  diagnosis, 21
  general, 21
  treatment, 21
Vascular abnormalities, 275–276
  cherry angioma, 275–276
  telangiectasia, 276
Vascular claudication, 93t
Vascular disease, 18–21
  acute rheumatic fever, 18
  aortic aneurysm, 18–19
  aortic dissection, 19
  arterial embolism/thrombosis, 19
  chronic/acute arterial occlusion, 19–20
  giant cell arteritis, 20
  phlebitis/thrombophlebitis, 20
  varicose veins, 21
  venous thrombosis, 20–21
Vascular disorders, 136–137
  of neurologic system, 168–172
    arteriovenous malformation, 168–169
    cerebral aneurysm, 169
    normal-pressure hydrocephalus, 169
    stroke, 170–171
    subarachnoid hemorrhage, 169–170
    syncope, 171–172
  retinal vascular occlusion, 136–137
Vasectomy, 187
Venereal warts, 262–263
Venlafaxine, 249–251t
Venous thrombosis, 20–21
  clinical manifestations, 21
  diagnosis, 21
  general, 20
  treatment, 21

Ventricular fibrillation, 8, 8f
  EKG findings, 8
  general, 8
  treatment, 8
Ventricular flutter, 8–9
  EKG findings, 9
  general, 8
  treatment, 9
Ventricular septal defect, 334–335
Ventricular tachycardia (VT), 8, 8f
  EKG findings, 8
  general, 8
  treatment, 8
Verapamil, 27–29t, 367t
Verrucae, 265
Vertigo, 140–141
  central, 141t
  peripheral, 141t
Vesicoureteral reflux, 306
Vesiculobullous disease, 276
  pemphigoid, 276
  pemphigus, 276
Vincristine, 376–377t, 377t
Viral disease, 218–225
  cytomegalovirus infections, 218
  of dermatologic system, 262–265
    condyloma acuminatum, 262–263
    herpes simplex, 263–264
    molluscum contagiosum, 264
    varicella-zoster virus infections, 264–265
    verrucae, 265
  Epstein-Barr virus infections, 218
  erythema infectiosum, 218–219
  hand-foot-and-mouth disease, 224
  herpangina, 224
  herpes simplex, 219
  human immunodeficiency virus infection, 220
  human papillomavirus infections, 220–222
  influenza, 222

Viral disease (Continued)
  mumps, 222–223
  rabies, 223
  roseola, 223
  rubella, 223–224
  rubeola (measles), 224
  varicella-zoster virus infections, 224
  Zika virus, 224–225
Viral disease infections, 225t
Virazole. see Ribavirin
Vision abnormalities, 137–138
  amaurosis fugax, 137
  amblyopia, 137
  glaucoma, 137–138
  scleritis, 138
  strabismus, 138
Vitamins
  A, 80t
  B$_{12}$
    deficiency, 285–286
    normal values for, 407–410t
  C, 80t
  D, 80t
  K, 80t
Vitiligo, 272–273
Voltaren. see Diclofenac
Volume depletion, 318
  causes of, 318t
Volume excess, 318
  causes of, 318t
Volvulus, 343
Von Gierke's disease, 341
Von Willebrand's disease, 297
VT. see Ventricular tachycardia (VT)
Vulva, 199

**W**
Warfarin, 21, 374–375
  drug effects with, 375t
Warts, 265

WBC. see White blood cell (WBC)
Weight-associated health risks, 238t
Wellbutrin. see Bupropion
Wernicke's encephalopathy, 155–156
Westermark's sign, 405t
White blood cell (WBC), 381
Wickham's striae, in lichen planus, 271
Wilms' tumor, 348
Wilson's disease, 63t
Wolff-Parkinson-White syndrome, 6f
Wrist
  disorders of, 87–89
  fractures of, 98–99
  sign, 405t

**X**
X-linked recessive inheritance, 330t
X-ray
  abdominal, of pancreatitis, 66f
  of edematous epiglottis, 149f
  of pneumonia, 34f
  of sinus infection, 146f
  of skull, with multiple myeloma, 293f
Xanax. see Alprazolam

**Y**
Yeast infection, 200, 200f

**Z**
Zafirlukast, 41–42t
Zanamivir, 361
Zarontin. see Ethosuximide
Zenker's diverticulum, 56
Zidovudine, 271t
Zika virus, 224–225
Zoloft. see Sertraline
Zyban. see Bupropion
Zyprexa. see Olanzapine